Phospholipid Spectrum Disorder in Psychiatry

Phospholipid Spectrum Disorder in Psychiatry

Edited by

Malcolm Peet
*University Department of Psychiatry,
Northern General Hospital, Sheffield, UK.*

Iain Glen
*Highland Psychiatric Research Group,
Craig Dunain Hospital, Inverness, Scotland, UK.*

and

David F. Horrobin
Laxdale Research, Stirling, Scotland, UK

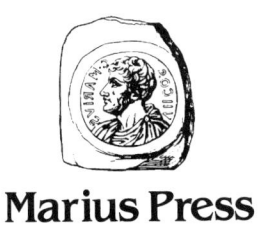

Marius Press

Marius Press, 1999
PO Box 15, Carnforth, Lancashire LA6 1HW, UK

All rights reserved. No part of this publication may be translated into other languages, stored in a retrieval system, or transmitted in any form or by any means, electronic, mechanical, photocopying, recording or otherwise, without the prior permission in writing of the publisher.

No responsibility is assumed by the publisher for any injury and/or damage to persons or property as a matter of products liability, negligence or otherwise, or from any use or operation of any methods, products, instructions or ideas contained in the material herein. Every effort has been made to ensure that the details given in this book regarding the choice, dosage and administration practices relating to drugs discussed in the text, are in accordance with the recommendations and practices current at the time of publication. However, because new research constantly leads to such recommendations and practices being updated, the reader should obtain independent verification of diagnoses and check the maker's instructions carefully regarding dosage, administration procedures, indications and contraindications, before using any of the agents mentioned in this book.

The opinions expressed in each of the chapters are those of the author or authors of the chapter, and do not necessarily reflect the views of the editors, the publisher, or the company or companies which manufacture and/or market any of the pharmaceutical agents or other products referred to.

ISBN: 1-871622-10-7

Typeset by The Drawing Room, Carnforth, UK
Printed and bound by Polestar Wheatons Ltd, Exeter, UK.

Contents

Preface ... ix

List of Contributors ... x

Part I: INTRODUCTION

1. The phospholipid concept of psychiatric disorders and its relationship to the neurodevelopmental concept of schizophrenia
   David F. Horrobin ... 3

Part II: SCHIZOPHRENIA: PHOSPHOLIPID METABOLISM

2. Brain and blood phospholipase activity in psychiatric disorders
   Brian M. Ross ... 23

3. Phospholipase A_2 gene polymorphism and associated biochemical alterations in schizophrenia
   C. N. Ramchand, J. Wei, K. H. Lee, and Malcolm Peet ... 31

4. Phospholipase A_2 and the hypofrontality hypothesis of schizophrenia
   Wagner F. Gattaz, and Jürgen Brunner ... 39

5. ^{31}P Magnetic resonance spectroscopy in the assessment of brain phospholipid metabolism in schizophrenia
   Peter C. Williamson and Dick J. Drost ... 45

6. Red blood cell and platelet fatty acid metabolism in schizophrenia
   Jeffrey K. Yao ... 57

Part III: SCHIZOPHRENIA: MEMBRANE ABNORMALITIES

7. Membrane-protective strategies in schizophrenia: conceptual and treatment issues
   Ravinder Reddy and Jeffrey K. Yao ... 75

8. Membrane abnormalities in schizophrenia as revealed by tyrosine transport
   Lars Bjerkenstedt, Gunnar Edman and Frits-Axel Wiesel ... 89

9. Membrane peroxidation and the neuropathology of schizophrenia
   Sahebarao P. Mahadik, Sandhya Sitasawad, and Meena Mulchandani ... 99

10. The effects of antipsychotic drugs on membrane phospholipids: a possible novel mechanism of action of clozapine
    David F. Horrobin ... 113

Part IV: SCHIZOPHRENIA: RETINAL FUNCTION

11. Retinal function in schizophrenia
    Fiona K. Skinner, Lois E. F. MacDonell and Iain Glen — 121

12. Essential fatty acids and the electroretinogram in schizophrenia
    R. W. Warner and Malcolm Peet — 133

Part V: SCHIZOPHRENIA: NIACIN FLUSH TEST

13. Oral and topical niacin flush testing in schizophrenia
    Pauline E. Ward and Iain Glen — 139

14. Family studies of schizophrenia
    Iain Glen — 145

Part VI: SCHIZOPHRENIA: DIETARY INFLUENCES AND TREATMENT

15. Breastfeeding, neurodevelopment, and schizophrenia
    Malcolm Peet, Jacqui Poole and Jonathon D. E. Laugharne — 159

16. Cultural and socioeconomic differences in dietary intake of essential fatty acids and antioxidants: effects on the course and outcome of schizophrenia
    Sahebarao P. Mahadik, Meena Mulchandani, Mahabaleshwar V. Hegde and Prabhakar K. Ranjekar — 167

17. Sustained remission of symptoms following treatment with eicosapentaenoic acid in a case of schizophrenia with dyslexia
    Alexandra J. Richardson and Basant K. Puri — 181

18. New strategies for the treatment of schizophrenia: omega-3 polyunsaturated fatty acids
    Malcolm Peet — 189

Part VII: DEPRESSION

19. Membrane lipids in relation to depression
    Joseph R. Hibbeln — 195

20. Essential fatty acid intake in relation to depression
    Rhian W. Edwards and Malcolm Peet — 211

Part VIII: DYSLEXIA AND DYSPRAXIA

21. Essential fatty acids in dyslexia: theory, evidence and clinical trials
    Alexandra J. Richardson, Terese Easton, Ann Marie McDaid, Jacqueline A. Hall, Paul Montgomery, Christine Clisby and Basant K. Puri   225

22. Brain phospholipid metabolism in dyslexia assessed by magnetic resonance spectroscopy
    Basant K. Puri and Alexandra J. Richardson   243

23. Essential fatty acids in the management of dyslexia and dyspraxia
    B. Jacqueline Stordy   251

Part IX: OTHER NEUROPSYCHIATRIC DISORDERS

24. Essential fatty acids in children with attention-deficit/hyperactivity disorder
    Laura J. Stevens and John R. Burgess   263

25. A possible role for phospholipases in autism and Asperger's syndrome
    David F. Horrobin   271

26. Decreased brain and platelet phospholipase A_2 activity in Alzheimer's disease
    Wagner F. Gattaz, Nigel J. Cairns, Raymond Levy, Hans Förstl, Dieter F. Braus and Athanasios Maras   275

27. Phospholipids and abnormal involuntary movements in the general male population
    Agneta Nilsson, David F. Horrobin and Annika Rosengren   279

28. Essential fatty acids and movement disorders
    Krishna Vaddadi   285

Part X: THE EVOLUTIONARY CONTEXT

29. A speculative overview: the relationship between phospholipid spectrum disorder and human evolution
    David F. Horrobin   299

Index   319

Preface

Psychiatric disorders, because they cause so much distress to sufferers, their relatives and friends, and because they may persist for many years, cause more damage than any other group of illnesses. The World Health Organisation now estimates that depression is the illness causing the greatest total disease burden. Schizophrenia is not far behind.

Yet, as Robert Kendell recently emphasised in his plenary welcoming lecture to 3000 psychiatrists and psychopharmacologists at the 1998 Glasgow CINP conference, there has been no improvement in the efficacy of drugs for schizophrenia and depression for 40 years. Adverse effects of newer drugs may be less, but their effects on symptoms are no better than they were in the late 1950s.

Our modern concepts of psychiatric diseases have almost all been derived from exploring the mechanisms of drugs which were found to work on the basis of accidental clinical observation. Thus antidepressants enhance the function of catecholamine systems, so depression must be caused by inadequate catecholamine activity. Or antipsychotic drugs block dopamine receptors, and so schizophrenia must be caused by dopaminergic excess. Evidence for these hypotheses, which is truly independent of drug actions, is scanty and rarely convincing. We have thus become locked into a cycle where drug actions provide the best evidence of mechanisms, and where all we can do is discover variants of existing drugs. This is because the drug discovery models are all ultimately based on the actions of drugs which empirically have been found to work, and not on a truly independent model of disease mechanism, which is derived from evidence other than that supplied by drugs.

The lecture by Kendell indicates that dissatisfaction with current biochemical models of psychiatric disorders is growing. New concepts are required which will allow new questions to be asked and new treatments developed.

One such concept is the idea that psychiatric disorders may be related to abnormalities in phospholipid metabolism. Phospholipids make up the bulk of all internal and external neuronal membranes. Most neuronal proteins are embedded in, or attached to phospholipid membranes. Protein quaternary structure, and therefore function, depends on the precise composition of the immediate phospholipid environment. Neuronal signal transduction processes depend on diacylglycerols, inositols, and fatty acids and their derivatives, which are released from membrane phospholipids during neuronal activation. Phospholipid biochemistry is therefore central in brain function.

There is now evidence, from many different laboratories, that phospholipid abnormalities are involved in several psychiatric disorders. If this is the case, then new avenues of investigation and new approaches to treatment can be opened up. This book summarises much of the evidence available. We believe that it may prove to be an important stage in redirecting psychiatric research into more productive channels.

Malcolm Peet, Iain Glen and David Horrobin, 1999

List of Contributors

Lars Bjerkenstedt	*Department of Psychiatry, Danderyds Hospital, Karolinska Institute, S-18288, Danderyd, Sweden.*
Dieter F. Braus	*Central Institute of Mental Health, Mannheim, Germany.*
Jürgen Brunner	*Central Institute of Mental Health, Mannheim, Germany.*
John R. Burgess	*Department of Foods and Nutrition, Purdue University, West Lafayette, Indiana 47907-1264, USA.*
Nigel J. Cairns	*MRC Alzheimer's Disease Brain Bank, Institute of Psychiatry, De Crespigny Park, Denmark Hill, London, UK.*
Christine Clisby	*University Laboratory of Physiology, Parks Road, Oxford OX1 3PT, UK.*
Dick J. Drost	*Department of Medical Biophysics and Department of Diagnostic Radiology and Nuclear Medicine, St Joseph's Health Centre, 268 Grosvenor Street, London, Ontario, Canada N6A 4V2.*
Terese Easton	*Division of Neurosciences and Psychological Medicine, Imperial College School of Medicine, Charing Cross Campus, St Dunstan's Road, London W6 8RP, UK.*
Gunnar Edman	*Department of Psychiatry, Danderyds Hospital, Karolinska Institute, S-18288, Danderyd, Sweden.*
Rhian W. Edwards	*University Department of Psychiatry, Northern General Hospital, Herries Road, Sheffield S5 7AU, UK.*
Hans Förstl	*Central Institute of Mental Health, Mannheim, Germany.*
Wagner F. Gattaz	*Central Institute of Mental Health, Mannheim, Germany, and Laboratory of Neurosciences (LIM-27), Department and Institute of Psychiatry, Faculty of Medicine, University of São Paulo 05403-010, PO Box 3671, São Paulo, SP, Brazil.*
Iain Glen	*Highland Psychiatric Research Foundation, Craig Dunain Hospital, Inverness IV3 6JU, Scotland, UK.*
Jacqueline A. Hall	*University Laboratory of Physiology, Parks Road, Oxford OX1 3PT, UK.*
Mahabaleshwar V. Hegde	*Division of Biochemical Sciences, National Chemical Laboratory, Pune, Maharashtra State 411 008, India.*
Joseph R. Hibbeln	*National Institute on Alcohol Abuse and Alcoholism, 12420 Parklawn Drive, Rockville, MD 20852, USA*

David F. Horrobin	*Laxdale Research, Kings Park House, Laurelhill Business Park, Stirling FK7 9JQ,, Scotland, UK.*
Jonathon D.E. Laugharne	*University Department of Psychiatry, Northern General Hospital, Herries Road, Sheffield S5 7AU, UK.*
K. H. Lee	*University Department of Psychiatry, Northern General Hospital, Herries Road, Sheffield S5 7AU, UK.*
Raymond Levy	*MRC Alzheimer's Disease Brain Bank, Institute of Psychiatry, De Crespigny Park, Denmark Hill, London, UK.*
Lois E.F. MacDonell	*Highland Psychiatric Research Foundation, Craig Dunain Hospital, Inverness IV3 6JU, Scotland, UK.*
Sahebarao Mahadik	*Department of Psychiatry and Health Behavior, Medical College of Georgia and Veterans Affairs Medical Center, 1 Freedom Way, Augusta, GA 30904-6285, USA.*
Athanasios Maras	*Central Institute of Mental Health, 68072 Mannheim, Germany.*
Ann Marie McDaid	*Division of Neurosciences and Psychological Medicine, Imperial College School of Medicine, Charing Cross Campus, St Dunstan's Road, London W6 8RP, UK.*
Paul Montgomery	*University Section of Child and Adolescent Psychiatry, Park Hospital, Old Road, Headington, Oxford OX3 7LQ, UK.*
Meena Mulchandani	*Division of Biochemical Sciences, National Chemical Laboratory, Pune, Maharashtra State 411 008, India.*
Agneta Nilsson	*Karsuddens Sjukhus, S-641 96, Katrineholm, Sweden.*
Malcolm Peet	*University Department of Psychiatry, Northern General Hospital, Herries Road, Sheffield S5 7AU, UK.*
Jacqui Poole	*University Department of Psychiatry, Northern General Hospital, Herries Road, Sheffield S5 7AU, UK.*
Basant K. Puri	*MRI Unit, MRC Clinical Sciences Centre, Imperial College School of Medicine, Hammersmith Hospital, Du Cane Road, London W12 0HS, UK.*
C.N. Ramchand	*University Department of Psychiatry, Northern General Hospital, Herries Road, Sheffield S5 7AU, UK.*
Prabhakar K. Ranjekar	*Division of Biochemical Sciences, National Chemical Laboratory, Pune, Maharashtra State 411 008, India.*

Ravinder Reddy	*Western Psychiatric Institute and Clinic, University of Pittsburgh School of Medicine, 3811 O'Hara Street, Pittsburgh, PA 15213, USA.*
Alexandra J. Richardson	*Division of Neurosciences and Psychological Medicine, Imperial College School of Medicine, Charing Cross Campus, St Dunstan's Road, London W6 8RP, and University Laboratory of Physiology, Parks Road, Oxford OX1 3PT, UK.*
Annika Rosengren	*Section of Preventive Cardiology, Department of Medicine, Östra University Hospital, Göteborg, Sweden*
Brian M. Ross	*Human Neurochemical Pathology Laboratory, Centre for Addiction and Mental Health, 250 College Street, and Department of Psychiatry, University of Toronto, Toronto, Ontario, M5T 1R8 Canada.*
Sandhya Sitasawad	*National Center for Cell Sciences, Pune University Campus, Ganeshkind, Pune, Maharashtra State 411 007, India.*
Fiona K. Skinner	*Highland Psychiatric Research Foundation, Craig Dunain Hospital, Inverness IV3 6JU, Scotland, UK.*
Laura J. Stevens	*Department of Foods and Nutrition, Purdue University, West Lafayette, Indiana 47907-1264, USA.*
B. Jacqueline Stordy	*Stordy Jones Nutrition Consultants, Manor House, Puttenham Heath Road, Puttenham, Guildford, Surrey GU3 1AP, UK.*
Krishna Vaddadi	*Department of Psychological Medicine, Monash Medical Centre, 246 Clayton Road, Clayton, Victoria 3168, Australia.*
Pauline E. Ward	*Highland Psychiatric Research Foundation, Craig Dunain Hospital, Inverness IV3 6JU, Scotland, UK.*
R. W. Warner	*Community Mental Health Care Directorate, Argyll House, 9 Williamson Road, Sheffield S11 9AR, UK.*
J. Wei	*Institute of Biological Psychiatry, Schizophrenia Association of Great Britain, Bryn Hyffrid, Upper Bangor, UK.*
Frits-Axel Wiesel	*Department of Neuroscience, Psychiatry, Ulleråker, Uppsala University Hospital, S-750 17 Uppsala, Sweden.*
Peter C. Williamson	*Departments of Psychiatry and Medical Biophysics, Faculty of Medicine, University of Western Ontario, London Health Sciences Center, 339 Windermere Road, London, Ontario N6A 5A5, Canada.*
Jeffrey K. Yao	*Pittsburgh Healthcare System, Department of Veterans Affairs and Western Psychiatric Institute and Clinic, University of Pittsburgh Medical Center, 7180 Highland Drive, Pittsburgh, PA 15206, USA.*

Part I

INTRODUCTION

The Phospholipid Concept of Psychiatric Disorders and its Relationship to the Neurodevelopmental Concept of Schizophrenia

D. F. Horrobin

INTRODUCTION

For the past 40 years, the dominant theme governing research into schizophrenia, the affective disorders, and other central nervous system diseases, has related these conditions to neurotransmitter system abnormalities. The idea has been that these disorders are caused by some abnormality in the synthesis, release, reuptake or receptor responses to dopamine, noradrenaline, serotonin, acetylcholine or excitatory amino acids. Therapeutic research has been directed towards finding agents which will, in some way, modulate these neurotransmitter systems at an appropriate step.

There is a substantial body of evidence in favour of the neurotransmitter concept, and it has successfully guided the development of drugs for schizophrenia, affective disorders, Parkinson's disease and Alzheimer's disease. There is, however, an emerging consensus that something else is required, that the neurotransmitter-based drugs are not quite achieving the successes that have been hoped for. There have been improvements in terms of reducing adverse effects, but it is not immediately apparent that, in terms of efficacy, the modern antidepressants are better than those which became available in the 1950s, the modern neuroleptics better than clozapine (first introduced 25 years ago), or the modern anti-Parkinson drugs substantially better than L-DOPA. Nor is it apparent that improvements in neurotransmitter-based drugs are part of a successful research paradigm which is steadily improving our knowledge base.

There is an uneasy feeling that something else is required. This volume brings together chapters by investigators who believe that an important component of that 'something else' will be provided by an understanding of phospholipid metabolism in neuronal membranes. All neuronal membranes are made up of lipids in which phospholipids, cholesterol and cholesteryl esters play the major roles. This is true of neuronal outer membranes, of nuclear membranes, of mitochondrial membranes, of membranes enclosing intracellular stores of calcium, and of synaptic vesicle membranes. It is particularly true of membranes of dendrites and synapses, which are up to 80% lipid by weight and where the enzymes which modulate lipid metabolism are strongly expressed. All substances moving across the neuronal membrane, or moving within the neurone, must cross these phospholipid-rich membranes.

Most of the proteins in neurones are embedded in, or are attached to, phospholipid-rich membranes. The phospholipid structures are not uniform throughout the membrane but are locally diferent and precisely determined. The specific phospholipid structure in the vicinity of a protein will determine the quaternary folding, and hence the function, of that protein. Many key neuronal proteins are palmitoylated, myristoylated, prenylated or farnosylated, in part to facilitate their interactions with phospholipids. Many of the cell signalling systems within cells are regulated by lipid products which are derived from the phospholipids of the neuronal membranes. Diacylglycerols released during the phosphatidyl–inositol cycle, free fatty acids released by phospholipases, hydroxyacids, prostaglandins, leukotrienes and other eicosanoids derived from the free fatty acids, are all important components of postreceptor signalling systems. This is true of dopamine, serotonin, acetylcholine, noradrenaline and excitatory amino acid systems.

It is therefore apparent that the phospholipid-related mechanisms associated with neuronal membranes of all types are in a position to interact with the neurotransmitter systems which, to date, have provided the dominant theme in biological psychiatry research. Of particular interest is the fact that the phospholipids provide a biochemical basis for the interaction between genetic and environmental factors in psychiatric disorders (Horrobin et al., 1995). The enzymes regulating phospholipid metabolism are, of course, genetically determined, whereas the fatty acids with which these enzymes must work are largely provided by the environment. The chapters in this book offer many examples of possible interactions between phospholipid mechanisms and other themes of biological psychiatry research.

The phospholipid concept enriches and amplifies these other research areas. It should not be seen as being in conflict with, for example, neurotransmitter research, but rather as expanding the explanatory power of other theories by making them more complex and more flexible.

One of the ideas which has been gaining strength in recent years is the neurodevelopmental concept of schizophrenia, the view that events in early development produce changes in brain function which may not be fully expressed until much later when the brain finally matures around and after puberty. This is an attractive concept, the major drawback of which is that it lacks a biochemical basis which might draw all the observations together. The purpose of the present chapter is to demonstrate that the phospholipid hypothesis of schizophrenia could provide the biochemical basis for the neurodevelopmental concept. The two approaches, far from being incompatible, are complementary. Each amplifies the explanatory power of the other.

THE NEURODEVELOPMENTAL CONCEPT OF SCHIZOPHRENIA

A neurodevelopmental approach to schizophrenia proposes that interaction between genetic and early environmental factors influences the ways in which nerve cells originate, migrate, are differentiated, culled by apoptosis, and remodelled by the selective expansion and retraction of dendrites and synaptic connections (Nasrallah, 1993; Falkai and Bogerts, 1995; Weinberger, 1995a). The factors begin to operate during neurodevelopment in the foetus and are often influenced by traumatic perinatal events; their effects become fully expressed, however, only in early adulthood when the brain finally matures and its myelination is completed. The key pieces of evidence are summarised below. In order to avoid an inordinately long reference list, only selected papers are cited in support of each point.

Evidence for a neurodevelopmental approach

Brain morphology

In schizophrenic patients there is increased ventricular size and there are abnormalities in brain morphology (Nasrallah, 1993; Falkai and Bogerts, 1995; Weinberger, 1995a). Some of these differences from normal occur well before the development of overt schizophrenic symptoms. Abnormalities in the hippocampus are particularly consistent and pronounced (Suddath et al., 1990; Shenton et al., 1992).

Childhood functional abnormalities

There are behavioural and neuromotor abnormalities which occur in childhood and which are to some degree predictive of later schizophrenia. These include: low IQ (David et al., 1997); poor motor skills (Marcus, 1974; Jones et al., 1994); poor development of language and word skills (Crow, 1995b, 1996b); lack of normal attention (Rieder and Nichols, 1979); and poor social development (Fish, 1987). In many individuals who later become frankly schizophrenic, behavioural precursors are detectable in childhood and adolescence.

Pregnancy and perinatal events

A number of events which can occur during pregnancy and the perinatal period have been found to be associated with an increased risk of later schizophrenia. These include: obstetric complications, particularly ones related to low birth weight and perinatal hypoxia (McNeil and Kaij, 1978; O'Callaghan et al., 1992; McGrath and Murray, 1995); starvation during pregnancy (Susser and Lin, 1992); low head circumference in otherwise normal individuals (McNeil et al., 1993); and viral infections, especially in the second trimester (O'Callaghan et al., 1991b; Sham et al., 1992). Schizophrenic patients often have minor physical abnormalities, of a type believed to originate in the second trimester of pregnancy and thus indicative of developmental problems around that time (Green et al., 1989; O'Callaghan et al., 1991a). In contrast to these factors which increase risk, breast feeding, especially when prolonged, appears to be protective (McCreadie, 1997; Peet et al., 1997b).

Sex differences

There are sex differences in the onset and clinical course of schizophrenia, with females usually falling ill later, and being less severely affected than males, but also showing a second, late post-menopausal, peak in incidence (Iacano and Beiser, 1992; Murray et al., 1992).

Season of birth

There is a small variation in the risk of schizophrenia related to the season of birth. In both hemispheres the risk of developing schizophrenia seems higher in babies born during the winter months than in those born at other times (Dalen, 1975; Yakley and Murray, 1995).

Biochemical basis of neurodevelopmental effects

These various pieces of evidence may be interpreted in different ways, but in general they suggest that there may be a genetic basis for schizophrenia, the expression of which is influenced by events during pregnancy, in the perinatal period and around puberty. However, none of these developmental influences seems individually to account for more than a small percentage of the total number of schizophrenia patients in society.

Whilst, in general terms, the neurodevelopmental concept of schizophrenia is appealing, the main problem is the lack of a biochemical basis through which the genetic and neurodevelopmental influences can be expressed. Glutamate receptor hypofunction has been proposed as a biochemical substrate for developmental problems, but cannot fully explain all the known neurodevelopmental influences (Olney and Farber, 1995). It is the thesis of the present chapter that the observations consistent with the neurodevelopmental hypothesis can, for the most part, be explained on the basis of disturbed phospholipid metabolism (Horrobin et al., 1994; Mahadik and Evans, 1997; Horrobin, 1998a). This is even true of glutamate receptor hypofunction, since the normal functioning of glutamate receptors requires normal levels of arachidonate in membrane phospholipids. The phospholipid hypothesis, as one of its core tenets, argues that normal amounts of arachidonic acid (AA) are not available for cell signalling, and that this will lead to glutamate receptor system hypofunction.

NEURONAL PHOSPHOLIPIDS AND THEIR IMPORTANCE

As already mentioned, all external and internal neuronal membranes are largely made up of phospholipids (Horrobin et al., 1994). Phospholipids are particularly important in cell signalling and in the formation and remodelling of dendrites and synapses (Horrobin, 1998a,b; Horrobin et al., 1994). Neurodevelopment is, in large part, a story of the development of the phospholipid structures of the brain.

The basics of phospholipid structure, syntheses, remodelling and breakdown are well described in several standard texts (e.g., Mead et al., 1986; Gurr and Harwood, 1991). All phospholipids have a 3-carbon glycerol backbone. Attached to the Sn3 position

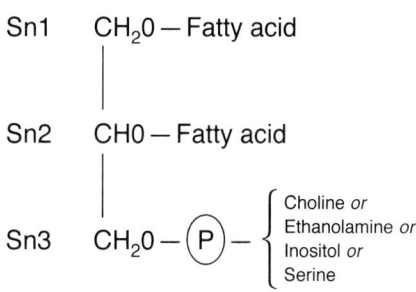

Figure 1.1. The general structure of a phospholipid. The three carbon atoms of the glycerol backbone are designated Sn1, Sn2 and Sn3.

(Figure 1.1) is a phosphorus atom, and to this is attached one of several possible 'head groups', usually choline, ethanolamine, inositol or serine. The functional behaviour of neuronal membranes largely depends on the ways in which individual phospholipids are aligned, are interspersed with cholesterol, and are associated with proteins.

There are many thousands of types of phospholipid in neurones. As with proteins, although the numbers of basic building blocks are relatively limited, final functional properties depend on which of these building blocks are present and how they are arranged. The properties of each phospholipid molecule are dependent both upon the nature of the head group, and on the natures of the other molecules attached to the Sn1 and Sn2 positions. These other molecules are commonly fatty acids – known as acyl groups – which may be of many different types. Saturated fatty acids, made up of a chain of single carbon–carbon bonds, are straight and rigid, but may have different chain lengths. Unsaturated fatty acids have one or more double carbon–carbon bonds and a range of chain lengths. The double bonds are angled and flexible and make the carbon chain more mobile. The more double bonds there are, the more fluid, flexible and apparently disordered does the phospholipid molecule become.

The brain phospholipids are uniquely rich in highly unsaturated fatty acids with three to six double bonds. These fatty acids are important in allowing rapid changes in membrane shape and in allowing membrane fusion, as, for instance, occurs during the making and breaking of synaptic connections and the release of neurotransmitters. These unsaturated fatty acids fall under the general class of essential fatty acids (EFAs) which cannot be manufactured *de novo* by the mammalian body (Horrobin and Manku, 1990; British Nutrition Foundation, 1992; Horrobin, 1992a). There are two types of unsaturated fatty acid, the n-6 and n-3 (or, alternatively, ω-6 and ω-3), named because of the position of the first double bond in the carbon chain, starting at the methyl end of the molecule. EFAs of both types are required for the normal structure and functioning of the mammalian nervous system.

Phospholipid synthesis

Phospholipid synthesis (Mead et al., 1986; Gurr and Harwood, 1991) involves a complex series of reactions, which can be abbreviated as shown in Figure 1.2. The usual intermediate is diacylglycerol (DAG), glycerol with one fatty acid (acyl group) attached to one outer carbon atom (Sn1) and a second fatty acid attached to the middle carbon atom (Sn2). Phosphorylated choline or ethanolamine may then be added to the third (Sn3) carbon atom giving phosphatidylcholine or phosphatidylethanolamine. DAG may be phosphorylated at the Sn3 position and myoinositol attached to it, to give phosphatidylinositol. Phosphatidylserine is usually made by exchanging serine for the ethanolamine in P-ethanolamine. P-choline may also be formed from P-ethanolamine *via* a reaction mediated by S-adenosylmethionine (SAM).

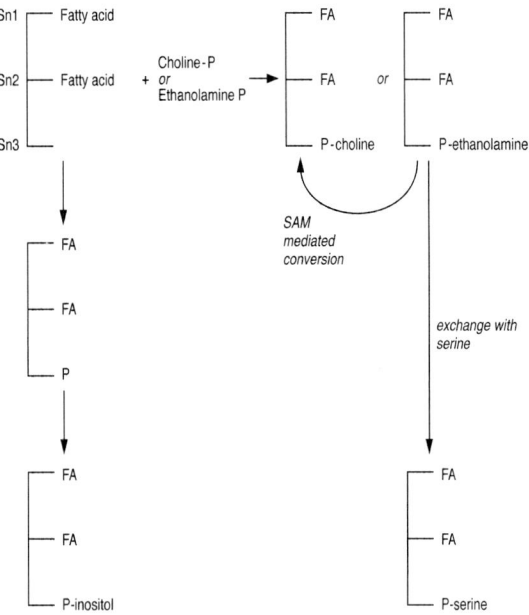

Figure 1.2. An outline of the basics of phospholipid synthesis, starting with glycerol with fatty acids (acyl groups) attached to the Sn1 and Sn2 positions.

Phospholipid breakdown

The phospholipids may be broken down by several classes of phospholipase (Mead et al., 1986; Gurr and Harwood, 1991). Within each class there are multiple individual enzymes, each of which appears likely to have a specific role in cellular biochemistry. The main ones are shown in Figure 1.3.

Phospholipases A_1 and A_2

Phospholipases A_1 (PLA$_1$) remove fatty acids (acyl groups) from the Sn1 position of all phospholipid classes, while phospholipases A_2 (PLA$_2$) remove fatty acids from the middle (Sn2) position of all phospholipids. The products of phospholipase A reactions are known as lysophospholipids.

Phospholipases B

Though less well defined than PLA$_1$ and PLA$_2$, phospholipases B may be able to remove fatty acids from both Sn1 and Sn2 positions.

Phospholipases C

Phospholipases C split the bond between the Sn3 carbon atom and phosphorus leaving DAG. DAG may then be further metabolized by DAG lipases to release fatty acids from the Sn2 position.

Phospholipases D

Phospholipases D split the bond between the phosphorus and the phospholipid head group, leaving the phosphorus attached to the glycerol backbone and giving phosphatidic acid.

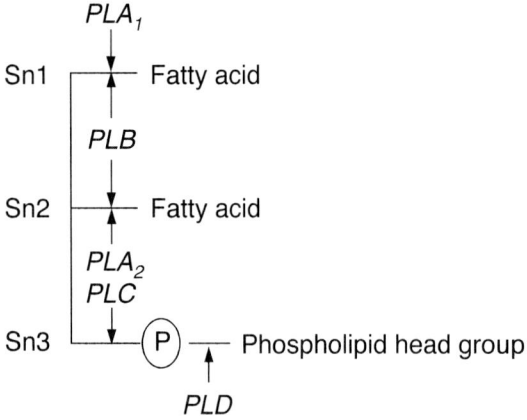

Figure 1.3. The points of action of the major groups of phospholipases. Within each group there are many different specific phospholipases. PLA$_1$ = phospholipase A$_1$; PLA$_2$ = phospholipase A$_2$; PLB = phospholipase B; PLC = phospholipase C; PLD = phospholipase D.

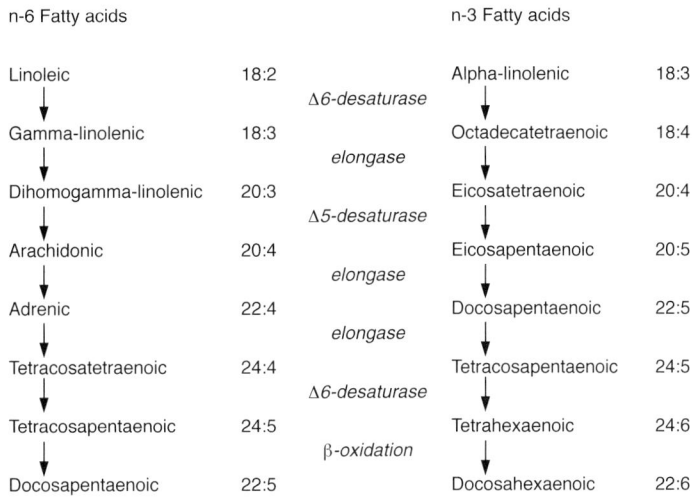

Figure 1.4. Summary of the synthesis of essential fatty acids from the dietary precursors, linoleic acid of the n-6 series and α-linolenic acid of the n-3 series. In mass and also functional terms, arachidonic acid (AA) and docosahexaenoic acid (DHA) are the most important fatty acids. Dihomo-γ-linolenic acid (DGLA) and eicosapentaenoic acid (EPA) are also important as cell signalling and enzyme-regulating molecules and as precursors of eicosanoids.

Phospholipid remodelling

The enzymes involved in phospholipid synthesis are highly specific with regard to the fatty acids attached to the Sn1 and Sn2 positions of the phospholipids, although there is a strong trend for unsaturated fatty acids with two or more carbon–carbon double bonds to be attached at the Sn2 position. Correspondingly, saturated and monounsaturated fatty acids tend to be attached at the Sn1 position. However, the final specific structures of phospholipids required for particular membranes at particular geographical sites in cells in particular tissues demand much more precision. This precision is achieved by the actions of cell- and tissue-specific PLA$_1$ and PLA$_2$ and C, and by acyltransferase enzymes which then attach fatty acid coenzyme A derivatives to the vacant Sn1 and Sn2 positions. Other acyl transferase enzymes may transfer fatty acids from one phospholipid to another, or between phospholipids and cholesteryl esters. These various enzymes therefore produce the final structured phospholipids required for each cell (Mead et al., 1986; Gurr and Harwood, 1991).

Phospholipids and neuronal structure and function

In neurones, the outstanding feature of the phospholipids is that, in contrast to other tissues, there are only small amounts of the parent essential fatty acids (EFAs), linoleic and α-linolenic acids (LA and ALA) (Figure 1.4). However, there are large amounts of AA and docosahexaenoic acid (DHA) in the Sn2 position, together with smaller, but still important, amounts of dihomo-γ-linolenic acid (DGLA), adrenic acid (AdrA), eicosapentaenoic acid (EPA) and docosapentaenoic acid (DPA). It is this rich structure of highly unsaturated fatty acids which gives the membranes of neurones their specific properties in relation to cell signalling and to modulation of the structures and functions of membrane-bound and membrane-associated proteins. Neuronal growth, modelling and remodelling represent the growth, modelling and remodelling of the phospholipids of which the neurones are made up.

The supply of fatty acids for phospholipids

The saturated and monounsaturated fatty acids can be provided by their synthesis from simple molecules by the body itself. This is impossible for the EFAs. EFAs can be interconverted along the pathways shown in Figure 1.4, but cannot be synthesized *de novo*. If EFAs are unavailable they will be replaced by nonessential fatty acids, thus changing the behaviour of the phospholipid molecules.

Brain phospholipids

Within the brain, four EFAs are particularly important, with two being overwhelmingly dominant. They are DGLA and AA of the n-6 series, and EPA and DHA of the n-3 series. Between them, they make up 15–30% of the dry weight of neuronal and retinal tissue, AA and DHA constituting 80–90% of that total. These EFAs have two broad roles within the neuronal membrane: structural and functional.

EFAs and membrane structures

The EFAs noted above are absolutely required for the normal structure of all plasma and other membranes within the neurone. The neurone cannot grow and develop, nor can it regress, without the involvement of the synthesis and breakdown of the EFA-rich phospholipids. Moreover, these phospholipids create the physicochemical environment of the membrane within which the proteins, such as receptors and ion channels, are embedded. The phospholipid environment determines the final tertiary and quaternary structure of these proteins; by doing so, it may modify their function in either direction, making the protein more or less functionally active in a quantitative way, depending on the precise nature of the lipid environment (Witt and Nielsen, 1994; Witt et al., 1996). Furthermore, all neurotransmitters, and calcium are wrapped up in phospholipid vesicles. The release and reuptake of such transmitters and of calcium depends on the realignment of phospholipid molecules. The nature of the phospholipid is a factor in determining how much transmitter or metal ion will pass out of a vesicle, or be taken back in.

EFAs and neuronal functioning

The phospholipids and their fatty acid components play a central role in most of the cell-signalling systems within the neurone. The following are just some of the ways in which they may function.

Fatty acid release from Sn2. The fatty acids may be released from the Sn2 position, usually by activation of one of the PLA_2 group of enzymes. They may then themselves regulate various cell functions, for example protein kinases, the nature of the regulation depending on the particular fatty acid molecule and on its geographical location within the cell (Nunez, 1993; Goodfriend and Elliot, 1995). The fatty acids may also be converted to an array of signalling molecules known by the general name of eicosanoids. These include prostaglandins, leukotrienes and hydroxyacids, among many others. They have a huge array of direct actions, as well as indirect actions mediated *via* cyclic nucleotides, calcium, and protein kinases. The range of effects produced depends on the chemical nature of the specific fatty acids, as well as upon the geographical location in the neurone where that fatty acid is released cell (Nunez, 1993; Goodfriend and Elliot, 1995).

Splitting of the phosphate from Sn3. Phospholipase C may split the phosphate from the Sn3 position of phosphatidylinositol, leaving a glycerol with two fatty acids attached in the 1 and 2 positions (DAG) and a phosphorylated inositol molecule (Vance, 1991; Thompson, 1992). Both components may have important cell signalling actions, and again the effects of the DAG will depend precisely on which fatty acids are attached to it. AA and DHA may then be released from DAG by further lipase action.

Phospholipids as the substrate for gene–environment interaction

Phospholipids are fundamental to neuronal structure, growth, remodelling and function. They are unique, in that environment and genes interact in an intimate way to determine the final phospholipid composition of the neuronal membrane. The various enzymes which are involved in phospholipid synthesis and breakdown have been summarised in the figures. Each of these enzymes is under genetic control, and abnormalities will produce varying degrees of abnormality in neuronal phospholipid structure.

The enzymes cannot, however, make EFAs *de novo*. The key EFAs of neuronal phospholipids must come from the diet, either directly or *via* conversion of dietary LA and ALA to the EFAs critical for neuronal structure. If they are not available they will be replaced by other, less desirable, fatty acids. The final phospholipid structure of the neurone, and thus its function and its capacity for remodelling, depend in a unique way on environment–gene interactions (Horrobin et al., 1995).

Supply of EFAs to the brain

It is important to understand the way in which the EFAs get to the brain from the food (Figure 1.5). The stages, starting at the neurone, are as follows:

Cellular uptake

EFAs in the extracellular fluid are rapidly taken up into cells, possibly partly by specific transport mechanisms involving fatty acid transport proteins (FATPs), but also by simple diffusion through the membrane

The Phospholipid Concept of Psychiatric Disorders

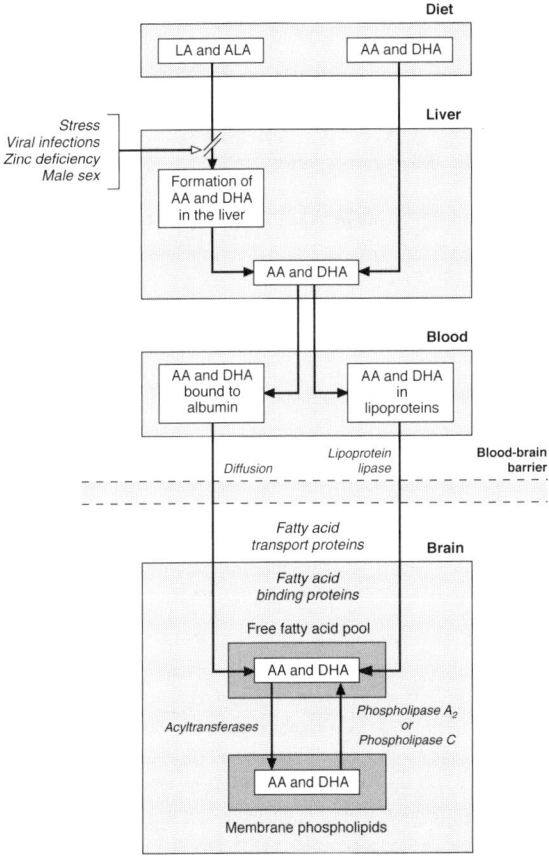

Figure 1.5. The routes whereby the essential fatty acids required for normal brain function reach the brain phospholipids. The formation of AA and DHA in the liver is blocked by stress, viral infections, zinc deficiency and male sex.

(Robert et al., 1983; Spector and Yorek, 1985; Thompson, 1992). They are then available for incorporation into phospholipids. Neurones probably normally require the four key EFAs to have been preformed, though some neurones may have a limited capacity for making DGLA and AA from LA, and EPA and DHA from ALA. Glial cells may also be involved in these reactions and may supply the EFAs to neurones (Robert et al., 1983). Within neurones and glial cells, fatty acid trafficking is regulated by at least three fatty acid binding proteins (FABPs). These FABPs appear to be very important in neuronal development since some or all of them are strongly expressed wherever neuronal growth and development are taking place (Owada et al., 1996; Rousselot et al., 1997; Utsunomiya et al., 1997).

Transport across the blood–brain barrier

EFAs diffuse across the blood–brain barrier, again in some cases assisted by specific transport mechanisms.

Release from blood transport mechanisms

The fatty acids are transported in the blood, either bound to albumin, or in the form of triglycerides associated with lipoproteins. The fatty acids may be released from albumin by diffusion, possibly depending on concentration gradients created by FABPs in the various tissues. In the case of the lipoprotein triglycerides, the fatty acids must be released by the action of lipoprotein lipase in the endothelial cells of the capillaries of the relevant tissue (Ben Zeev et al., 1990; Vilaro et al., 1990; Nunez et al., 1995). Lipoprotein lipase is one of the fundamental controllers of the overall rate of supply of fatty acids to the brain (Ben Zeev et al., 1990; Vilaro et al., 1990; Nunez et al., 1995). Lipoprotein lipase levels are considerably higher in the hippocampus than in other brain areas, and are also relatively high in the neocortex (Ben Zeev et al., 1990; Vilaro et al., 1990; Nunez et al., 1995). Hippocampal lipoprotein lipase activities are highest in the neonatal period, indicating that this is a particularly important time for the incorporation of fatty acids into hippocampal phospholipids. Lipoprotein lipase is also adversely affected by ovarian and testicular steroids, and its activity can be substantially inhibited at puberty (Bucher et al., 1997). It is therefore of considerable interest that the gene for lipoprotein lipase is located on chromosome 8p22 (Sparkes et al., 1987; Horrobin, 1997), one of the hot spots where there is the strongest evidence for a gene predisposing to a high risk of schizophrenia. Lipoprotein lipase therefore becomes a strong candidate for a modulating action in schizophrenia (Horrobin, 1997).

Entry of EFAs into the blood

The two main points at which EFAs may enter the blood are the liver or the gastrointestinal tract. The brain-specific EFAs are mostly made in the liver from their common dietary precursors, LA and ALA. However, this is a strongly rate-limited process, with less than 5% of the dietary LA being metabolised down to AA, or of dietary ALA being converted to DHA, even in young, healthy adults (Cunnane, 1996). Factors which are of interest in the context of schizophrenia may interfere with the rates of conversion of LA and ALA, and therefore with the formation of the EFAs required for brain phospholipids (Brenner, 1981; Horrobin, 1990a; 1992a).

Factors affecting LA and ALA conversion

The extremes of life. The very young may not be able to make AA and DHA at an adequate rate. Equally, the rate falls off with age (Horrobin, 1981; Takahashi et al., 1991).

Stress. Both catecholamines and glucocorticoids have a powerful inhibitory effect on the conversions of LA and ALA to AA and DHA (Brenner, 1981).

Viral infections. Viral infections inhibit the formation of AA and DHA (Horrobin, 1990b). This may be because interferon utilizes AA to achieve its antiviral effects (Chandrabose et al., 1981). As a defence against the action of interferon, many viruses appear to have developed a strategy of interfering with AA formation.

Sex differences. Females convert LA and ALA more rapidly than males, and, under conditions of EFA deficiency, retain AA and DHA within membrane phospholipids to a greater extent than males (Huang and Horrobin, 1987; Marra and de Alaniz, 1989; Huang et al., 1990). These effects are partly dependent on oestrogen.

Brain EFAs from food

If conversion of LA and ALA to AA, DGLA, EPA and DHA is impaired, then the only way for the brain to obtain the EFAs it requires is directly from the food. This is probably why human breast milk is rich in the EFAs required for the brain; until recently, however, most formula milks contained only LA and ALA. It is increasingly recognized that these EFA differences are major contributors to the differences between breast-fed and bottle-fed babies (Koletzko, 1992; Lucas et al., 1992; Carlson et al., 1993; Makrides et al., 1995). Other foods relatively rich in the brain EFAs are egg yolks, seafood and meat from wild, but not domesticated, animals.

Importance of antioxidants

The ease with which a fatty acid can be oxidized increases with the number of double bonds in the chain. Thus the brain EFAs are exceptionally susceptible to oxidation. This can occur even when the fatty acid is in situ in a membrane phospholipid, but it is liable to take place at a much higher rate when the EFA is in a free form. EFAs may therefore be particularly vulnerable when being liberated by phospholipases. It is important that there should be a supply of appropriate antioxidants (Mahadik and Gowda, 1996; Mahadik and Mukherjee, 1996). These are of three main types: the primary lipophilic antioxidants (such as vitamin E), which work in membranes; the hydrophilic antioxidants (such as ascorbic acid), which work in the aqueous compartments of the cell and the extracellular fluid; and a variety of cofactors which assist in limiting oxidation in various ways and which include β-carotene, lipoic acid, ubiquinone zinc, selenium, pyridoxine and nicotinamide. All these factors work together to limit the access of pro-oxidant radicals to the double bonds of the EFAs and to remove oxidized materials which may be formed. If the EFAs do become oxidized they lose their ability to function physiologically. There is considerable evidence that excessive oxidation may be involved in the pathogenesis of tardive dyskinesia (Rotrosen et al., 1996), in aging (Harman, 1994), and possibly in schizophrenia (Phillips et al., 1993; Mahadik and Scheffer, 1996). Traditional neuroleptic drugs may act as pro-oxidants (Mahadik and Scheffer, 1996).

Overall comment: phospholipid metabolism

An array of genetic and environmental factors may modulate the composition of brain phospholipids and therefore modulate brain function. The phospholipids provide a focal point for the interaction of genetic and environmental factors in the development of psychiatric disorders.

THE MEMBRANE PHOSPHOLIPID HYPOTHESIS OF SCHIZOPHRENIA

The membrane phospholipid hypothesis suggests that disturbed phospholipid metabolism is the fundamental cause of schizophrenia. Specifically, it is postulated that, in individuals who develop schizophrenia, there is an accelerated rate of loss of unsaturated fatty acids, notably AA, DHA, EPA and DGLA, from the Sn2 position of phospholipids (Glen et al., 1994; Horrobin et al., 1994, 1995; Peet et al., 1994, 1996; Ward et al., 1997). When present to a mild degree, this increased rate of loss will be compensated by an increased role of incorporation, with no change in phospholipid composition, but when present to a greater degree, or when associated with problems of incorporation, there will be an actual change in membrane composition (Horrobin et al., 1995).

An increased rate of loss of these key fatty acids will lead to changes in functioning of membrane-associated proteins and of various cell signalling systems. A possible enzymatic basis for such increased loss is the overactivity of one or more of the PLA_2 group of enzymes which remove the unsaturated fatty acids from the Sn2 position. This could result from the presence of an abnormal enzyme variant or from overexpression of the normal enzyme. Another possibility would be the sequential action of a phospholipase C and of a DAG lipase. Either way, the increased rate of removal from phospholipids would make the free acids more susceptible to oxidation. There is a substantial body of evidence for this concept.

Evidence for increased rate of loss of key fatty acids

Increased PLA_2 activity

There are increased levels of functional PLA_2 activity detectable in the blood of patients with schizophrenia (Gattaz et al., 1990; Gattaz and Brunner, 1996; Ross et al., 1997).

Changed AA and DHA levels

Patients with schizophrenia frequently exhibit reduced levels of AA and DHA in membrane phospholipids (Glen et al., 1994; Peet et al., 1994, 1996). Increased oxidation of the highly unsaturated fatty acids may be a part explanation for this (Ramchand et al., 1996). Clozapine, unlike typical neuroleptics, has recently been found to raise red cell phospholipid AA and DHA levels in schizophrenic patients (Glen et al., 1996; Horrobin et al., 1997). This mechanism could contribute to the unusual therapeutic efficacy of clozapine which is difficult to explain in full on the basis of the drug's receptor-blocking profile.

Magnetic resonance imaging

Magnetic resonance imaging provides results consistent with an increased rate of phospholipid breakdown in the frontal cortex of unmedicated schizophrenic patients (Pettegrew et al., 1991, 1993; Williamson et al., 1996).

Flushing response of niacin

Schizophrenic patients may show a reduced flushing response to oral or topical niacin. With a topical test, involving the application of niacin to forearm skin, about 70% of patients show values below the bottom end of the normal range. This test depends on the mobilization of AA and its conversion to prostaglandin D_2, and is a marker of the availability of AA for cell signalling (Ward et al., 1997, 1998). The reduced flushing indicates that the availability of AA is reduced, possibly explaining the hypofunction of glutamate receptors in schizophrenia (Olney and Farber, 1995).

Reduced maximal electroretinogram response

The retina is particularly rich in DHA and the maximum amplitude of the electroretinogram (ERG) depends on the availability of DHA for cell signalling. Schizophrenic patients show a significantly reduced maximal ERG response to a light stimulus (Warner and Peet, 1999), indicating that the availability of DHA, like AA, for cell signalling is reduced.

Genetic abnormalities

Two different genetic abnormalities have now been found in schizophrenic patients in the vicinity of the gene for PLA_2 on chromosome 1. These abnormalities may lead to differential expression of the gene and suggest that a variety of changes in the gene may be involved in schizophrenia, possibly accounting for different subtypes of the disease (Hudson et al., 1996; Peet et al., 1998).

Other observations

There are several other observations in schizophrenia which are ignored by receptor-based hypotheses, but which can be explained by the phospholipid concept. These include the resistance to pain, the resistance to arthritis and other inflammatory diseases, and the improvement in psychosis which may occur in response to fever (Horrobin, 1979, 1997; Horrobin et al., 1978, 1994, 1995).

Modulation of the phospholipid disorder by other factors

Several factors are able to modulate the effects of abnormalities of fatty acid removal from, or incorporation into, membrane phospholipids.

The relative availability of the EFAs and of other fatty acids from the diet

The EFAs on the one hand, and saturated and monounsaturated fatty acids on the other, compete with each other for incorporation into phospholipids. An increased intake of saturated fats, and/or a reduced intake of EFAs, would be expected to exacerbate a situation where there are reduced amounts of EFAs in brain phospholipids. Conversely, an increased availability of dietary EFAs should attenuate the problem.

The specific availability of the EFAs important in the brain

AA, DHA, EPA and DGLA may be supplied by the diet, as in breast milk or in foods from the sea or algal-rich fresh water (Gibson and Kneebone, 1981; Birch et al., 1992; Broadhurst et al., 1998). They may also be manufactured within the body by synthesis from dietary LA and ALA. The rates of synthesis and of incorporation of these brain EFAs into membrane phospholipids are reduced by viral infections, male sex, stress, and old age, and are attenuated by female sex and female sex hormones. Insulin is a potent stimulator of the conversion of LA to AA and of ALA to DHA (Brenner, 1981), which makes one wonder whether insulin therapy for schizophrenia might have influenced this system.

The activities of lipoprotein lipase and fatty acid binding proteins

Lipoprotein lipase is a key enzyme determining the availability of all fatty acids for the brain. Its activity is substantially modified by general hormones at puberty (Bucher et al., 1997), and is enhanced by prolactin, the blood levels of which are elevated by all typical neuroleptics. A variant of lipoprotein lipase is associated with a reduced risk of inflammatory disorders as occurs in schizophrenia (Wallberg-Jonsson et al., 1996). FABPs which bind long-chain fatty acids also play important roles in regulating the supply of EFAs such as AA and DHA to the brain. They are strongly expressed whenever brain development, reorganization and remodelling are taking place (Owada et al., 1996; Rousselot et al., 1997; Utsunomiya et al., 1997).

Fatty acid oxidation

Increased rates of fatty acid oxidation will exacerbate the problem, while reduced rates will attenuate it. The balance between oxidant and antioxidant systems will therefore influence the severity of the abnormality.

The rate of incorporation of fatty acids into phospholipids

A reduced rate of fatty acid incorporation will exacerbate the consequences of an enhanced rate of removal. In dyslexia, which is associated with schizotypal disorders, there seems to be a reduced rate of fatty acid incorporation (Horrobin et al., 1995; Stordy, 1995). This view is now supported by evidence of reduced brain phospholipid synthesis in dyslexia found on ^{31}P magnetic resonance imaging (Richardson et al., 1997). In schizophrenia, there is direct evidence of reduced uptake of fatty acids into platelet phospholipids (Mahadik et al., 1996; Yao et al., 1996).

THE PHOSPHOLIPID CONCEPT AS AN EXPLANATION OF THE BIOCHEMISTRY BEHIND THE NEURODEVELOPMENTAL HYPOTHESIS OF SCHIZOPHRENIA

The majority of the observations which support the neurodevelopmental concept can be biochemically explained on the basis of the phospholipid hypothesis.

Brain morphology

Since phospholipids form the bulk of the brain, a genetic abnormality in phospholipid metabolism would be expected to lead to abnormal brain morphology. The processes involved in the formation of neurones and of their synaptic connections are dependent on phospholipid synthesis and remodelling. PLA$_2$ and cyclooxygenase 2 (COX-2), the latter being the enzyme which catalyses the first step in conversion of fatty acids to eicosanoids, are both highly expressed in sprouting nerve endings (Kaufmann et al., 1994; Negre-Aminou et al., 1996; Smalheiser et al., 1996). Selective apoptosis plays an important role in brain development. EFAs are required for normal control of apoptosis (de Kock et al., 1996), raising the possibility that, in the absence of normal EFA metabolism, regulation of the pruning of brain connections may be defective. Neuronal cell adhesion molecules (N-CAMs) are important in the regulation of brain micromorphology, and are elevated in schizophrenia (Poltorak et al., 1996; Van Kammen et al., 1997). The synthesis of CAMs in other tissues can be regulated by AA and EPA (Huang et al., 1997; Hughes et al., 1996). The excess N-CAM production in schizophrenia could therefore be explained by reduced availability of AA and EPA.

Effects of puberty, aging and sex

A problem facing the neurodevelopmental hypothesis is an explanation for the delay between presumed events *in utero* or in the perinatal period, and their delayed full expression in schizophrenia after puberty. There is a surge of synaptic remodelling and myelination around and after puberty, and the hypothesis is that such remodelling will allow the expression of deficits laid down earlier (Waddington, 1993; Weinberger, 1995b). Phospholipids are of crucial importance in remodelling and myelination, and these processes would be expected to be abnormal in the presence of a genetic abnormality in phospholipid metabolism. COX-2 expression is linked to phospholipase expression, and in animals there is an explosion of COX-2 expression in nerve endings at the time of puberty, when synapses are being remodelled (Kaufman et al., 1996). Lipoprotein lipase function is also changed at puberty (Bucher et al., 1997). The delay until puberty of the full expression of the schizophrenic phenotype is therefore reasonably explicable by the phospholipid concept.

The sex differences in the time of onset and in the severity of schizophrenia, as well as the existence of a second, later, period of increased risk in females, are also explicable on the basis of the importance of phospholipid AA and DHA. These EFAs are more readily synthesized from their precursors, more readily incorporated into phospholipids, and their depletion more strongly resisted, in females than in males (Pudelkewicz et al., 1968; Huang and Horrobin, 1987; Marra and de Alaniz, 1989; Huang et al., 1990). Thus females would be expected to be more resistant than males to a defect in phospholipid-related metabolism.

The effect of being female on EFA metabolism is partly dependent on oestrogen. Schizophrenic women with higher oestrogen levels have milder psychiatric symptoms than do these with lower oestrogen levels (Hoff et al., 1997). The postmenopausal onset of schizophrenia in females could therefore be explained by the effects of oestrogen loss on AA and DHA phospholipid metabolism.

In both sexes, there can be emergence in old age of a schizophrenic-like syndrome (Castle and Murray, 1993). The rate of formation of AA and DHA from dietary precursors falls in old age (Horrobin, 1981; Takahashi et al., 1991). This would exacerbate any marginal problem relating to incorporation or retention of AA and DHA in brain phospholipids. In animals, there is an age-related fall in brain AA levels which is associated with loss of normal glutamate-related neurotransmission and long-term potentiation: normal brain AA levels, long-term potentiation, and glutamatergic transmission can all be restored by administration of AA (McGahon et al., 1997).

Pregnancy and perinatal events

The pregnancy and perinatal events which have been found to be related to later schizophrenia can for the most part be readily explained by their effects on the availability of normally-structured phospholipids.

Breast feeding

Two studies have found that breast feeding is significantly less common among infants who, in later life, develop schizophrenia than in those who go on to develop normally (McCreadie, 1997; Peet et al., 1997a). These observations are consistent with a protective effect of breast feeding, which is predicted by the phospholipid hypothesis. This is because breast milk, but not infant formula, is rich in DGLA, AA, EPA and DHA. Infants, especially premature ones, are not able to make AA and DHA from dietary LA and ALAs at an adequate rate to serve the needs of the brain (Koletzko, 1992; Lucas et al., 1992; Carlson et al., 1993; Makrides et al., 1995). Formula feeding would therefore be expected to exacerbate schizophrenia-related problems in phospholipid metabolism, whereas breast feeding should attenuate them.

Starvation during pregnancy

Starvation during pregnancy increases the risk of schizophrenia (Susser and Lin, 1992). Such starvation will lead to EFA deficiency during brain development. Sinclair's experience in the Dutch famine of 1944–45 was one of the reasons for his understanding of the importance of EFAs for humans (Sinclair, 1956). The strongest evidence for the impact of maternal food deprivation on later schizophrenia comes from that famine.

Head circumference

Low head circumference in otherwise normal individuals is a risk factor for schizophrenia (McNeil et al., 1993). The supply of AA to the developing foetus is a determinant of brain growth (Crawford, 1992; Koletzko, 1992). A low head circumference could therefore be an indicator of reduced availability of AA to the foetus which would exacerbate any tendency towards reduced AA levels in phospholipids.

Obstetric complications

There is a small but consistent increase in the risk of schizophrenia in association with obstetric complications, particularly prematurity and perinatal hypoxia (McNeil and Kaij, 1978; O'Callaghan et al., 1992; McGrath and Murray, 1995). Hypoxia causes mobilization of EFAs from brain phospholipids (Rordorf et al., 1991), which would exacerbate any tendency towards low AA and DHA levels in neuronal membranes.

Stress

Stress during pregnancy is associated with a small, but significant, increased risk of schizophrenia in the offspring (Selten et al., 1997). Stress leads to elevation of cortisol and catecholamines, both of which are known to reduce the rate of formation of AA and DHA from dietary precursors (Brenner, 1981; Horrobin, 1990a,

1992a; Mills, 1991). Stress could therefore lead to reduced availability of brain-specific EFAs for the foetus.

Viral infections

There is disputed evidence of a modestly increased risk of schizophrenia in the offspring of mothers who experience viral infections during pregnancy, especially during the second trimester (O'Callaghan et al., 1991b; Sham et al., 1992). Viral infections are also known to inhibit the formation of AA and DHA from their dietary precursors (Chandrabose et al., 1981; Horrobin, 1981). Viral infections would thus be expected to exacerbate any impairment in EFA-phospholipid metabolism resulting from a genetic abnormality.

Season of birth

Infants born in the late winter months are at increased risk of schizophrenia in comparison with those born at other times. During the winter months, the incorporation of EFAs into ectodermal lipids in the skin is greatly reduced (Conti et al., 1996). If a similar change were to take place in ectodermal brain lipids, it would put at risk those already vulnerable because of a genetic abnormality in phospholipid metabolism.

Minor physical abnormalities

There is an increased frequency of minor physical abnormalities among schizophrenic individuals (Green et al., 1989; O'Callaghan et al., 1991a). Such minor defects are likely to involve abnormalities of cell remodelling, migration, adhesion and apoptosis. Phospholipids, the EFAs and their metabolites play important roles in the these processes (Kaufmann et al., 1994, 1996; Weinberger, 1995b; de Kock et al., 1996; Hughes et al., 1996; Poltorak et al., 1996; Smalheiser et al., 1996; Huang et al., 1997; Van Kammen et al., 1997). Impairment of normal phospholipid metabolism would be likely to be associated with minor physical abnormalities.

Childhood behaviour and later schizophrenia

Many studies have attempted to identify features of childhood behaviour and performance which might allow prediction as to which individuals will later develop schizophrenia.

IQ

The risk of later schizophrenia increases with reduction in IQ (David et al., 1997). The EFA-rich phospholipids are required for the normal pattern and richness of neuronal interconnections and so it is reasonable to suppose that phospholipid metabolism and the EFA supply might be related to intelligence. There is evidence in support of this suggestion. In a study of premature infants, none of whom was breast fed, half were given breast milk containing the EFAs needed for brain development, and half were given formula milk containing the EFA precursors, LA and ALA. At the age of 8 years, the infants given breast milk had IQs that were eight points higher than those of the formula-fed infants, a highly significant increase (Lucas et al., 1992). There are several possible explanations, but one is that the difference was attributable to the availability of the EFAs required for the brain. Direct evidence of such an effect from a randomized study comes from an investigation of visual acuity in bottle-fed infants (Makrides et al., 1995). All were given the same basic formula, but the infants were randomized on a double-blind basis to receive a brain EFA supplement or a placebo supplement added to the formula. At the age of 30 weeks, the EFA supplemented infants could, on average, detect squares 0.7 cm in size, whereas the mean square size detectable by the placebo-fed infants was 2.0 cm. This indicates an effect of the brain-related EFAs on brain and eye development. The association of schizophrenia with low IQ could be due to an EFA-phospholipid effect on both IQ and risk of schizophrenia.

Language and verbal skills

Poor language and verbal skills indicate children at risk of schizophrenia. Such poor skills are also indicative of dyslexia which is associated with impaired EFA incorporation into phospholipids (Horrobin et al., 1995; Stordy, 1995; Richardson et al., 1997). Impaired language skills may therefore be associated with impaired phospholipid metabolism.

Motor coordination

Poor motor coordination is predictive of an increased risk of later schizophrenia (Marcus, 1974; Jones et al., 1994). Dyspraxia, which is a severe form of motor incoordination, is associated with EFA abnormalities and is correctable with EFA treatment (Stordy, 1996).

Attention

Defects in attention are associated with increased risk of schizophrenia (Rieder and Nichols, 1979). Children with attention deficit hyperactivity disorder (ADHD) have normal LA and ALA blood levels, but reduced concentrations of the brain-related EFAs. These reduced levels cannot be explained by defective diet (Colquhoun and Bunday, 1981; Mitchell et al., 1987; Stevens et al., 1995, 1996). A strong inverse relationship has been reported between the blood levels of EPA and DHA and the severity of the attention deficits and other behavioural problems (Stevens et al., 1996).

Social skills

Impaired social skills are predictive of increased later schizophrenia risk. Dyslexia, which is associated with impaired EFA incorporation into phospholipids, is associated with schizotypal personality and reduced social skills (Richardson, 1994).

INTERACTION BETWEEN PHOSPHOLIPID AND NEURO-DEVELOPMENTAL HYPOTHESES

The basic premise of the phospholipid hypothesis is that normal neuronal phospholipid metabolism is required for the normal development of brain architecture *in utero* and in childhood, for the normal modulation of that architecture around the time of puberty, and for normal functioning of the adult nervous system. The hypothesis proposes that in schizophrenia there is a modest, genetically-based increase in the rate of AA and DHA loss from neurones, and that this leads to abnormalities in thought and behaviour. The abnormality is described as being only modest because, for long stretches of time, some schizophrenic patients behave near normally, because identical twins are often discordant for schizophrenia, and because a small elevation in brain temperature can produce a near normalization of function (Horrobin et al., 1978, 1995).

The proposed increase in the rate of DHA and AA removal is likely to relate to increased activity of one or more phospholipases. This could be due to a variant in phospholipase structure or to increased expression of a normal phospholipase. Several different genotypic variations could lead to similar phenotypic end results. The phospholipases involved are likely to be from the A_2 and C groups since it these which lead to release of AA and DHA from the Sn2 position.

It is further proposed that the consequences of the abnormality in removal of EFAs from phospholipids will be exacerbated by the simultaneous presence of an abnormality of phospholipid synthesis and remodelling, such that the rate of incorporation of AA and DHA into phospholipids is reduced. This type of abnormality has been postulated both in dyslexia (Horrobin et al., 1995; Horrobin, 1996; Richardson et al., 1997) and in schizophrenia (Mahadik et al., 1996; Yao et al., 1996). The severity of the impact of such an abnormality of EFA incorporation will be modified by variations in the rate of supply of EFAs or incorporation into neuronal phospholipids. This will depend on the rate of conversion of the main dietary EFAs to the brain-related EFAs, on the direct intake of brain-related EFAs, on the activities of brain lipoprotein lipase and FABPs, and on the rate of formation of coenzyme A derivatives of the EFAs, which are required for the transfer step to the phospholipids.

Thus it is proposed that the basic abnormality in phospholipid metabolism in schizophrenia creates a vulnerable state which may be exacerbated by starvation, viral infections, perinatal hypoxia, the absence of breast feeding, variations in diet, and the presence of a second abnormality similar to that in some patients with dyslexia. The sex of the individual and changes in hormone levels involved in the life cycle, will also have important influences. These observations are consistent with, and able to explain, most of the features of the neurodevelopmental hypothesis. They may also help to explain the genetic susceptibility loci on chromosome 8 and chromosome 6. The lipoprotein lipase gene is in the region identified on chromosome 8, while the dyslexia gene is close to one of the high risk loci on chromosome 6 (Grigorenko et al., 1997).

The phospholipid hypothesis therefore proposes that in schizophrenia there are two major primary abnormalities in phospholipid metabolism and that the impact of these may be modified by other lipid-related genes and by environmental factors. The two primary abnormalities are an increased rate of removal of EFAs, especially AA and DHA, from membrane phospholipids, coupled with a reduced rate of incorporation into phospholipids of these same fatty acids. Both abnormalities may need to be present simultaneously to produce a full schizophrenic syndrome. One highly speculative possibility is that the problem of incorporation when present alone may produce dyslexia and schizotypy, whereas the problem of excess removal by increased PLA_2 or C activity when present alone may produce bipolar disorder (Horrobin et al., 1995; Horrobin, 1996, 1997, 1998a,b). Recently, it has been shown that therapeutically relevant concentrations of lithium inhibit PLA_2 *in vivo*, so strengthening the case for the involvement of this enzyme in manic-depression (Chang et al., 1996).

The overall impact of these two abnormalities will be exacerbated or attenuated by the rate at which key EFAs enter the brain. This will be dependent on dietary supply, on rate of formation of brain-related EFAs in the liver, on transport in the blood by lipoproteins and albumin and related proteins, and on entry into the brain mediated by FABPs and lipoprotein lipase. Lipoprotein lipase is of particular interest because it is found in very high concentrations in the hippocampus, one of the most vulnerable parts of the brain both in schizophrenia and following ischaemic or traumatic damage. The supply of EFAs, and especially of AA, to the brain is one of the main determinants of brain size (Crawford, 1992; Koletzko, 1992; Oloyede et al., 1992). FABPs, as discussed earlier, are also of great interest because of their expression wherever neurodevelopment is occurring.

There has been much interest in brain asymmetry, or the relative lack of it, in schizophrenia. Brain phospholipid metabolism is asymmetric: this asymmetry is phylogenetically old and can be demonstrated in mice (Pediconi and Rodriguez de Turco, 1984; Ginobili de Martinez et al., 1985; Ginobili de Martinez and Barrantes, 1988). Basal levels of free EFAs, which are substantially determined by acyltransferase activity, and the massive release of EFAs which occurs in ischaemia and which is dependent on PLA_2 activity (Rordorf et al., 1991), both show large right/left differences in mice. Crow (1995a, 1996a) has discussed the possibility that increased brain asymmetry in normal individuals may have been related to the development of language, and that some abnormality in the development of that asymmetry may be involved in schizophrenia. Such asymmetry could be related to a mutation in brain lipoprotein lipase which produced a more effective supply of EFAs for brain phospholipid and so drove brain growth. Acting against a pre-existing background of cerebral asymmetry in acyltransferase and phospholipase activities, such a change in lipoprotein lipase could have been responsible for enhancing the development of asymmetry in hemisphere size and structure in humans (Horrobin, 1998a,b).

CONCLUSIONS

The overall concept is illustrated in Figure 1.5. Two main groups of enzymes, the phospholipases and acyltransferases, determine the fine structure of brain phospholipids. These enzymes have to work with fatty acids provided to them by the blood and whose entry to the brain will be dependent either on diffusion from albumin and other FABPs, or on release from lipoproteins by lipoprotein lipase. The availability of the brain EFAs will depend partly on dietary supply, and partly on liver metabolism. Liver synthesis requires many cofactors, including insulin, zinc and various vitamins, whereas it can be blocked by factors such as stress, viral infections or a high intake of saturated or *trans* fatty acids.

At all points, the highly unsaturated brain fatty acids are susceptible to oxidation and so their supply will also be modified by oxidants and antioxidants.

This model provides a paradigm for research into schizophrenia which allows for the interaction between a limited number of major genes, a larger number of modifying genes, and a wide range of nutritional, biochemical, psychological and social environmental factors. It is therefore flexible enough to allow for the complexity of schizophrenia, but precise enough to allow specific questions to be asked and answered. The model is consistent with much of what we know about the genetics of schizophrenia, and also with the neurodevelopmental and neurotransmitter hypotheses.

The ultimate test of the usefulness of the model will be whether it leads to improved treatment. There is evidence from epidemiological studies and clinical trials that modifying the intake of EFAs can change the outcome of schizophrenia (World Health Organisation, 1979; Christensen and Christensen, 1988; Horrobin, 1992b; Mellor et al., 1995, 1996; Peet et al., 1997a). The chapters which follow in this volume suggest that we may be on the right track to improve outcomes in this devastating illness, and give reasonable hope that we may be able to provide, for a range of other behavioural disturbances, biochemical explanations which could then offer new and effective treatment options.

ACKNOWLEDGEMENT

This paper is based on a paper which appeared in Schizophrenia Research in 1998 (Horrobin, 1998a).

REFERENCES

Ben Zeev O, Doolittle MH, Singh N, Chang CH, Schotz MC. Synthesis and regulation of lipoprotein lipase in the hippocampus. J Lipid Res 1990; 31: 1307–1313.

Birch EE, Birch DG, Hoffman DR, Uauy R. Dietary essential fatty acid supply and visual acuity development. Invest Ophthalmol Vis Sci 1992: 33; 3242–3253.

Brenner RR. Nutritional and hormonal factors influencing desaturation of essential fatty acids. Prog Lipid Res 1981; 20: 41–47.

British Nutrition Foundation. Unsaturated fatty acids: nutritional and physiological significance. London: Chapman and Hall, 1992.

Broadhurst CL, Cunnane SC, Crawford MA. Rift Valley lake fish and shellfish provided brain-specific nutrition for early *Homo*. Br J Nutr 1998; 79: 3–21.

Bucher H, Rampini S, James RW et al. Marked changes of lipid levels during puberty in a patient with lipoprotein lipase deficiency. Eur J Paediatr 1997; 156: 121–125.

Carlson SE, Werkman SH, Peeples JM, Cooke RJ, Tolley EA. Arachidonic acid status correlates with first year growth in preterm infants. Proc Natl Acad Sci USA 1993; 90: 1073–1077.

Castle DJ, Murray RM. The epidemiology of late-onset schizophrenia. Schizophr Bull 1993; 19: 691–700.

Chandrabose KA, Cuatrecasas P, Pottathil R, Lang DJ. Interferon-resistant cell line lacks cyclooxygenase activity. Science 1981; 212: 329–331.

Chang MCJ, Grange E, Rabin O, Bell JM, Allen DD, Rapoport SI. Lithium decreases turnover of arachidonate in several brain phospholipids. Neurosci Lett 1996; 220: 171–174.

Christensen O, Christensen E. Fat consumption and schizophrenia. Acta Psychiatr Scand 1988; 78: 587–591.

Colquhoun I, Bunday S. A lack of essential fatty acids as a possible cause of hyperactivity in children. Med Hypotheses 1981; 7: 673–679.

Conti A, Rogers J, Verdejo P, Harding CR, Rawlings AV. Seasonal influences on stratum corneum ceramide 1 fatty acids and the influence of topical essential fatty acids. Int J Cosmet Sci 1996; 18: 1–12.

Crawford MA. The role of dietary fats in biology: their place in the evolution of the human brain. Nutr Rev 1992; 50: 3–11.

Crow TJ. A Darwinian approach to the origins of psychosis. Br J Psychiatry 1995a; 167: 12–25.

Crow TJ. Constraints on concepts of pathogenesis. Language and the speciation process as the key to the etiology of schizophrenia. Arch Gen Psychiatry 1995b; 52: 1011–1014.

Crow TJ. Language and psychosis: common evolutionary origins. Endeavour 1996a; 20: 105–109.

Crow TJ. Sexual selection as the mechanism of evolution of Machiavellian intelligence: a Darwinian theory of the origins of psychosis. J Psychopharmacol 1996b; 10: 77–87.

Cunnane SC. Recent studies on the synthesis beta-oxidation and deficiency of linoleate and alpha-linoleate: are essential fatty acids more aptly named dispensable or conditionally dispensable fatty acids. Can J Physiol Pharmacol 1996; 74: 629–639.

Dalen P. Season of birth: a study of schizophrenia and other mental disorders. Amsterdam: North Holland, 1975.

David AS, Malmberg A, Lewis G, Allebeck P. Psychiatric morbidity, social development and cognition and later schizophrenia: premorbid adjustment or prodrome? Schizophr Res 1997; 24: 249.

de Kock M, Lottering M-L, Grobler CJS, Viljoen TC, le Roux M, Seegers JC. The induction of apoptosis in human cervical carcinoma (HeLa) cells by gamma-linolenic acid. Prostagland Leukotr Essent Fatty Acids 1996; 55: 403–411.

Falkai P, Bogerts B. The neuropathology of schizophrenia. In: Hirsch SR, Weinberger DR, eds. Schizophrenia. Oxford: Blackwell, 1995: 275–292.

Fish B. Infant predictors of the longitudinal course of schizophrenic development. Schizophr Bull 1987; 13: 395–409.

Gattaz WF, Brunner J. Phospholipase A_2 and the hypofrontality hypothesis of schizophrenia. Prostagland Leukotr Essent Fatty Acids 1996; 55: 109–113.

Gattaz WF, Hübner CK, Nevalainen TJ, Thuren T, Kinnunen PKJ. Increased serum phospholipase-A_2 activity in schizophrenia: a replication study. Biol Psychiatry 1990; 28: 495–501.

Gibson RA, Kneebone GM. Fatty acid composition of human colostrum and mature breast milk. Am J Clin Nutr 1981; 34: 252–257.

Ginobili de Martinez MS, Barrantes FJ. Ca2+ and phospholipid-dependent protein kinase activity in rat cerebral hemispheres. Brain Res 1988; 440: 386–390.

Ginobili de Martinez MS, Rodriguez de Turco EB, Barrantes FJ. Endogenous asymmetry of rat brain lipids and dominance of the right cerebral hemisphere in free fatty acid response to electroconvulsive shock. Brain Res 1985; 339: 315–321.

Glen AIM, Glen EMT, Horrobin DF et al. A red cell membrane abnormality in a subgroup of schizophrenic patients: evidence for two diseases. Schizophr Res 1994; 12: 53–61.

Glen AIM, Cooper SJ, Rybakowski J, Vaddadi K, Brayshaw N, Horrobin DF. Membrane fatty acids, niacin flushing and clinical parameters. Prostagland Leukotr Essent Fatty Acids 1996; 15: 9–15.

Goodfriend TL, Elliot ME. Fatty acids in cell signalling. Prostagland Leukotr Essent Fatty Acids 1995; 52: 75–211.

Green MF, Satz P, Gaier DJ, Ganzell S, Kharabi F. Minor physical anomalies in schizophrenia. Schizophr Bull 1989; 15: 91–99.

Grigorenko EL, Wood FB, Meyer MS et al. Susceptibility loci for distinct components of developmental dyslexia on chromosomes 6 and 15. Am J Hum Genet 1997; 60: 27–39.

Gurr MI, Harwood JL. Lipid biochemistry. London: Chapman and Hall, 1991.

Harman D. Aging: prospects for further increases in the functional life span. Age 1994; 17: 119–146.

Hoff AL, Wieneke M, Horon R et al. Estrogen levels relate to neurophysiological function in female schizophrenics. Schizophr Res 1997; 24: 107.

Horrobin DF. Schizophrenia: reconciliation of the dopamine, prostaglandin and opioid concepts and the role of the pineal. Lancet 1979; i: 529–531.

Horrobin DF. Loss of delta-6-desaturase activity as a key factor in aging. Med Hypotheses 1981; 7: 1211–1220.

Horrobin DF. Gamma-linolenic acid: an intermediate in essential fatty acid metabolism with potential as an ethical pharmaceutical and as a food. Rev Contemp Pharmacother 1990a; 1: 1–41.

Horrobin DF. Post-viral fatigue syndrome viral infections in atopic eczema and essential fatty acids. Med Hypotheses 1990b; 32: 211–217.

Horrobin DF. Nutritional and medical importance of gamma-linolenic acid. Prog Lipid Res 1992a; 31: 163–194.

Horrobin DF. The relationship between schizophrenia and essential fatty acids and eicosanoid metabolism. Prostagland Leukotr Essent Fatty Acids 1992b; 46: 71–77.

Horrobin DF. A possible relationship between dyslexia and schizophrenia, two disorders in which membrane phospholipid (PL) metabolism is disturbed. Schizophr Res 1996; 18: 156.

Horrobin DF. Overview: the role of brain lipid metabolism in schizophrenia. Prostagland Leukotr Essent Fatty Acids 1997; 57: 208.

Horrobin DF. The membrane phospholipid hypothesis as a biochemical basis for the neurodevelopmental concept of schizophrenia. Schizophr Res 1998a; 30: 193–208.

Horrobin DF. Schizophrenia: the illness that made us human. Med Hypotheses 1998b; 50: 269–288.

Horrobin DF, Manku MS. Clinical biochemistry of essential fatty acids. In: Horrobin DF, ed. Omega-6 essential fatty acids, pathophysiology and roles in clinical medicine. New York: Wiley-Liss, 1990: 21–53.

Horrobin DF, Ally AI, Karmali RA, Karmazyn M, Manku MS, Morgan RO. Prostaglandins and schizophrenia: further discussion of the evidence. Psychol Med 1978; 8: 43–48.

Horrobin DF, Glen AIM, Vaddadi K. The membrane hypothesis of schizophrenia. Schizophr Res 1994; 13: 195–207.

Horrobin DF, Glen AIM, Hudson CJ. Possible relevance of phospholipid abnormalities and genetic interactions in psychiatric disorders: the relationship between dyslexia and schizophrenia. Med Hypotheses 1995; 45: 605–613.

Horrobin DF, Glen AIM, Cantrill RC. Clozapine: elevation of membrane unsaturated lipid levels as a new mechanism of action. Schizophr Res 1997; 24: 214.

Huang Y-S, Horrobin DF. Sex differences in n-3 and n-6 fatty acid metabolism in EFA-depleted rats. Proc Soc Exp Biol Med 1987; 185: 291–296.

Huang Y-S, Horrobin DF, Watanabe Y, Bartlett ME, Simmons VA. Effects of dietary linoleic acid on growth and liver phospholipid fatty acid composition in intact and gonadectomized rats. Biochem Arch 1990; 6: 47–54.

Huang ZH, Bates EJ, Ferrante JV et al. Inhibition of stimulus-induced endothelial cell intercellular adhesion molecule-1 E-selectin and vascular cellular adhesion molecule-1 expression by arachidonic acid and its hydroxy and hydroperoxy derivatives. Circ Res 1997; 80: 149–158.

Hudson CJ, Kennedy JL, Gotowiec A et al. Genetic variant near cytosolic phospholipase A_2 associated with schizophrenia. Schizophr Res 1996; 21: 111–116.

Hughes DA, Southon S, Pinder AC. (n-3) Polyunsaturated fatty acids modulate the expression of functionally associated molecules on human monocytes *in vitro*. J Nutr 1996; 126: 603–610.

Iacano WG, Beiser M. Where are the women in first-episode studies of schizophrenia? Schizophr Bull 1992; 18: 471–480.

Jones P, Rodgers B, Murray R, Marmot M. Child developmental risk factors for adult schizophrenia in the British 1946 birth cohort. Lancet 1994; 344: 1398–1402.

Kaufmann WE, Yamagata K, Andreasson KI, Worley PF. Rapid response genes as markers of cellular signaling during cortical histogenesis: their potential in understanding mental retardation. Int J Dev Neurosci 1994; 12: 263–271.

Kaufmann WE, Worley PF, Pegg J, Bremer M, Isakson P. COX-2, a synaptically induced enzyme, is expressed by excitatory neurons at postsynaptic sites in rat cerebral cortex. Proc Natl Acad Sci USA 1996; 93: 2317–2321.

Koletzko B. Fats for brains. Eur J Clin Nutr 1992; 46 (Suppl 1): S51–S62.

Lucas A, Morley R, Cole TJ, Lister G, Leeson-Payne C. Breast milk and subsequent intelligence quotient in children born pre-term. Lancet 1992; 339: 261–264.

Mahadik SP, Evans DR. Essential fatty acids in the treatment of schizophrenia. Drugs Today 1997; 33: 5–17.

Mahadik SP, Gowda S. Antioxidants in the treatment of schizophrenia. Drugs Today 1996; 32: 553–565.

Mahadik SP, Mukherjee S. Free radical pathology and antioxidant defense in schizophrenia: a review. Schizophr Res 1996; 19: 1–17.

Mahadik SP, Scheffer RE. Oxidative injury and potential use of antioxidants in schizophrenia. Prostagland Leukotr Essent Fatty Acids 1996; 55: 45–54.

Mahadik SP, Shendarkar NS, Scheffer R, Mukherjee S, Correnti EE. Utilization of precursor essential fatty acids in culture by skin fibroblasts from schizophrenic patients and normal controls. Prostagland Leukotr Essent Fatty Acids 1996; 55: 65–70.

Makrides M, Neumann M, Simmer K, Pater J, Gibson R. Are long-chain polyunsaturated fatty acids essential nutrients in infancy? Lancet 1995; 345: 1463–1468.

Marcus J. Cerebral functioning in offspring of schizophrenics: a possible genetic factor. Int J Ment Health 1974; 3: 57–73.

Marra CA, de Alaniz MJ. Influence of testosterone administration on the biosynthesis of unsaturated fatty acids in male and female rats. Lipids 1989; 24: 1014–1019.

McCreadie RG. The Nithsdale Schizophrenia Surveys. 16. Breastfeeding and schizophrenia: preliminary results and hypotheses. Br J Psychiatry 1997; 170: 334–337.

McGahon B, Clements MP, Lynch MA. The ability of aged rats to sustain long term potentiation is restored when the age-related decrease in membrane arachidonic acid concentration is reversed. Neuroscience 1997; 81: 9–16.

McGrath J, Murray R. Risk factors for schizophrenia: from conception to birth. In: Hirsch SR, Weinberger DR, eds. Schizophrenia. Oxford: Blackwell, 1995: 187–205.

McNeil TF, Cantor-Graae E, Nordstrom LG, Rosenlund T. Head circumference in 'preschizophrenic' and control neonates. Br J Psychiatry 1993; 162: 517–523.

McNeil TF, Kaij L. Obstetric factors in the development of schizophrenia: complications in the births of preschizophrenics and in reproduction by schizophrenic patients. In: Wynne LC, Cromwell RL, Matthysee S, eds. The nature of schizophrenia. New York: John Wiley and Sons, 1978: 401–429.

Mead JF, Alfin-Slater RB, Howton DR, Popjak G. Lipids: chemistry, biochemistry and nutrition. New York: Plenum Press, 1986.

Mellor JE, Laugharne JDE, Peet M. Schizophrenic symptoms and dietary intake of n-3 fatty acids. Schizophr Res 1995; 18: 85–86.

Mellor JE, Laugharne JDE, Peet M. Omega-3 fatty acid supplementation in schizophrenia patients. Hum Psychopharmacol 1996; 11: 39–46.

Mills DE. Dietary omega-3 and omega-6 fatty acids and cardiovascular responses to pressor and depressor stimuli. World Rev Nutr Diet 1991; 66: 349–357.

Mitchell EA, Aman MG, Turbott SH, Manku M. Clinical characteristics and serum essential fatty acid levels in hyperactive children. Clin Pediatr 1987; 26: 406–411.

Murray RM, O'Callaghan E, Castle DJ, Lewis SW. A neurodevelopmental approach to the classification of schizophrenia. Schizophr Bull 1992; 18: 319–332.

Nasrallah HA. Neurodevelopmental pathogenesis of schizophrenia. Psychiatr Clin North Am 1993; 16: 269–280.

Negre-Aminou P, Nemenoff RA, Wood MR, de la Houssaye BA, Pfenninger KH. Characterization of phospholipase A_2 activity enriched in the nerve growth cone. J Neurochem 1996; 67: 2599–2608.

Nunez EA, ed Fatty acids and cell signalling. Prostagland Leukotr Essent Fatty Acids 1993; 48: 1–122.

Nunez M, Peinado Onsurbe J, Vilaro S, Llobera M. Lipoprotein lipase activity in developing rat brain areas. Biol Neonate 1995; 68: 119–127.

O'Callaghan E, Larkin C, Kinsella A, Waddington JL. Familial obstetric and other clinical correlates of minor physical anomalies in schizophrenia. Am J Psychiatry 1991a; 148: 479–483.

O'Callaghan E, Sham P, Takei N, Glover G, Murray RM. Schizophrenia after prenatal exposure to 1957 A$_2$ influenza epidemic. Lancet 1991b; 337: 1248–1250.

O'Callaghan E, Gibson T, Colohan HA et al. Risk of schizophrenia in adults born after obstetric complications and their association with early onset of illness: a controlled study. Br Med J 1992; 305: 1256–1259.

Olney JW, Farber NB. Glutamate receptor dysfunction and schizophrenia. Arch Gen Psychiatry 1995; 52: 998–1007.

Oloyede OB, Folyan AT, Odutuga AA. Effects of low-iron status and deficiency of essential fatty acids on some biochemical constituents of rat brain. Biochem Int 1992; 27: 913–922.

Owada Y, Yoshimoto T, Kondo H. Spatio-temporally different expression of genes for three members of fatty acid binding proteins in developing and mature rat brains. J Chem Neuroanat 1996; 12: 113–122.

Pediconi MF, Rodriguez de Turco EB. Free fatty acid content and release kinetics as manifestations of cerebral lateralization in mouse brain. J Neurochem 1984; 43: 1–7.

Peet M, Laugharne JDE, Horrobin DF, Reynolds GP. Arachidonic acid: a common link in the biology of schizophrenia? Arch Gen Psychiatry 1994; 51: 665–666.

Peet M, Laugharne JDE, Mellor J, Ramchand CN. Essential fatty acid deficiency in erythrocyte membranes from chronic schizophrenic patients and the clinical effects of dietary supplementation. Prostagland Leukotr Essent Fatty Acids 1996; 55: 71–75.

Peet M, Laugharne JDE, Ahluwalia N, Mellor J. Fatty acid supplementation in schizophrenic patients. Schizophr Res 1997a; 24: 209.

Peet M, Poole J, Laugharne J. Infant feeding and the development of schizophrenia. Schizophr Res 1997b; 24: 255.

Peet M, Ramchand CN, Lee KH et al. Association of the Ban I dimorphic site at the human phospholipase A$_2$ gene with schizophrenia. Psychiatr Genet 1998; 3: 1–2.

Pettegrew JW, Keshavan MS, Panchalingam K et al. Alterations in brain high-energy phosphate and membrane phospholipid metabolism in first-episode drug-naïve schizophrenics. A pilot study of the dorsal prefrontal cortex by *in vivo* phosphorus-31 nuclear magnetic resonance spectroscopy. Arch Gen Psychiatry 1991; 48: 563–568.

Pettegrew JW, Keshavan MS, Minshew NJ. 31P nuclear magnetic resonance spectroscopy: neurodevelopment and schizophrenia. Schizophr Bull 1993; 19: 35–53.

Phillips M, Sabas M, Greenberg J. Increased pentane and carbon disulfide in the breath of patients with schizophrenia. J Clin Pathol 1993; 46: 861–864.

Poltorak M, Frye MA, Wright R et al. Increased neural cell adhesion molecule in the CSF of patients with mood disorder. J Neurochem 1996; 66: 1532–1538.

Pudelkewicz C, Seufert J, Holman RT. Requirements of the female rat for linoleic and linolenic acids. J Nutr 1968; 94: 138–146.

Ramchand CN, Davies JI, Tresman RL, Griffiths ICD, Peet M. Reduced susceptibility to oxidative damage of erythrocyte membranes from medicated schizophrenic patients. Prostagland Leukotr Essent Fatty Acids 1996; 55: 27–31.

Richardson AJ. Dyslexia, handedness and syndromes of psychosis-proneness. Int J Psychophysiol 1994; 18: 251–263.

Richardson AJ, Cox IJ, Sargentoni J, Puri BK. Abnormal cerebral phospholipid metabolism in dyslexia indicated by phosphorus-31 magnetic resonance spectroscopy. NMR Biomed 1997; 10: 309–314.

Rieder RO, Nichols PL. The offspring of schizophrenics. 3. Hyperactivity and neurological soft signs. Arch Gen Psychiatry 1979; 36: 665–674.

Robert J, Montaudon D, Hugues P. Incorporation and metabolism of exogenous fatty acids by cultured normal and tumoral glial cells. Biochim Biophys Acta 1983; 752: 383–395.

Rordorf G, Uemura Y, Bonventre JV. Characterization of phospholipase A$_2$ (PLA$_2$) activity in gerbil brain: enhanced activities of cytosolic mitochondrial and microsomal forms after ischemia and reperfusion. J Neurosci 1991; 11: 1829–1836.

Ross BM, Hudson C, Erlich J, Warsh JJ, Kish SJ. Increased phospholipid breakdown in schizophrenia: evidence for the involvement of a calcium-independent phospholipase A$_2$. Arch Gen Psychiatry 1997; 54: 487–494.

Rotrosen J, Adler L, Lohr J, Edson R, Lavori P. Antioxidant treatment of tardive dyskinesia. Prostagland Leukotr Essent Fatty Acids 1996; 55: 77–81.

Rousselot P, Heintz N, Nottebohm F. Expression of brain lipid binding protein in the brain of the adult canary and its implications for adult neurogenesis. J Comp Neurol 1997; 385: 415–426.

Selten JP, van Durursen R, van der Graaf C, Gispen-de Wied C, Kahn RS. Second-trimester exposure to maternal stress is a possible risk factor for psychotic illness in the child. Schizophr Res 1997; 24: 258.

Sham PC, O'Callaghan E, Takei N, Murray GK, Hare EH, Murray RM. Schizophrenia following pre-natal exposure to influenza epidemics between 1939 and 1960. Br J Psychiatry 1992; 160: 461–466.

Shenton ME, Kikinis R, Jolesz FA et al. Abnormalities of the left temporal lobe and thought disorder in schizophrenia. N Engl J Med 1992; 327: 604–612.

Sinclair HM. Deficiency of essential fatty acids and atherosclerosis *etcetera*. Lancet 1956; i: 381–383.

Smalheiser NR, Dissanayake S, Kapil A. Rapid regulation of neurite outgrowth and retraction by phospholipase A$_2$-derived arachidonic acid and its metabolites. Brain Res 1996; 721: 39–48.

Sparkes RS, Zollman S, Klisak I et al. Human genes involved in lipolysis of plasma lipoproteins: mapping of loci for lipoprotein lipase to 8p22 and hepatic lipase to 15q21, Genomics 1987; 1: 138–143.

Spector AA, Yorek MA. Membrane lipid composition and cellular function. J Lipid Res 1985; 26: 1015–1035.

Stevens LJ, Zentall SZ, Deck JL, Abate ML, Lipp SR, Burgess JR. Essential fatty acid metabolism in boys with attention-deficit hyperactivity disorder. Am J Clin Nutr 1995; 62: 761–768.

Stevens LJ, Zentall SS, Abate ML, Kuczek T, Burgess JR. Omega-3 fatty acids in boys with behavior, learning, and health problems. Physiol Behav 1996; 59: 915–920.

Stordy BJ. Benefit of docosahexaenoic acid supplements to dark adaptation in dyslexics. Lancet 1995; 346: 385.

Stordy BJ. Dark adaption, docosahexaenoic acid and dyslexia. International Conference on highly unsaturated fatty acids in nutrition and disease prevention. Barcelona, Spain, 4–6 November, 1996.

Suddath RL, Christison GW, Torrey EF, Casanova MF, Weinberger DR. Anatomical abnormalities in the brains of monozygotic twins discordant for schizophrenia. N Engl J Med 1990; 322: 789–794.

Susser ES, Lin SP. Schizophrenia after prenatal exposure to the Dutch Hunger Winter of 1944–1945. Arch Gen Psychiatry 1992; 49: 983–988.

Takahashi R, Ito H, Horrobin DF. Fatty acid composition of serum phospholipids in an elderly institutionalized Japanese population. J Nutr Sci Vitaminol (Tokyo) 1991; 37: 401–409.

Thompson GA, ed. The regulation of membrane lipid metabolism. 2nd edn. Boca Raton: CRC Press, 1992.

Utsunomiya A, Owada Y, Yoshimoto T, Kondo H. Localisation of mRNA for fatty acid transport protein in developing and mature brain of rats. Mol Brain Res 1997; 46: 217–222.

Van Kammen DP, Poltorak M, Kelley ME et al. CSF neuronal cell adhesion molecule (N-CAM) in schizophrenia. Schizophr Res 1997; 24: 68.

Vance DE. Phospholipid metabolism and cell signalling in eucaryotes. In: Vance DE, Vance J, eds. Biochemistry of lipids lipoproteins and membranes. Amsterdam: Elsevier, 1991: 205–240.

Vilaro S, Camps L, Reina M, Perez Clausell J, Llobera M, Olivecrona T. Localization of lipoprotein lipase to discrete areas of the guinea pig brain. Brain Res 1990; 506: 249–253.

Waddington JL. Schizophrenia: developmental neuroscience and pathobiology. Lancet 1993; 341: 531–536.

Wallberg-Jonsson S, Dahlen G, Johnson O, Olivecrona G, Rantapaa-Dahlqvist S. Lipoprotein lipase in relation to inflammatory activity in rheumatoid arthritis. J Int Med 1996; 240: 373–380.

Ward P, Sutherland J, Glen E, Glen AIM, Horrobin DF. Skin flushing in response to graded doses of topical niacin: a new test which distinguishes schizophrenics from controls. Schizophr Res 1997; 24: 70.

Ward PE, Sutherland J, Glen EMT, Glen AIM. Niacin skin flush in schizophrenia: a preliminary report. Schizophr Res 1998; 29: 269–274.

Warner RW, Peet M. Essential fatty acids and the electroretinogram in schizophrenia. In: Glen I, Peet M, Horrobin DF, eds. Phospholipid spectrum disorder in psychiatry. Carnforth: Marius Press, 1999: 133–136.

Weinberger DR. Schizophrenia as a neurodevelopmental disorder. In: Hirsch SR, Weinberger DR, eds. Schizophrenia. Oxford: Blackwell, 1995a: 293–323.

Weinberger DR. Schizophrenia: from neuropathology to neurodevelopment. Lancet 1995b; 346: 552–557.

Williamson PC, Brauer M, Leonard S, Thompson T, Drost D. 31P magnetic resonance spectroscopy studies in schizophrenia. Prostagland Leukotr Essent Fatty Acids 1996; 55: 115–118.

Witt MR, Nielsen M. Characterization of the influence of unsaturated free fatty acids on brain GABA/benzodiazepine receptor binding in vitro. J Neurochem 1994; 62: 1432–1439.

Witt MR, WesthHansen SE, Rasmussen PB, Hastrup S, Nielsen M. Unsaturated free fatty acids increase benzodiazepine receptor agonist binding depending on the subunit composition of the GABA(A) receptor complex. J Neurochem 1996; 67: 2141–2145.

World Health Organization. Schizophrenia: an international follow-up study. New York: Wiley, 1979.

Yakley J, Murray RM. Genetic and environmental risk factors for schizophrenia. In: Brunello N, Racagni G, Langer SZ, Mendlewicz J, eds. Critical issues in the treatment of schizophrenia. Basel: Karger, 1995; 10: 9–34.

Yao JK, Van Kammen DP, Gurklis JA. Abnormal incorporation of arachidonic acid into platelets of drug-free patients with schizophrenia. Psychiatry Res 1996; 60: 11–21.

Part II

SCHIZOPHRENIA: PHOSPHOLIPID METABOLISM

Brain and Blood Phospholipase Activity in Psychiatric Disorders

Brian M. Ross

PERIPHERAL AND CNS STUDIES OF PHOSPHOLIPID METABOLISM IN SCHIZOPHRENIA

The results of studies carried out over a period of three decades have indicated that schizophrenia may be associated with abnormal metabolism of membrane phospholipid and fatty acids. Numerous, though not all, investigators have observed that levels of the major membrane phospholipids, phosphatidylcholine and phosphatidylethanolamine are decreased in erythrocytes, platelets and skin fibroblasts of patients with schizophrenia (Table 2.1). Moreover, the abundance in blood of the phospholipid breakdown product lysophosphatidylcholine is increased (Table 2.1). Complementing these findings are reports of elevated turnover of platelet phosphatidylinositol (Yao et al., 1992) and arachidonic acid (Demisch et al., 1987) in patients with schizophrenia, whilst levels of specific fatty acid species are reduced (Glen et al., 1994). Taken together, these findings suggest that the rate of phospholipid breakdown may be increased, in peripheral tissues at least, in the disorder. Recently, such peripheral tissue findings have been extended by studies utilizing ^{31}P magnetic resonance spectroscopy (MRS), which allows the abundance of phosphorus-containing compounds to be measured *in vivo* within the brain of the patient. Several independent investigators have reported increased levels of brain phosphodiesters in the frontal and temporal cortices of drug-naïve (Pettegrew et al., 1991; Keshavan et al., 1993; Stanley et al., 1995) and medicated (Fujimoto et al., 1992; Fukazako et al., 1994) schizophrenic subjects. Since a major portion of the total phosphodiester signal is comprised of glycerophosphodiesters, compounds formed during phospholipid catabolism, such data have been interpreted as indicating that the rate of brain phospholipid breakdown is increased in schizophrenia, suggesting that the earlier peripheral tissue findings can be extended to the CNS. Furthermore, the abundance of metabolites utilized in membrane synthesis (phosphomonoesters) has consistently been found to be decreased in the frontal cortex of both medicated and drug-naïve patients (Pettegrew et al., 1991; Williamson et al., 1991; Shioiri et al., 1994; Stanley et al., 1994, 1995; Kato et al., 1995), suggesting more rapid utilization of these compounds for membrane biosynthesis. Thus, a substantial body of evidence suggests that the rate of membrane turnover is accelerated in schizophrenia, an abnormality that may, by means of altered production of phospholipid-derived second messengers (e.g., prostaglandins, leukotrienes, inositol-phosphates), lead to aberrant neurodevelopment and/or interneuronal communication within the brain, ultimately resulting in the behavioural abnormalities observed in the disorder.

Table 2.1. Alterations in membrane phospholipid levels in peripheral tissues of patients with schizophrenia.

Compartment and study	PC	PE	LPC
Erythrocytes			
Stevens (1972)	↓	↓	nd
Lautin et al. (1982)	–	–	nd
Tolbert et al. (1983)	↓	↓	nd
Hitzemann et al. (1984)	↓	–	nd
Hitzemann et al. (1985)	↓	nd	nd
Keshaven et al. (1993)	–	↓	nd
Platelets			
Pangerl et al. (1991)	–	–	↑
Platelets, erythrocytes			
Sengupta et al. (1981)	↑	↓	nd
Skin fibroblasts			
Mahadik et al. (1994)	–	↓	nd

PC = phosphatidylcholine; PE = phosphatidylethanolamine; LPC = lysophosphatidylcholine; ↑ = increased; ↓ = decreased; – = unchanged; nd = not done.

PHOSPHOLIPASE A$_2$ ACTIVITY IN SCHIZOPHRENIA

The observations described in the preceding section suggest that schizophrenia may be associated with a systemic abnormality in phospholipid metabolism. It is, however, unclear as to what the underlying molecular cause(s) of such a deficiency may be. A candidate mechanism currently receiving much interest is abnormal activity of the phospholipid metabolizing enzyme, phospholipase A$_2$ (PLA$_2$). PLA$_2$ catalyses the hydrolysis of the Sn2 ester bond of the phospholipid molecule, resulting in the formation of free fatty acid and lysophospholipid. This reaction, besides being important for general membrane phospholipid turnover and repair, is also the source of the polyunsaturated fatty acid precursors of eicosanoid biosynthesis. Furthermore, PLA$_2$ is the rate-limiting reaction of a two-step process (the second reaction being catalyzed by lysophospholipase) which results in the formation of the glycerophosphodiester metabolites detected using ^{31}P MRS. With this in mind, it is apparent that increased PLA$_2$ activity could result in reduced levels of the enzyme's phospholipid/fatty acid substrate, with concomitant increases in the abundance of PLA$_2$-derived metabolites, lysophospholipids and glycerophosphodiesters, changes consistent with those which occur in schizophrenia.

Peripheral measures

As summarized in Table 2.2, the hypothesis of increased PLA$_2$ activity in schizophrenia initially received support from Gattaz et al. (1987, 1990) who reported that, in two independent studies, both serum and plasma PLA$_2$ activity were increased in patients with schizophrenia, results consistent with the later study of Noponen et al. (1993). Gattaz et al. (1995) subsequently reported that platelet PLA$_2$ activity was also increased in the disorder, although the increase was of a smaller magnitude than that in either plasma or serum. However, a third research group found blood PLA$_2$ activity to be normal in patients with schizophrenia (Albers et al., 1993). A possible explanation for such conflicting findings may relate to the fact that PLA$_2$ is not a single protein species, but a family of different enzymes (Mayer and Marshall, 1993) having varied regulatory and functional properties, many of which possess distinct substrate preferences. Examination of the various investigations of PLA$_2$ activity in blood of patients reveals that each research group utilized a different assay system (Table 2.2). Thus, different investigators, employing various assay procedures, may be detecting different PLA$_2$ subtypes. This notion is supported by work (Ross et al., 1997) which showed that, using the substrate employed by Gattaz et al. (1987, 1990) (C28-O-PHPM), serum PLA$_2$ activity is increased by approximately 50% in patients with schizophrenia, whereas when the enzyme is reassayed in the same patients, employing the bacterial membrane substrate employed by Albers et al. (1993), activity is found to be normal. Subsequent investigations determined that using C28-O-PHPM as substrate detected a calcium-independent form of PLA$_2$ in blood, whereas the bacterial membrane substrate results in the assay of a calcium-dependent isoform (Ross et al., 1997). Thus, one may conclude that, in blood at least, PLA$_2$ activity is indeed increased in schizophrenia, but that this occurs in a subtype-specific manner. Such findings emphasize the need to consider the heterogeneous nature of PLA$_2$

Table 2.2. Phospholipase A$_2$ activity in blood of patients with schizophrenia.

Compartment and study	Assay substrate	Change (%)[a]	Neuroleptic-free[b]
Plasma			
Gattaz et al. (1987)	C28-O-PHPM	+147	Yes
Serum			
Gattaz et al. (1990)	C28-O-PHPM	+94	Yes
Albers et al. (1993)	Bacterial membranes	No change	Yes
Noponen et al. (1993)	PC vesicles	+26	Yes
Ross et al. (1997)	C28-O-PHPM	+49	No
	Bacterial membranes	No change	No
Platelets			
Gattaz et al. (1995)	PC vesicles	+18	Yes

[a]With respect to controls (only changes which were statistically significant are shown); [b]patients who had not received neuroleptics for at least 1 week before testing; PC = phosphatidylcholine.

activity when investigating the role of these enzymes in pathological states.

Although the Ross et al. (1997) study is largely in agreement with that of Gattaz (1987, 1990), the findings of each group do contrast in the apparent influence of neuroleptic drug-treatment upon blood PLA$_2$ activity, with Gattaz et al. (1987, 1990) reporting that PLA$_2$ activity is increased in drug-free subjects, returning to normal following neuroleptic therapy, whilst Ross et al. (1997) observed PLA$_2$ activity to be increased in patients actively receiving neuroleptic therapy. Although the reason for the contrasting findings of each study is unclear, one may speculate that any reduction in blood PLA$_2$ activity following neuroleptic treatment is transient, with increased PLA$_2$ activity returning in long-term chronically treated patients.

Activity in the CNS

Despite the positive nature of the blood PLA$_2$ studies, with the exception of the circumstantial evidence provided by the ^{31}P MRS studies, the crucial question of whether PLA$_2$ activity is altered in the brain of patients with schizophrenia has received little attention, perhaps due to the difficulty in obtaining clinically well characterized autopsy brain specimens from patients with this disorder. To answer this question my co-workers and I recently undertook a study of the status of PLA$_2$ in the autopsied brain of patients with schizophrenia. The diagnosis of schizophrenia according to DSM-IV criteria was confirmed post-mortem from case histories by two independent psychiatrists. The autopsied temporal and prefrontal cortices, and putamen, were obtained from 10 patients with paranoid-type schizophrenia (five males and five females, aged 46 ± 5 years, post-mortem interval 12 ± 2 h), all of whom had received long-term neuroleptic treatment, and from 12 neurologically and psychiatrically normal healthy controls matched with the patients for age, post-mortem-interval and sex (seven males and five females, aged 48 ± 5 years, post-mortem interval 14 ± 2 h). PLA$_2$ activity was radiometrically assayed in tissue homogenates, utilizing the substrate 1-palmitoyl, 2-^{14}C-arachidonyl phosphatidylethanolamine under calcium-stimulated and calcium-independent conditions (Ross et al., 1996). Calcium-independent PLA$_2$ activity was significantly increased by 45% in the temporal cortex of patients with schizophrenia relative to controls ($p < 0.05$), but was normal in the prefrontal cortex and putamen (Figure 2.1). In contrast, calcium-stimulated PLA$_2$ activity (Figure 2.1) was decreased by 27–29% in the temporal cortex and

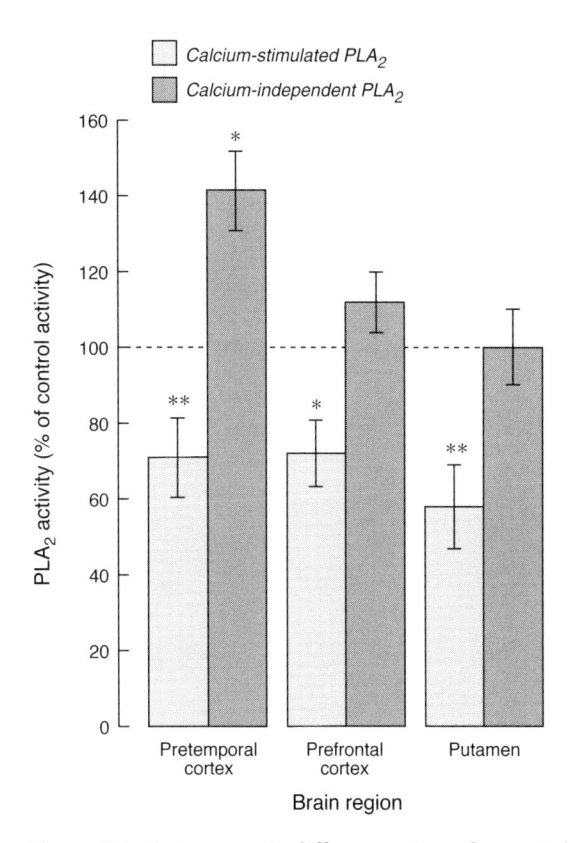

Figure 2.1. PLA$_2$ activity in different regions of autopsied brains of patients with schizophrenia ($n = 10$) compared to that in normal controls ($n = 12$). Values are percentages of control activity; means ± SEM. With respect to control group activity, $p <$: *0.05; **0.01 (Student's unpaired, two-tailed t test).

prefrontal cortices ($p < 0.05$) and by 44% in the putamen, relative to controls ($p < 0.01$).

Thus, in a similar manner to that of blood PLA$_2$ activity, calcium-independent and calcium-stimulated PLA$_2$ forms are differentially altered in the brain of patients with schizophrenia. In both tissues, this probably occurs as a consequence of the varied regulatory and functional properties of different PLA$_2$ subtypes. Indeed, no significant reciprocal relationship existed between calcium-stimulated and calcium-independent PLA$_2$ activity in the temporal cortex of patients with schizophrenia ($r = +0.22$; $p > 0.05$), suggesting that the alterations may not be directly related.

The underlying cause of altered PLA$_2$ activity in the brain of patients with schizophrenia is at present unclear. However, two, not necessarily mutually exclusive, possibilities seem likely: namely morphological brain changes, and alterations of a purely biochemical nature, e.g., changes in PLA$_2$ expression and/or activity. We reported recently that calcium-stimulated PLA$_2$ activity is markedly decreased in degenerating brain regions of patients with Alzheimer's disease, indicating that reduced neuronal volume and/or synaptic loss, as might occur in schizophrenia (Weinberger and Lipska, 1995), may be associated with PLA$_2$ deficiency (Ross et al., 1998b). Indeed, PLA$_2$ activity is particularly high in neuronal processes (Negre-Aminou and Pfenninger, 1993). However, whereas in schizophrenia the activity of calcium-independent PLA$_2$ is either increased or normal, in Alzheimer's disease calcium-independent PLA$_2$ activity is decreased (Ross et al., 1998b), suggesting the possibility that altered PLA$_2$ activity in schizophrenia may be due to membrane metabolic alterations. This appears especially likely in the case of calcium-independent PLA$_2$ activity, since the activity of this PLA$_2$ type is increased in both blood (Ross et al., 1997) and at least one brain region of patients with schizophrenia. Such an alteration may relate to the key role calcium-independent PLA$_2$ may play in the control of fatty acid incorporation into the cell membrane *via* production of lysophospholipid acceptors required for fatty acid esterification (Balsinde et al., 1995). Thus, increased calcium-independent PLA$_2$ activity may be mechanistically related to the decreased abundance of specific fatty acid types in peripheral tissue of patients with schizophrenia. Interestingly, chronic oxidative stress, a condition associated with damage to, and increased turnover of, fatty acids, also results in increased activity of calcium-independent, but not calcium-stimulated PLA$_2$ activity (Kuo et al., 1995). This, combined with reports of elevated oxidative stress in schizophrenia (reviewed in Mahadik and Scheffer, 1996), has led to the recent proposal (Smalheiser and Swanson, 1998) that calcium-independent PLA$_2$ activity, decreased fatty acid abundance, and elevated oxidative stress in schizophrenia, are related phenomena. However, it should be noted that increased calcium-independent PLA$_2$ activity in brain was limited to a single cortical area, indicating that this may not be a systemic change, especially since calcium-independent PLA$_2$ possesses a relatively homogeneous regional distribution in the human brain (Ross et al., 1998a).

In principle, increased temporal cortex calcium-independent PLA$_2$ activity could explain elevated brain phosphodiester levels in this brain region in patients with schizophrenia (Fukazako et al., 1994). However, phosphodiester levels are also reported to be increased in the frontal cortex of patients (Keshavan et al., 1993; Stanley et al., 1995), an area in which calcium-independent PLA$_2$ activity is normal and calcium-stimulated PLA$_2$ activity is decreased. Thus, the PLA$_2$ activity changes in schizophrenic brain do not appear consistent with the hypothesis that elevated brain phosphodiesters in schizophrenia are due to increased PLA$_2$ activity.

PHOSPHOLIPASE A$_2$ ACTIVITY CHANGES IN COCAINE USERS AND THEIR RELATIONSHIP TO SCHIZOPHRENIA

Since calcium-dependent activity is unaltered in the blood of patients with schizophrenia, decreased calcium-stimulated PLA$_2$ activity in the brain of patients may be a CNS-specific occurrence. In addition to the possible effect that structural alterations in the brain of patients with schizophrenia have upon the activity of this PLA$_2$ type, a neural plastic mechanism may be at work, given that calcium-stimulated, but not calcium-independent, PLA$_2$ activity is reduced in the striatum of chronic human cocaine (a dopamine uptake blocker) users (Ross et al., 1996), parallelling the changes in schizophrenia. Importantly, only one of the patients with schizophrenia used in the autopsied brain study had a history of substance abuse, thereby making it unlikely that concomitant drug use is responsible for the reduced striatal PLA$_2$ activity we observed. Instead, altered dopaminergic signalling in the brain of persons with the disorder may lead to reduced calcium-stimulated PLA$_2$ activity. In this regard, both dopamine D$_2$ and D$_4$ receptors potentiate arachidonic acid release in Chinese hamster ovary (CHO) cells (McAllister et al., 1993; Chio et al., 1994), *via* activation of a calcium-stimulated form of PLA$_2$, cPLA$_2$ (Vial and Piomelli, 1995). Interestingly, Hudson et al. (1996) recently reported an association between schizophrenia and the size of a poly-A repeat in the 5′-upstream region of the gene encoding cPLA$_2$. Taken together, these data suggest that overstimulation of the brain's dopamine system, as occurs in cocaine use, and which may also take place in schizophrenia, as evidenced by recent brain ^{11}C-raclopride imaging studies (Breier et al., 1997), leads to reduced striatal calcium-stimulated PLA$_2$ activity. Importantly, however, unlike patients with schizophrenia, calcium-stimulated PLA$_2$ activity is normal in the cerebral cortex of cocaine users (Ross et al., 1996), indicating that a hyperdopaminergic state is not solely responsible for the changes in brain PLA$_2$ observed in schizophrenia. Animal models suggest that diminished brain PLA$_2$ activity, especially within the basal ganglia, by means of limiting prostaglandin production, should have dopaminergic potentiating effects. For example, the prostaglandin synthesis inhibitor indomethacin antagonizes haloperidol-induced catalepsy (Bala-Lall et al.,

1984) and potentiates the operant suppressor activity of amphetamine (Nielsen and Sparber, 1984), whereas intraventricular injection of prostaglandins inhibits amphetamine- and apomorphine-induced circling in 6-hydroxydopamine lesioned mice (Schwarz et al., 1982a,b). Consistent with these observations are the clinical, largely anecdotal, reports of indomethacin-induced transient psychosis in humans (reviewed in Hoppmann et al., 1991), an observation which could be explained by enhancement of dopaminergic neurotransmission *via* prostaglandin synthesis inhibition. Thus, reduced striatal PLA$_2$ activity in schizophrenia may lead to a potentiation of dopaminergic neurotransmission, increasing the risk of psychosis. Moreover, in cocaine users, repeated dopaminergic stimulation, leading to downregulation of PLA$_2$ activity, may result in the development of sensitization to the drug (sensitization being the process by which repeated administration of cocaine or amphetamine results, somewhat counter-intuitively, in a heightened response to the drug). A role for PLA$_2$ in sensitization has also been suggested by the observations that systemic administration of the PLA$_2$ inhibitor, quinacrine, inhibits sensitization, whereas brain injections of the PLA$_2$ stimulatory peptide, mellitin, produce sensitization (Reid et al., 1996). Such results suggest that activation of PLA$_2$ should increase dopaminergic activity, which would appear contradictory to the findings of those studies in which prostaglandin synthesis inhibitors have been used, suggesting, in turn, that activating PLA$_2$ should inhibit dopamine function. However, it is presently unknown as to how or whether the two processes are related. Indeed, the primary brain anatomical site of action of both quinacrine and prostaglandin synthesis inhibitors in their role as modulators of dopaminergic activity has yet to be determined.

PHOSPHOLIPASE ACTIVITY IN OTHER PSYCHIATRIC DISORDERS

With the exception of cocaine use, investigation of phospholipase activity in other psychiatric disorders has been minimal. Indeed, PLA$_2$ activity measures in disorders other than schizophrenia have involved small numbers of patients having heterogeneous disorders, defined mainly in terms of their not having schizophrenia. Moreover, such studies have yielded contradictory results, with Gattaz et al. (1987, 1990, 1995) reporting that PLA$_2$ activity is normal in their psychiatric control group, whereas Noponen et al. (1993) observed PLA$_2$ activity to be increased in a similar group. Clearly, the use of homogeneous, well-defined, psychiatric disorders in such studies would be beneficial, especially since similar ^{31}P MRS findings to those noted in schizophrenia have recently been observed in patients with bipolar affective disorder (Kato et al., 1994; Deicken et al., 1995a,b).

SUMMARY

In summary, it appears likely that the activity of one or more forms of PLA$_2$ is abnormal in patients with schizophrenia, and that altered activity of this enzyme may play a role in the mechanism of action of dopaminergic drugs such as cocaine. In addition, preliminary evidence also suggests a possible involvement of altered membrane metabolism in bipolar disorder. Ultimately, the importance or otherwise of such alterations awaits the development, and clinical trials in psychiatric disorders, of compounds which modulate the activity of one or more forms of brain PLA$_2$.

REFERENCES

Albers MA, Meurer H, Märki F, Klotz J. Phospholipase A$_2$ activity in serum of neuroleptic-naïve psychiatric inpatients. Pharmacopsychiatry 1993; 26: 94–98.

Bala-Lall S, Tekur U, Sen P. Effect of drugs influencing synthesis of prostaglandins on haloperidol-induced catalepsy in rats. Indian J Physiol Pharmacol 1984; 28: 219–222.

Balsinde J, Bianco ID, Ackermann E, Conde-Frieboes K, Dennis EA. Inhibition of calcium-independent phospholipase A$_2$ prevents arachidonic incorporation and phospholipid remodeling in P388D$_1$ macrophages. Proc Natl Acad Sci USA 1995; 92: 8527–8531.

Breier A, Su TP, Saunders R et al. Schizophrenia is associated with elevated amphetamine-induced synaptic dopamine concentrations: evidence from a novel positron tomography method. Proc Natl Acad Sci USA 1997; 94: 2569–2574.

Chio CL, Drong RE, Riley DT, Gill GS, Slightom JL, Huff RM. D$_4$ dopamine receptor-mediated signaling events determined in transfected chinese hamster ovary cells. J Biol Chem 1994; 269: 11813–11819.

Deicken RF, Weiner MW, Fein G. Decreased temporal lobe phosphomonoesters in bipolar disorder. J Affective Disord 1995a; 33: 195–199.

Deicken RF, Fein G, Weiner MW. Abnormal frontal lobe phosphorus metabolism in bipolar disorder. Am J Psychiatry 1995b; 152: 915–918.

Demisch L, Gerbaldo H, Gebhart P, Georgi K, Bochnik HJ. Incorporation of ^{14}C-arachidonic acid into platelet phospholipids of untreated patients with schizophreniform or schizophrenic disorders. Psychiatry Res 1987; 22: 275–282.

Fujimoto T, Nakano T, Takano T, Hokazano Y, Asakura T, Tsuji T. Study of chronic schizophrenics using ^{31}P magnetic resonance chemical shift imaging. Acta Psychiatr Scand 1992; 86: 455–462.

Fukazako H, Takeuchi K, Ueyama K et al. ^{31}P magnetic resonance spectroscopy of the medial temporal lobe of schizophrenic patients with neuroleptic-resistant marked positive symptoms. Eur Arch Psychiatry Clin Neurosci 1994; 244: 236–240.

Gattaz WF, Köllisch M, Thuren T, Virtanen JA, Kinnunen PKJ. Increased plasma phospholipase-A_2 activity in schizophrenic patients: reduction after neuroleptic therapy. Biol Psychiatry 1987; 22: 421–426.

Gattaz WF, Hübner CK, Nevalainen TJ, Thuren T, Kinnunen PKJ. Increased serum phospholipase-A_2 activity in schizophrenia: a replication study. Biol Psychiatry 1990; 28: 495–501.

Gattaz WF, Schmitt A, Maras AM. Increased platelet phospholipase A_2 activity in schizophrenia. Schizophr Res 1995; 16; 1–6.

Glen AIM, Glen EMT, Horrobin DF et al. A red cell membrane abnormality in a subgroup of schizophrenic patients: evidence for two diseases. Schizophr Res 1994; 12: 53–61.

Hitzemann R, Hirschowitz J, Garver D. Membrane abnormalities in the psychoses and affective disorders. J Psychiatry Res 1984; 18: 319–326.

Hitzemann RJ, Mark C, Hirschowitz J, Garver DL. Characteristics of phospholipid methylation in human erythrocyte ghosts: relationship(s) to the psychoses and affective disorders. Biol Psychiatry 1985; 20: 297–307.

Hoppmann RA, Peden JG, Over SK. Central nervous system side effects of non-steroidal anti-inflammatory drugs. Arch Int Med 1991; 151: 1309–1313.

Hudson CJ, Kennedy JL, Gotowiec A et al. Genetic variant near cytosolic phospholipase A_2 associated with schizophrenia. Schizophr Res 1996; 21: 111–116.

Kato T, Shioiri T, Murashita J, Hamakawa H, Inubushi T, Takahashi S. Phosphorus-31 magnetic resonance spectroscopy and ventricular enlargement in bipolar disorder. Psychiatry Res Neuroimaging 1994; 55: 41–50.

Kato T, Shioiri T, Murashita J, Hamakawa H, Inubushi T, Takahashi S. Lateralized abnormality of high-energy phosphate and bilateral reduction of phosphomonoester measured by phosphorus31 magnetic resonance spectroscopy of the frontal lobes in schizophrenia. Psychiatry Res Neuroimaging 1995; 61: 151–160.

Keshavan MS, Mallinger AG, Pettegrew JW, Dippold C. Erythrocyte membrane phospholipids in psychotic patients. Psychiatry Res 1993; 49: 89–95.

Keshavan MS, Sanders RD, Pettegrew JW, Dombrowsky SM, Panchalingam KS. Frontal lobe metabolism and cerebral morphology in schizophrenia: ^{31}P MRS and MRI studies. Schizophr Res 1993; 10: 241–246.

Kuo CF, Cheng S, Burgess JR. Deficiency of vitamin E and selenium enhances calcium-independent phospholipase A_2 activity in rat lung and liver. J Nutr 1995; 125: 1419–1429.

Lautin A, Mandio CD, Segarnick DJ, Wod L, Mason MF, Rotrosen J. Red cell phospholipids in schizophrenia. Life Sci 1982; 31: 3051–3056.

Mahadik SP, Scheffer RE. Oxidative injury and potential use of antioxidants in schizophrenia. Prostagland Leukotr Essent Fatty Acids 1996; 55: 45–54.

Mahadik SP, Mukherjee S, Correnti EE et al. Plasma membrane phospholipid and cholesterol distribution of skin fibroblasts from drug-naïve patients at the onset of psychosis. Schizophr Res 1994; 13: 239–247.

Mayer RJ, Marshall LA. New insights on mammalian phospholipase A_2(s); comparison of arachidonyl-selective and -nonselective enzymes. FASEB J 1993; 7: 339–348.

McAllister G, Knowles MR, Patel S et al. Characterization of a chimeric D_3/D_2 dopamine receptor expressed in CHO cells. FEBS Lett 1993; 324: 81–86.

Negre-Aminou P, Pfenninger KH. Arachidonic acid turnover and phospholipase A_2 activity in neuronal growth cones. J Neurochem 1993; 60: 1126–1136.

Nielsen JA, Sparber SB. Indomethacin potentiates the operant behavior suppressant and rectal temperature lowering effects of low doses of d-amphetamine in rats. Pharmacol Biochem Behav 1984; 21: 219–224.

Noponen M, Sanfilipo M, Samanich K et al. Elevated PLA_2 activity in schizophrenics and other psychiatric disorders. Biol Psychiatry 1993; 34: 641–649.

Pangerl AM, Steudle A, Jaroni HW, Rufer R, Gattaz WF. Increased platelet membrane lysophosphatidylcholine in schizophrenia. Biol Psychiatry 1991; 30: 837–840.

Pettegrew JW, Keshavan MS, Panchalingam K et al. Alterations in brain high-energy phosphate and membrane phospholipid metabolism in first-episode drug-naïve schizophrenics. A pilot study of the dorsal prefrontal cortex by in vivo phosphorus-31 nuclear magnetic resonance spectroscopy. Arch Gen Psychiatry 1991; 48: 563–568.

Reid MS, Hsu K, Tolliver BK, Crawford CA, Berger SP. Evidence for the involvement of phospholipase A_2 mechanisms in the development of stimulant sensitisation. J Pharmacol Exp Ther 1996; 276: 1244–1256.

Ross BM, Moszczynska A, Kalasinsky K, Kish SJ. Phospholipase A_2 activity is selectively decreased in the striatum of chronic cocaine users. J Neurochem 1996; 67: 2620–2623.

Ross BM, Hudson C, Erlich J, Warsh JJ, Kish SJ. Increased phospholipid breakdown in schizophrenia: evidence for the involvement of a calcium-independent phospholipase A_2. Arch Gen Psychiatry 1997; 54: 487–494.

Ross BM, Moszczynska A, Erlich J, Kish SJ. Low activity of key phospholipid catabolic and anabolic enzymes in human substantia nigra: possible implications for Parkinson's disease. Neuroscience 1998a; 83: 791–798.

Ross BM, Moszczynska A, Erlich J, Kish SJ. Phospholipid-metabolising enzymes in Alzheimer's disease: increased lysophospholipid acyltransferase activity and decreased phospholipase A_2 activity. J Neurochem 1998b; 70: 786–793.

Schwarz RD, Uretsky NJ, Bianchine JR. Prostaglandin inhibition of amphetamine-induced circling in mice. Psychopharmacology 1982a; 78: 317–321.

Schwarz RD, Uretsky NJ, Bianchine JR. Prostaglandin inhibition of apomorphine induced circling in mice. Pharmacol Biochem Behav 1982b; 17: 1233–1237.

Sengupta N, Datta SC, Sengupta D. Platelet and erythrocyte membrane lipid and phospholipid patterns in different types of mental patients. Biochem Med 1981; 25: 267–275.

Shioiri T, Kato T, Inubushi T, Murashita J, Takahashi S. Correlations of phosphomonoesters measured by phosphorus-31 magnetic resonance spectroscopy in the frontal lobes and negative symptoms in schizophrenia. Psychiatry Res 1994; 55: 223–235.

Smalheiser NR, Swanson DR. Calcium-independent phospholipase A_2 and schizophrenia. Arch Gen Psychiatry 1998; 55: 753.

Stanley JA, Williamson PC, Drost DJ et al. Membrane phospholipid metabolism and schizophrenia: an *in vivo* ^{31}P-MR spectroscopy study. Schizophr Res 1994; 13: 209–215.

Stanley JA, Williamson PC, Drost DJ et al. An *in vivo* study of the prefrontal cortex of schizophrenic patients at different stages of illness *via* phosphorus magnetic resonance spectroscopy. Arch Gen Psychiatry 1995; 52: 399–406.

Stevens JD. The distribution of phospholipid fractions in the red cell membranes of schizophrenics. Schizophr Bull 1972; 6: 60–61.

Tolbert LC, Monti JA, O'Shields H, Walter-Ryan W, Meadows D, Smythies JR. Defects in transmethylation and membrane lipids in schizophrenia. Psychopharmacol Bull 1983; 19: 594–599.

Vial D, Piomelli D. Dopamine D_2 receptors potentiate arachidonate release *via* activation of cytosolic, arachidonic-specific phospholipase A_2. J Neurochem 1995; 64: 2765–2772.

Weinberger DR, Lipska BK. Cortical maldevelopment, antipsychotic drugs, and schizophrenia: a search for common ground. Schizophr Res 1995; 16: 87–110.

Williamson PC, Drost D, Stanley J, Carr T, Morrison S, Merskey H. Localized phosphorus-31 magnetic resonance spectroscopy in chronic schizophrenic patients and normal controls. Arch Gen Psychiatry 1991; 48: 578.

Yao JK, Yasaei P, van Kammen DP. Increased turnover of platelet phosphatidylinositol in schizophrenia. Prostagland Leukotr Essent Fatty Acids 1992; 46: 39–46.

Phospholipase A$_2$ Gene Polymorphism and Associated Biochemical Alterations in Schizophrenia

C. N. Ramchand, J. Wei, K. H. Lee and Malcom Peet

PHOSPHOLIPIDS AND SCHIZOPHRENIA

There is now compelling evidence to support the view that there is a generalized membrane abnormality in schizophrenia (Hitzemann et al., 1984). Converging evidence implicating cell membrane pathology in schizophrenia arises from studies in many different areas, such as: *in vivo* NMR spectroscopy (Pettegrew et al., 1991); the lipid profile of platelets and red cell membranes (Horrobin et al., 1991; Kaiya et al., 1991; Pangerl et al., 1991; Bates et al., 1992); *in vitro* investigations on the fatty acid composition of neuronal membranes (Horrobin et al., 1991); biopsied muscle tissue (Borg et al., 1987); phospholipase A$_2$ (PLA$_2$) activity (Noponen et al., 1993; Brunner and Gattaz, 1995; Gattaz et al., 1995; Gattaz and Brunner, 1996) and gene polymorphism (Hudson et al., 1996; Peet et al., 1998); abnormal prostaglandin metabolism (Horrobin et al., 1978); altered antioxidant enzyme levels and membrane peroxidation (Ramchand et al., 1996a); altered cellular transport process (Weisel et al., 1994; Ramchand et al., 1996b); altered glucose metabolism (Ramchand et al., 1995) and polyamine levels (Ramchand et al., 1994); decreased niacin flushing (Hudson et al., 1997); and the therapeutic efficacy of some of the polyunsaturated fatty acids (Peet et al., 1996).

It is well known that, for the optimal performance of any functional protein, it is necessary for that protein to have a specific three-dimensional conformation. This specific conformation can be altered by an addition, deletion or specific alteration of amino acids, such as is seen in genetic abnormality, which alters the kinetics of the protein in question. Many functional proteins, such as enzymes, ionic channels, receptors, and proteins involved in transduction mechanisms, are embedded in the membranes, which are made up mainly of phospholipids. These membrane constituents are in constant interaction with each other, thus creating a specific physico-chemical environment. Under normal circumstances, these interactions are in a constant dynamic equilibrium (synthesis and breakdown of membrane constituents), thereby providing a stable physico-chemical environment and thus facilitating optimal performance of the functional proteins.

About 20% by dry weight of brain consists of highly unsaturated fatty acids, such as arachidonic acid (AA), eicosapentaenoic acid (EPA) and docosahexaenoic acid (DHA), which possess several double bonds in the carbon backbone. This SP2 hybridized double bond (C=C) has a specific localized electronic environment which is in constant interaction with its wider environment. A minor change in the electronic environment can have a profound effect on the functional molecules due to molecular interactions, especially on proteins, as the C–C single bond conformation can be easily altered, resulting in changed activity. Alteration of the physico-chemical properties of synaptic membranes can cause changes in transmembrane and surface potentials and in lipid bilayer microviscosity (Erin et al., 1985). For example, Witt and Nielsen (1994) have shown that, in the isolated diazepam receptor, incubation with various saturated fatty acids had no effect, whereas the incubation of a double-bonded fatty acid doubled the receptor binding profile. Perhaps the observed multi-neurotransmitter dysfunction in schizophrenia results from alteration of some of the membrane fatty acids.

SCHIZOPHRENIA, PHOSPHOLIPIDS AND ESSENTIAL FATTY ACIDS

Several studies have shown that the levels of essential fatty acids which form the major part of phospholipids, and hence of the membranes which are made up, in large part, of those fatty acids, are altered in schizophrenics (Horrobin et al., 1994; Horrobin, 1996; Peet et al., 1996). These studies were carried out mainly in erythrocytes/plasma from patients and matched controls and, in some instances, from post-mortem brains (Horrobin et al., 1991). Most of the reports show depleted fatty acid levels in schizophrenics.

Horrobin et al. (1989) have shown a significant depletion of 18:2n-6 and 20:4n-6 and increased n-3 fatty acids in the plasma of schizophrenia. Erythrocyte membrane fatty acid analyses from patients have shown more consistent results. Studies conducted by Vaddadi et al. (1989), Glen et al. (1994) and Peet et al. (1995, 1996), have all shown depleted fatty acids in schizophrenics. Dietary deficiency or the effects of drugs could be implicated in these findings. However, in a recent study (unpublished) we have found that patients who have been drug-free in the long term (15 years; samples obtained from Malaysia), and drug-naïve patients (from India), show significantly altered membrane composition compared to control subjects matched for socioeconomic and dietary status. Several recent studies (Gattaz et al., 1990, 1995; Noponen et al., 1993) have shown that, compared to controls, schizophrenic patients exhibit elevated PLA$_2$ activity in plasma, serum and platelets. Thus it is possible that the observed fatty acid abnormalities in schizophrenics may be attributed to a genetic defect in PLA$_2$, although the dietary pattern and drug levels may be playing their parts too.

PLA$_2$ AND LIPIDS IN TRANSDUCTION MECHANISMS

There are four groups of PLA$_2$ enzymes, referred to as types I, II, III and IV, which vary with regard to function, localization, regulation, mechanism, sequence, and requirement for Ca^{2+} ions. Types I, II and III are secreted and Ca^{2+}-dependent, whereas type IV is cytosolic with one subgroup Ca^{2+}-dependent and the other subgroup Ca^{2+}-independent (Dennis, 1994). PLA$_2$ enzymes catalyze the hydrolysis of the Sn2 fatty acyl bond of phospholipids to free fatty acid and the lysophospholipid. The major fatty acid released is AA, which is the major source of production of prostaglandins and leukotrienes. The role of prostaglandins in the disease process of schizophrenia is well recognized (Horrobin, 1977). Platelet activating factor (PAF), a potent cellular mediator, is produced from the lysophospholipid (Dennis, 1987).

All types of PLA$_2$ are involved in essentially similar cellular reactions, such as playing an important role in central phospholipid metabolism. They also participate in several physiological functions. Specific cell surface PLA$_2$ receptors have been identified (Hanasaki and Arita, 1992). Elevated expression of PLA$_2$ (type II) in several inflammatory diseases suggests that it is involved in host defence mechanisms (Dennis, 1994). PLA$_2$ enzymes are involved in the initial steps in the eicosanoid cascades and therefore in its production and control (Dennis, 1994); they are more importantly involved in several signal transduction mechanisms, being specific to the release of AA and the Ca^{2+}-dependent phospholipid-binding domain. Both Ca^{2+}-dependent and Ca^{2+}-independent types of PLA$_2$ are involved in cellular signal transductions (Dennis et al., 1991). In neuronal membranes the PLA$_2$ enzymes play an essential role in signal transduction by affecting the physico-chemical properties of synaptic membranes (Farooqui et al., 1992); they have been shown to modulate dopamine (DA) synthesis, release and DA receptor sensitivity (Anand-Srivastava and Johnson, 1981; Oliveira et al., 1984). In neurones, many of the second messenger systems depend on lipids, such as free fatty acids, diacyl glycerols, prostaglandins, leukotrienes and hydroxy-fatty acids.

PLA$_2$ IN SIGNAL TRANSDUCTION AND SCHIZOPHRENIA

The large class (i.e., types I, II and III) of the secretory forms of PLA$_2$ (sPLA$_2$) is prevalent in digestive enzymes, requiring millimolar concentrations of Ca^{2+} for optimal activity, and showing no selectivity among the fatty acids in the Sn2 position of phospholipids (Schalkwijk et al., 1990). Type IV, i.e., cytosolic PLA$_2$ (cPLA$_2$), has been shown specifically to cleave arachidonyl phosphatidylcholine to release AA and to initiate eicosanoid and PAF production (Ramesha and Pickett, 1986; Suga et al., 1990). Several ligands that couple to GTP-binding proteins have been shown to stimulate cPLA$_2$ and to initiate the biosynthesis of potent inflammatory mediators (Irvine, 1982; Burch et al., 1986; Hanahan, 1986; Jelsema and Axelrod, 1987; Gupta et al., 1990). It has been reported that, for the activation of cPLA$_2$, submicromolar concentrations of Ca^{2+} are required (Channon and Leslie, 1990) and many of the known ligands that activate cPLA$_2$ are also Ca^{2+}-mobilisers in the cytosol.

From the literature, it is clear that cPLA$_2$ enzymes are major mediators of diverse biochemical mechanisms (Clark et al., 1991). Several recent studies have suggested that there may be a defect in neurotransmitter signal transduction, particularly in the generation of second messengers derived from membrane phospholipids, such as inositol phosphates (IPs), diacylglycerols (DAG), and AA, in schizophrenia (Horrobin et al., 1994). The major enzymes involved in the production of these second messengers are those in the type IV group (cPLA$_2$); thus a genetic abnormality leading to altered cPLA$_2$ activity may be a major contributory factor in the pathophysiology of schizophrenia.

PLA$_2$ ACTIVITY IN SCHIZOPHRENIA

The results of several studies suggest the existence of disordered phospholipid metabolism in schizophrenics, an abnormality possibly attributable to dietary deficiency and drug effects, as well as to a metabolic abnormality arising from a genetic factor. In a recent unpublished study using drug-naïve patients and controls matched for age, sex, socioeconomic status and diet, we have shown that the levels of both n-6 and n-3 fatty acids are significantly altered in schizophrenic patients. From these results it can be postulated that the observed difference in fatty acids in erythrocytes in schizophrenic patients can be attributed to a metabolic defect rather than to environmental factors, though the latter may also be contributory. The various types of PLA$_2$ are key enzymes involved in phospholipid metabolism and are enriched in neuronal membrane. Gattaz et al. (1987) found PLA$_2$ levels in schizophrenics and nonschizophrenic psychiatric controls to be significantly elevated in comparison with the levels in normal controls. Similar results were found in drug-free schizophrenics (Gattaz et al., 1990). These studies were confirmed by Noponen et al. (1993). Gattaz et al. (1995) also found elevated levels of PLA$_2$ activity in platelets from schizophrenics. In addition to this, *in vivo* measurement of phospholipid metabolism in the central nervous system (CNS) has provided indirect evidence that levels of cPLA$_2$ activity are elevated in schizophrenics (Pettegrew et al., 1991; Stanley et al., 1995).

cPLA$_2$ GENE STUDIES IN SCHIZOPHRENIA

The findings discussed above suggest that cPLA$_2$ enzymes play an important role in the development and manifestation of schizophrenia. Since a genetic component is likely to be involved in schizophrenia, it is important to examine whether the cPLA$_2$ abnormality is related to defects in its gene locus. Recently, Horrobin et al. (1995) hypothesized that polymorphism of the cPLA$_2$ gene may be associated with schizophrenia. The human genome mapping project has provided the possibility of studying the genetic aetiology of schizophrenia at the DNA level. The cPLA$_2$ gene has been mapped to the chromosome 1q25 in humans (Tay et al., 1994). The human cPLA$_2$ gene has also been isolated and sequenced (Clark et al., 1991). Tay et al. (1995) reported two simple sequence repeats, i.e., the poly(A) or (dA)n mononucleotide repeat and the (CA)n dinucleotide repeat, at the human cPLA$_2$ locus. The poly(A) simple sequence repeat is located at the 5′ end of an inverted Alu repeat near the promotor region, and its predicted DNA fragment should contain the (dA)43 repeat sequence. The analysis of length polymorphism within this marker, using a polymerase chain reaction (PCR) method, showed 10 individual alleles with about 76% of heterozygosity due to the poly(A) repeat among unrelated individuals (Tay et al., 1995). Hudson et al. (1996) have examined the association of the poly(A) simple sequence repeat in the human cPLA$_2$ gene with schizophrenia, in 65 patients and 65 matched healthy controls. They found that the distribution of allele frequencies for the subjects with schizophrenia was significantly different from that of healthy control subjects. Out of 10 alleles (A1–A10), the frequency of A1–A6 was significantly lower in patients with schizophrenia than in control subjects. They also reported that a halotype relative risk study in 44 nuclear families typed for the cPLA$_2$ poly(A) repeat revealed a significant association between the A8 allele and schizophrenia (Hudson et al., 1996). A similar study was conducted in 58 patients with schizophrenia and 56 control subjects by Price et al. (1997), but they failed to find the allelic association of the poly(A) repeat polymorphism with schizophrenia.

Tay et al. (1995) also reported that the (CA)n simple sequence repeat was located in the promoter of the human cPLA$_2$ gene, and four individual alleles were identified among the human population. Unfortunately, the human (CA)n repeat was not highly informative, as one of the alleles showed a frequency of 0.96. To assess the functional polymorphism of the (CA)n repeat for schizophrenia, we have undertaken a further study comparing the allelic distribution of the (CA)n repeat between patients with schizophrenia and healthy control subjects. Genomic DNA was extracted from whole blood taken from unrelated patients with schizophrenia who fulfilled DSM-IIIR criteria, and from healthy subjects. The fragments containing the polymorphic (CA)n repeat were amplified by a PCR-based process with a pair of primers, 5′ GACAAGTAGCAATTTCA-GACG3′ (sense strand) and 5′ CTGTTGGGATTTCT-GTGTG3′ (antisense strand). The predicted length of the PCR product should be 80 bp, according to the sequence data. The results showed four individual alleles in patients and two among controls. The sizes of allelic fragments were 82 bp (A1), 80 bp (A2), 78 bp (A3) and 74 bp (A4). As shown in Table 3.1, we failed to find a significant difference in allelic frequencies of the (CA)n repeat between schizophrenic patients and the control subjects.

Table 3.1. Allelic frequencies of the (CA)n repeat of cPLA$_2$ gene among schizophrenic patients (n = 52) and controls (n = 48).

	Allelic fragment			
Group	A1	A2	A3	A4
Patients	1	99	2	6
Controls	0	93	3	0

There was no statistically significant difference between the allelic frequencies in patients and controls.

Table 3.2. Allelic frequency of the Ban I dimorphic site in the human cPLA$_2$ gene among schizophrenics and unrelated controls (number of chromosomes shown in parentheses).

	Allelic fragment	
Group	A1	A2
Patients	0.305 (22)	0.695 (50)
Controls	0.481 (26)	0.536 (30)

$\chi^2(df,1) = 4.050; p = 0.044$.

Table 3.3. Genotypic frequency of the Ban I dimorphic site in the human cPLA^2 gene among schizophrenics (n = 36) and unrelated controls (n = 27).

	Genotype		
Group	A1/A1	A2/A2	A1/A2
Patients	0.111	0.500*	0.389
Controls	0.185	0.222	0.593

*In comparison with controls, $\chi^2(df,1) = 5.048; p = 0.024$.

In spite of the results obtained in the studies mentioned above, the findings reported for the cPLA$_2$ gene have not yet been sufficiently clear to indicate a significant association between the polymorphic cPLA$_2$ gene and schizophrenia. Recently, we have utilized a long PCR combined with restriction length fragment polymorphism analysis to search a polymorphic restriction site on the human cPLA$_2$ gene in patients with schizophrenia and in healthy control subjects; preliminary data from this study have recently been published (Peet et al., 1998). We found that there was a dimorphic site in the first intron of the cPLA$_2$ gene with Ban I digestion. The Ban I dimorphic site is highly informative and can be used as a genetic marker to undertake an association study on schizophrenia.

Thirty six drug-naïve patients were recruited, all of whom fulfilled DSM-IV criteria for schizophrenia; 27 unrelated, ethnically matched healthy subjects were used as controls. The controls had no personal or family history of schizophrenia. All the subjects were from India and all gave informed consent to the study, which had been approved by the local ethical committee. Overnight fasting blood was drawn from the antecubital vein between 08:00 and 09:00 and immediately cooled to 2–4°C. Genomic DNA was extracted from whole blood by using Micromix 200 kits (Talent, Trieste, Italy). The sequence spanning from the 5'-flanking region to the 3' end of the first intron of the cPLA$_2$ gene (EMBL accession No. U11239) was amplified by using a PCR with a pair of primers: 5' GACAAGTAG-CAATTTCAGACA3') (sense strand) and 5' TCTGC-TTATGGTGAGCATTGAGTTG3' (antisense strand). The PCR products were respectively digested with the following restriction enzymes: Taq I, Rsa I, Xba I, Hae III, Hha I, BamH I, Pst I, Dra I, Alu I, Msp I and Ban I. The digested PCR products were electrophoresed on agarose gels. Polymorphic sites were determined according to the presence of additional restriction sites or the absence of predicted restriction sites.

As shown in Table 3.2, Ban I digestion gave two individual alleles, A1 and A2. There was a statistically significant difference in allelic frequencies between schizophrenic patients and control subjects ($p < 0.05$).

Our study has also shown that schizophrenic patients have a significant excess of A2/A2 homozygotic genotype as compared with controls (Table 3.3). The goodness-of-fit test demonstrated that genotypic frequencies among both patients and controls were in Hardy-Weiberg equilibrium.

These results suggest that the Ban I polymorphic site in the first intron of the human cPLA$_2$ may be in linkage disequilibrium with a faulty locus responsible for schizophrenia. The faulty locus may be within the cPLA$_2$ gene or nearby (usually less than a million base pairs of distance). However, distribution of allelic or genotypic frequencies may vary among different subgroups of differing geographic origins. It is therefore necessary to replicate the work in geographically different individuals.

Genetic alteration in the cPLA$_2$ gene may be manifested as a membrane abnormality throughout the body. Since a major proportion of neuronal membrane is made up of unsaturated fatty acids this abnormality will be most pronounced in the brain. As discussed earlier, this abnormality can be manifested as neurotransmitter dysfunction and abnormalities of signal transduction.

The fatty acid composition of the erythrocytes from these patients was analyzed and the erythrocytes were separated according to genotype. Fatty acids from red blood cell membranes were obtained from samples separated for between 30 and 60 min by centrifugation ($1000 \times g$) for 15 min, washed twice with cold saline and centrifuged again. RBC were frozen at –70°C until used for analysis. Fatty acid analysis, carried out at Scotia Pharmaceuticals, Canada, used the method described by Manku et al. (1982). The lipid fraction extracted from each sample was separated by TLC and the fatty acid composition analyzed by gas–liquid chromatography. The results are shown in Table 3.4.

Adrenic acid (22:4n-6) and docosahexaenoic acid (22:6n-3) are altered in patients, compared to controls. As discussed earlier, the Ban I dimorphic site is highly informative and can be used for association studies. Alteration in the levels of fatty acids found among genotypes of the Ban I site in patients, compared to controls, may be responsible for altered signal transduction through altered cytokine production (Konieczkowski and Sedor, 1993).

Table 3.4. Essential fatty acid levels (mg/100 mg phospholipid) among genotypes of Ban I dimorphic site, in schizophrenic patients (total $n = 36$) and controls (total $n = 27$); the number of cases of each genotype is shown in parentheses; means ± SEM.

Group and fatty acid	A1/A1	A2/A2	A1/A2
Patients			
n-6			
18:2	14.4 ± 4.9	16.0 ± 5.2	13.8 ± 4.3
20:2	0.38 ± 0.1	0.37 ± 0.1	0.38 ± 0.06
20:3	1.65 ± 1.14	1.81 ± 0.64	1.83 ± 0.81
20:4	15.4 ± 6.86	14.8 ± 3.71	14.3 ± 5.95
22:4	2.78 ± 1.2	2.55 ± 0.74**	2.00 ± 0.79*
22:5	0.72 ± 0.32	0.63 ± 0.14	0.75 ± 0.09
n-3			
20:5	0.31[a]	0.25 ± 0.09	0.46 ± 0.38
22:5	0.95 ± 0.50	1.28 ± 0.51	1.31 ± 0.62
22:6	2.28 ± 0.71	2.10 ± 0.80	2.57 ± 1.10*
Controls			
n-6			
18:2	20.7 ± 5.3	16.7 ± 4.6	15.6 ± 5.4
20:2	0.35 ± 0.09	0.31 ± 0.06	0.34 ± 0.07
20:3	2.24 ± 0.54	1.70 ± 0.67	1.47 ± 0.64
20:4	16.7 ± 2.09	15.2 ± 1.21	14.1 ± 5.8
22:4	2.45 ± 1.03	3.61 ± 0.88	2.9 ± 1.3
22:5	0.55 ± 0.14	0.64 ± 0.12	0.71 ± 0.21
n-3			
20:5	0.22 ± 0.14	0.34 ± 0.62	0.27 ± 0.12
22:5	1.17 ± 0.30	1.26 ± 0.49	0.98 ± 0.32
22:6	1.78 ± 0.54	1.75 ± 0.65	1.75 ± 0.62

In comparison with the corresponding value for controls, $p <$: *0.05; **0.01. [a] Single value.

REFERENCES

Anand-Srivastava MB, Johnson RA. Role of phospholipids in coupling of adenosine and dopamine receptors to striatal adenylate cyclase. J Neurochem 1981; 36: 1819–1828.

Bates C, Horrobin DF, Ellis K. Fatty acids in plasma phospholipids and cholesterol esters from identical twins concordant and discordant for schizophrenia. Schizophr Res 1992; 6: 1–7.

Borg J, Edström L, Bjerkenstet L, Wiesel FA, Farde L, Hagenfeldt L. Muscle biopsy findings, conduction velocity and refractory period of single motor nerve fibres in schizophrenia. J Neurol Neurosurg Psychiatry 1987; 50: 1644–1655.

Brunner J, Gattaz WF. Intracerebral injection of phospholipase A_2 inhibits dopamine mediated behaviour in rats. Possible implications for schizophrenia. Eur Arch Psychiatry Clin Neurosci 1995; 246: 13–16.

Burch RM, Luini A, Axelrod J. Phospholipase A_2 and phospholipase C are activated by distinct GTP binding proteins in response to α_1-adrenergic stimulation in FTRL5 thyroid cells. Proc Natl Acad Sci USA 1986; 83: 7201–7205.

Channon JY, Leslie CC. A calcium-dependent mechanism for associating a soluble arachidonyl-hydrolyzing phospholipase A_2 with membrane in the macrophage cell line RAW. J Biol Chem 1990; 265: 5409–5413.

Clark JD, Lin LL, Kriz RW et al. A novel arachidonic acid-selective cytosolic PLA_2 contains a Ca^{2+} dependent translocation domain with homology to PKC and GAP. Cell 1991; 65: 1043–1051.

Dennis EA. Regulation of eicosanoid production. Role of phospholipases and inhibitors. Biol Technol 1987; 5: 1294–1300.

Dennis EA. Diversity of group types, regulation and function of phospholipase A_2. J Biol Chem 1994; 269: 13057–13060.

Dennis EA, Rhee SG, Billah MM, Hannun YA. Role of phospholipases in generating lipid second messengers in signal transduction. FASEB J 1991; 5: 2068–2077.

Erin AN, Tyurin VA, Brusovanil VI et al. Change in the physicochemical parameters of synaptosomal membranes under the action of PLA_2. Biochem USSR 1985; 50: 431–436.

Farooqui AA, Hirashima Y, Horrocks LA. Brain phospholipases and their role in signal transduction. In: Bazán NG, Murphy MG, Tofano G, eds. Neurobiology of essential fatty acids. New York: Plenum Press, 1992: 11–26.

Gattaz WF, Brunner J. Phospholipase A_2 and the hypofrontality hypothesis of schizophrenia. Prostagland Leukotr Essent Fatty Acids 1996; 55: 109–113.

Gattaz WF, Kollisch M, Thuren T, Virtanen JA, Kinnunen PKJ. Increased plasma phospholipase-A_2 activity in schizophrenic patients: reduction after neuroleptic therapy. Biol Psychiatry 1987; 22: 421–426.

Gattaz WF, Hübner CK, Nevalainen TJ, Thuren T, Kinnunen PKJ. Increased serum phospholipase-A_2 activity in schizophrenia: a replication study. Biol Psychiatry 1990; 28: 495–501.

Gattaz WF, Schmitt A, Maras AM. Increased platelet phospholipase A_2 activity in schizophrenia. Schizophr Res 1995; 16: 1–6.

Glen AIM, Glen EMT, Horrobin DF et al. A red cell membrane abnormality in a subgroup of schizophrenic patients: evidence for two diseases. Schizophr Res 1994; 12: 53–61.

Gupta SK, Diez E, Heasley LE, Osawa S, Johnson GL. A G-protein mutant that inhibits thrombin and purinergic receptor activation of phospholipase A_2. Science 1990; 249: 662–666.

Hanahan DJ. Platelet activating factor: a biologically active phosphoglyceride. Ann Rev Biochem 1986; 55: 483–509.

Hanasaki K, Arita H. Characterisation of a high affinity binding site for pancreatic type phospholipase A_2 in the rat. Its cellular and tissue distribution. J Biol Chem 1992; 267: 6414–6420.

Hitzemann R, Hirschowitz J, Garver D. Membrane abnormalities in the psychoses and affective disorders. J Psychiatry Res 1984; 18: 319–326.

Horrobin DF. Schizophrenia as a prostaglandin deficiency disease. Lancet 1977; i: 936–937.

Horrobin DF. Schizophrenia as a membrane lipid disorder which is expressed throughout the body. Prostagland Leukotr Essent Fatty Acids 1996; 55: 3–7.

Horrobin DF, Ally AI, Karmali RA, Karmazyn M, Manku MS, Morgan RO. Prostaglandins and schizophrenia: further discussion of the evidence. Psychol Med 1978; 8: 43–48.

Horrobin DF, Manku MS, Morse-Fisher N, Vaddadi KS. Essential fatty acids in plasma phospholipids in schizophrenics. Biol Psychiatry 1989; 25: 562–568.

Horrobin DF, Manku MS, Hillman H, Glen AIM. Fatty acid levels in the brains of schizophrenics and normal controls. Biol Psychiatry 1991; 30: 795–805.

Horrobin DF, Glen AIM, Vaddadi K. The membrane hypothesis of schizophrenia. Schizophr Res 1994; 13: 195–207.

Horrobin DF, Glen AIM, Hudson CJ. Possible relevance of phospholipid abnormalities and genetic interactions in psychiatric disorders: the relationship between dyslexia and schizophrenia. Med Hypotheses 1995; 6: 605–613.

Hudson CJ, Kennedy JL, Gotowiec A et al. Genetic variant near cytosolic phospholipase A_2 associated with schizophrenia. Schizophr Res 1996; 21: 111–116.

Hudson CJ, Lin A, Cogan S, Cashman F, Warsh JJ. The niacin challenge test: clinical manifestation of altered transmembrane signal transduction in schizophrenia. Biol Psychiatry 1997; 41: 507–513.

Irvine RF. How is the level of free arachidonic acid controlled in mammalian cells? Biochem J 1982; 204: 3–16.

Jelsema CL, Axelrod J. Stimulation of phospholipase A_2 activity in bovine rod outer segments by the $\beta\gamma$ subunits of transducin and its inhibition by the α subunit. Proc Natl Acad Sci USA 1987; 84: 3623–3627.

Kaiya H, Horrobin DF, Manku MS, Morse-Fisher N. Essential and other fatty acids in plasma in schizophrenics and normal individuals from Japan. Biol Psychiatry 1991; 30: 357–362.

Konieczkowski M, Sedor JR. Cell specific regulation of type II phospholipase A_2 expression in rat mesangial cells. J Clin Invest 1993; 92: 2524–2532.

Manku MS, Horrobin DF, Morse N et al. Reduced levels of prostaglandin precursors in the blood of atopic patients. Defective delta-6 desaturase functions as a biochemical basis for atopy. Prostagland Leukotr Med 1982; 9: 615–628.

Noponen M, Sanfilipo M, Samanich K et al. Elevated PLA_2 activity in schizophrenics and other psychiatric patients. Biol Psychiatry 1993; 34: 641–649.

Oliveira CR, Duarte EP, Carvalho AP. Effects of phospholipase digestion and lysophosphatydylcholine on dopamine receptor binding. J Neurochem 1984; 43: 455–465.

Pangerl AM, Steudle A, Jaroni HW, Rüfer R, Gattaz WF. Increased platelet membrane lysophosphatydylcholine in schizophrenia. Biol Psychiatry 1991; 30: 837–840.

Peet M, Laugharne JDE, Rangarajan N, Horrobin DF, Reynolds G. Depleted red cell membrane essential fatty acids in drug-treated schizophrenic patients. J Psychiatr Res 1995; 29: 227–232.

Peet M, Laugharne JDE, Mellor J, Ramchand CN. Essential fatty acid deficiency in erythrocyte membranes from chronic schizophrenic patients and the clinical effect of dietary supplementation. Prostagland Leukotr Essent Fatty Acids 1996; 55: 71–75.

Peet M, Ramchand CN, Lee KH et al. Association of the Ban I dimorphic site at the human phospholipase A_2 gene with schizophrenia. Psychiatr Genet 1998; 3: 1–2.

Pettegrew JW, Keshavan MS, Panchalingam K et al. Alterations in brain high-energy phosphate and membrane phospholipid metabolism in first-episode drug-naïve schizophrenics. A pilot study of the dorsal prefrontal cortex by in vivo phosphorus-31 nuclear magnetic resonance spectroscopy. Arch Gen Psychiatry 1991; 48: 563–568.

Price SA, Fox H, St Clair D, Shaw DJ. Lack of association between schizophrenia and a polymoprhism close to the cytosolic phospholipase A_2 gene. Psychiatr Genet 1997; 7: 111–114.

Ramchand CN, Das I, Gliddon A, Hirsch SR. Role of polyamines in the membrane pathology of schizophrenia. A study using fibroblasts from schizophrenic patients and normal controls. Schizophr Res 1994; 13: 249–253.

Ramchand CN, Clark AE, Gliddon AE, Hemmings GP. Glucose oxidation and monoamine oxidase activity from the fibroblasts of schizophrenic patients and controls. Life Sci 1995; 56: 1639–1646.

Ramchand CN, Davies JI, Tresman RL, Griffiths ICD, Peet M. Reduced susceptibility to oxidative damage of erythrocyte membranes from medicated schizophrenic patients. Prostagland Leukotr Essent Fatty Acids 1996a; 55: 27–31.

Ramchand CN, Peet M, Clark AE, Gliddon AE, Hemmings GP. Decreased tyrosine transport in fibroblasts from schizophrenics: implications for membrane pathology. Prostagland Leukotr Essent Fatty Acids 1996b; 55: 59–64.

Ramesha CS, Pickett WC. Platelet activating factor and leucotriene biosynthesis is inhibited in polynuclear leucocytes depleted of arachidonic acid. J Biol Chem 1986; 261: 7592–7595.

Schalkwijk CG, Marki F, van den Bosch H. Studies on the acyl chain selectivity of cellular phospholipase A_2. Biochim Biophys Acta 1990; 1044: 139–146.

Stanley JA, Williamson PC, Drost DJ et al. An in vivo study of the prefrontal cortex of schizophrenic patients at different stages of illness via phosphorus magnetic resonance spectroscopy. Arch Gen Psychiatry 1995; 52: 399–406.

Suga K, Kawasaki T, Blank ML, Snyder F. An arachidonyl (polyenoic)-specific phospholipase A_2 activity regulates the synthesis of platelet-activating factor in granulocyte HL-60 cells. J Biol Chem 1990; 265: 12363–12371.

Tay A, Maxwell P, Li ZG, Goldberg H, Skorecki K. Isolation of promoter for cytosolic phospholipase A_2 ($cPLA_2$). Biochim Biophys Acta 1994; 1217: 345–347.

Tay A, Simon JS, Squire J, Jacob HJ, Skorecki K. Cytosolic phospholipase A_2 gene in human and rat chromosomal localization and polymorphic markers. Genomics 1995; 26: 138–141.

Vaddadi KS, Courtney P, Gilleard CJ, Manku MS, Horrobin DF. A double-blind trial of essential fatty acid supplementation in patients with tardive dyskinesia. Psychiatry Res 1989; 27: 313–323.

Weisel FA, Venizelos N, Bjerkensedt L, Hagenfeldt L. Tyrosine transport in schizophrenia. Schizophr Res 1994; 13: 255–258.

Witt MR, Nielsen M. Characterization of the influence of the unsaturated free fatty acids on brain GABA/benzodiazepine receptor binding in vitro. J Neurochem 1994; 62: 1432–1439.

Phospholipase A₂ and the Hypofrontality Hypothesis of Schizophrenia

Wagner F. Gattaz and Jürgen Brunner

INTRODUCTION

The intracellular enzyme phospholipase A_2 (PLA_2) catalyzes the hydrolysis of membrane phospholipids to release fatty acids and cytotoxic products such as lysophosphatidylcholine. In neuronal membranes, PLA_2 plays an essential role in signal transduction by influencing the physicochemical properties of synaptic membranes (Farooqui et al., 1992). *In vitro* studies show that increased PLA_2 activity modulates dopamine (DA) synthesis and release (Bradford et al., 1983; Ohmichi et al., 1989) and DA-receptor sensitivity (Anand-Srivastava and Johnson, 1981; Oliveira et al., 1984).

In schizophrenic patients, PLA_2 activity has been reported to be increased in plasma (Gattaz et al., 1987; Ross et al., 1997), serum (Gattaz et al., 1990; Noponen et al., 1993), and platelet membranes (Gattaz et al., 1995). In platelets of schizophrenics, phosphatidylcholine concentration (a substrate of PLA_2) was found to be decreased (Rotrosen and Wolkin, 1987) and lysophosphatidylcholine concentration (a breakdown product of PLA_2 hydrolysis) elevated (Pangerl et al., 1991). These data suggest an accelerated breakdown of membrane phospholipids in schizophrenia.

Disordered phospholipid metabolism has also been reported in the brains of schizophrenics by means of *in vivo* NMR-spectroscopy studies. Phosphomonoesters (PME) are the precursors, and phosphodiesters (PDE) are the breakdown products, of membrane phospholipids in the brain. PME were found to be decreased, and PDE to be elevated, in the frontal lobe of schizophrenic patients (Williamson et al., 1991; Deicken et al., 1993; Pettegrew et al., 1993), suggesting that an accelerated phospholipid breakdown may be found in some schizophrenic brains.

Because increased PLA_2 activity is one mechanism that accelerates the breakdown of membrane phospholipids, and because PLA_2 modulates dopaminergic neurotransmission, we investigated the effects of intracerebral injections of the enzyme on DA-mediated behaviour in rats. To our knowledge, there is only one *in vivo* investigation of the effects of intracerebral PLA_2 injection on DA-mediated behaviour (Cadet et al., 1989). These authors investigated the effects of intranigral PLA_2 application on DA-mediated rotational behaviour in rats. In the first part of our study (Experiment 1) we were able to replicate and to extend the previous data obtained by Cadet et al. (1989). We adopted the rotational model presented by Ungerstedt and Arbuthnott (1970) because it is an easily quantifiable and well-validated approach to monitoring dopaminergic activity *in vivo*. In the second part of our study (Experiment 2) we investigated the effects of intracerebroventricular (i.c.v.) injections of PLA_2 on DA-mediated behaviour in rats, such as locomotion and stereotyped behaviour. To our knowledge, this is the first report on behavioural changes induced by i.c.v. PLA_2 application.

EXPERIMENTAL PROCEDURES
Experiment 1. Intranigral PLA₂ application

Stereotaxic surgery

Adult female Sprague Dawley rats (Charles River/Wiga, Sulzfeld), weighing 223 ± 10 g (mean ± SD), were anaesthetized with 10 mg ketamine (Ketavet®) s.c. per animal and 30 mg/kg pentobarbital (Nembutal®) i.p., and mounted in a David Kopf stereotaxic frame with the incisor bar 5 mm above horizontal zero. The substances were injected unilaterally into the substantia nigra pars compacta (SNC) in a volume of $4\,\mu l$ at a constant rate of $1\,\mu l$/min, using a Hamilton microlitre syringe (22 gauge). After completion of the injections, cannulas were left in place for an additional 3 min. The stereotaxic coordinates of the SNC (AP, 2.2 mm; L, 1.6 mm; DV, 2.5 mm from interaural line) were taken from the atlas of De Groot (1959). To validate stereotaxis precision, nine rats received a unilateral intranigral injection of $8\,\mu g$

6-hydroxydopamine (6-OHDA, Sigma) in 4 μl of saline with 0.2 μg/μl ascorbic acid added. These animals were pretreated with 10 mg/kg desipramine (Thomae) p.o. 60 min prior to surgery to protect noradrenergic nigral neurones. With these stereotaxic coordinates, the results of Ungerstedt and Arbuthnott (1970) could be replicated. Methamphetamine (5 mg/kg s.c.) induced an ipsilateral rotational asymmetry ($p < 0.01$) with 871 ± 69 ipsilateral and 4 ± 1 contralateral turns/h (means ± SEM).

Low-dose intranigral PLA$_2$ application

PLA$_2$, isolated and purified from bovine pancreas (Sigma), with an enzymatic activity of 6.8 U/mg, was unilaterally injected into the SNC in three different doses: 1, 3 and 5 μg ($n = 6$ for each dose). 1 U hydrolyzes 1 μmol L-α-phosphatidylcholine to L-α-lysophosphatidylcholine and a free fatty acid per min at pH 8.0 and 37°C. The control group ($n = 6$) received unilateral intranigral vehicle injection (4 μl of saline). Seven days after stereotaxic surgery, rotational behaviour induced by 0.5 mg/kg apomorphine (APO) s.c. was recorded for 60 min.

High-dose intranigral PLA$_2$ application

PLA$_2$ from bovine pancreas (Sigma) with higher enzymatic activity (12 U/mg) was unilaterally injected into the SNC in two different doses: 20 μg ($n = 11$) and 100 μg ($n = 12$), dissolved in 4 μl of saline. The control group ($n = 11$) received a unilateral intranigral injection of the vehicle (4 μl of saline). Twenty-one days after stereotaxis surgery, rotational behaviour induced by 0.5 mg/kg APO s.c. was recorded for 60 min.

Rotational assessments

Rotational behaviour was recorded automatically with a rotometer. Only complete turns (360°) in each direction were counted.

Statistics

Data were analyzed by nonparametric tests. The Mann-Whitney rank sum test was used for comparisons between different treatment groups. Rotational asymmetries (number of ipsilateral versus contralateral turns) within the same group were analyzed using the Wilcoxon matched pairs signed rank test.

Experiment 2. Intracerebroventricular PLA$_2$ application

Stereotaxic surgery

Twenty-four adult male Wistar rates (Charles River/Wiga, Sulzfeld) weighing 287 ± 12 g (mean ± SD) were anaesthetized with 30 mg/kg pentobarbital (Nembutal®) i.p. and 10 mg ketamine (Ketavet®) s.c. per animal and mounted in a David Kopf stereotaxic frame with the incisor bar set 3.3 mm below the horizontal zero. PLA$_2$, isolated and purified from bovine pancreas (Sigma) with an enzymatic activity of 12 U/mg, was used for i.c.v. injections. PLA$_2$ was unilaterally injected in the lateral ventricle at a constant rate of 1 μl/min, using a Hamilton microlitre syringe (22 gauge), in three different doses; i.e., 30, 60 and 120 μg PLA$_2$ dissolved in 5 μl of saline; there were six animals in each dosage group. The placebo group ($n = 6$) received i.c.v. saline injections (5 μl). Right/left positions were counterbalanced. After completion of the injections, cannulas were left *in situ* for an additional 2 min. Stereotaxic coordinates of the lateral ventricle with bregma as the reference point were: AP, –0.9; L, ± 1.5; and DV, 3.5 mm, according to Paxinos and Watson (1986).

Behavioural assessments

Each animal was individually placed in a standardized Plexiglas cage (42 × 26 × 15 cm). Each cage was placed in a soundproof box where the rats were observed. Oral stereotypies (licking, sniffing, chewing) and sitting were scored (present or absent) every 20 s, so that during 60 min 180 observations were scored for each animal. We used the number of sittings to assess locomotion indirectly. Under standardized conditions the duration of sitting correlates close to –1 with locomotion. The observer was blind with regard to the drug status of the animal. On days 1, 3 and 21, postoperatively, spontaneous behaviour was monitored for 30 min. On day 6, each animal was given 2 mg/kg methamphetamine (AMPH) s.c. On days 10 and 27, the rats received 0.25 mg/kg APO s.c. The behavioural changes were assessed for 60 min following the DA-agonist injections.

Statistics

Data were analyzed by Student's *t*-tests (two-tailed).

EFFECTS ON ROTATIONAL SYMMETRY AND LOCOMOTION

Experiment 1. Intranigral PLA$_2$ application

After unilateral intranigral injection of PLA$_2$ in low and high doses, APO induced an ipsilateral asymmetry. No APO-induced asymmetry was observed in animals pretreated with intranigral saline injections. As no significant differences were found among the three low-dose PLA$_2$ groups (1 μg PLA$_2$ – ipsilateral 47 ± 20, contra-

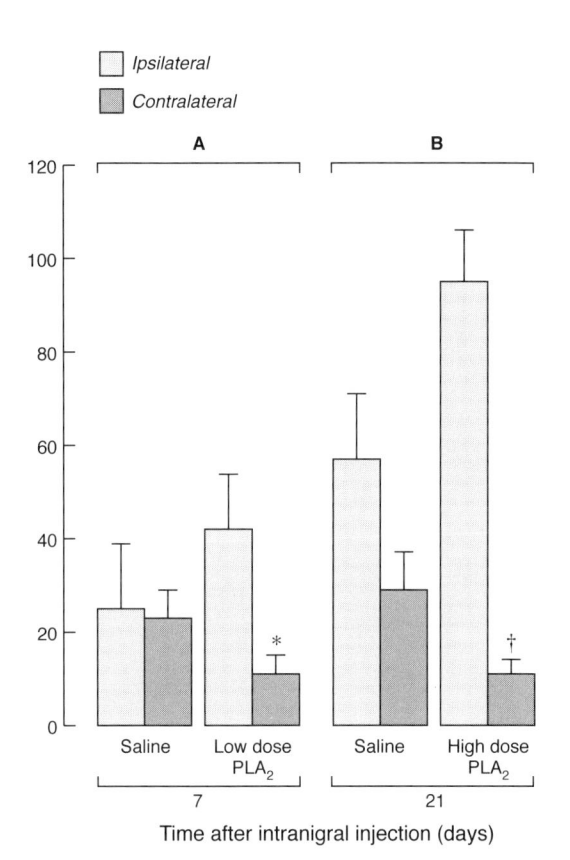

Figure 4.1. Rotational behaviour induced by 0.5 mg/kg apomorphine. A: 7 days after intranigral injection of low-dose PLA$_2$ (pooled data 1, 3 and 5 µg) or saline. B: 21 days after intranigral injection of high-dose PLA$_2$ (pooled data, 20 and 100 µg), or saline. Means ± SEM. In comparison with the corresponding score for ipsilateral rotations, $p <$: *0.05; †0.001.

lateral 5 ± 3; 3 µg PLA$_2$ – ipsilateral 30 ± 17, contralateral 7 ± 2; 5 µg PLA$_2$ – ipsilateral 48 ± 24, contralateral 22 ± 8 rotations/h; means ± SEM), the data were pooled as presented in Figure 4.1A. As no significant differences were found between the two high-dose PLA$_2$ groups (20 µg PLA$_2$ – ipsilateral 92 ± 15, contralateral 15 ± 5; 100 µg PLA$_2$ – ipsilateral 96 ± 17, contralateral 7 ± 2 rotations/h), the data were pooled as presented in Figure 4.1B.

Experiment 2. Intracerebroventricular PLA$_2$ application

Ten days after i.c.v. injection, PLA$_2$ inhibited APO-induced locomotion: sitting was enhanced by 94% in

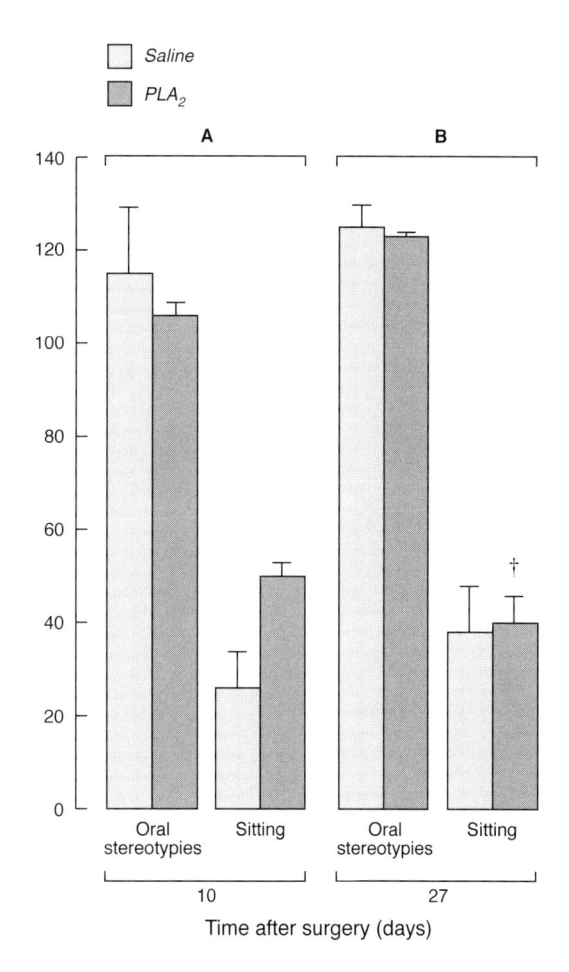

Figure 4.2. Apomorphine-induced behavioural changes in rats pretreated with intracerebroventricular PLA$_2$ (pooled data, 30, 60 and 120 µg) or saline injections; means ± SEM. A: 10 days after surgery. B: 27 days after surgery. †In comparison with the corresponding score for saline treatment, $p < 0.001$

rats pretreated with PLA$_2$ as compared to the placebo group ($p < 0.001$). As no significant differences were found among the three PLA$_2$ dose-groups, the data were pooled as presented in Figure 4.2A. The differences in APO-induced locomotion between PLA$_2$ and saline-pretreated animals disappeared 27 days after stereotaxis surgery (Figure 4.2B). No intergroup differences were found in APO-induced stereotypies 10 and 27 days after surgery. No differences were found between PLA$_2$ and saline-pretreated rats regarding spontaneous behaviour on days 1, 3 and 21 after surgery, and no differences were found regarding AMPH-induced behaviour on day 6 after surgery.

DISCUSSION

Intranigral PLA$_2$ application

In the rotational model used in the present study, the direction of circling is ipsilateral to the hemisphere with the lower nigrostriatal dopaminergic activity (Zetterström et al., 1986; Carman et al., 1991). After unilateral intranigral injection of PLA$_2$ in low and high doses, the direct DA-agonist APO induced an ipsilateral asymmetry. This effect was specific for PLA$_2$, because no asymmetry was induced by APO in the saline-pretreated animals. Our findings are in line with the results of Cadet et al. (1989) who also observed APO-induced ipsilateral circling behaviour after intranigral injection of PLA$_2$. The results from these animal experiments indicate that intranigral injection of PLA$_2$ reduced dopaminergic activity *in vivo*. This assumption is supported by the findings of Cadet et al. (1989) who reported a reduction of the striatal concentrations of DA and its metabolites, diphenylacetic acid (DOPAC) and homovanillic acid (HVA), on the side where PLA$_2$ was injected.

Intracerebroventricular PLA$_2$ application

APO increases locomotion in rats by a direct agonism of postsynaptic DA-receptors. In our experiment, i.c.v. PLA$_2$ application antagonized the APO-induced increase of locomotion, suggesting inhibition of postsynaptic DA-receptors by PLA$_2$.

Taken together, the results from our animal experiments and data from the literature suggest that intracerebral application of PLA$_2$ inhibits dopaminergic neurotransmission *in vivo*. An inhibitory effect of PLA$_2$ on dopaminergic neurotransmission has also been observed in *in vitro* experiments: PLA$_2$ inhibits the activation of DA-sensitive adenylate cyclase in striatal tissue (Anand-Srivastava and Johnson, 1981) and reduces [^{3}H]spiperone binding to DA-receptors (Oliveira et al., 1984).

How could this inhibitory effect of PLA$_2$ on dopaminergic neurotransmission be involved in the pathophysiology of schizophrenia? In schizophrenic patients, increased PLA$_2$ activity and an accelerated breakdown of membrane phospholipids have been observed in platelet membranes. Recent NMR-spectroscopy studies showed disordered phospholipid metabolism in the prefrontal cortex of drug-naïve schizophrenic patients, which correlated with a deficit of neuropsychological functions (Deicken et al., 1995). Further studies should clarify whether this accelerated phospholipid metabolism is caused by increased PLA$_2$ activity in the brain of schizophrenics, as observed in platelet membranes (Gattaz et al., 1995). A reduced dopaminergic activity in the prefrontal cortex has been hypothesized in the hypofrontality hypothesis of schizophrenia (Weinberger, 1987). In the light of the present findings, it is conceivable that increased PLA$_2$ activity may be related to the postulated hypodopaminergic activity in the prefrontal system in schizophrenia.

We speculate that increased PLA$_2$ activity in the prefrontal cortex of schizophrenic patients could contribute to the accelerated breakdown of membrane phospholipids and to the hypodopaminergic activity as postulated in the hypofrontality hypothesis of schizophrenia. This conclusion is highly speculative and can only be understood as a preliminary working hypothesis for the development of new studies. The profound effects of PLA$_2$ on the membrane phospholipid bilayer suggest that these effects are probably not specific for dopaminergic neurone. It is likely that increased PLA$_2$ activity in the brains of schizophrenics will influence the function of virtually all membrane-bound receptors, thereby disrupting normal brain function.

SUMMARY

PLA$_2$ catalyzes the hydrolysis of membrane phospholipids to release cytotoxic products, such as lysophosphatidylcholine. In schizophrenia, increased PLA$_2$ activity and an accelerated breakdown of membrane phospholipids have been reported. In neuronal membranes, PLA$_2$ modulates DA release and DA-receptor sensitivity.

Using two different animal models, inhibition of dopaminergic activity is shown *in vivo* by intracerebral PLA$_2$ application: unilateral stereotaxic injection of PLA$_2$ into the SNC causes an apomorphine-induced ipsilateral rotational asymmetry; and intracerebroventricular PLA$_2$ application reduces apomorphine-induced locomotion.

NMR spectroscopy studies show disordered phospholipid metabolism in the prefrontal cortex (PFC) of schizophrenics. The hypofrontality hypothesis of schizophrenia postulates hypodopaminergic activity in the PFC. Increased PLA$_2$ activity in the PFC of schizophrenics may be related to both abnormalities and could thus contribute to hypofrontality in schizophrenia.

ACKNOWLEDGEMENTS

This study was supported by the Deutsche Forschungsgemeinschaft, SFB 258, Project S4. We are indebted to Dr Gross and Dr Teschendorf (Knoll AG, Ludwigshafen) for valuable support to the experimental work.

REFERENCES

Anand-Srivastava MB, Johnson RA. Role of phospholipids in coupling of adenosine and dopamine receptors to striatal adenylate cyclase. J Neurochem 1981; 36: 1819–1828.

Bradford PG, Marinetti GV, Abood LG. Stimulation of phospholipase A_2 and secretion of catecholamines from brain synaptosomes by potassium and A23187. J Neurochem 1983; 41: 1684–1693.

Cadet JL, Hu M, Jackson-Lewis V. Behavioural and biochemical effects of intranigral injection of phospholipase-A_2. Biol Psychiatry 1989; 26: 106–110.

Carman LS, Gage FH, Shults CW. Partial lesion of the substantia nigra: relation between extent of lesion and rotational behavior. Brain Res 1991; 553: 275–283.

De Groot J. The rat forebrain in stereotaxic coordinates. Verhandeligen der koninklijke Nederlandse Akademie van Wetenschappen, afd. Natuurkunde. Amsterdam: N.V. Noord-Hollandische Uitgevers Maatschappij, 1959.

Deicken RF, Merrin E, Calabrese G, Dillon W, Weiner MW, Fein G. [31]Phosphorous MRSI of the frontal and parietal lobes in schizophrenia. Biol Psychiatry 1993; 33: 46A.

Deicken RF, Merrin EL, Floyd TC, Weiner MW. Correlation between left frontal phospholipids and Wisconsin Card Sort Test performance in schizophrenia. Schizophr Res 1995; 14: 177–181.

Farooqui AA, Hirashima Y, Horrocks LA. Brain phospholipases and their role in signal transduction. In: Bazán NG, Murphy MG, Tofano G, eds. Neurobiology of essential fatty acids. New York: Plenum Press, 1992: 11–26.

Gattaz WF, Köllisch M, Thuren T, Virtanen JA, Kinnunen PKJ. Increased plasma phospholipase-A_2 activity in schizophrenic patients: reduction after neuroleptic therapy. Biol Psychiatry 1987; 22: 421–426.

Gattaz WF, Hübner CK, Nevalainen TJ, Thuren T, Kinnunen PKJ. Increased serum phospholipase-A_2 activity in schizophrenia: a replication study. Biol Psychiatry 1990; 28; 495–501.

Gattaz WF, Steudle A, Maras A. Increased platelet phospholipase A_2 activity in schizophrenia. Schizophr Res 1995; 16: 1–6.

Noponen M, Sanfilipo M, Samanich K et al. Elevated PLA_2 activity in schizophrenics and other psychiatric patients. Biol Psychiatry 1993; 34: 641–649.

Ohmichi M, Hirota K, Koike K et al. Involvement of extracellular calcium and arachidonate in [3H]dopamine release from rat tuberoinfundibular neurons. Neuroendocrinology 1989; 50: 481–487.

Oliveira CR, Duarte EP, Carvalho AP. Effects of phospholipase digestion and lysophosphatidylcholine on dopamine receptor binding. J Neurochem 1984; 43: 455–465.

Pangerl AM, Steudle A, Jaroni HW, Rüfer R, Gattaz WF. Increased platelet membrane lysophosphatidylcholine in schizophrenia. Biol Psychiatry 1991; 30: 837–840.

Paxinos G, Watson C. The rat brain in stereotaxic coordinates. 2nd edn. San Diego: Academic Press, 1986.

Pettegrew JW, Keshavan MS, Minshew NJ. [31]P nuclear magnetic resonance spectroscopy: neurodevelopment and schizophrenia. Schizophr Bull 1993; 19: 35–53.

Ross BM, Hudson C, Erlich J, Warsh JJ, Kish SJ. Increased phospholipid breakdown in schizophrenia: evidence for the involvement of a calcium-independent phospholipase A_2.. Arch Gen Psychiatry 1997; 54: 487–494.

Rotrosen J, Wolkin A. Phospholipid and prostaglandin hypotheses of schizophrenia. In: Meltzer HY, ed. Psychopharmacology: the third generation of progress. New York: Raven Press, 1987: 759–764.

Ungerstedt U, Arbuthnott GW. Quantitative recording of rotational behavior in rats after 6-hydroxydopamine lesions of the nigrostriatal dopamine system. Brain Res 1970; 24: 485–493.

Weinberger DR. Implications of normal brain development for the pathogenesis of schizophrenia. Arch Gen Psychiatry 1987; 44: 660–669.

Williamson PC, Drost D, Stanley J, Carr T, Morrison S, Merskey H. Localized phosphorus-31 magnetic resonance spectroscopy in chronic schizophrenic patients and normal controls. Arch Gen Psychiatry 1991; 48: 578.

Zetterström T, Herrera-Marschitz M, Ungerstedt U. Simultaneous measurement of dopamine release and rotational behaviour in 6-hydroxydopamine denervated rats using intracerebral dialysis. Brain Res 1986; 376: 1–7.

^{31}P Magnetic Resonance Spectroscopy in the Assessment of Brain Phospholipid Metabolism in Schizophrenia

5

Peter C. Williamson and Dick J. Drost

INTRODUCTION

It has been proposed that phospholipid metabolism is altered in schizophrenic patients (Ryer and Rotrosen, 1989; Horrobin et al., 1994). Most, but not all, investigators have observed increased levels of phosphatidylserine and decreased levels of phosphatidylcholine and phosphatidylethanolamine, the main constituents of cell membranes, in the red blood cells, platelets or fibroblasts of schizophrenic patients (Stevens, 1972; Sengupta et al., 1981; Lautin et al., 1982; Hitzemann et al., 1984; Pangerl et al., 1991; Keshavan et al., 1993; Tolbert et al., 1993; Mahadik et al., 1994). Increased turnover of platelet phosphatidylinositol (Yao et al., 1992) and arachidonic acid (Demisch et al., 1987), as well as increased levels of serum phospholipase A$_2$, a phospholipid catabolizing enzyme, in schizophrenic patients suggest elevated phospholipid breakdown in schizophrenia (Gattaz et al., 1987, 1990; Ross et al., 1997). However, all of these studies have examined peripheral tissue which may not be relevant to brain membrane metabolism.

^{31}P magnetic resonance spectroscopy allows direct assessment of membrane phospholipid and high energy phosphate metabolism in localized regions of the brains of living schizophrenic patients (Pettegrew et al., 1995a; Williamson et al., 1995). The technique, its limitations, and findings resulting from its use in patients with schizophrenia and other neuropsychiatric disorders will be discussed in this chapter.

^{31}P MAGNETIC RESONANCE SPECTROSCOPY

Techniques

The phosphorus (^{31}P) nucleus is one of several that have been utilized in nuclear magnetic resonance (NMR) techniques for more than three decades in *in vitro* cellular physiology studies (Gorenstein, 1984; Cohen, 1987; Cady, 1990). However, investigators have been limited to small *in vitro* preparations of small animals by the small size of the magnet, this being due to both cost and technological constraints. With the advent of whole-body magnetic resonance imaging (MRI), and the recent availability of magnetic resonance spectroscopy (MRS) option packages for these imagers, *in vivo* human MRS has become a clinical research tool, though not yet a diagnostic test (Bottomley et al., 1988; Lenkinski, 1989; Cady, 1990).

A ^{31}P nucleus resonates at a frequency which is dependent on the molecular electron structure which shields the ^{31}P nucleus from the large static magnetic field. Therefore, different ^{31}P-containing molecules will resonate, or have peaks, at a unique frequency in a spectrum. The height or, more specifically, the peak area, will be proportional to the concentration for that molecule. Major signals in a ^{31}P brain spectrum are from adenosine triphosphate (ATP), phosphocreatine (PCr) and inorganic phosphorus (Pi), which reflect metabolic activity generally, and from phosphomonoesters (PME) and phosphodiesters (PDE) which reflect phospholipid synthesis and breakdown, respectively (Gadian and Radda, 1981; Pettegrew et al., 1986, 1987; Cady, 1990). The metabolism of these pathways is shown in Figure 5.1. Intracellular magnesium and pH can be calculated indirectly from the frequency separation between metabolite peaks (Gupta et al., 1984; Pettegrew et al., 1988a). These components are not currently quantifiable by other imaging techniques. However, the levels of free metabolites measured include both physiologically active and inactive molecules (Eastwood et al., 1985).

There are some inherent differences between ^{31}P-containing molecules and ^{1}H in water which add complexities to ^{31}P MRS compared to ^{1}H MRI. The magnetic resonance signal per nucleus from ^{31}P nuclei is one-fifteenth that of ^{1}H nuclei, and the concentration of ^{31}P metabolites is less than 10 mM, compared to

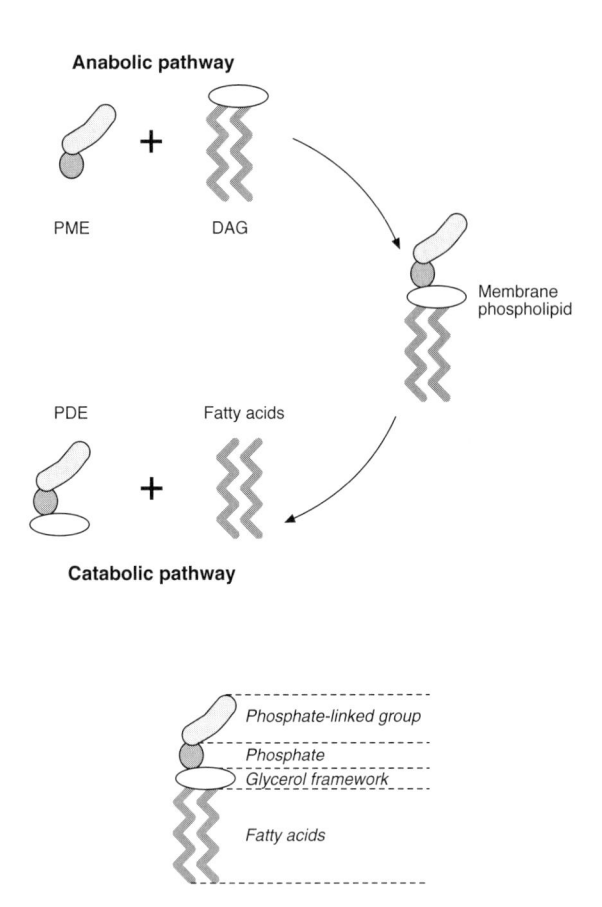

Figure 5.1. A simplified outline of the anabolic and catabolic pathways of membrane phospholipid metabolism. The phosphate-linked group may be choline, ethanolamine, serine, etc. Phosphocholine and phosphoethanolamine can be quantified with proton decoupled ^{31}P magnetic resonance spectroscopy, as seen in Figure 5.3. PME = phosphomonoesters; DAG = diacylglycerol; PDE = phosphodiesters.

55 M for water (^{1}H). The resulting lower signal:noise ratio limits the resolution for ^{31}P-MRS to approximately 10 cm^3 voxels, whereas for ^{1}H-magnetic resonance imaging it is approximately 1 mm^3 voxels. Since the signal:noise ratio is also linearly proportional to the static magnetic field strength, *in vivo* ^{31}P spectroscopy has been performed at a static field strength of 1.5 tesla (T), or greater, to even achieve this limited spatial resolution.

Also, since ^{31}P resonates at a different frequency from ^{1}H (25.7 MHz *versus* 63.6 MHz at 1.5 T), additional hardware, including rf coils, is required along with software for ^{31}P MRS. The rf coils (antennae which both excite the nuclei and receive the NMR signals) can range from linearly polarized surface coils to more complex circularly polarized (quadrature) volume coils, analogous to what is used for standard ^{1}H imaging. As in MR imaging, small surface coils will produce higher signal:noise ratios than volume coils at the cost of a more limited field of view. Usually, the rf MRS coils are doubly tuned, or switchable, between ^{31}P and ^{1}H, which allows the same rf coil both to image with ^{1}H for localization and to acquire the ^{31}P spectra, without having to change the coil and/or move the patient. In addition, the static magnetic field homogeneity can be improved *in vivo* by shimming on the ^{1}H signal, a critical step for optimum spectra quality. However, there are currently no doubly tuned ^{1}H/^{31}P quadrature head coils operating above 2 T, because rf design problems increase with higher frequencies and coil size.

Spatial localization in ^{31}P MRS can be performed with rf localization with surface coils and/or gradients with advantages and disadvantages for different techniques (Aue, 1986). Utilized techniques include single-pulse excitation with a surface coil for localization (Ackerman et al., 1980), rotating-frame methods (Garwood and Ugurbil, 1992), depth-resolved surface coil spectroscopy (DRESS) (Bottomley et al., 1984), stimulated echo acquisition mode (STEAM) localization techniques (Merboldt et al., 1990), image-selected *in vivo* spectroscopy (ISIS) (Ordidge et al., 1986), and fast rotating gradient spectroscopy (FROGS) (Sauter et al., 1987). Another technique, called chemical shift imaging (CSI), which has become standard on most manufacturers' software, allows the acquisition of spectroscopy data from several voxels within one slab at a time (2D-CSI) or several slabs concurrently (3D-CSI), encoding the spatial information with the magnetic field gradients employed in MRI (Brown et al., 1982; Hugg et al., 1992; Moonen et al., 1992; Lara et al., 1993). This technique is very similar to 3D volume imaging in MRI and has the advantage that the voxel grid can be shifted after acquiring the data, allowing one to centre a voxel over the desired region of interest, as shown in Figure 5.2. Spatial localization techniques can also be combined.

All these techniques can be combined with proton decoupling to provide very high resolution ^{31}P MR spectra (Bachert-Baumann et al., 1990; Potwarka et al., 1999a). With ^{1}H decoupling, the ^{1}H nuclei are continuously saturated with low rf power both before and during the ^{31}P signal readout. This increases both signal:noise ratio and spectral resolution for some ^{31}P molecules. However, this technique does require a second rf transmit channel, a feature not supplied by the MR manufacturer. Further, subject rf power deposition

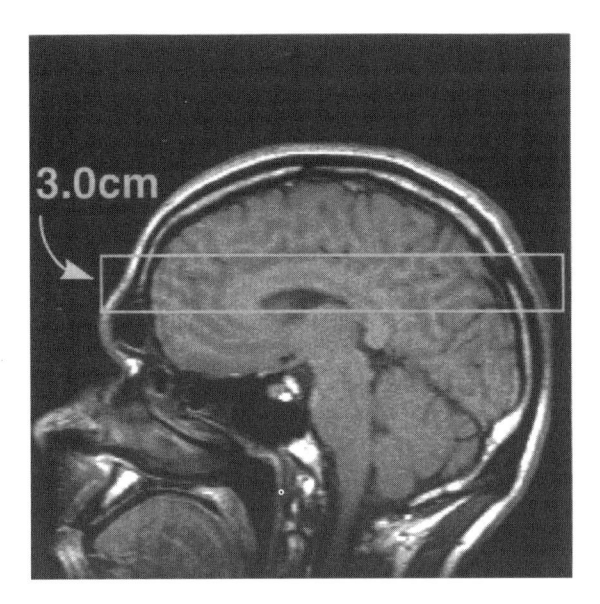

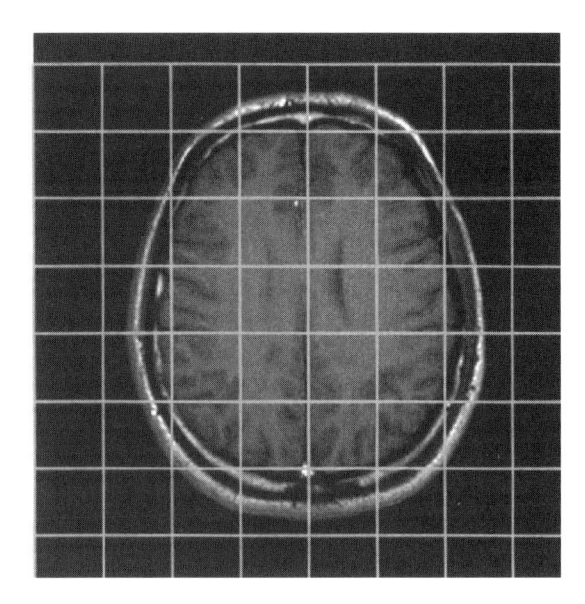

Figure 5.2. Sagittal and transverse ^{1}H MR images showing the location of the 2D CSI ^{31}P acquisition. The transverse ^{1}H image is centred on the 3 cm thick slab, and the overlying grid shows the locations of the 3 × 3 × 3 cm^3 CSI voxels. Note that the grid has been shifted approx 1 cm from anterior to posterior during postprocessing of the data to get ^{31}P spectra from the prefrontal region without contamination from the skull.

is a problem, and since rf power deposition increases as the square of the rf frequency, this will most likely limit ^{1}H decoupling in the brain to MR systems below 2 T. With decoupling, the main constituents of the PME peak, phosphocholine (PCh) and phosphoethanolamine (PEth), and the main constituents of the PDE peak, glycerol-3-phosphocholine (GPCh) and glycerol-3-phosphoethanolamine (GPEth), can be resolved (Pettegrew et al., 1986). Figure 5.3 shows a proton decoupled ^{31}P spectrum from a voxel in the parieto-occipital cortex. The data were acquired with 2D-CSI using a ^{31}P/^{1}H quadrature head coil (Murphy-Boesch et al., 1994) and a second rf transmit channel on a 1.5 T clinical MR system.

Limitations

A considerable amount of processing of spectra is required before quantitative information (peak areas) can be obtained. Even with the relatively small number of peaks seen in *in vivo* ^{31}P spectra, this can be a difficult process because of low signal:noise ratios and overlapping peaks. Most groups have used curve fitting with Lorentzian functions after the time domain signal has been zero filled, Fourier transformed, phased and baseline corrected. Another approach is to fit damped exponential functions to the complex time domain data, equivalent to fitting Lorentzian functions in the frequency domain since the two domains are related by the Fourier transform. With time domain fitting, a Fourier transform is not required, and hence there is no necessity for phasing or baseline correction, steps which can be subject to operator bias (Haselgrove et al., 1987). Regardless of the domain chosen, time or frequency, the low signal:noise ratio and broad peaks in *in vivo* spectroscopy require the incorporation of prior knowledge in the spectra model before fitting this model to the data. Lack of, or incorrect, prior knowledge will result in poor fits which, in turn, will lead to very high coefficients of variation (>100%) in the quantified spectra metabolites, making it difficult to detect differences in metabolite levels between patients and normals.

Differences in metabolite relaxation times, T1 and T2, can also result in apparent changes in metabolite levels when the repetition time is too short or the echo time is too long (Bottomley, 1991). In ^{31}P MRS, the echo time is usually nonexistent or very short, so T2 decay [exp(–TE/T2), with TE < 2 ms in this case] is not a problem. However, full T1 relaxation requires a repetition time (TR) of about 20 s, leading to an unrealistically long time (>1 h) for *in vivo* 2D-CSI acquisitions in the brain. *In vivo* repetition times are normally 0.5 s to several seconds and therefore changes in metabolite T1 relaxation between patients and normal controls can cause apparent differences in metabolite levels.

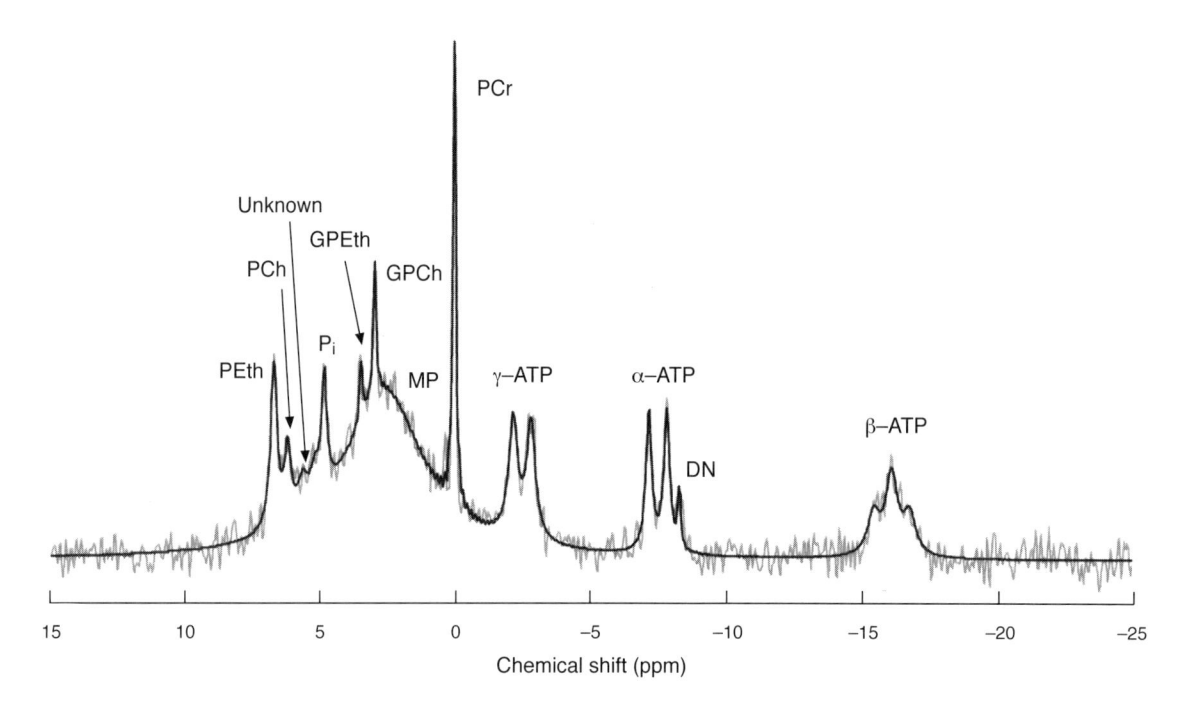

Figure 5.3. Proton decoupled ^{31}P spectrum from the parieto-occipital cortex. The fitted spectrum is shown in the frequency domain, although all data were fitted in the time domain. ATP = adenosine triphosphate; DN = dinucleotides; GPCh = glycerol-3-phosphocholine; GPEth = glycerol-3-phosphoethanolamine; MP = mobile phospholipid; PCh = phosphocholine; PCr = phosphocreatine; PEth = phosphoethanolamine; Pi = inorganic orthophosphate. PCh and PEth are phosphomonoesters (PME), while GPEth, GPCh, and MP are phosphodiesters (PDE).

Accurate spatial localization of *in vivo* spectra remains a problem. Any localization technique which combines frequency selective rf pulses with gradients (which includes most current spectroscopy techniques as well as ^{1}H imaging), has spatial misregistration due to the chemical shift artefact (Elster, 1994). For a typical rf select bandwidth of 4 kHz, the chemical shift between β-ATP and PME (590 Hz at 1.5 T) will cause the PME slice to be offset 15% from the β-ATP slice in the direction perpendicular to the slice. Since the typical *in vivo* ^{31}P slice thickness is 3 cm, this corresponds to a 0.5 cm offset between the 'PME slice' and the 'β-ATP slice.' Chemical shift increases proportionally with field strength and inversely with the rf selective gradient strength. A second problem specific to CSI techniques, which incorporate phase encoding, is the point spread function of each voxel in the slice plane due to the limited number of phase encode steps. This causes signal contamination from surrounding voxels into the selected voxel of interest, effectively making each voxel larger than illustrated by the grid in Figure 5.2 (Koch et al., 1993). This second effect contributes to the partial volume problem.

Because fairly large regions of interest are examined in ^{31}P spectroscopy, there could be differences between the proportions of grey and white matter in normals *versus* schizophrenics. Since levels of both PME and PDE tend to be higher by about 40% in white matter (Buchli et al., 1994), and CSF appears to contain almost no signal from ^{31}P metabolites (Hugg et al., 1992), differences in ^{31}P metabolites between normals and schizophrenics could arise from partial volume effects. This issue is discussed later in this chapter.

FINDINGS IN SCHIZOPHRENIC PATIENTS

Drug-naïve patients

The first ^{31}P magnetic phosphorus study was done by Pettegrew et al. (1991) (Table 5.1). In this pilot study, membrane phospholipid and high energy phosphate metabolism were studied in the dorsolateral prefrontal cortex utilizing a surface coil technique at 1.5 T. Eleven drug-naïve, first-episode schizophrenic patients were compared to ten healthy control volunteers of comparable age, education and parental education. The schizophrenic patients had significantly reduced levels

Table 5.1. ³¹P Magnetic resonance spectroscopy studies in schizophrenia.

Study	Subjects	Technique	Region	Findings
Pettegrew et al. (1991)	11 dn 10 c	SC	DPF	↓PME, ↑PDE ↓Pi, ↑ATP
Williamson et al. (1991)	10 m 7 c	FROGS + SC	LPF	↓PME, ↑PCr ↑Mg²⁺, ↑Pi
O'Callaghan et al. (1991)	1 um 17 m 10 c	SC	LTP	No significant differences
Calabrese et al. (1992)	2 um 9 m 9 c	ISIS	LRT	PCr/β-ATP higher on right
Fujimoto et al. (1992)	16 m 20 c	CSI	FP T BG	↓PCr on left ↑PDE, ↓ATP on left ↑PME on right ↓PDE both sides ↑β-ATP on right
Shiori et al. (1994)	6 um 20 m 26 c	DRESS + SC	F	↓PME in subjects high on –ve symptoms ($n = 12$) *versus* subjects low on –ve symptoms ($n = 14$)
Deicken et al. (1994)	6 um 14 m 16 c	CSI	F P	↑PDE, ↓PCr on right and left, ↓Pi on left No differences
Stanley et al. (1994)	19 m 18 c	FROGS + SC	LPF	↓PME in patient group ↑PDE in newly diagnosed ($n = 7$)
Kato et al. (1995a)	10 um 17 m 26 c	CSI	LRF	↓PME both sides, ↑β-ATP on left ↑PCr on left in patients high on –ve symptoms
Stanley et al. (1995)	11 dn 10 c	FROGS	LPF	↓PME, ↑PDE ↓Pi, ↑Mg²⁺
Volz et al. (1997)	13 m 14 c	ISIS	LRF	↓PDE
Potwarka et al. (1999b)	11 m 11 c	pd-CSI	PF	↓PCh, ↑PDE ↑MP, ↓Pi

Subject abbreviations: c = controls; dn = drug-naïve; m = medicated; um = unmedicated.

Technique abbreviations: CSI = chemical shift imaging; pd-CSI = proton decoupled chemical shift imaging; DRESS = depth-resolved surface coil spectroscopy; FROGS = fast-rotating gradient spectroscopy; ISIS = image selected *in vivo* spectroscopy; SC = surface coil.

Region abbreviations: BG = basal ganglia; DFP = dorsal prefrontal; F = frontal; FP = frontoparietal; LPF = left prefrontal; LTP = left temporoparietal; LRF = left and right frontal; LRT = left and right temporal; P = parietal; PF = prefrontal; T = temporal.

Findings abbreviations: ATP = adenosine triphosphate; Mg²⁺ = calculated intracellular magnesium; MP = mobile phospholipid; PCh = phosphocholine; PCr = phosphocreatine; PDE = phosphodiesters; Pi = inorganic orthophosphate; PME = phosphomonoesters; ↑ = increased; ↓ = reduced.

of PME and Pi, and significantly increased levels of PDE and ATP, compared to the controls. Levels of PCr and adenosine diphosphate did not differ between the two groups. The investigators suggested that the findings indicated hypoactivity of the dorsal prefrontal cortex, possibly caused by premature aging or exaggeration of neuronal pruning.

Pettegrew et al. (1991) argued that decreased levels of PMEs could be due to decreased kinase activity, decreased phospholipase C activity, decreased PDE phosphodiester activity, increased phosphatase activity, or increased chemical exchange with divalent cations leading to decreased NMR observability. The PDEs are products of phospholipase A_1 and A_2 activity and are converted to their respective PMEs by PDE phosphodiesterase activity. Thus, Pettegrew et al. (1991) suggested that increased PDEs could be accounted for by decreased PDE phosphodiesterase activity, in keeping with *in vitro* studies (Gattaz et al., 1987, 1990; Ross et al., 1997). Decreased chemical exchange with divalent cations could also account for this observation.

The only other study to examine exclusively drug-naïve patients was conducted by Stanley et al. (1995). In this study, 11 drug-naïve, eight newly diagnosed medicated, and ten chronic-medicated patients were compared with controls of similar sex, education, parental education and handedness. [31]P MR spectra were collected with a FROGS surface coil technique at 2.0 T from the left prefrontal region. Compared to controls, drug-naïve, newly diagnosed medicated and chronic-medicated patients had significantly decreased levels of PME. Significantly increased levels of PDE were seen in drug-naïve patients. There were no significant differences in the levels of high energy phosphate metabolites between groups, except for a significant decrease in Pi levels in newly diagnosed medicated patients. A significant increase in the calculated intracellular magnesium concentration was observed in drug-naïve, newly diagnosed medicated and chronic-medicated patients, compared to the controls.

The findings from both studies seemed to suggest that there was a decrease in PMEs and an increase in PDEs early on in illness. The findings could not be accounted for on the basis of neuroleptic medication since the subjects were drug-naïve. The effects of age, sex, education and parental education levels were also controlled for. However, both examined the prefrontal region with surface coil techniques. So far, no other study has utilized other imaging techniques or examined other parts of the brain in drug-naïve patients.

Chronic patients

A number of studies have examined the prefrontal region in chronic patients (Table 5.1). Williamson et al. (1991) studied ten chronic-medicated schizophrenics and seven controls of comparable age, sex and handedness. [31]P MR spectra were acquired from the left prefrontal region with a FROGS surface coil technique at 2.0 T. Schizophrenic patients had lower levels of PMEs than the controls, but there was no difference between the groups in terms of PDE levels. Levels of PCr and calculated intracellular magnesium were increased in patients compared to controls.

Stanley et al. (1994) used the same techniques to study a larger series of newly diagnosed medicated, and chronic-medicated patients. Decreased levels of PME were found in both groups of patients compared with controls, as in the earlier report. PDE levels did not differ between chronic-medicated patients and controls, but there was a significant increase in PDE levels in newly diagnosed medicated patients compared to controls.

Shioiri et al. (1994), using a DRESS surface coil technique at 1.5 T, found significantly decreased levels of PME in the prefrontal region of 12 schizophrenic patients who had high scores on negative symptoms, compared with 14 patients with low negative symptom scores. However, the relative signal intensities of phosphorus metabolites did not differ between the entire group of 26 schizophrenic patients and 26 age- and sex-matched control subjects. Subsequently, Kato et al. (1995a) used one-dimensional chemical shift imaging at 1.5 T to examine membrane phospholipid and high energy phosphate metabolism in the left and right frontal lobes of 27 unmedicated and medicated schizophrenic patients compared to 26 age-matched normal subjects. PMEs were found to be decreased bilaterally in the frontal lobes compared to the controls. Levels of β-ATP were increased in the left frontal lobe of schizophrenic patients compared to the controls. PCr levels were also observed to be increased in the left frontal lobe of schizophrenic patients with high ratings of negative symptoms. No differences were noted on PDE.

In contrast to these findings, two CSI studies (Fujimoto et al., 1992; Deicken et al., 1994) and one ISIS study (Volz et al., 1997) failed to reveal differences in PMEs in the prefrontal region. Deicken et al. (1994) observed an increase in PDE in frontal regions but Volz et al. (1997) observed a decrease in PDEs. It is possible that these different results were due to the differences in localization technique and region of interest which could alter the grey:white ratio. This is especially true when making a comparison with surface coil techniques which are biased towards signals from the brain surface, i.e., grey matter. Also, different methods of spectral quantification were used in these studies. This may have been a particular problem in the study of Volz et al. (1997), in which a convolution difference filter was applied to the time domain signal. Since this filter attenuates broad components of the frequency spectrum, such as PDE, it is possible that components which differ between groups were removed with this procedure.

Studies in the temporal and parietal regions have not been consistent. O'Callaghan et al. (1991) and Calabrese et al. (1992), using surface coil techniques at 1.5 T and 2.0 T, respectively, failed to observe any differences in PME or PDE between unmedicated and medicated schizophrenic patients compared with controls. However, Calabrese et al. (1992) did observe an increase in the PCr:β-ATP ratio on the right side. Negative findings were reported by Deicken et al. (1994) in the parietal region. The only positive finding in the temporal region has been the report of Fujimoto et al. (1992) of increased levels of PDE but not PME, along with a decreased level of ATP on the left side. These investigators also observed an increase in PME on the right side and a decrease in PDE on both sides in chronic-medicated patients compared to controls. No other studies have examined basal ganglia regions.

Thus, the results of studies of chronic patients have been far from consistent. While there are several reports of decreased levels of PME in the prefrontal region, there are also negative reports which may, in part, be accounted for by technical considerations. Similarly, levels of PDE have been found to be increased, and in some cases decreased, by various investigators. Findings in other regions appear to be negative or unreplicated at the present time.

Proton decoupled ^{31}P MRS

Potwarka et al. (1999b) have reported the only proton decoupled CSI study done to date in schizophrenic patients. Volumes (Figure 5.2) were examined in the prefrontal, motor and parieto-occipital regions of 11 chronic-medicated schizophrenic patients compared with 11 healthy controls of comparable age, handedness, sex, education and parental educational levels. The proton decoupled technique allowed the assessment of levels of PEth, PCh within the PME peak, and GPEth, GPCh and a mobile phospholipid (MP) within the PDE peak. This study also used an operator-independent time domain spectra quantification with no convolution difference or other filters applied (Potwarka et al., 1999a). Schizophrenic patients were found to have lower levels of PCh and increased levels of MP and PDE in the prefrontal but not other regions. Levels of Pi were also found to be lower in the schizophrenic patients than in the controls but no differences were observed on ATP or PCr.

These findings suggest that the increased PDE in schizophrenic patients may have arisen from the MP and not the GPEth or GPCh peaks as previously suspected. The majority of the MP peak can be attributed to the more mobile phospholipids than those found in the membrane layer. This MP signal originates from either vesicles or macromolecules containing phospholipids, such as proteolipids (Murphy et al., 1989; Kilby et al., 1991; McNamara et al., 1994). In keeping with this suggestion is a recent post-mortem study (Gabriel et al., 1997) which found higher concentrations of presynaptic proteins in the anterior cingulate cortex of schizophrenic subjects than in controls. Alternatively, an increase in the relative MP area in schizophrenic patients may be related to an increase in the proportion of myelin in the prefrontal cortex, as proteolipids are particularly abundant in myelin. An increased number of vertical axons has also been reported post-mortem in the prefrontal region of schizophrenic patients (Benes et al., 1987).

CORRELATIONS WITH SYMPTOMS

The strongest evidence of a connection between PME and negative symptoms comes from the study by Shioiri et al. (1994). In this study, subjects high on negative symptoms measured by the Brief Psychiatric Rating Scale (BPRS) (Overall and Gorham, 1962) were found to have low levels of PMEs compared to those subjects with low ratings of negative symptoms. However, no differences were noted on levels of PME within the entire group. Schizophrenic patients with high scores on the Scale for the Assessment of Negative Symptoms (SANS) (Andreasen, 1984a) were found by Kato et al. (1995a) to have high levels of PCr in the left frontal lobe. No significant differences in PME were found in this study between patients with low and high ratings of negative symptoms.

Diecken et al. (1994) found that right frontal PDE and right frontal PCr were highly correlated with scores on the hostility–suspiciousness and anxiety–depression subscales of the BPRS. The only other significant correlation between ^{31}P MRS parameters and symptom scores was reported by Calabrese et al. (1992) who found significant correlations between total BPRS scores and PCr:β-ATP ratio in both the left and right temporal lobes.

Three studies have reported no correlation between ^{31}P MRS parameters and symptomatology. Volz et al. (1997) found no correlation between either PME or PDE and BPRS, SANS, or Scale for Assessment of Positive Symptoms (SAPS) (Andreasen, 1984b) scores. Stanley et al. (1995) and Potwarka et al. (1999b) also reported no significant correlation between SANS or SAPS and PME or PDE. Some of these discrepancies might be explained by the different techniques used. The subject groups also varied from drug-naïve patients to chronic-medicated patients. Consequently, no consistent correlations have been established between ^{31}P MR metabolites and symptomatology.

PARTIAL VOLUME CONSIDERATIONS

Although it has been widely recognized that different proportions of grey and white matter can influence measures of ^{31}P MR metabolites, relatively few investigators have directly assessed this problem in their evaluation of schizophrenic patients. One exception is Hinsberger et al. (1997). ^{31}P MRS parameters and MRI volumetric data were collected in the left prefrontal region in ten patients with schizophrenia and ten healthy subjects of comparable age, handedness, sex, education and parental education levels. Amounts of grey and white matter were quantified anterior to the genu of the corpus callosum on both sides. PME decreased significantly with age but was not significantly correlated with left prefrontal grey matter in the schizophrenic patients, normals, or both groups combined. No other ^{31}P MR metabolite correlated with left anterior grey or white matter volumes. Although the volumetric measurements were not taken from exactly the same volume as the MRS measurements, these data indicate that ^{31}P MRS metabolite differences in schizophrenic patients are not likely to be related to differences in the proportion of grey and white matter volumes.

Potwarka et al. (1999b) further examined this issue. Assuming a grey:white matter ratio of 1.8–1.0, with a 7% reduction in grey matter reported in some schizophrenic patients (Zipursky et al., 1992) and a 40% greater PDE in cerebral white than in grey matter (Buchli et al., 1994), only 1.5% of the 13% increase in PDE could be accounted for by partial volume effects. In addition, the 4% deficit in the parieto-occipital grey matter in schizophrenics found by Zipursky et al. (1992) should correspond to increases in PDE, which were not observed in this region. Therefore, different proportions of grey or white matter in the subject groups are unlikely to explain the ^{31}P differences found in many studies.

SPECIFICITY OF FINDINGS

^{31}P MRS metabolites have been reported to be different in a number of other neuropsychiatric conditions. Williamson et al. (1996) reported lower levels of PME and a tendency to increased levels of PDE in a small series of patients suffering from psychotic depression. Patients with bipolar affective disorder have been reported to show increased levels of PME (Kato et al., 1994, 1995b). Patients in the manic state have fairly consistently been found to show increased levels of PME (Kato et al., 1991, 1993, 1994), while bipolar patients in the euthymic state have been found to have either normal (Kato et al., 1994) or decreased levels of PME (Kato et al., 1993).

Patients with panic disorder have not been found to show any abnormalities in PME or PDE levels (Shioiri et al., 1996). Autistic patients also have not been found to show any abnormalities in these metabolites, but a number of correlations were noted between both high energy phosphate and membrane phospholipid measures and neuropsychological test performance (Minshew et al., 1993).

There have been a number of reports of increased levels of PME in Alzheimer's disease (Pettegrew et al., 1988b, 1995b; Brown et al., 1989). In some cases, these changes seem to precede the onset of symptoms (Pettegrew et al., 1995b). However, other reports have failed to demonstrate differences from normal control groups (Murphy et al., 1993; Gonzalez et al., 1996).

While a number of differences have been reported in other neuropsychiatric disorders, the pattern of these differences appears to be much different than that in schizophrenia. In bipolar disorders, some patients with psychotic depression have been found to have decreased levels of PME, but other patients with bipolar depression have actually been found to have increased levels. Patients with manic symptoms have fairly consistently been found to have increased, rather than decreased, levels of PME. Findings in panic disorder, autism and Alzheimer's disease have not been consistent but, if anything, have suggested increased, rather than decreased, levels of PME in these conditions. Consequently, it appears that the pattern of decreased levels of PME and increased levels of PDE is specific to schizophrenia.

IMPLICATIONS FOR THE MEMBRANE HYPOTHESIS IN SCHIZOPHRENIA

^{31}P MRS offers a unique opportunity to examine membrane phospholipids in the brains of living schizophrenic patients rather than in peripheral tissues. In keeping with the studies done in red blood cells, platelets or fibroblasts, a number of membrane phospholipid abnormalities have been found.

The most consistent finding is that of lower levels of PME in drug-naïve patients (Pettegrew et al., 1991; Stanley et al., 1995). Findings in chronic patients have been less consistent; this is probably explained by the different acquisition or spectral quantification techniques used. The lower PME is entirely consistent with the observation of decreased levels of PCh and PEth in peripheral tissue in schizophrenic patients (Stevens, 1972; Sengupta et al., 1981; Lautin et al., 1982; Hitzemann et al., 1984; Pangerl et al., 1991; Keshavan et al., 1993; Tolbert et al., 1993; Mahadik et al., 1994).

Proton decoupled ^{31}P MRS studies are only in preliminary stages of development. Although the first study in this area (Potwarka et al., 1999b) has confirmed a decrease in PCh, the peripheral tissue studies would have also predicted a difference in PEth. Larger studies including drug-naïve patients will be necessary to evaluate this possibility.

Almost all replicated findings seem to be localized to the prefrontal region. This would not be expected if there were a generalized phospholipid metabolic abnormality. However, it is possible that early neurodevelopmental lesions to the ventral hippocampus (Lipska et al., 1992) or mediodorsal thalamus (Rajakumar et al., 1996), which would affect afferents to this region, could make prefrontal neurones more vulnerable to any underlying metabolic defect. Both of these lesions in animals lead to dopaminergic hyperresponsivity at maturity and make the animals more reactive to stress, which can also affect phospholipid metabolism.

Do ^{31}P MRS studies support increased turnover of membrane phospholipids? The finding of increased levels of PDE in drug-naïve patients and some chronic schizophrenic patients is in keeping with earlier observations of increased levels of serum phospholipase A$_2$ (Gattaz et al., 1987; 1990, Ross et al., 1997). However, Potwarka et al. (1999b) failed to demonstrate a difference in GPCh or CPEth in their proton decoupled study, which would be predicted by an increase in this phospholipid catabolizing enzyme. Rather, most of the difference in the PDE peak was attributed to the MP component of PDE. An increase in this component could be related to membrane phospholipid abnormalities in these patients involving proteolipids, or could reflect a higher density of vesicles. Further work is necessary to evaluate these possibilities.

In summary, ^{31}P MRS studies have confirmed a number of abnormalities seen in studies of peripheral tissue in these patients. The most consistent of these has been a decrease in PME likely to be related to PCh and an increase in PDE likely to be related to MP. These findings appear to be specific to schizophrenia and to be localized to the prefrontal region, but do not appear to be correlated with particular symptoms.

REFERENCES

Ackerman JJ, Grove TH, Wong GG, Gadian GG, Radda GK. Mapping of metabolites in whole animals by P-31 NMR using surface coils. Nature 1980; 283; 167–170.

Andreasen NC. Scale for the assessment of negative symptoms (SANS). Iowa City, Iowa: University of Iowa, 1984a.

Andreasen NC. Scale for the assessment of positive symptoms (SAPS). Iowa City, Iowa: University of Iowa, 1984b.

Aue WP. Localization methods for *in vivo* nuclear magnetic resonance spectroscopy. Rev Magn Reson Med 1986; 1: 21–72.

Bachert-Baumann P, Ermark F, Zabel H-J, Sauter R, Semmler W, Lorenz WJ. In vivo nuclear overhauser effects in ^{31}P-[^{1}H] double-resonance experiments in a 1.5-T whole-body MR system. Magn Reson Med 1990; 15: 165–172.

Benes FM, Majocha R, Bird ED, Marotta CA. Increased vertical axon numbers in cingulate cortex of schizophrenics. Arch Gen Psychiatry 1987; 44: 1017–1021.

Bottomley PA. The trouble with spectroscopy papers. Radiology 1991; 181: 344–530.

Bottomley PA, Foster TB, Darrow RD. Depth-resolved surface-coil spectroscopy (DRESS) for *in vivo* 1H, ^{31}P and ^{13}C NMR. J Magn Reson 1984; 59: 338–342.

Bottomley PA, Charles HC, Roemer PB et al. Human *in vivo* phosphate metabolite imaging with ^{31}P NMR. Magn Reson Med 1988; 7: 319–336.

Brown GG, Levine SR, Gorell JM et al. *In vivo* ^{31}P NMR profiles of Alzheimer's disease and multiple subcortical infarct dementia. Neurology 1989; 39: 1423–1426.

Brown TR, Kincaid BM, Ugurbil K. NMR chemical shift imaging in three dimensions. Proc Natl Acad Sci USA 1982; 79: 3523–3526.

Buchli R, Duc CO, Martin E, Boesizer P. Assessment of absolute metabolite concentrations in human tissue by ^{31}P MRS *in vivo*. Part 1: cerebrum, cerebellum, cerebral grey and white matter. Magn Reson Med 1994; 32: 447–452.

Cady EB. Clinical magnetic resonance spectroscopy. New York, NY: Plenum, 1990.

Calabrese G, Deicken RF, Fein G, Merrin EL, Schoenfeld F, Weiner MW. ^{31}Phosphorus magnetic resonance spectroscopy of the temporal lobes in schizophrenia. Biol Psychiatry 1992; 32: 26–32.

Cohen SM. Physiological NMR spectroscopy: from isolated cells to man. Ann N Y Acad Sci 1987; 508: 1–537.

Deicken RF, Calabrese G, Merrin EL et al. ^{31}Phosphorus magnetic resonance spectroscopy of the frontal and parietal lobes in chronic schizophrenia. Biol Psychiatry 1994; 36: 503–510.

Demisch L, Gerbaldo H, Gebhart P, Georgi K, Bochnik HJ. Incorporation of ^{14}C-arachidonic acid into platelet phospholipids of untreated patients with schizophreniform or schizophrenic disorders. Psychiatry Res 1987; 22: 275–282.

Eastwood LM, Hutchinson JMS, Besson JAO. Nuclear magnetic resonance (NMR): imaging biochemical change. Br J Psychiatry 1985; 146: 26–31.

Elster DE. Questions and answers in magnetic resonance imaging. St Louis: Mosby, 1994.

Fujimoto T, Nakano T, Takano T, Hokazono Y, Asakura T, Tsuji T. Study of chronic schizophrenics using ^{31}P magnetic resonance chemical shift imaging. Acta Psychiatr Scand 1992; 86: 455–462.

Gabriel SM, Haroutunian V, Powchik P et al. Increased concentrations of presynaptic proteins in the cingulate cortex of subjects with schizophrenia. Arch Gen Psychiatry 1997; 54: 559–566.

Gadian DG, Radda GK. NMR studies of tissue metabolism. Ann Rev Biochem 1981; 50: 69–83.

Garwood M, Ugurbil K. B_1 insensitive adiabatic RF pulses. In: Diehl P, Fluck E, Günther H, Kosfeld R, Seelig J, eds. NMR: basic principles and progress. New York: Springer-Verlag, 1992; 26: 109–147.

Gattaz WF, Köllisch M, Thuren T, Virtanen JA, Kinnunen PKJ. Increased plasma phospholipase-A_2 activity in schizophrenic patients: reduction after neuroleptic therapy. Biol Psychiatry 1987; 22: 421–426.

Gattaz WF, Hübner CK, Nevalainen TJ, Thuren T, Kinnunen PKJ. Increased serum phospholipase-A_2 activity in schizophrenia: a replication study. Biol Psychiatry 1990; 28: 495–501.

González RG, Guimaraes AR, Moore GJ, Crawley A, Cupples LA, Growden JH. Quantitative in vivo ^{31}P magnetic resonance spectroscopy of Alzheimer's disease. Alzheimer Dis Assoc Disord 1996; 10: 46–52.

Gorenstein DG. Phosphorus-31 NMR: principals and applications. Orlando: Academic Press, 1984.

Gupta RK, Gupta P, Moore RD. NMR studies of intracellular metal ions in intact cells and tissues. Ann Rev Biophys Bioeng 1984; 13: 221–246.

Haselgrove JC, Subramanian VH, Christen R, Leigh JS. Analysis of in vivo NMR spectra. Rev Magn Reson Med 1987; 2: 167–222.

Hinsberger AD, Williamson PC, Carr TJ et al. Magnetic resonance imaging volumetric and phosphorus 31 magnetic resonance spectroscopy measurements in schizophrenia. J Psychiatry Neurosci 1997; 22: 111–117.

Hitzemann R, Hirschowitz J, Garver D. Membrane abnormalities in the psychoses and affective disorders. J Psychiatr Res 1984; 18: 319–326.

Horrobin DF, Glen AIM, Vaddadi K. The membrane hypothesis of schizophrenia. Schizophr Res 1994; 13: 195–207.

Hugg JW, Matson GB, Twieg DB, Maudsley AA, Sappey-Marinier D, Weiner MW. Phosphorus-31 MR spectroscopic imaging (MRSI) of normal and pathological brains. Magn Reson Imaging 1992; 10: 227–243.

Kato T, Shioiri T, Takahashi S, Inubushi T. Measurement of brain phosphoinositide metabolism in bipolar patients using in vivo ^{31}P-MRS. J Affective Disord 1991; 22: 185–190.

Kato T, Takaihashi S, Shioiri T, Inubushi T. Alterations in brain phosphorus metabolism in bipolar disorder detected by in vivo ^{31}P and ^{7}Li magnetic resonance spectroscopy. J Affective Disord 1993; 27: 53–60.

Kato T, Takaihashi S, Shioiri T, Murashita J, Hamakawa H, Inubushi T. Reduction of brain phosphocreatine in bipolar II disorder detected by phosphorus-31 magnetic resonance spectroscopy. J Affective Disord 1994; 31: 125–133.

Kato T, Shioiri T, Murashita j, Hamakawa H, Inubushi T, Takahashi S. Lateralized abnormality of high-energy phosphate and bilateral reduction of phosphomonoester measured by phosphorus-31 magnetic resonance spectroscopy of the frontal lobes in schizophrenia. Psychiatry Res Neuroimaging 1995a; 61: 151–160.

Kato T, Shioiri T, Murashita J et al. Lateralized abnormality of high energy phosphate metabolism in the frontal lobes of patients with bipolar disorder detected by phase-encoded ^{31}P-MRS. Psychol Med 1995b; 25: 557–566.

Keshavan MS, Mallinger AG, Pettegrew JW, Dippold C. Erythrocyte membrane phospholipids in psychotic patients. Psychiatry Res 1993; 49: 89–95.

Kilby PM, Bolas NM, Radda GK. ^{31}P-NMR study of brain phospholipid structures in vivo. Biochim Biophys Acta 1991; 1085: 257–264.

Koch T, Brix G, Lorenz W. Theoretical description, measurement and correction of localisation errors in ^{31}P chemical shift imaging. J Magn Reson Ser B 1993; 104: 199–211.

Lara RS, Matson GB, Hugg JW, Maudsley AA, Weiner MW. Quantitation of in vivo phosphorus metabolites in human brain with magnetic resonance spectroscopic imaging (MRSI). Magn Reson Imaging 1993; 11: 273–278.

Lautin A, Mandio CD, Segarnick DJ, Wod L, Mason MF, Rotrosen J. Red cell phospholipids in schizophrenia. Life Sci 1982; 31: 3051–3056.

Lenkinski RE. Clinical magnetic resonance spectroscopy: a critical evaluation. Invest Radiol 1989; 24: 1034–1038.

Lipska BK, Jaskiw GE, Chrapasta S, Karoum F, Weinberger DR. Ibotenic acid lesion of the ventral hippocampus differentially affects dopamine and its metabolites in the nucleus accumbens in prefrontal cortex. Brain Res 1992; 585: 1–6.

Mahadik SP, Mukherjee S, Correnti EE et al. Plasma membrane phospholipid and cholesterol distribution of skin fibroblasts from drug-naïve patients at the onset of psychosis. Schizophr Res 1994; 13: 239–247.

McNamara R, Arias-Mendoza F, Brown TR. Investigation of broad resonances in ^{31}P NMR spectra of the human brain in vivo. NMR Biomed 1994; 7: 237–242.

Merboldt KD, Chien D, Hanicke W, Gyngell ML, Bruhn H, Frahm J. Localized ^{31}P NMR spectroscopy of the adult human brain in vivo using stimulated-echo (STEAM) sequences. Magn Reson Med 1990; 89: 343–361.

Minshew NJ, Goldstein G, Dombrowski SM, Panchalingam K, Pettegrew J. A preliminary ^{31}P MRS study of autism: evidence for undersynthesis and increased degradation of brain membranes. Biol Psychiatry 1993; 33: 762–773.

Moonen CTW, Sobering G, van Zijl PCM, Gillen J, von Kienlin M, Bizzi A. Proton spectroscopic imaging of human brain. J Magn Reson 1992; 98: 556–575.

Murphy DGM, Bottomley PA, Salerno JA et al. An in vivo study of phosphorus and glucose metabolism in Alzheimer's disease using magnetic resonance spectroscopy and PET. Arch Gen Psychiatry 1993; 50: 341–349.

Murphy EJ, Rajagopalan B, Brindle KM, Radda K. Phospholipid bilayer contribution to ^{31}P NMR spectra *in vivo*. Magn Reson Med 1989; 12: 282–289.

Murphy-Boesch J, Srinivasan R, Carvagal L, Brown T. Two configurations of the four-ring birdcage coil for ^{1}H imaging and ^{1}H decoupled ^{31}P spectroscopy of the human head. J Magn Reson Ser B 1994; 103: 103–114.

O'Callaghan E, Redmond O, Ennis R et al. Initial investigation of the left temporoparietal region in schizophrenia by ^{31}P magnetic resonance spectroscopy. Biol Psychiatry 1991; 29: 1149–1152.

Ordidge RJ, Connelly A, Lohman JAB. Image-selected *in vivo* spectroscopy (ISIS): a new technique for spatially selective NMR spectroscopy. J Magn Reson 1986; 66: 283–294.

Overall JE, Gorham DR. The brief psychiatric rating scale. Psychol Rep 1962; 10: 799–812.

Pangerl AM, Steudle A, Jaroni HW, Rüfer R, Gattaz WF. Increased platelet membrane lysophosphatidylcholine in schizophrenia. Biol Psychiatry 1991; 30: 837–840.

Pettegrew JW, Kopp SJ, Dadok J et al. Chemical characterization of a prominent phosphomonoester resonance from mammalian brain. ^{31}P and ^{1}H NMR analysis at 4.7 and 14.1 Tesla. J Magn Reson 1986; 67: 443–450.

Pettegrew JW, Withers G, Panchalingam K, Post JFM. ^{31}P nuclear magnetic resonance (NMR) spectroscopy of brain in aging and Alzheimer's disease. J Neural Transm Suppl 1987; 24: 261–268.

Pettegrew JW, Withers G, Panchalingam K, Post JF. Considerations for brain pH assessment by ^{31}P NMR. Magn Reson Imaging 1988a; 6: 135–142.

Pettegrew JW, Moossy J, Withers G, McKeag D, Panchalingam K. ^{31}P nuclear magnetic resonance study of the brain in Alzheimer's disease. J Neuropathol Exp Neurol 1988b; 47: 235–248.

Pettegrew JW, Keshavan MS, Panchalingam K et al. Alterations in brain high-energy phosphate and membrane phospholipid metabolism in first-episode drug-naïve schizophrenics. A pilot study of the dorsal prefrontal cortex by *in vivo* phosphorus-31 nuclear magnetic resonance spectroscopy. Arch Gen Psychiatry 1991; 48: 563–568.

Pettegrew JW, Keshavan MS, Minshew NJ, McClure RJ. ^{31}P-MRS of metabolic alterations in schizophrenia and neurodevelopment. In: Nasrallah HA, Pettegrew JA, eds. NMR spectroscopy in psychiatric brain disorders. Washington, DC: American Psychiatric Press, 1995a: 45–77.

Pettegrew JW, Klunk WE, Kanal E, Panchalingam K, McClure RJ. Changes in brain membrane phospholipid and high-energy phosphate metabolism precede dementia. Neurobiol Aging 1995b; 6: 973–975.

Potwarka JJ, Drost DJ, Williamson PC. Quantifying ^{1}H decoupled *in vivo* ^{31}P brain spectra. Nucl Magn Reson Biomed 1999a; 12: 8–14.

Potwarka JJ, Drost DJ, Williamson PC. A ^{1}H-decoupled ^{31}P chemical shift imaging study with of medicated schizophrenic patients and healthy controls. Biol Psychiatry, 1999b; 45: 687–693.

Rajakumar N, Williamson P, Stoessl J, Flumerfelt B. Neurodevelopmental pathogenesis of schizophrenia. Proc Soc Neurosci Mtg, Washington, DC, USA, 1996; 2: 1187.

Ross BM, Hudson C, Erlich J, Warsh JJ, Kish SJ. Increased phospholipid breakdown in schizophrenia: evidence for the involvement of a calcium-independent phospholipase A_2. Arch Gen Psychiatry 1997; 54: 487–494.

Ryer H, Rotrosen J. Phospholipids and schizophrenia. In: Bazan NG, Horrocks LA, Toffano G, eds. Phospholipids in the nervous system: biochemical and molecular pathology. Padova: Liviana Press, 1989: 177–182.

Sauter R, Mueller S, Weber H. Localization *in vivo* ^{31}P NMR spectroscopy by combining surface coils and slice selective saturation. J Magn Reson 1987; 75: 167–173.

Sengupta N, Datta SC, Sengupta D. Platelet and erythrocyte membrane lipid and phospholipid patterns in different types of mental patients. Biochem Med 1981; 25: 267–275.

Shioiri T, Kato T, Inubushi T, Murashita J, Takahashi S. Correlations of phosphomonoesters measured by phosphorus-31 magnetic resonance spectroscopy in the frontal lobes and negative symptoms in schizophrenia. Psychiatry Res 1994; 55: 223–235.

Shioiri T, Kato T, Murashita J, Hamakawa H, Inubushi T, Takahashi S. High-energy phosphate metabolism in the frontal lobes of patients with panic disorder detected by phase-encoded ^{31}P-MRS. Biol Psychiatry 1996; 40: 785–793.

Stanley JA, Williamson PC, Drost DJ et al. Membrane phospholipid metabolism and schizophrenia: an *in vivo* ^{31}P-MR spectroscopy study. Schizophr Res 1994; 13: 209–215.

Stanley JA, Williamson PC, Drost DJ et al. An *in vivo* study of the prefrontal cortex of schizophrenic patients at different stages of illness *via* phosphorus magnetic resonance spectroscopy. Arch Gen Psychiatry 1995; 52: 399–406.

Stevens JD. The distribution of phospholipid fractions in the red cell membranes of schizophrenics. Schizophr Bull 1972; 6: 60–61.

Tolbert LC, Monti JA, O'Shields H, Walter-Ryan W, Meadows D, Smythies JR. Defects in transmethylation and membrane lipids in schizophrenia. Psychopharmacol Bull 1993; 19: 594–599.

Volz H-P, Rzanny R, May S et al. ^{31}P magnetic resonance spectroscopy in the dorsolateral prefrontal cortex of schizophrenics with a volume selective technique – preliminary findings. Biol Psychiatry 1997; 441: 644–648.

Williamson PC, Drost D, Stanley J, Carr T, Morrison S, Merskey H. Localized phosphorus-31 magnetic resonance spectroscopy in chronic schizophrenic patients and normal controls. Arch Gen Psychiatry 1991; 48: 578.

Williamson PC, Drost DJ, Stanley JA, Carr TJ. ^{31}P-MRS in the study of schizophrenia. In: Nasrallah HA, Pettegrew JA, eds. NMR spectroscopy in psychiatric brain disorders. Washington: American Psychiatric Press, 1995; 107–129.

Williamson PC, Brauer M, Leonard S, Thompson T, Drost D. ^{31}P magnetic resonance spectroscopy studies in schizophrenia. Prostagland Leukotr Essent Fatty Acids 1996; 55: 115–118.

Yao JK, Yasaei P, van Kammen DP. Increased turnover of platelet phosphatidylinositol in schizophrenia. Prostagland Leukotr Essent Fatty Acids 1992; 46: 39–46.

Zipursky RB, Lim KO, Sullivan EV, Brown BW, Pfefferbaum A. Widespread cerebral gray matter volume deficits in schizophrenia. Arch Gen Psychiatry 1992; 49: 195–205.

Red Blood Cell and Platelet Fatty Acid Metabolism in Schizophrenia

Jeffrey K. Yao

INTRODUCTION

A multiplicity of pathophysiological theories for schizophrenia have been proposed over the years, including alterations in central neurotransmitter systems, neuropeptides, viral infections, autoimmune dysfunctions, abnormal synthesis of prostaglandins, and many others. The dopamine hypothesis remains the most widely studied conceptualization. None of the above hypotheses can, however, fully explain the aetiology and manifold manifestations of schizophrenia, perhaps due to the aetiopathogenetic heterogeneity of the condition (Meltzer, 1987). Furthermore, a recent comprehensive review of neurochemical and neuroendocrine studies of schizophrenia found an extensive but fragmentary body of data which provide neither consistent nor conclusive evidence for any specific aetiopathophysiological theory (Lieberman and Koreen, 1993).

A point of convergence for many theoretical models occurs at the level of the neuronal membrane, which is the site of neurotransmitter receptors, ion channels, signal transduction, and drug effects. Membrane damage, specifically free radical-mediated, can significantly alter a broad range of membrane functions. A putative role for free radicals in some domains of schizophrenic pathophysiology has thus been proposed (Cadet and Lohr, 1987; Lohr, 1991; Cadet and Kahler, 1994; Mahadik and Mukherjee, 1996; Reddy and Yao, 1996). Membrane dysfunction can be secondary to free radical-mediated pathology, and may contribute to specific aspects of schizophrenic symptomatology and complications of its treatment. Specifically, free radical-mediated abnormalities may contribute to the development of a number of clinically significant consequences, including prominent negative symptoms, tardive dyskinesia, neurological 'soft' signs, and Parkinsonian symptoms. Our previous results showing altered membrane dynamics and antioxidant defense system in schizophrenia, and findings from other investigators, are consistent with the notion of membrane defects and free radical pathology in schizophrenia. This chapter will focus upon recent findings of structural and metabolic defects of fatty acids in red blood cell (RBC) and platelet membranes of schizophrenic patients.

POLYUNSATURATED FATTY ACID (PUFA) DEFECTS IN RBC MEMBRANES

Earlier findings of diverse abnormalities

Although fatty acid abnormalities were noted in patients with schizophrenia and other psychiatric disorders more than 20 years ago, there are very few published and consistent reports. Ellis and Sanders (1977) first reported an increase of eicosapentaenoic acid (20:5n-3) and docosahexaenoic acid (22:6n-3), but not of dihomo-γ-linolenic acid (20:3n-6) and arachidonic acid (20:4n-6) (AA), in plasma phosphatidylcholine (PC) of patients with endogenous depression. Obi and Nwanze (1979) later found a significant increase of linolenic acid (18:3n-3), in both plasma and RBC of schizophrenic patients. Hitzemann and Garver (1982) also showed, in PC of RBC ghost membranes from patients with schizophrenia or schizophreniform disorder, that a significant decrease of the linoleic acid (18:2n-6), associated with an increase of 20:4n-6, was found only in patients with a normal intra/extra cellular Li^+ ratio ($n = 9$) and not in those patients with a high Li^+ ratio ($n = 7$). Their results may explain an abnormal synthesis of prostaglandin (PG), i.e., decreased PGE_1 in platelets (Abdulla and Hamadah, 1975) and increased PGE_2 in cerebrospinal fluid (Horrobin, 1980; Mathé et al., 1980). However, Vaddadi et al. (1989) have demonstrated significantly lower levels of both 18:2n-6 and 20:4n-6 in schizophrenics than in controls. On the other hand, Rudin (1981) hypothesized that schizophrenia may be related to a deficiency of the metabolites of the linolenic acid series. The above studies were carried out many years ago using patients with neuroleptic treatment as well as methods with insufficient resolution of fatty acid separation. With today's advancements in gas chromatography, i.e., capillary column, there is obviously a need for re-evaluation of fatty acid composition in psychotic disorders under rigid experimental and clinical conditions.

Recent findings in abnormal n-6 PUFA pathway

Using a within subject, repeated measures, on-off-on antipsychotic drug treatment design, we have systematically compared RBC fatty acid concentrations of schizophrenic patients to those of age- and sex-matched normal control subjects (Yao et al., 1994b). The concentrations (nmol/ml packed RBC) of polyenoic acids including 18:2n-6, 20:4n-6, and 22:6n-3 were significantly lower in both haloperidol-treated (HT) and drug-free (DF) patients than in normal control subjects (Table 6.1). Similarly, the mean percentages of 18:2n-6 and 20:4n-6 to total fatty acids were also significantly lower in both HT and DF patients than in normal control subjects. Concomitantly, a significant decrease in total polyenoic fatty acids was associated with significant increases in both saturated and monoenoic fatty acids. The resultant fatty acid profile consequently lowers the fatty acid unsaturation index, which represents the average number of double bonds per fatty acid molecule, of RBC ghost membranes in schizophrenic patients (Table 6.1). No significant differences in RBC fatty acid composition were demonstrated in patients on- and off-haloperidol treatment. Our findings are in accordance with those data reported by Vaddadi et al. (1989) and by Peet et al. (1994, 1995).

A similar decrease of n-6 PUFAs was also found in plasma (Horrobin et al., 1989). They found a significant reduction of both 18:2n-6 and 20:4n-6, associated with an increase of total n-3 fatty acids, in three schizophrenic patient groups from England ($n = 45$), Scotland ($n = 19$) and Ireland ($n = 20$), respectively. Their findings were later replicated in plasma total phospholipids of schizophrenic patients ($n = 59$) from Japan (Kaiya et al., 1991), although no significant decrease of 20:4n-6 was demonstrated in the Japanese patient group. In analysis of autopsied brain tissues ($n = 7$), Horrobin et al. (1991) have further shown a decrease of 18:2n-6 and 20:4n-6 in phosphatidylethanolamine (PE) of the frontal cortex from schizophrenic patients. Recently, we have also found a significant reduction of 20:4n-6 in PE of postmortem caudate from schizophrenic patients relative to normal and psychiatric controls (Yao et al., unpublished data). Therefore, decreased levels of 18:2n-6 and 20:4n-6 in schizophrenic patients appear to be a general consensus from the above studies.

Possible metabolic blocks during fatty acid desaturation and elongation

The ratio of 20:4n-6/18:2n-6 provides a biochemical index of the product-substrate relationship in the n-6 polyenoic pathology. The n-6 pathway consists of a series of desaturations (Δ6, Δ5, and Δ4 reactions) and elongations (Figure 6.1). In normal RBC membranes, the levels of 18:3n-6 and 22:5n-6 are minute. 20:4n-6 is the major metabolic product of 18:2n-6. Recently, we have demonstrated a decreased ratio of 20:4n-6/20:3n-6 associated with a normal ratio of 22:4n-6/20:4n-6 in schizophrenic patients, suggesting a defect in the Δ5 desaturation (Yao et al., 1994a) (Table 6.2).

On the other hand, 22:6n-3 and 22:5n-6 are formed by a final desaturation at Δ4 (Figure 6.1). These reactions follow elongations and Δ5 desaturations in both n-3 and n-6 series. The ratio of 22:6n-3/22:5n-3 was not significantly different between schizophrenic patients and normal control subjects (Table 6.2). Therefore, decreases in 22:5n-3 and 22:6n-3 may be caused, at least in part, by the diminished formation of 20:5n-3, which is derived from 20:4n-3 by the Δ5 reaction.

The increase in products of Δ9 desaturase, as indicated by the ratio of 24:1n-9/18:0 and 18:1n-9/18:0 (Table 6.2), may be a compensatory increase in endogenously synthesized monounsaturated fatty acids. These increases partially substitute for the n-6 and n-3 PUFA normally present. Despite the increase in Δ9 products,

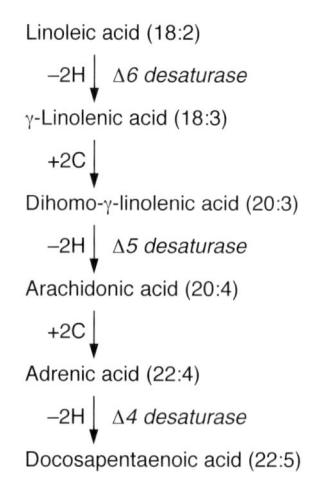

Linoleic acid (18:2)
−2H ↓ Δ6 desaturase
γ-Linolenic acid (18:3)
+2C ↓
Dihomo-γ-linolenic acid (20:3)
−2H ↓ Δ5 desaturase
Arachidonic acid (20:4)
+2C ↓
Adrenic acid (22:4)
−2H ↓ Δ4 desaturase
Docosapentaenoic acid (22:5)

Figure 6.1. Metabolic pathway of the n-6 family of polyunsaturated fatty acids.

Table 6.1. Levels of polyunsaturated fatty acids (PUFAs) in red blood cells of schizophrenic patients, either under treatment with haloperidol ($n = 24$) or drug-free for less than ($n = 19$) or more than ($n = 10$) 5 weeks, compared with normal control subjects ($n = 22$). Also shown are values for the unsaturation index for each group. Means ± SD. Data from Yao et al. (1994b).

		Schizophrenics		
		Haloperidol-	Drug-free	
PUFAs	Normals	treated	<5 weeks	>5 weeks
Levels of PUFAs (nmol/ml packed red blood cells)				
18:2n-6	218 ± 69	167 ± 77*	164 ± 93*	165 ± 42*
20:3n-6	33 ± 16	25 ± 12	26 ± 17	26 ± 11
20:4n-6	301 ± 125	190 ± 97*	208 ± 135*	216 ± 87*
22:4n-6	70 ± 35	46 ± 25*	51 ± 31	56 ± 23
22:5n-3	36 ± 17	21 ± 11*	29 ± 20	28 ± 13
22:6n-3	58 ± 33	32 ± 19*	39 ± 27*	47 ± 29
Total[a]	733 ± 282	493 ± 231*	535 ± 324*	557 ± 190*
Unsaturation index[b] (%)	41 ± 4	33 ± 6*	36 ± 8*	35 ± 8*

[a]The total is greater than the sum of listed fatty acids in each case, because some small amounts of PUFAs were omitted from the final tabulation; [b]unsaturation index is the average number of double bonds per fatty acid molecule. *In comparison with the corresponding value for control subjects, $p < 0.05$.

Table 6.2. Comparison of fatty acid elongation and desaturation in red blood cells of schizophrenic patients, either under treatment with haloperidol ($n = 24$) or drug-free for less than ($n = 19$) or more than ($n = 10$) 5 weeks, compared with normal control subjects ($n = 22$). Means ± SD. Data from Yao et al. (1994b).

		Schizophrenics		
		Haloperidol-	Drug-free	
PUFAs	Normals	treated	<5 weeks	>5 weeks
n family				
18:0/16:0	0.79 ± 0.07	0.67 ± 0.13*	0.71 ± 0.10*	0.68 ± 0.13*
24:0/22:0	2.08 ± 0.35	2.09 ± 0.31	2.07 ± 0.25	2.26 ± 0.35
n-3 family				
22:6/22:5	1.60 ± 0.60	1.53 ± 0.42	1.47 ± 0.77	1.60 ± 0.82
n-6 family				
20:4/18:2	1.36 ± 0.29	1.16 ± 0.30*	1.24 ± 0.35	1.28 ± 0.37
20:4/20:3	9.48 ± 2.21	7.81 ± 2.08*	8.05 ± 2.46	8.04 ± 1.86
22:4/20:4	0.23 ± 0.04	0.24 ± 0.03	0.25 ± 0.03	0.26 ± 0.03*
n-9 family				
24:1/18:0	0.20 ± 0.07	0.25 ± 0.10*	0.26 ± 0.06*	0.25 ± 0.08
18:1/18:0	0.95 ± 0.13	1.07 ± 0.23*	1.03 ± 0.08*	0.95 ± 0.13

*In comparison with the corresponding value for control subjects, $p < 0.05$ (Student's two-tailed t test).

the total degree of unsaturation of the RBC fatty acids decreased significantly (Table 6.1), suggesting that RBC membranes are less unsaturated in schizophrenic patients, than in normal controls.

As indicated by the ratio of 18:0/16:0, but not 24:0/22:0 (Table 6.2), the product of chain elongation was also significantly less in both HT and DF patients than in the normal control subjects. This decrease, however, could be partially due to an increased turnover of 18:0 through the desaturase reaction.

Effect of PUFA alterations on membrane dynamics

Biological membranes are highly dynamic structures composed predominately of lipids and proteins. The dynamic state, or 'fluidity', of the cell membrane is dependent upon its composition and, in the intact cell, is also influenced by motion imposed by the cytoskeleton. Using chemical labels, phospholipases and phospholipid exchange proteins, it has been demonstrated that the phospholipid constituents are asymmetrically distributed over both sides of the membrane (Op den Kamp, 1979). In human RBC, the outer monolayer contains predominantly choline-containing phospholipids, i.e., PC and sphingomyelin, while the inner monolayer contains predominantly aminophospholipids, i.e., PE and phosphatidylserine (PS). Despite the highly asymmetric location of the phospholipid in the membrane, the lipid bilayer exhibits a remarkably high degree of stability (Van Meer et al., 1980). Selective modification of the molecular species of PC in the outer monolayer may destabilize the structural matrix of the RBC membrane (Roelofsen et al., 1981). It is also apparent that small changes in fatty acid turnover may accompany changes in membrane function and morphology (Dise et al., 1980).

Using the fluorescent probe 1,6-diphenyl-1,3,5-hexatriene (DPH), we have determined steady-state anisotropy (r_s) values in RBC ghost membranes of schizophrenic patients before and after haloperidol (HPD) withdrawal, as well as of age-matched normal male controls (Yao and van Kammen, 1994). Although the mean r_s value of HT patients was not significantly different from that of either the DF patients or the normal controls, a small but significant increase (two-tailed $p < 0.05$) of the mean r_s value was observed in DF schizophrenic patients as compared to that of controls. Furthermore, the increases in 'structure order' of RBC ghost membranes as measured by r_s were significantly correlated to the decreases in the fatty acid unsaturation index in DF normal controls and schizophrenic patients

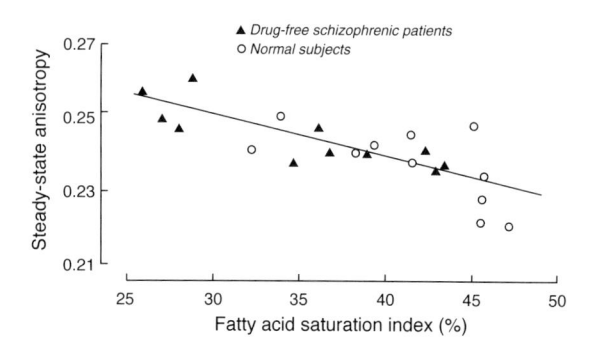

Figure 6.2. Relationships of the steady-state anisotropy (r_s) of 1,6-diphenyl-1,3,5-hexatriene-labelled RBC ghost membranes to fatty acid unsaturation index of RBC membrane phospholipids from normal subjects and drug-free schizophrenic patients; $n = 23$; $r = -0.75$; $p < 0.0001$. After Yao and van Kammen (1994) and Yao et al. (1994b).

(Figure 6.2). Thus, a decreased fatty acid unsaturation may be, at least in part, responsible for the decreased RBC membrane fluidity in DF schizophrenic patients.

Using a similar approach to assay r_s of DPH-labelled RBC ghost membranes, Hitzeman et al. (1986) have demonstrated a significant increase in r_s values from patients with schizophreniform disorder as compared to control subjects. In addition, three of eight manic patients and five of eight schizophrenic patients had r_s values higher than the highest control values, although the differences are not statistically significant. All patients in their study were medication-free for at least 30 days prior to the study. Therefore, there appears to be a similar trend of increased 'structure order' of RBC ghost membranes in DF schizophrenic patients.

Effect of antipsychotic drugs

To test whether PUFAs in RBC membranes were affected by the antipsychotic drug treatment, we have compared the levels of 18:2n-6, 20:4n-6, and fatty acid unsaturation index between HT schizophrenic patients and the same individuals after HPD withdrawal (Yao et al., 1994a). Patients on HPD were treated with doses between 5 and 20 mg/day (11 ± 4 mg/day, mean ± SD). The average days on medication and drug-free period were 52 and 40 days, respectively. No significant differences were demonstrated in either absolute concentration (Table 6.1) or percentage distribution of RBC PUFAs between HT and DF patients. However, there was a positive correlation between 18:2n-6 level (but not 20:4) and HPD dose level, although the correlation was not quite statistically significant ($r = 0.45, p = 0.06$).

No significant correlation was demonstrated between RBC PUFAs and plasma HPD levels.

Fatty acid defects and clinical states

Correlation between PUFA defects and behavioural rating scores

To test whether the levels of PUFAs and the degree of fatty acid unsaturation in RBC ghost membranes of schizophrenic patients are related to the severity of psychopathology, we (Yao et al., 1994a) have previously compared the levels of 18:2n-6, 20:4n-6, total PUFAs or the fatty acid unsaturation index (FAUI) with various behavioural ratings, including the Bunney-Hamburg psychosis ratings (BHPR), the Brief Psychiatric Rating Scale (BPRS), and the Scale for the Assessment of Negative Symptoms (SANS). In the DF group, both 18:2n-6 and FAUI are correlated significantly with the BHPR scores (Figure 6.3). Furthermore, a negative correlation was consistently demonstrated between biochemical variables and behaviour (BHPR and total BPRS, but not total SANS) scores, although these correlations were not quite statistically significant. On the other hand, in the HT group, only 18:2n-6 was correlated significantly with total BPRS. Such an increase may be related to the dose of HPD, although the correlation was not quite statistically significant (see above).

Effect of relapse on RBC membrane fatty acids

When schizophrenic patients were divided into relapsed and clinically stable groups, the mean values (%) of 20:4n-6, total PUFAs or FAUI were consistently higher in the clinically stable than in the relapsed schizophrenic patients, although the difference between the groups was not statistically significant (Yao et al., 1994a). No significant difference was found in the level of 18:2n-6 between relapsed and clinically stable schizophrenic patients. Furthermore, there were no significant differences between patients before and after HPD withdrawal in either relapsed or clinically stable groups.

Bimodal distribution of PUFAs in patients with negative symptoms

Recently, Glen et al. (1994) demonstrated a bimodal distribution of PUFAs with 20 and 22 carbons in RBC membranes of schizophrenic patients, but not in normal subjects. Furthermore, they related the decreased PUFAs and increased saturated fatty acids to patients with negative syndromes, whereas the reverse trend was associated with positive symptom patients (Figure 6.4). Such a bimodal distribution was later confirmed by Peet et al. (1994, 1996), although psychiatric rating scales were not determined to differentiate positive from negative symptom patients in their study. Nevertheless, the wide variations in the RBC PUFA levels of schizophrenic patients may have contributed, in part, to the discrepancies of RBC membrane phospholipid abnormalities obtained from schizophrenic patients in different studies (see review by Rotrosen and Wolkin, 1987).

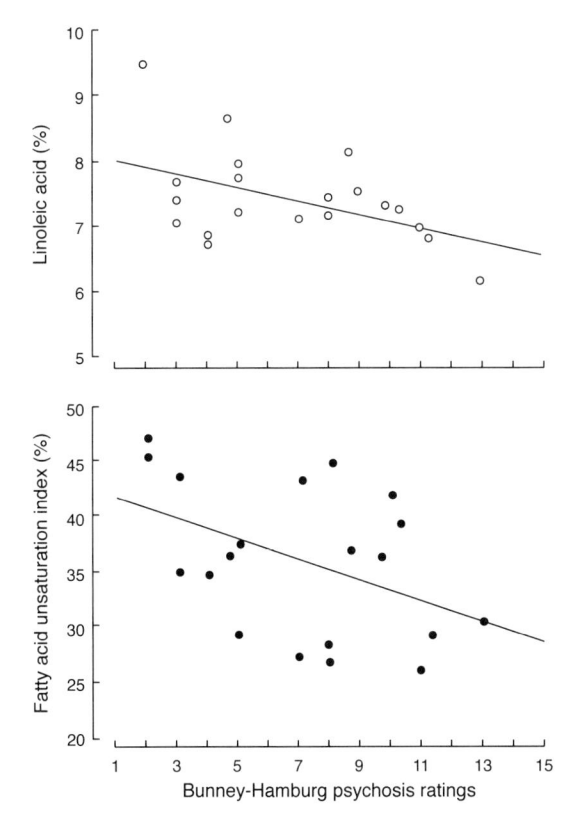

Figure 6.3. Relationships of linoleic acid and fatty acid unsaturation index of red blood cell membrane phospholipids to Bunney-Hamburg psychosis ratings (3-day mean) in drug-free schizophrenic patients. For linoleic acid: $n = 20$; $r = -0.49$; $p < 0.05$. For the fatty acid unsaturation index: $n = 20$; $r = -0.46$; $p < 0.05$. After Yao et al. (1994a).

Biochemical mechanisms underlying the decreased n-6 PUFAs

There are several known mechanisms that can lead to the type of RBC fatty acid defects that have been identified in schizophrenia. They include: decreased fatty

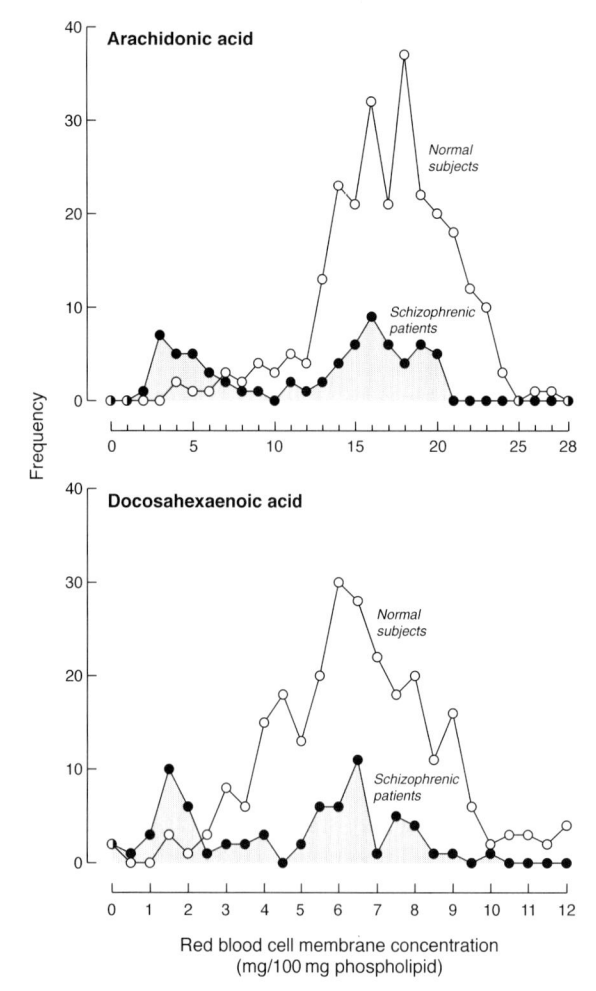

Figure 6.4. Frequency distribution of arachidonic acid and docosahexaenoic acid in red blood cell membrane phospholipids of schizophrenic patients and normal subjects. After Glen et al. (1994).

acid incorporation into phospholipids; increased phospholipid degradation; oxidative stress; and/or low dietary intake of essential fatty acids. The most compelling evidence in schizophrenia exists for decreased incorporation of AA and increased phospholipid degradation, which will be systematically examined below.

Decreased fatty acid incorporation

Demisch et al. (1987, 1992) have shown that incorporation of [^{14}C]AA into platelet phospholipids was significantly lower in untreated patients (>6 months) with a schizophreniform or schizoaffective disorder than in normal control subjects. The incorporation rates were only slightly, but not significantly, reduced in chronic schizophrenic patients. Thus, they suggested that the rate of AA incorporation was related to the type and time course of the disorder. However, their study was not carried out in schizophrenic patients both on and off neuroleptic treatment, although they have reported an increased rate of [^{14}C]AA incorporation by HPD in their earlier report (Demisch et al., 1985). We have recently demonstrated that the total incorporation of [^{3}H]AA in DF patients was significantly lower than in the same individuals on HPD treatment as well as in normal controls (Yao et al., 1996): details are given later in this chapter. No significant difference of [^{3}H]AA incorporation was demonstrated between relapsed and clinically stable DF patients. Thus, it is unlikely that changes in AA incorporation are related to a specific syndrome or its intensity.

Increased degradation of phospholipids

Phospholipase A$_2$ (PLA$_2$) is a key enzyme responsible for turnover of membrane phospholipids (Figure 6.5). PLA$_2$ is enriched in the neuronal membranes. Most of the agonists that provoke inositol phospholipid hydrolysis can also activate PLA$_2$ (Dennis et al., 1991; Weiss and Insel, 1991). Free fatty acids and lysophospholipids are the major products of PLA$_2$ reaction. Several cis unsaturated fatty acids enhance the diacylglycerol (DAG)-dependent activation of protein kinase C (PKC) (Seifert et al., 1988; Shinomura et al., 1991; Chen and Murakami, 1992), particularly in the presence of membrane-permeant DAG (Yoshida et al., 1992). The other metabolite of PLA$_2$ reaction, lysophosphatidylcholine (LPC), potentiates long-term cellular response (e.g., cell proliferation and differentiation) in the presence of DAG (Asaoka et al., 1991), suggesting a role of LPC in the signal transduction. Moreover, LPC can affect a series of other second messengers, such as phospholipase C (PLC), PKC, cGMP, Ca^{2+}, and neurotransmitters. Therefore, the agonist-induced activation of PLA$_2$ appears to play a pivotal role in the phospholipids turnover and signal transduction mechanism.

Increased cytoplasmic PLA$_2$ activity has been found in the serum of DF schizophrenic patients (Gattaz et al., 1987; Gattaz, 1992; Noponen et al., 1993). Such increases in serum PLA$_2$ activity, however, were also found in patients with other psychiatric disorders (Noponen et al., 1993), questioning the specificity of this finding to schizophrenia. Moreover, Albers et al. (1993) found no significant differences of serum PLA$_2$ activity between six neuroleptic-naïve schizophrenics and 10 normal controls. These discrepancies may be due

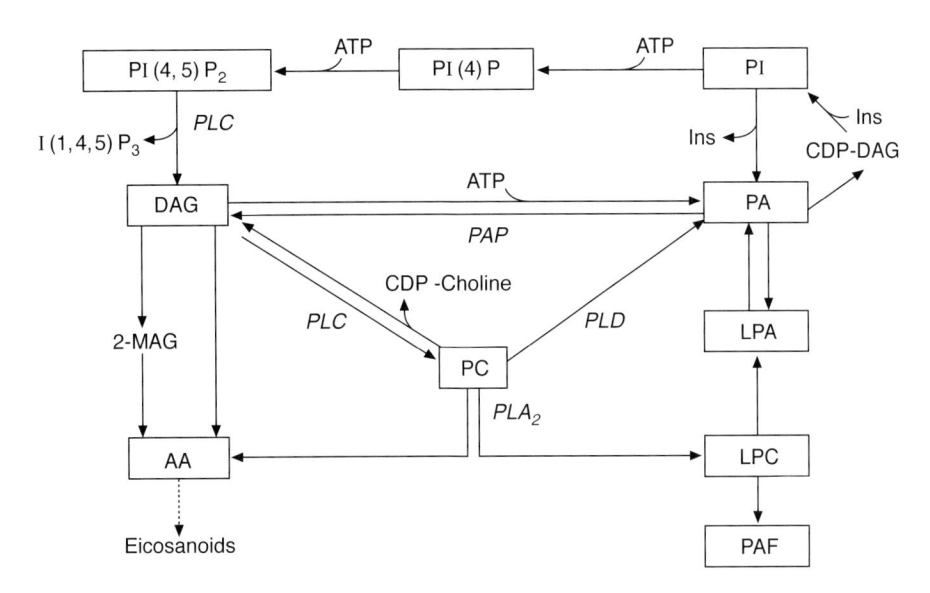

Figure 6.5. Metabolic pathways of lipid derived messengers. Abbreviations: PI, phosphatidylinositol; PI-4-P, phosphatidylinositol 4-phosphate; PI-4,5-P$_2$, phosphatidylinositol 4,5-bisphosphate; I-1,4,5-P$_3$, inositol 1,4,5-triphosphate; PC, phosphatidylcholine; PA, phosphatidic acid; AA, arachidonic acid; MAG, monoacylglycerol; DAG, diacylglycerol; LPA, lysophosphatidic acid; LPC, lysophosphatidylcholine; PAF, platelet activating factor; PLA$_2$, phospholipase A$_2$; PLC, phospholipase C; PLD, phospholipase D; PAP, phosphatidic acid phosphohydrolase; CDP, cytidine diphosphate; Ins, inositol.

to the differences in assay procedure and the heterogeneous class of extracellular PLA$_2$ (Ross et al, 1997). Recently, Gattaz et al. (1995) showed that the intracellular membrane-bound PLA$_2$ activity was significantly higher in platelets of schizophrenic patients than in normal and psychiatric controls, with no significant differences between the latter two groups. It is therefore unlikely that the increased platelet PLA$_2$ activity in schizophrenia results from nonspecific stressors. Furthermore, HPD treatment reduced platelet PLA$_2$ activity to control levels. Other neuroleptics also inhibit PLA$_2$ activity (Schroder et al., 1981; Aarsman et al., 1985; Taniguchi et al., 1988).

Further support for elevated PLA$_2$ activity in schizophrenia comes from the findings of increased LPC (the break-down product of the PLA$_2$ reaction) found in platelets of schizophrenic patients (Pangerl et al., 1991; Steudle et al., 1994). Moreover, the increase in LPC was significantly correlated with the duration of illness in neuroleptic-naïve but not previously treated patients, suggesting an accelerated breakdown of membrane phospholipids after the onset of disease. Such a correlation is consistent with the finding that the duration of illness before treatment in first-episode, drug-naïve patients is significantly associated with time to remission (Wyatt, 1986; Loebel et al., 1992).

The clinical significance of PLA$_2$ alterations in schizophrenia has been less systematically examined. Recently, Ross et al. (1997) found positive relations between calcium-independent PLA$_2$ and general psychopathology scores and positive symptoms, but not with negative symptoms. They examined PLA$_2$ activity in chronic schizophrenic patients who were receiving long-term antipsychotic treatment, and exhibited significant positive symptoms. Although they were not characterized as poor outcome patients, the clinical characteristics of these patients are suggestive of an unfavourable outcome. Whether the relations between PLA$_2$ and AA in first-episode schizophrenic patients will be the same or different from that observed in chronic schizophrenic patients remains to be determined.

Increased lipid peroxidation

PUFAs are highly susceptible to free radical insult and autoxidation to form peroxy-radicals and lipid peroxide intermediates, the existence of which within cell membranes results in unstable membrane structure, altered membrane fluidity and permeability, and impaired signal transduction. The brain, which is rich in PUFAs, is particularly vulnerable to free radical-mediated damage (reviewed in Reddy and Yao, 1996). Thus, lipid peroxidation can lead to decreased membrane AA content.

Low intake of essential fatty acids

AA is mainly synthesized from linoleic acid by desaturation and elongation (Figure 6.1). Linoleic acid, a so-called essential fatty acid (EFA), can not be synthesized by mammals and must be obtained from plant sources. A dietary deficiency of linoleic acid usually leads to a higher content of trienoic acids of the n-9 group, which can be synthesized endogenously (Holman, 1973). An increased level of 20:3n-9 was not demonstrated either in RBC ghost membranes of our schizophrenic patients (Yao et al., 1994b) or in plasma samples of other schizophrenic patient groups (Horrobin et al., 1989; Kaiya et al., 1991). In addition, all patients in our study were placed in the low-monoamine, alcohol-free and caffeine-restricted diet. It is thus reasonable to exclude a dietary deficiency of EFA in our schizophrenic patients.

On the other hand, it is possible that a person who has a low dietary intake of EFA may have a higher risk and/or poorer outcome for schizophrenia. There is an indication that outcome is better in those countries (India and Nigeria) that have a relatively high intake of EFA-rich foods and low intake of saturated fats, while countries with poorer outcome have the opposite ratios of EFA to saturated fats (Christensen and Christensen, 1988). Thus, there is a close correlation between a good lifetime outcome for schizophrenia and a high ratio of unsaturated to saturated fat intake (Horrobin, 1992).

ALTERED METABOLIC PATHWAYS OF PLATELET ARACHIDONIC ACID

Since it is impossible to study the metabolic turnover of brain phospholipids in living patients, it is reasonable to use a peripheral model comparable to that of central neurones. Platelets not only show similarities to serotonergic pre- and postsynaptic membranes (Passenon, 1968; Stahl, 1977; Pletscher, 1978; Paul et al., 1981) and have similar intracellular calcium dynamics (Erne et al., 1984; O'Rourke et al., 1985; Avdonin et al., 1987; Bowden et al., 1988), but they are also comparable to catecholaminergic neurones (Sneddon, 1973; Pletscher, 1981). In addition, platelets have proven to be a rich source of information for studies regarding the interrelationship between phospholipid fatty acid metabolism and other cellular events, including receptor function, receptor-coupled intracellular signal generation, and secretion (Laychock and Putney, 1982). Thus, platelets provide us with a convenient model of a neurosecretory cell with which to study membrane-related functions, even though some differences do exist between platelets and central neurones (Hallam et al., 1984; Doyle and Ruegg, 1985; Sage and Rink, 1986; Young, 1986).

Recently, we have evaluated receptor-stimulated turnover of membrane phospholipids by incorporating [^{3}H]AA into resting platelets from a carefully diagnosed group of schizophrenic patients on and off HPD treatment, as well as age- and sex-matched normal control subjects (Yao and van Kammen, 1996; Yao et al., 1996). The prelabelled platelets were then activated by thrombin for various periods of time, so that the resulting second messenger (Figure 6.5) and eicosanoids cascade (Figure 6.6) could be assessed in neuroleptic-stabilized and DF schizophrenic patients. Over 85% of incorporated [^{3}H]AA was found in the phospholipid subclasses of normal resting platelets. Minute amounts of ^{3}H-labelling were found in free AA, DAG, and

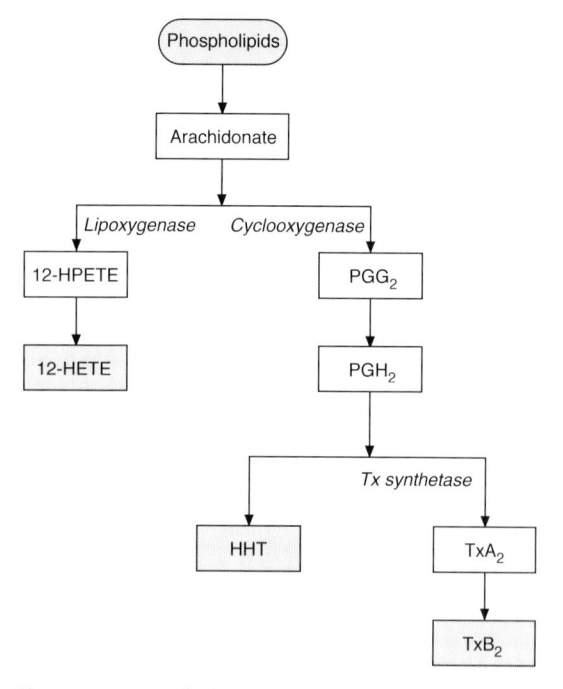

Figure 6.6. Arachidonic acid metabolism in platelets. Abbreviations: 12-HPETE, 12-hydroperoxy-5,8,10,14-eicosatetraenoic acid; 12-HETE, 12-hydroxy-5,8,10,14-eicosatetraenoic acid; HHT, 12-hydroxy-5,8,10-heptadecatrienoic acid; PG, prostaglandin; PGH$_2$, prostaglandin H$_2$; PGG$_2$, prostaglandin G$_2$; Tx, thromboxane; TxA$_2$, thromboxane A$_2$; TxB$_2$, thromboxane B$_2$.

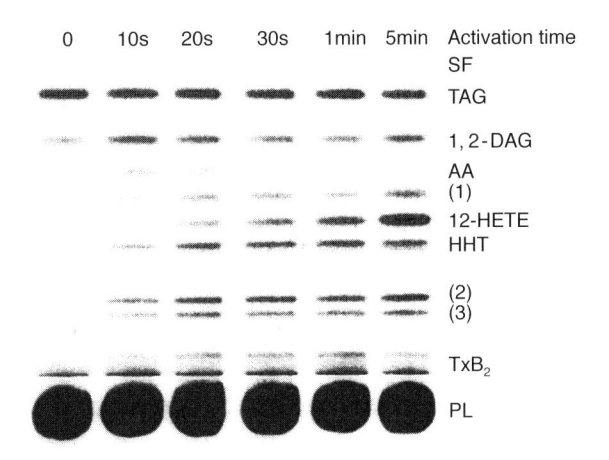

Figure 6.7. Separation of ^{3}H-labelled lipids on oxalate-impregnated high-performance thin-layer chromatogram. Following incorporation of [^{3}H]arachidonic acid into normal platelets, which were subsequently activated by thrombin for various time periods, approximately 5×10^4 cpm/sample were applied to thin-layer plate. After development, the plate was exposed to Kodak X-Omat S film at $-70°C$ for 1 month. SF, solvent front; TAG, triacylglycerol; 1,2-DAG, 1,2-diacylglycerol; AA, arachidonic acid; 12-HETE, 12-hydroxyeicosatetraenoic acid; HHT, hydroxyhepta-decatrienoic acid; TxB$_2$, thromboxane B$_2$; PL, phospholipids; and (1), (2), (3), unidentified metabolites. After Yao et al. (1996).

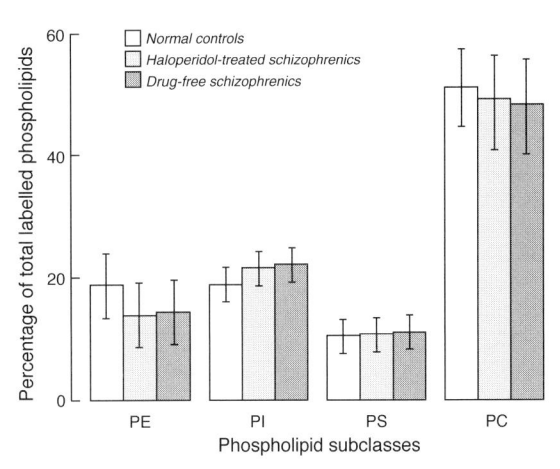

Figure 6.8. Percentage distribution of ^{3}H-labelled phospholipid subclasses following incorporation of [^{3}H]arachidonic acid into resting platelets from normal control subjects and schizophrenic patients on and off haloperidol treatment. PE, phosphatidylethanolamine; PI, phosphatidylinositol; PS, phosphatidylserine; PC, phosphatidylcholine. Group means ($\pm$ SD) were compared by one-way analysis of variance, using Friedman's nonparametric and Dunn's multiple comparison tests. Only PI showed a significant difference among the group means ($F = 8.08$; $df = 2,24$; $p < 0.001$). After Yao and van Kammen (1996).

triacylglycerol as well in AA metabolites derived from cyclooxygenase and lipoxygenase pathways. Following thrombin activation, however, there was increased formation of AA metabolites which can be separated and identified by high-performance thin-layer chromatography in conjunction with fluorography. Increased ^{3}H-labelling was found in three major AA metabolites of thrombin-activated platelets (Figure 6.7).

Phosphatidylinositol turnover and increased production of second messenger

The interaction of an agonist such as thrombin with its platelet receptor leads to the activation of various phospholipases (Liscovitch, 1991). In human platelets, DAG can be produced from phosphatidylinositol (PI) by PLC within 5 s of thrombin-activation (Bell et al., 1979; Rittenhouse-Simmons, 1979). The resulting DAG and AA may serve as second messengers for the sustained activation of PKC (Nishizuka, 1992).

Following incorporation of [^{3}H]AA into resting platelets, we have demonstrated that the percentage distribution of labelled PI to total labelled phospholipids was significantly higher in schizophrenic patients (both on and off haloperidol) than in normal subjects (Yao and van Kammen, 1996) (Figure 6.8). Variations of other ^{3}H-labelled phospholipid subclasses (PC, PE, and PS), however, were minimal following thrombin activation. Demisch et al. (1992) have also found a highly significant decrease in the rate of esterification of [^{14}C]AA into platelet PC, PE, and PI/PS from patients with schizophreniform, schizoaffective or major depressive disorders, but not with chronic schizophrenia. In their study, however, the ^{14}C-labelled PI was not separated from ^{14}C-labelled PS.

In addition, we have reported an increased formation of DAG but not AA release in thrombin-activated platelets of both HT and DF schizophrenic patients (Figure 6.9), which is in accordance with the results of Kaiya et al. (1989). It is particularly prominent during the first minute of thrombin-activation. Thus, the increased ^{3}H-labelling in PI may indicate an increased substrate concentration for PLC reaction, leading to DAG accumulation. Following thrombin activation, decreased ^{3}H-labelling is expected to be present in PI in response to an increase in DAG production.

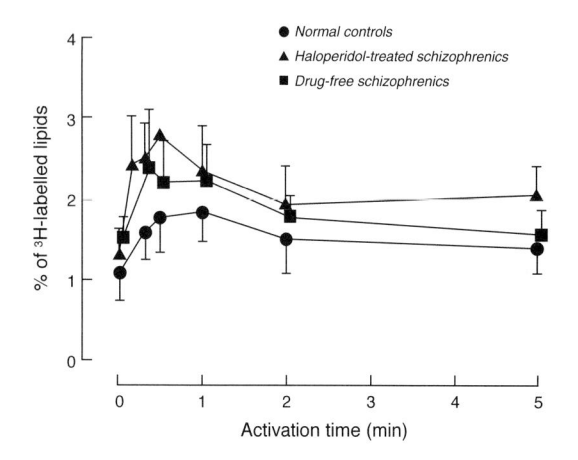

Figure 6.9. Thrombin-induced formation of ³H-labelled diacylglycerol following incorporation of [³H]arachidonic acid into platelets of normal subjects and schizophrenic patients with and without haloperidol treatment. After Yao et al. (1996).

However, our data demonstrate that the ³H-labelling in PI was higher in schizophrenic patients than in normal control subjects (Figure 6.10). The increased PI labelling may be derived from the newly released AA following thrombin activation, since the thrombin-induced AA released was not reduced in schizophrenic patients both on and off haloperidol treatment (Yao et al., 1996).

Using [³²P]orthophosphate as a precursor, we have previously demonstrated that thrombin-induced platelet phosphatidic acid (PA) is significantly higher in schizophrenic patients than in normal controls (Yao et al., 1992). Thus, the increase in thrombin-induced DAG may be due, at least in part, to an increased PI turnover in schizophrenic patients (Kaiya et al., 1989; Essali et al., 1990; Yao et al., 1992). Such an increase in second messengers may reflect an increase in PLC reaction in schizophrenia, since thrombin-induced platelet activation is mediated by PLC activity through G-protein regulated hydrolysis of polyphosphoinositides. It is unclear, however, whether such an abnormality is related to neuroleptic treatment, stress, or the pathophysiology of the psychotic state. Several neurotransmitters have been shown to stimulate PLC and generate second messengers *via* PI pathways (Baraban et al., 1989). It is possible that increased second messenger production may be associated with increased release of specific neurotransmitters such as 5HT$_2$ in schizophrenia.

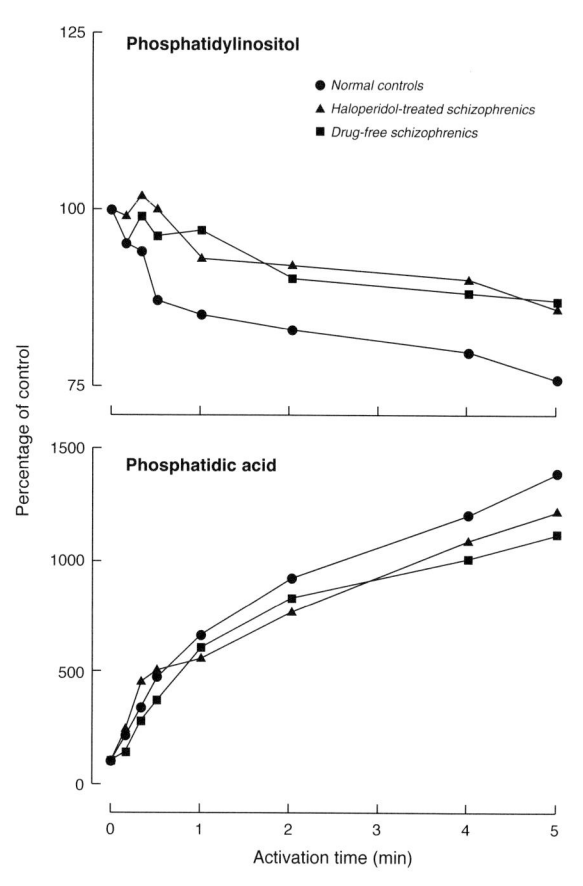

Figure 6.10. Changes in the ³H-labelled phosphatidylinositol and phosphatidic acid incorporated from [³H]arachidonic acid at various times after thrombin activation. After Yao and van Kammen (1996).

Phosphorylation of diacylglycerol

[³H]AA was mainly incorporated into PE, PC, PI, and PS in resting human platelets. Minute amounts of ³H-labelling were found in the PA fraction. Following thrombin activation, however, substantial amounts of ³H-labelling were demonstrated in PA. The newly synthesized PA gradually increased with activation time up to 5 min (Figure 6.10). PA is produced by a rapid phosphorylation of DAG through DAG kinase (Lapetina and Hawthorne, 1971; Billah et al., 1979). It has been hypothesized that a reduced activity of DAG kinase is responsible for the increased DAG accumulation (Kaiya et al., 1989). Our data, however, have shown a similar thrombin-stimulated increase of PA in platelets among normal control subjects and schizophrenic patients both on and off HPD treatment. Using [³²P]orthophosphate as a precursor, we have additionally shown that the

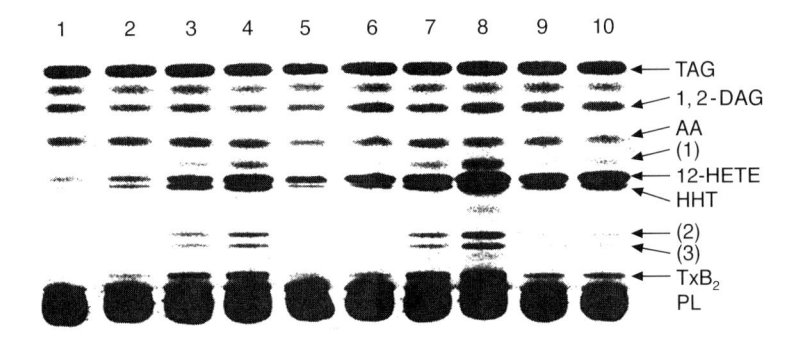

Figure 6.11. Effect of phospholipase inhibitors and activators on thrombin-induced metabolic turnover of arachidonic acid following incorporation of [^{3}H]arachidonic acid into platelet lipids. Lane 1, resting platelet lipids; lanes 2–4, platelet lipids following thrombin activation for 1, 2 and 5 min, respectively; lanes 5–6, in the presence of compound 48/80 (phosphatidylinositol-specific phospholipase C inhibitor) following thrombin activation for 2 and 5 min, respectively; lanes 7–8, in the presence of neomycin sulphate (phospholipase A$_2$ activator) following thrombin activation for 2 and 5 min, respectively; lanes 9–10, in the presence of aristolochic acid (phospholipase A$_2$ inhibitor) following thrombin activation for 2 and 5 min, respectively. For abbreviations, see Figure 6.7.

thrombin-induced PA formation was higher in schizophrenic patients than in normal controls (Yao et al., 1992). Taken together, these findings imply that DAG kinase activity was not reduced in schizophrenic individuals as compared to normal controls. Also, an inhibitory action of DAG kinase activity was not demonstrated by HPD treatment. The pharmacological action of HPD on PI response is thus somewhat different from that of other antipsychotic drugs, such as chlorpromazine, demonstrating an inhibition of DAG kinase that leads to the thrombin-induced DAG accumulation (Wakatabe et al., 1991).

Arachidonic acid metabolism and outcome

It has been suggested that the reduced esterification of AA into platelet phospholipids may be an indicator of a favourable course of episode of an endogenous pyschosis (Demisch et al., 1987). Subsequently, Kaiya et al. (1989) have found that schizophrenic patients with an impaired platelet PI pathway had a better outcome of their present episode. Demisch et al. (1992) also observed that patients with atypical phasic psychosis, characterized by a good prognosis and the symptomatic termination of each episode without any deficit symptoms (Gerbaldo et al., 1989), had the greatest reduction of [^{14}C]AA esterification into platelet PI/PS fractions. Further investigations are needed to establish such a role of membrane phospholipids in the prognosis of psychotic episodes.

Altered biosynthesis of eicosanoids

In addition to the formation of second messengers, the newly released AA from membrane phospholipids can be converted to endoperoxides and thromboxane A$_2$ (TXA$_2$) through the concerted reactions of cyclooxygenase and thromboxane synthetase (Lapetina, 1990). Using high-performance thin-layer chromatography (TLC) and fluorography (Figure 6.7), we have identified three major AA metabolites, 12-hydroxy-5,8,10,14-eicosatetraenoic acid (12-HETE), 12-hydroxy-5,8,10-heptadecatrienoic acid (12-HHT) and thromboxane B$_2$ (TxB$_2$, stable metabolite of TxA$_2$), in thrombin-stimulated platelets. Following activation of prelabelled platelets by thrombin, three other unknown bands were also labelled from [^{3}H]AA (Figure 6.7). These three AA metabolites were not revealed by Lapetina and Cuatrecasas (1979) using the identical TLC developing solvent system. By applying the EN^{3}HANCE to the TLC plate prior to radioautography, the increased sensitivity of radioactivity detection may account for such differences. These three unknown compounds are tentatively identified as cyclooxygenase products, since their syntheses are completely inhibited by the presence of indomethacin, imidazole (Yao et al., 1996) or phospholipase inhibitors (Figure 6.11). Further investigations are needed to study the structural and metabolic roles of these AA metabolites.

In schizophrenic patient groups, the thrombin-induced formation of eicosanoids was found to be

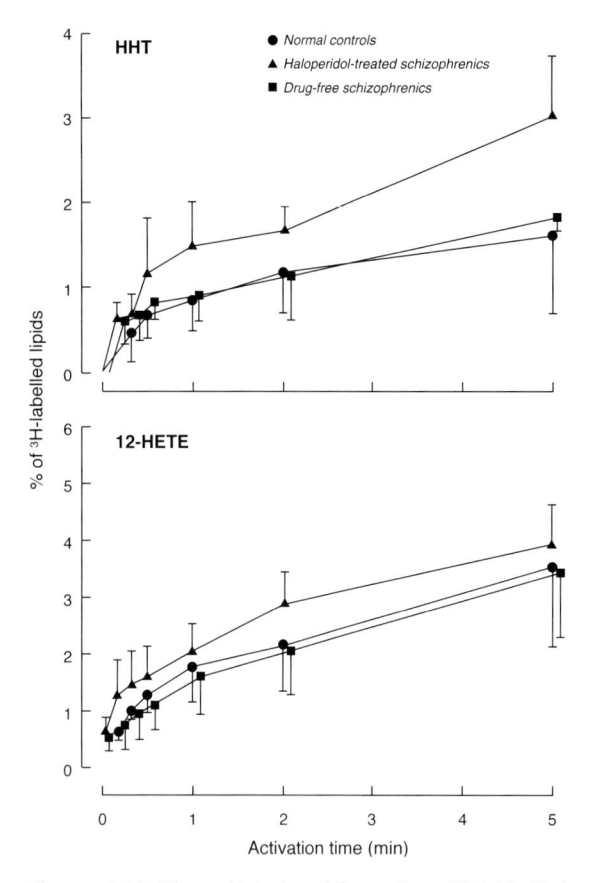

Figure 6.12. Thrombi-induced formation of ³H-labelled HHT and 12-HETE following incorporation of [³H]arachidonic acid into platelets of normal subjects and schizophrenic patients with and without haloperidol treatment. Abbreviations: HHT, hydroxyheptadecatrienoic acid; 12-HETE, 12-hydroxyeicosatetraenoic acid. After Yao et al. (1996).

significantly ($p < 0.05$) higher in HT patients (8106 ± 3574 dpm/10^8 platelets/min) than in normal controls (4310 ± 1914 dpm/10^8 platelets/min). Such an increase is probably associated with an increased turnover of platelet phospholipids (see above). Following withdrawal of HPD treatment, however, the ³H-labelling in 12-HETE, HHT, TxB$_2$ and the three unidentified AA metabolites were reduced in thrombin-activated platelets of DF patients. Figure 6.12 shows the time course of thrombin-induced formation of platelet eicosanoids, demonstrating a continuous increase of HHT and 12-HETE during the first 5 min of the activation period. The thrombin-induced formation of ³H-labelled HHT and 12-HETE was significantly higher in HT schizophrenic patients than in normal controls after 2 min of activation.

Previously, Piomelli et al. (1989) showed that 12-HPETE and its metabolites, 12-keto-5,8,10,14-eicosatetraenoic acid (12-KETE) and hepoxilin-A$_3$, but not 12-HETE, can act as second messengers at the synapse. If there is a parallelism between the platelets and brain regarding AA metabolic pathways in schizophrenic patients, the present data in neuroleptic regulated increase of 12-HETE in activated platelets may reflect a decreased availability of other 12-lipoxygenase products. Thus, it is possible that one of the pharmacological effects of HPD is to regulate the second messenger function *via* the AA pathways.

CONCLUSIONS

Recent findings provide evidence that altered membrane structure and function of RBCs and platelets are unequivocally present in chronic schizophrenic patients. Specifically, decreased contents of the linoleic acid and AA in RBC membranes were demonstrated in both neuroleptic treated and drug-free conditions, as well as low incorporation of AA in platelets in the drug-free condition. These membrane defects were associated with psychosis severity in the drug-free state. Further, defects in polyunsaturated fatty acids have also been found in plasma and brain tissue. Since the dynamic state of all membranes, including neuronal, is dependent on their composition, even small changes in key polyunsaturated fatty acids that make up phospholipids, such as AA, can lead to a broad range of membrane dysfunctions involving receptor binding, neurotransmission, signal transduction, and prostaglandin synthesis. Thus, deficits of membrane AA may explain many biological, physiological, and clinical phenomena observed in schizophrenia (see review by Horrobin, 1996). The findings of altered cortical phospholipid metabolism (reviewed in Keshavan and Pettegrew, 1997), suggest that deficits identified in peripheral membranes may also be present in the brain. However, it is not known whether the membrane defect identified in chronic schizophrenic patients is also present early in the course of illness, and whether it is associated with a less favourable clinical outcome. Thus, future studies are needed to shed light on whether the membrane defect detected peripherally, hypothesized to be present early in illness, is also associated with alterations in central phospholipid metabolism. Further, these studies will help clarify relations between peripheral and central membrane defects and early outcome. The findings reviewed above suggest that membrane

AA decreases are associated with clinical features of the illness that are typically associated with an unfavourable outcome, and that a number of putative mechanisms have been identified to explain the decreased AA levels. In light of this, the question arises whether there are any interventions available that modify AA levels and whether such interventions are associated with behavioural change.

ACKNOWLEDGEMENT

This work was supported by research grants from the Department of Veterans Affairs Research and Development Service (Merit Review), National Institute of Mental Health, and the Highland Drive VA Pittsburgh Healthcare System.

REFERENCES

Aarsman AJ, Roosenboom CFP, van Geffen GEW, van den Bosch H. Some aspects of rat platelet and serum phospholipase A_2 activities. Biochim Biophys Acta 1985; 837: 88–95.

Abdulla YH, Hamadah K. Effect of ADP on PGE formation in blood platelets from patients with depression, mania and schizophrenia. Br J Psychiatry 1975; 127: 591–595.

Albers M, Meurer H, Märki F, Klotz J. Phospholipase A_2 activity in serum of neuroleptic-naïve psychiatric inpatients. Pharmacopsychiatry 1993; 26: 94–98.

Asaoka Y, Oka M, Yoshida K, Sasaki Y, Nishizuka Y. Role of lysophosphatidylcholine in T lymphocyte activation: involvement of phospholipase A_2 in signal transduction through protein kinase C. Proc Natl Acad Sci USA 1991; 88: 8681–8685.

Avdonin PV, Cheglakov IB, Boogry EM, Svitina-Ulitina IV, Mazaev AV, Tkachuk VA. Evidence for the receptor-operated calcium channels in human platelet plasma membrane. Thromb Res 1987; 46: 29–37.

Baraban JM, Worley PF, Snyder SH. Second messenger psychoactive drug action: focus on the phosphoinositide system and lithium. Am J Psychiatry 1989; 146: 1251–1260.

Bell RL, Kennerly DA, Stanford N, Majerus PW. Diglyceride lipase: a pathway for arachidonate release from human platelets. Proc Natl Acad Sci USA 1979; 76: 3238–3241.

Billah MM, Lapetina EG, Cuatrecasas P. Phosphatidylinositol-specific phospholipase C of platelets: association with 1,2-diacylglycerol kinase and inhibition by cyclic AMP. Biochem Biophys Res Commun 1979; 90: 92–98.

Bowden CL, Huang LG, l Javors MA et al. Calcium function in affective disorders and healthy controls. Biol Psychiatry 1988; 23: 367–376.

Cadet JL, Kahler LA. Free radical mechanisms in schizophrenia and tardive dyskinesia. Neurosci Biobehav Rev 1994; 18: 457–467.

Cadet JL, Lohr JB. Free radicals and the developmental pathophysiology of schizophrenic burnout. Integr Psychiatry 1987; 5: 40–48.

Chen SG, Murakami K. Synergistic activation of type III protein kinase C by cis-fatty acid and diacylglycerol. Biochem J 1992; 282: 33–39.

Christensen O, Christensen E. Fat consumption and schizophrenia. Acta Psychiatr Scand 1988; 78: 587–591.

Demisch L, Gerbaldo H, Gebbart P, Schushter N, Bochnik HJ. Treatment with haloperidol or fluperlapine increases the incorporation of ^{14}C-arachidonic acid into blood platelets in patients with schizophrenic or schizoaffective disorders: relationship to clinical improvement. IVth World Congress of Biological Psychiatry; Abstracts, 1985: 206.

Demisch L, Gerbaldo H, Gebbart P, Georgi K, Bochnik HJ. Incorporation of ^{14}C-arachidonic acid into platelet phospholipids of untreated patients with schizophreniform or schizophrenic disorders. Psychiatry Res 1987; 22: 275–282.

Demisch L, Heinz K, Gerbaldo H, Kirsten R. Increased concentrations of phosphatidylinositol and decreased esterification of arachidonic acid into phospholipids in platelets from patients with schizoaffective disorders or atypic phasic psychoses. Prostagland Leukotr Essent Fatty Acids 1992; 46: 47–52.

Dennis EA, Rhee SG, Billah MM, Hannun YA. Role of phospholipases in generating lipid second messengers in signal transduction. FASEB J 1991; 5: 2068–2077.

Dise CA, Goodman DBP, Fasmussen H. Definition of the pathway for membrane phospholipid fatty acid turnover in human erythrocytes. J Lipid Res 1980; 21: 292–300.

Doyle VM, Ruegg UR. Lack of evidence for voltage dependent calcium channels on platelets. Biochem Biophys Res Commun 1985; 127: 161–167.

Ellis FR, Sanders TAB. Long-chain polyunsaturated fatty acids in endogenous depression. J Neurol Neurosurg Psychiatry 1977; 40: 168–169.

Erne P, Bolli P, Burgisser E, Buhler FR. Correlation of platelet calcium with blood pressure: effect of antihypertensive therapy. N Engl J Med 1984; 310: 1084–1088.

Essali MA, Das I, de Belleroche J, Hirsch SR. The platelet phosphoinositide system in schizophrenia: the effects of neuroleptic treatment. Biol Psychiatry 1990; 28: 475–487.

Gattaz WF. Phospholipase A_2 in schizophrenia. Biol Psychiatry 1992; 31: 209–216.

Gattaz WF, Kπllisch M, Thuren T, Virtanen JA, Kinnunen PKJ. Increased plasma phospholipase-A_2 activity in schizophrenic patients: reduction after neuroleptic therapy. Biol Psychiatry 1987; 22: 421–426.

Gattaz WF, Schmitt A, Maras AM. Increased platelet phospholipase A_2 activity in schizophrenia. Schizophr Res 1995; 16: 1–6.

Gerbaldo H, Demisch L, Bochnik HJ. Phasic and process psychosis: a polydiagnostic comparison among the Frankfurt Classification System, DSM III, RDC, Feighner Criteria and ICD-9. Psychopathology 1989; 22: 14–27.

Glen AIM, Glen EMT, Horrobin DF et al. A red cell membrane abnormality in a subgroup of schizophrenic patients: evidence for two diseases. Schizophr Res 1994; 12: 53–61.

Hallam TJ, Thompson NT, Serutton MD, Rink TJ. The role of cytoplasmic free calcium in the responses of Quin2 loaded human platelets to vasopressin. Biochem J 1984; 221: 897–901.

Hitzemann R, Garver D. Membrane abnormalities in schizophrenia. Psychopharmacol Bull 1982; 18: 190–193.

Hitzemann R, Hirschowitz J, Garver D. On the physical properties of red cell ghost membranes in the affective disorders and psychoses. A fluorescence polarization study. J Affective Disord 1986; 10: 227–232.

Holman RT. Essential fatty acid deficiency in humans. In: Galli C, Jacini G, Pecile A, eds. Dietary lipids and postnatal development. New York: Raven Press, 1973: 127–143.

Horrobin DF. Prostaglandins and schizophrenia. Lancet 1980; i: 706–707.

Horrobin DF. The relationship between schizophrenia and essential fatty acids and eicosanoid metabolism. Prostagland Leukotr Essent Fatty Acids 1992; 46: 71–77.

Horrobin DF. Schizophrenia as a membrane lipid disorder which is expressed throughout the body. Prostagland Leukotr Essent Fatty Acids 1996; 55: 3–7.

Horrobin DF, Manku MS, Morse-Fisher N, Vaddadi KS. Essential fatty acids in plasma phospholipids in schizophrenics. Biol Psychiatry 1989; 25: 562–568.

Horrobin DF, Manku MS, Hillman S, Glen AIM. Fatty acid levels in the brains of schizophrenics and normal controls. Biol Psychiatry 1991; 30: 795–805.

Kaiya H, Nishida A, Imai A et al. Accumulation of diacylglycerol in platelet phosphoinositide turnover in schizophrenia: a biological marker of good prognosis? Biol Psychiatry 1989; 26: 669–676.

Kaiya H, Horrobin DF, Manku MS, Morse-Fisher N. Essential and other fatty acids in plasma in schizophrenics and normal individuals from Japan. Biol Psychiatry 1991; 30: 357–362.

Keshaven MS, Pettegrew JW. Magnetic resonance spectroscopy in schizophrenia and psychotic disorders. In: Krishnan KRR, Doraiswamy PM, eds. Brain imaging in clinical psychiatry. New York: Marcell-Dekker Inc., 1997: 381–400.

Lapetina EG. The signal transduction induced by thrombin in human platelets. FEBS Lett 1990; 268: 400–404.

Lapetina EG, Cuatrecasas P. Stimulation of phosphatidic acid production in platelets precedes the formation of arachidonate and parallels the release of serotonin. Biochim Biophys Acta 1979; 573: 394–402.

Lapetina EG, Hawthorne JN. The diglyceride kinase of rat cerebral cortex. Biochemistry 1971; 122: 171–179.

Laychock SG, Putney JW, Jr. Role of phospholipid metabolism in secretory cells. In: Conn M, ed. Cellular regulation of secretion and release. New York: Academic Press, 1982: 53–60.

Lieberman JA, Koreen AR. Neurochemistry and neuroendocrinology of schizophrenia: a selective review. Schizophr Bull 1993; 19: 371–429.

Liscovitch M. Signal-dependent activation of phosphatidylcholine hydrolysis: role of phospholipase. Biochem Soc Trans 1991; 19: 402–407.

Loebel AD, Lieberman JA, Albin JMJ et al. Duration of psychosis and outcome in first episode schizophrenia. Am J Psychiatry 1992; 149: 1183–1188.

Lohr JB. Oxygen radicals and neuropsychiatric illness: some speculations. Arch Gen Psychiatry 1991; 48: 1097–1106.

Mahadik SP, Mukherjee S. Free radical pathology and antioxidant defense in schizophrenia: a review. Schizophr Res 1996; 19: 1–17.

Mathé AA, Sedwall G, Wiesel FA, Nyback H. Increased content of immunoreactive prostaglandin E in cerebrospinal fluid of patients with schizophrenia. Lancet 1980; i: 16–17.

Meltzer HY. Biological studies in schizophrenia. Schizophr Bull 1987; 13: 77–111.

Nishizuka Y. Intracellular signaling by hydrolysis of phospholipids and activation of protein kinase C. Science 1992; 258: 607–614.

Noponen M, Sanfilipo M, Samanich K et al. Elevated PLA_2 activity in schizophrenics and other psychiatric patients. Biol Psychiatry 1993; 34: 641–649.

Obi FO, Nwanze EAC. Fatty acid profiles in mental disease. J Neurol Sci 1979; 43: 447–454.

Op den Kamp JAF. Lipid symmetry in membranes. Annu Rev Biochem 1979; 48: 47.

O'Rourke FA, Halenda SP, Zavacco GB, Feinstein MB. Inositol 1,4,5-triphophate releases Ca^{2+} from a Ca^{2+}-transporting membrane vesicle fraction derived from human platelets. J Biol Chem 1985; 260: 956–962.

Pangerl AM, Steudle A, Jaroni HW, RŸfer R, Gattaz WF. Increased platelet membrane lysophosphatidylcholine in schizophrenia. Biol Psychiatry 1991; 30: 837–840.

Passenon MK. Platelet 5-hydroxtryptamine as a model in pharmacology. Ann Med Exp Biol Fenn 1968; 46: 416–422.

Paul SM, Rehavi M, Rice KC, Ittah Y, Skolnick P. Does high-affinity ^{3}H-imipramine binding label serotonin reuptake sites in brain and platelet? Life Sci 1981; 28: 2753–2760.

Peet M, Laugharne JDE, Horrobin DF, Reynolds GP. Arachidonic acid: a common link in the biology of schizophrenia? Arch Gen Psychiatry 1994; 51: 665–666.

Peet M, Laugharne JDE, Rangarajan N, Horrobin DF, Reynolds G. Depleted red cell membrane essential fatty acids in drug-treated schizophrenic patients. J Psychiatr Res 1995; 29: 227–232.

Peet M, Laugharne JDE, Mellor J, Ramchand CN. Essential fatty acid deficiency in eyrthrocyte membranes from chronic schizophrenic patients, and the clinical effects of dietary supplementation. Prostagland Leukotr Essent Fatty Acids 1996; 55: 71–75.

Piomelli D, Feinmark S, Shapiro E, Schwartz JH. Formation and biological activity of 12-ketoeicosatetraenoic acid in the nervous system of Apland action of 8-hydroxy-11, 12-epoxy-5, 9, 14-eicosatrienoic acid in *Aplysia*: a possible second messenger in neurones. Proc Natl Acad Sci USA 1989; 86: 1721–1725.

Pletscher A. Platelets as models for monographic neurons. In: Youdim MBH, Lovenberg W, Sharman DF, Lagnado JR, eds. Essays in neurochemistry and neuropharmacology. Vol 13. New York: John Wiley and Sons, 1978: 48–54.

Pletscher A. Liberation of catecholamines from blood platelets. Br J Pharmacol 1981; 72: 349.

Reddy R, Yao JK. Free radical pathology in schizophrenia: a review. Prostagland Leukotr Essent Fatty Acids 1996; 55: 33–43.

Rittenhouse-Simmons S. Production of diglyceride from phosphatidylinositol in activated human platelets. J Clin Invest 1979; 63: 580–587.

Roelofsen B, Van Meer G, Op den Kamp JAF. The lipids of red cell membranes. Scan J Clin Lab Invest 1981; 41 (Suppl 156): 111–115.

Ross BM, Hudson C, Erlich J, Warsh JJ, Kish SJ. Increased phospholipid breakdown in schizophrenia: evidence for the involvement of a calcium-independent phospholipase A_2. Arch Gen Psychiatry 1997; 54: 487–494.

Rotrosen J, Wolkin A. Phospholipid and prostaglandin hypotheses of schizophrenia. In: Meltzer NY, ed. Psychopharmacology: the third generation of progress. New York: Raven Press, 1987: 759–764.

Rudin DO. The major psychoses and neuroses as omega-3 essential fatty acid deficiency syndrome: substrate pellagra. Biol Psychiatry 1981; 16: 837–850.

Sage SO, Rink TJ. Effects of ionic substitution on [Ca^{2+}] irises evoked by thrombin and PAF in human platelets. Eur J Pharmacol 1986; 128: 99–107.

Schroder T, Lempinen M, Nordling S, Kinnunen PKJ. Chlorpromazine treatment of experimental acute fulminant pancreatitis in pigs. Eur Surg Res 1981; 13: 143–151.

Seifert R, Schachtele C, Rosenthal W, Schultz G. Activation of protein kinase C by cis-trans fatty acids and its potentiation by diacylglycerol. Biochem Biophys Res Commun 1988; 154: 20–26.

Shinomura T, Asaoka Y, Oka M et al. Synergistic action of diacylglycerol and unsaturated fatty acid for protein kinase C activation: its possible implications. Proc Natl Acad Sci USA 1991; 88: 5149–5153.

Sneddon JM. Blood platelets as a model for monoamine-containing neurons. Prog Neurobiol 1973; 1: 151–198.

Stahl SM. The human platelet: a diagnostic and research tool for the study of biogenic amines in psychiatric and neurologic disorders. Arch Gen Psychiatry 1977; 34: 509–561.

Steudle A, Maras A, Gattaz WF. Platelet membrane phospholipids in schizophrenia. Schizophr Res 1994; 11: 23.

Taniguchi K, Urakami M, Takanaka K. Effects of various drugs on superoxide generation, arachidonic acid release and phospholipase A_2 in polymorphonuclear leukocytes. Jpn J Pharmacol 1988; 46: 275–284.

Vaddadi KS, Courtney P, Gillard CJ, Manku MS, Horrobin DF. A double-blind trial of essential fatty acid supplementation in patients with tardive dyskinesia. Psychiatry Res 1989; 27: 313–323.

Van Meer G, De Kruijff B, Op de Kamp JAF, Deenen LLM. Preservation of bilayer structure in human erythrocytes and erythrocyte ghosts after phospholipase treatment. A ^{31}P-NMR study. Biochim Biophys Acta 1980; 596: 1.

Wakatabe H, Tsukahara T, Ishigooka J, Miura S. Effects of chlorpromazine on phosphatidylinositol turnover following thrombin stimulation of human platelets. Biol Psychiatry 1991; 29: 965–978.

Weiss BA, Insel PA. Intracellular Ca^{2+} and protein kinase C interact to regulate α_1-adrenergic and bradykinin receptor-stimulated phospholipase A_2 activation in madin-darby canine kidney cells. J Biol Chem 1991; 266: 2126–2133.

Wyatt RJ. The dopamine hypothesis: variations on a theme (11). Psychopharmacol Bull 1986; 22: 923–927.

Yao JK, van Kammen DP. Red blood cell membrane dynamics in schizophrenia. I. Membrane fluidity. Schizophr Res 1994; 11: 209–216.

Yao JK, van Kammen DP. Incorporation of [^{3}H]arachidonic acid into platelet phospholipids of patients with schizophrenia. Prostagland Leukotr Essent Fatty Acids 1996; 55: 21–26.

Yao JK, Yasaei P, van Kammen DP. Increased turnover of platelet phosphatidylinositol in schizophrenia. Prostagland Leukotr Essent Fatty Acids 1992; 46: 39–46.

Yao JK, van Kammen DP, Welker JA, Gurklis J. Red blood cell membrane dynamics in schizophrenia. III. Correlation of fatty acid abnormalities with clinical measures. Schizophr Res 1994a; 13: 227–232.

Yao JK, van Kammen DP, Welker JA. Red blood cell membrane dynamics in schizophrenia. II. Fatty acid composition. Schizophr Res 1994b; 13: 217–226.

Yao JK, van Kammen DP, Gurklis JA. Abnormal incorporation of arachidonic acid into platelets of drug-free patients with schizophrenia. Psychiatry Res 1996; 60: 11–21.

Yoshida J, Asaoka Y, Nishizuka Y. Platelet activation by simultaneous actions of diacylglycerol and unsaturated fatty acids. Proc Natl Acad Sci USA 1992; 89: 6443–6446.

Young WE. Human monoamine oxidase: lack of brain and platelet correlation. Arch Gen Psychiatry 1986; 43: 604–609.

Part III

SCHIZOPHRENIA: MEMBRANE ABNORMALITIES

Membrane-protective Strategies in Schizophrenia: Conceptual and Treatment Issues

Ravinder Reddy and Jeffrey K. Yao

INTRODUCTION

The challenge continues to uncover the pathophysiology of mental disorders so as to develop effective treatments. Significant progress, generally in step with technological advances, has been made in understanding brain function and dysfunction. However, this has translated less well to developing effective treatments, although there are exceptions. An increasing number of 'designer' psychotropic agents have been developed and some, such as olanzapine for the treatment of psychosis, are currently in use. These drugs essentially produce effects *via* neurotransmitter receptor binding through either agonist or antagonist effects. Because of the almost exclusive emphasis on neurotransmission, neurobiological research in psychiatry has largely been limited to measuring levels and binding of various neurotransmitters. Only lately has attention been paid to other mediators of brain function, such as the lipid environment of the neuronal membrane, the membrane microenvironment of neurotransmitter receptors, and the effects of membrane composition on signal transduction. Several chapters in this book illustrate the importance of lipids to normal neuronal functioning, and, by extension, the key role that abnormalities of membrane lipids can have on impairing neuronal function, and *ipso facto* on behaviour.

It is only a matter of time before the full scope of membrane disturbance in psychiatric and neuropsychiatric disorders becomes apparent. There already is an accumulating, and consistent, body of evidence for altered concentrations of phospholipids and key essential fatty acids in schizophrenia, in both blood and brain tissue. While the debate over the existence of membrane deficits in major psychiatric and neuropsychiatric disorders is almost over, the debate over the implications of these findings for the aetiology, illness presentation, course and treatment of these disorders continues. Further, mechanisms that can lead to the observed membrane deficits are being actively explored by many laboratories. This is an important area of investigation, predicated on two assumptions: (1) elucidating the aetiological implications of membrane dysfunction is likely to take longer than identifying pathogenic mechanisms that lead to membrane dysfunction; and (2) identifying these pathogenic mechanisms can rapidly lead to utilizing existing membrane-protective strategies or developing such approaches. One recent research approach has been aimed at examining the role of free radicals in inducing the observed membrane deficits.

In this chapter, we focus primarily on schizophrenia since this disorder has attracted the most attention among investigators exploring the 'membrane hypothesis' (Horrobin et al., 1994), as well as research on mechanisms that may underlie the observed membrane dysfunction. We will very briefly (since this has been extensively done elsewhere) examine the evidence for membrane dysfunction in schizophrenia and the possible mechanisms that can lead to some of the identified membrane abnormalities. Next we will review the general principles of membrane protection, and how some of these have been applied in schizophrenia. In one sense, a discussion regarding membrane-protective strategies is ahead of its time, given the state of the evidence for the clinical relevance of membrane abnormalities. On the other hand, we contend that any treatment approach, even when used adjunctively, to improve the outcome of serious psychiatric disorders is of value to patients, their families and the community, even if the underlying pathological mechanisms are yet to be fully elucidated.

MEMBRANE DEFICITS IN SCHIZOPHRENIA

The accumulating evidence for a broad range of membrane deficits in schizophrenia is extensively reviewed in other chapters in this book. The following is a brief overview of findings pertinent to the issue at hand.

Alterations in phospholipids and polyunsaturated fatty acids

Phospholipid abnormalities have been found in the plasma or red blood cell (RBC) membranes of patients with a variety of psychoses, primarily schizophrenia. These earlier findings, reviewed by Rotrosen and Wolkin (1987), included variable alterations in levels of phosphatidylcholine (PC), phosphatidylserine (PS) and phosphatidylinositol (PI), but consistent decreases in phosphatidylethanolamine (PE) levels. These results are diverse and inconsistent due primarily to differences in patient groups and methodology. Further, these results may be confounded by the more recent finding, in chronic schizophrenic patients, of a bimodal distribution of RBC arachidonic acid (AA) and docosahexaenoic acid (DHA) (Glen et al., 1994; Peet et al., 1994), in contrast to the unimodal distribution seen in normal controls. Previous studies were in chronic schizophrenic patients. However, even in a series of recent-onset schizophrenic patients, decreased RBC PE has been found (Keshavan et al., 1993), and decreases in all four key membrane phospholipids were found in fibroblasts from similar patients (Mahadik et al., 1996).

Peet et al. (1994) reported significant decrease in RBC AA concentration in hospitalized neuroleptic-treated schizophrenic patients, relative to normal controls. Significant decreases of both AA and LA, the precursor of AA, but an increase of total n-3 fatty acids, were reported in plasma of three schizophrenic patient groups from England, Scotland, and Ireland (Horrobin et al., 1989). A similar decrease of LA, but not of AA, was reported in plasma of schizophrenic patients from Japan (Kaiya et al., 1991). Such decreases in the polyunsaturated fatty acids (PUFA) were also demonstrated in RBC membranes of schizophrenic patients (Vaddadi et al., 1989; Glen et al., 1994; Laugharne et al., 1996; Peet et al., 1996). In a clinical trial of essential fatty acid (EFA) supplementation, Vaddadi et al. (1989) confirmed their previously reported low levels of PUFA in schizophrenic patients. More recently, Yao et al. (1994) reported a significant decrease of PUFA, particularly LA and AA, in the RBC ghost membranes of schizophrenic patients on and off haloperidol treatment. Thus, a decreased level of LA in the blood of schizophrenic patients appears to be a consistent finding. There are initial data of decreased AA from fibroblasts of first-episode schizophrenic patients (Mahadik et al., 1996) and chronic schizophrenic patients (Ramchand et al., 1997). This latter finding suggests that these abnormalities are present very early in the course of the illness and are not a consequence of neuroleptic treatment. In light of the various findings of membrane defects in a variety of peripheral cell types (platelets, RBC, and fibroblasts), it has been proposed that, in schizophrenia, membrane compositional defects may occur in all cell membranes in the body, thus being detectable in both extraneural tissues as well as in the central nervous system (CNS) (Horrobin, 1996).

Alterations of brain membrane lipids

With the introduction of magnetic resonance spectroscopy (MRS) it has become possible to carry out noninvasive study of *in vivo* phosphorus metabolism in humans. Pettegrew et al. (1991, 1993) demonstrated a significant reduction of phosphomonoesters (phospholipid precursors) and significantly increased levels of phosphodiesters (phospholipid breakdown products) in the frontal cortices of neuroleptic-naïve first-episode schizophrenic patients as compared to the controls. In addition, an increased level of ATP and a decreased inorganic orthophosphate were also found in the frontal cortex of schizophrenic patients. The authors (Pettegrew et al., 1993) suggested that changes in membrane phospholipids may be related to molecular changes that precede the onset of clinical symptoms and brain structural changes in schizophrenia, while changes in high energy phosphate metabolism may be state-dependent. Other groups (Williamson et al., 1991; Fukazako et al., 1992, 1996; Deicken et al., 1993; Stanley et al., 1995) also reported findings of membrane phospholipid perturbations in both acutely and chronically ill patients. Also based on ^{31}P MRS findings, Keshavan et al. (1991) suggested a possible familial basis for membrane phospholipid changes in schizophrenia. Keshavan and Pettegrew (1997) have comprehensively reviewed the MRS methodology and findings in schizophrenia.

Direct evidence of decreased fatty acid levels comes from postmortem study of frontal cortices of schizophrenic patients relative to normal controls (Horrobin et al., 1991). We recently conducted a preliminary study of the postmortem caudate from 10 normal controls, 11 schizophrenic patients, and five psychiatric control subjects (unpublished data). There were significant differences in the concentrations of membrane phospholipid subclasses among normal, schizophrenic, and psychiatric control groups. Both PE and PC concentrations are significantly reduced in schizophrenics. Consequently, total membrane phospholipids are also significantly lower in schizophrenic than in normal or psychiatric control groups. In addition, a small but significant increase of PI concentration was found in the schizophrenic group. A robust reduction of total PUFA was found in schizophrenic brains, relative to normal or psychiatric control brains. Specifically, the decrease of PUFA was largely attributable to reduction in AA concentration and, to some extent its precursor, LA. These findings are, in part, consistent with previous reports of decreased RBC membrane fatty acids (Glen et al., 1994; Yao et al., 1994). Further, these findings support the notion that decreased membrane fatty acids in peripheral tissue may be associated with similar changes in the brain.

Oxidative stress and membrane fatty acid defects

There is substantial evidence that oxidative stress can lead directly to the type of specific membrane defects reported, and that AA is particularly susceptible to oxidative damage (Katsuki and Okuda, 1995). There is an intriguing finding in schizophrenic patients of an inverse relationship between RBC AA concentration and thiobarbituric acid reactive substances (an index of lipid peroxidation) (Peet et al., 1994). There is abundant evidence that free radicals are involved in membrane pathology in the CNS (Halliwell, 1992), and may play a role in neuropsychiatric disorders, including schizophrenia (Lohr, 1991). Several independent lines of evidence indicate the presence of oxidative stress in schizophrenia, including measures of oxidative membrane damage products, elevations of which have been reported in first-episode and chronic schizophrenic patients (reviewed in Reddy and Yao, 1996). Below is a brief review of the findings in schizophrenia, preceded by a short outline of free radical biochemistry.

What is oxidative stress?

Oxidative stress is a state in which there is a dysequilibrium between pro-oxidant processes and the antioxidant defence system in favour of the former, and generally occurs as a consequence of increased production of free radicals, or when the antioxidant defence system is inefficient, or a combination of both events. Oxidative stress, regardless of the specific cause, can result in the initiation of a number of pathophysiological processes leading to cellular toxicity.

Free radicals target cellular components indiscriminately, including lipids, proteins, DNA, and carbohydrates. Protein oxidation can lead to loss of sulphhydryl groups, in addition to modifications of amino acids, leading to the formation of carbonyl moieties. Accumulation of oxidized proteins may be involved in losses of selected biochemical and physiological functions. Free radical-mediated damage can also affect cellular macromolecules, such as DNA, by destroying pathways critical to the maintenance of normal adenine and pyridine nucleotide status. These alterations can affect the viability of DNA and modify gene expression. Lipids, by virtue of their location in cell membranes, are particularly vulnerable to peroxidation.

The origins of free radicals

A consequence of aerobic metabolism is the generation of potentially toxic free radicals, which are chemical species with unpaired electrons (primarily the reactive oxygen species, superoxide and hydroxyl radicals). They are generated *in vivo* during many normal biochemical reactions involving oxygen, including the mitochondrial electron transfer chain, NADPH-dependent oxidases, and oxidation of PUFAs and catecholamines (Kalyanaraman, 1989; Cohen, 1994; Rice-Evans, 1994). The superoxide radical generated during these reactions is catalytically dismutated to hydrogen peroxide. Although hydrogen peroxide is itself not a free radical, it is susceptible to autoxidation to yield the highly reactive hydroxyl radical, particularly in the presence of iron which is present in significant concentrations in the CNS.

Neurotransmitters as contributors to free radical burden

It is well known that dopamine (DA) metabolism yields free radicals under normal physiological conditions (Cohen, 1994). DA is susceptible to autoxidation when the antioxidant defence system (AODS) is weak (Zhang and Dryhurst, 1994). Interestingly, it has been recognized that DA-mediated toxicity is also mediated through DA actions on the N-methyl-D-aspartate (NMDA) glutamate receptors (Michel and Hefti, 1990; Cadet and Kahler, 1994; Ben-Schachar et al., 1995). There is accumulating evidence that NMDA-mediated excitotoxicity involves free radicals, such as superoxide and nitric oxide (e.g., Coyle and Puttfarcken, 1993; Patel et al., 1996). Activation of NMDA by glutamate stimulates phospholipase A_2 (PLA_2) activity to release AA to act as a second messenger, which in turn can lead to the formation of free radicals (Iuliano et al., 1994).

Mitochondrial abnormalities

Mitochondria process most of the cellular oxygen to provide energy that drives almost all metabolic processes, and also are the site of significant free radical production. About 3% of all oxygen consumed is converted to superoxide, and subsequently to hydrogen peroxide (Floyd, 1996). Thus, there is an enormous and continuous free-radical burden. Antioxidant systems keep this in check. When the equilibrium between pro-oxidant and antioxidant systems are disturbed in favour of the former, mitochondrial damage can occur. Mitochondrial membranes, similar to neuronal membranes, are vulnerable to lipid peroxidation. Any impairment in mitochondrial oxidative phosphorylation can lead to a broad range of cellular disturbances, including decreased neurotransmission, decreased DNA repair, and finally cell death. Cytochrome-c oxidase (COX, Complex IV) is a key enzyme in the mitochondrial electron transport chain. Decreased activity of this enzyme has been reported in the frontal cortex and caudate nucleus of schizophrenic patients, which was unrelated to age or the amount of mitochondrial DNA (Cavelier et al., 1995). Interestingly, COX activity is maintained by cardiolipin, a key lipid in the mitochondrial membrane, which is highly susceptible to peroxidation during oxidative stress (Radi et al., 1997). Several lines of evidence suggest decreased oxidative metabolism in some brain areas in schizophrenia (Buchsbaum et al., 1990), and may be explained in part by mitochondrial dysfunction. We propose that this is secondary to oxidative stress due either to decreased antioxidant capacity and/or increased free radical burden. There is initial evidence for this proposition. Decreased activity of the scavenging enzyme manganese-containing superoxide dismutase (Mn-SOD) in schizophrenic brains has been reported (Loven et al., 1996). Mn-SOD is a key antioxidant in mitochondria.

Defences against free radicals: the antioxidant defense system

Biological systems have evolved complex protective strategies against free radical toxicity. Under physiological conditions, the potential for free radical-mediated damage is kept in check by the AODS, comprising a series of enzymatic and nonenzymatic components. The critical antioxidant enzymes include superoxide dismutases (SOD), catalase (CAT) and glutathione peroxidase (GSHPOD). These enzymes act cooperatively at different sites in the metabolic pathway of free radicals (see Figure 7.1).

Hydrogen peroxide produced by SOD is decomposed to water and oxygen by the heme protein, CAT, thereby preventing the formation of hydroxyl radicals. Failure of this first line antioxidant defence may lead to an initiation of lipid peroxidation, the key pathological process leading to membrane lipid loss. Selenium-dependent GSHPOD protects against lipid peroxidation by converting hydrogen peroxide to water, or more critically by converting toxic hydroperoxides to less toxic alcohols. Since SOD, CAT and GSHPOD are critical to different stages of free radical metabolism, altered activity of one enzyme without compensatory changes in other enzymes may leave membranes vulnerable to damage. Thus, the differential patterning of the antioxidant enzyme activities may provide important clues to the pathogenetic mechanisms of abnormal free radical metabolism (Sohal and Orr, 1992).

The nonenzymatic antioxidant components, that may be equally important in the overall AODS, consist of molecules that react with activated oxygen species and thereby prevent the propagation of free radical chain reactions. The most common nonenzymatic antioxidant molecules are glutathione, tocopherol (vitamin E), ascorbic acid (vitamin C), β-carotene, albumin and uric acid.

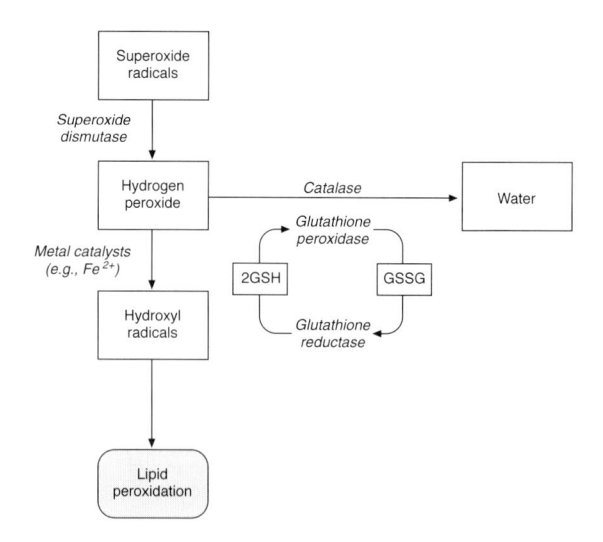

Figure 7.1. Schematic representation of the pathway leading from superoxide radicals to lipid peroxidation and the antioxidant scavenging enzymes that protect against pro-oxidant processes. Superoxide dismutase catalyses the conversion of superoxide radicals to hydrogen peroxide. Catalase and glutathione peroxidase convert hydrogen peroxide to water. Glutathione (GSH) is utilized by glutathione peroxidase in this process, yielding the oxidized form of glutathione (GSSG) which is converted back to GSH by glutathione reductase. Hydrogen peroxide is susceptible to autoxidation, particularly in presence of metal catalysts such as iron, yielding the highly reactive hydroxyl radicals that can attack membrane fatty acids, resulting in lipid peroxidation.

OXIDATIVE STRESS IN SCHIZOPHRENIA

Although a role for toxic radicals in the aetiology of schizophrenia was proposed over 40 years ago (Hoffer et al., 1954), the first study examining any index of free radical metabolism was conducted over 20 years later (Michelson et al., 1977). Subsequent studies have generally examined indirect measures of free radical activity, since direct measures of free radicals *in vivo* are difficult and cumbersome. The majority of studies have examined the activities of key antioxidant enzymes in plasma and RBC, based on the premise that alterations in enzyme activities, which are tightly coupled with free radical production, reflect oxidative stress. A few studies have examined levels of lipid peroxidation products that provide a more direct evidence of oxidative membrane damage.

Studies of antioxidant enzymes

Much of the focus has been on the key scavenging antioxidant enzymes: SOD, GSHPOD and CAT. Of these, SOD activity has been the most frequently examined. Increased SOD activity has been reported in RBC of schizophrenic patients (Michelson et al., 1977; Golse et al., 1978; Abdalla et al., 1986; Reddy et al., 1991; Wang, 1992; Vaiva et al., 1994; Khan and Das, 1997) but not by others (Sinet et al., 1983; Yao et al., 1998a). Neuroleptic-naïve first-episode schizophreniform and schizophrenic patients show both increased SOD activity (Khan and Das, 1997) and decreased SOD activity (Mukherjee et al., 1996). This discrepancy may be explained in part by the extremely short duration of illness in the study of Mukherjee et al. (1996). Alterations in SOD appear to be independent of neuroleptic treatment in some studies (Reddy et al., 1991; Yao et al., 1998a), but not others (Khan and Das, 1997). Several studies have examined the relationships between SOD activity and a variety of clinical dimensions. For example, SOD activity in chronic schizophrenic patients is inversely related to negative symptom severity (Yao et al., 1998d). On the other hand, a correlation between SOD activity and positive symptoms (SAPS score) has been observed in neuroleptic-naïve schizophrenic patients (Khan and Das, 1997). Decreased SOD activity is associated with deteriorating premorbid school functioning (Mukherjee et al., 1996) and tardive dyskinesia (Yamada et al., 1997).

GSHPOD activity was found to be lower, relative to normal controls, in neuroleptic-treated chronic schizophrenic patients (Stoklasova et al., 1986), in drug-free female schizophrenic patients (Abdalla et al., 1986) and in neuroleptic-naïve psychotic children (Golse et al., 1977). By contrast, Zhang et al. (1998) reported increased plasma GSHPOD in long-term neuroleptic-free, as well as neuroleptic-naïve, schizophrenic patients. Further, no differences were found in GSHPOD levels from skin fibroblasts of schizophrenic patients and normal controls (Zhang et al., 1998), suggesting that plasma GSHPOD elevations in patients may be state-dependent changes, and not a consequence of the course of the illness, treatment effects or neuroleptics. Human plasma GSHPOD (hpGSHPOD), an enzyme related to RBC GSHPOD, is not significantly different between schizophrenic patients and normal subjects, but is correlated with psychosis severity (Yao et al., 1999).

Decreased CAT activity has also been reported in some studies of schizophrenic patients (Glazov and Mamzev, 1976; Reddy et al., 1991, 1993), but not others (Mukherjee et al., 1996; Yao et al., 1998a). Although the above studies show abnormalities in individual antioxidant enzymes, the physiology of the AODS suggests that examining a single enzyme may have limited value for elucidating the role of abnormal free radical metabolism in disease processes (Sohal and Orr, 1992).

Studies of antioxidant molecules

Although the major contribution to the total antioxidant capacity comes from antioxidant molecules in plasma, little attention has been paid to this. McCreadie et al. (1995) found lower vitamin E:cholesterol ratios in patients compared with normal control subjects. Inpatients, whom the investigators commented were probably the most seriously disturbed, had the lowest levels. Brown et al. (1998) also found decreased lipid-corrected vitamin E levels in schizophrenic patients with tardive dyskinesia, relative to healthy controls, but not in patients without dyskinesia.

Vitamin C is widely distributed in all tissues, and is a potent antioxidant. Further, it is involved in the recycling of vitamin E. Many previous studies have found variable results. More recently, in a carefully conducted study, plasma and urinary vitamin C levels were found decreased, relative to normal controls, even after controlling for diet (Suboticanec et al., 1990). After vitamin C supplementation for one month, group differences were no longer significant. The authors suggested that vitamin C requirements for schizophrenic patients may be higher than for nonschizophrenics.

Antioxidant molecules such as albumin, uric acid, and ascorbic acid are known to account for the major contributions (>85%) to the total antioxidant capacity in human plasma. This predominance is largely due to their high concentrations relative to those of other antioxidants in blood, e.g., bilirubin, α-tocopherol, and β-carotene. The total antioxidant status (TAS) serves as an index for the state of balance from various antioxidants in plasma. Although individual antioxidants play a specific role in the AODS, these antioxidants may act cooperatively *in vivo* to provide synergistic protection to the organs against oxidative damage. We recently examined the TAS in male schizophrenic patients and matched normal controls. All patients were on regular hospital diets. TAS was significantly lower in schizophrenic patients (Yao et al., 1998b). Further, we found reductions in plasma uric acid (Yao et al., 1998c), as well as reductions in biliriubin and albumin levels in schizophrenic patients (Yao et al., 1998b).

Studies of peroxidative damage

Although there is robust evidence of altered AODS, this by itself does not indicate that membrane lipid damage has occurred. Evidence of peroxidative damage is required, and in schizophrenic patients the findings, while limited, have been consistent. Increased blood levels of malondialdehyde were found in schizophrenic patients relative to normal controls (Prilipko, 1984; Guliaeva et al., 1988; Sram and Binkova, 1992; McCreadie et al., 1995). Higher levels of thiobarbituric acid reactive substances (TBARS) and conjugated dienes (both lipid peroxidation byproducts) have been observed in patients with tardive dyskinesia (TD) (Lohr et al., 1990), and correlated with dyskinesia severity (Peet et al., 1993; Brown et al., 1998). More critically, there is evidence of plasma lipid peroxidation at the onset of psychosis in never-medicated, first-episode schizophrenic patients (Mahadik et al., 1998). These findings, if replicated, suggest that oxidative stress may be occurring very early in the course of illness, and independent of treatment. Increased concentrations of pentane, another marker of lipid peroxidation, have also been reported in schizophrenic patients relative to normal controls (Kovaleva et al., 1989; Phillips et al., 1993).

Findings in the brain

There have been, to date, two published accounts of the postmortem study of SOD activity in schizophrenia. A recent study found increased activity of manganese-SOD, a key antioxidant enzyme in mitochondria, in the temporal and frontal cortices (Loven et al., 1996). An earlier study, that examined only the diencephalon, found no differences between schizophrenic patients and control subjects (Wise et al., 1974). Indirect evidence, suggestive of oxidative stress, has been reported in electron microscope studies of brains from schizophrenics, including large amounts of lipofuscin-like material in oligodendrocytes (Miyakawa et al., 1972), abnormal pigment-laden neurones (Averback, 1981), and axonal deposits of lipofuscin-like bodies (Senitz and Winkelmann, 1981). Lipofuscin is a by-product of lipid peroxidation. While some studies have reported gliosis, a potential response to neuronal loss, in schizophrenic patients others have not (Roberts, 1991). However, cell death is not the only consequence of oxidative stress, which more often leads to sublethal membrane abnormalities, and subsequent neuronal dysfunction.

Clinical implications of oxidative stress in schizophrenia

The behavioural consequences of alterations in neuronal membranes, secondary to oxidative stress, have to be understood within the context of as yet undetermined specific neuronal substrates of behaviour. In one key brain area implicated in schizophrenia – the prefrontal cortex – there is evidence of both phospholipid abnormality (e.g., Pettegrew et al., 1993) and impaired free radical metabolism (Loven et al., 1996). Since PUFAs are preferentially vulnerable to free radical insult, it is conceivable that there also exists membrane pathology in the implicated areas. In spite of the absence of contemporaneous evidence of brain membrane deficits and oxidative stress, there exist highly suggestive associations between membrane abnormalities, oxidative stress and clinical phenomenon in schizophrenia (Reddy and Yao, 1996). We hypothesize that oxidative stress, primarily by inducing membrane dysfunction, leads to 'down-stream' behavioural disturbances (Figure 7.2). If the putative pathological events are indeed shown to be of clinical significance in schizophrenia, then the possibility exists of protecting neuronal membranes against free radical insults.

MEMBRANE-PROTECTIVE STRATEGIES: GENERAL PRINCIPLES

The recognition that free radical pathology occurs in schizophrenia, and that this may underlie membrane deficits, provides an opportunity for therapeutic interventions. The methods for such interventions already exist, either in the clinical armamentarium (e.g., vitamin E) or in the laboratory (e.g., lazaroids). The impetus for the use of antioxidants in the treatment of schizophrenia was initially based on the proposal that TD, a chronic movement disorder in schizophrenia, may be a consequence of free radical pathology (Cadet and Lohr, 1989). This has turned out to be a nice example of theory-driven treatment development. There are a number of approaches one can take to providing membrane

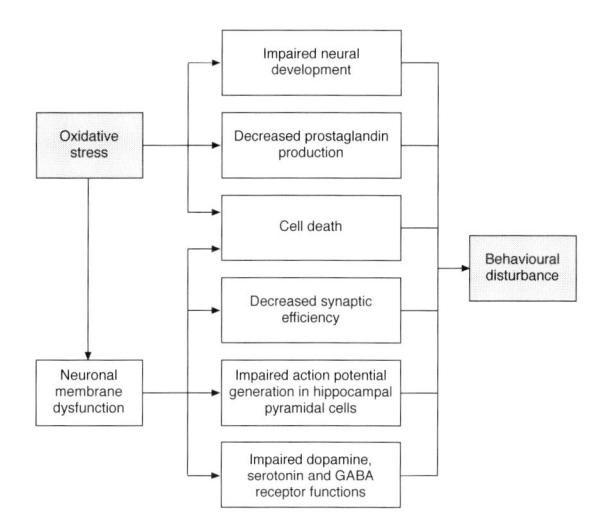

Figure 7.2. Scheme depicting mechanisms that may mediate neuronal dysfunction and subsequent behavioural disturbance.

protection, including decreasing free radical production, scavenging excess free radicals, and stabilizing membranes. Our focus is primarily on oxygen-derived radicals.

Decreasing free radical formation

Oxidative stress can be reduced by decreasing the substrates for free radical formation and by inhibiting enzymatic mechanisms that generate free radicals. Exogenous factors that modify free radical production and antioxidant status include diet, smoking, pollution, and possibly a sedentary lifestyle. It has been observed that caloric intake is correlated with oxidative stress, particularly in the brain (Sohal et al., 1994), and high caloric intake is associated with decreased maximal longevity, presumably due to oxidative stress. By contrast, decreased caloric intake in animals is associated with increased maximal longevity, and maintenance of cognitive and motor skills for longer duration. It is unclear whether total calorie intake or the origin of the calories makes a difference in the generation of free radicals. Diets high in fats and iron (e.g., from red meat) can increase free radical production. The role of alcohol in free radical production may be due to its adding to the total calorie intake; its direct pro-oxidant effects are probably also significant. Smoking is well known to induce oxidative stress, the effects of which are probably mediated through free radical generation (Bridges et al., 1993; Halliwell, 1993).

Free radical scavenging

Scavenging is the interception of free radicals. It involves both enzymatic and nonenzymatic mechanisms, as noted above. The key antioxidant enzyme is SOD, which converts two moles of superoxide to hydrogen peroxide. Exogenous SOD, in the form of polyethylene glycol-conjugated form (PEG-SOD), has been utilized in hypoxia–reperfusion models (e.g., Uyama et al., 1992). However, exogenous SOD cannot cross the blood–brain barrier, a fact that has limited its utility as a practical free radical scavenger (Hall, 1997).

Hydroxyl radicals are highly reactive, and will react with almost any chemical species with which they come in to contact. Therefore, achieving specificity of action as a hydroxyl radical scavenger is difficult. However, a group of compounds known as lazaroids have been shown to decrease hydroxyl radical levels in animal models of ischaemia (Hall et al., 1994). Lazaroids, such as tirilazad, are nonglucocorticoid 21-aminosteroids. The effectiveness of lazaroids as hydroxyl radical scavengers may lie in their ability to localize in areas where these radicals are produced (Hall et al., 1992).

Membrane stabilization

Once lipid peroxidation is initiated by free radicals, the only intervention available is to interrupt the chain reaction to limit its propagation along the membrane. This can be achieved by two mechanisms: scavenging peroxyl radicals and decreasing membrane fluidity. A key, and much investigated, peroxyl radical scavenger is vitamin E (α-tocopherol).

Vitamin E is a highly efficient lipid-soluble 'chain-breaking' antioxidant that acts to stabilize plasma membranes. It is located entirely within membranes, which may explain the high degree of scavenging efficiency. It appears to be a particularly effective membrane stabilizer of phospholipids with high concentrations of PUFAs, such as PE (Therond et al., 1996). Numerous studies in animals and humans have demonstrated protective effects of vitamin E against a large variety of free radical-mediated pathological insults (Burton and Ingold, 1989; Beuttner, 1993; Packer, 1994).

Combining approaches

Although our understanding of the mechanisms involved in free radical generation and defences against oxidative stress continues to evolve, our understanding of the specific free radical mechanisms mediating neuronal injury is limited. As shown in Figure 7.3,

Table 7.1. Controlled studies of vitamin E in schizophrenia and tardive dyskinesia.

Study and subjects	Study design	Vitamin E dose	Results and comments
Lohr et al. (1987) n = 25 11M; 4F 44 years (19–71) TD 2.6 ± 1.9 years	DB CO	400 IU/day to 1200 IU/day over 2 weeks, then 1200 IU/day for 2 weeks for each treatment	AIMS scores mean ↓43%; 7 patients ↓50%. Vitamin E plasma levels ↑100%. Some BPRS items improved. 50% improvement in patients with shorter TD duration and later age at illness onset.
Elkashef et al. (1990) n = 8 7M; 1F 57 years (18–75) TD 3.8 ± 2.8 years	DB CO	Week 1, 400 IU/day, week 2, 800 IU/day, weeks 3–4, 1200 IU/day, then crossover	AIMS score ↓6.75 (SD 3.9). >30% improvement in 5 patients. Most improvement in buccolingual movements and dystonia. No change in BPRS. Patients had neuroleptic treatment for >15 years.
Schmidt et al. (1991) n = 19 (inpatients) 9M; 10F 45 years (21–88) TD <2 months (2) <1 year (7) >1 year (10)	DB CO	1200 mg/day	No global differences in AIMS scores. ↓AIMS scores significant in group receiving Vitamin E before placebo. ↓Symptoms (unspecified) significant.
Shriqui et al. (1992) n = 27 22Sz; 5Bp 43 years (19–69) TD ?	DB CO	400 IU/day for 6 weeks	74% of patients had been ill for more than 10 years. No significant changes in AIMS scores or EPS.
Egan et al. (1992) n = 18 44 years TD 5.9 years	DB CO	Week 1, 400 IU/day; week 2, 800 IU/day; week 3, 1200 IU/day; weeks 4–6, 1600 IU/day	No significant changes in AIMS scores or other ratings (BPRS, SANS). ↑Vitamin E plasma levels. ↓18.5% in AIMS scores of patients with TD <5 years. Clinical improvements significant for individual patients.
Adler et al. (1993) n = 28 27Sz; 27M; 1F 58 years TD ?	DB PG	400 IU bid for 2 weeks, then 800 IU bid for 6–10 weeks	AIMS score ↓32.5% (SD 28). 55% improvement in patients with TD <5 years *versus* 27% in patients with TD ≥ 5 years. Diarrhoea in 1 patient.
Akhtar et al. (1993) n = 32 TD ?	DB PG	Week 1, 600 mg/day weeks 2–4, 1200 mg/day	↓TDRS score significant.
Peet et al. (1993) n = 14 11M; 3F Chronic Sz TD ?	OL(br)	400 IU/day for 1 month; 11 patients followed up with AIMS after 7–13 months	↓AIMS significant. Plasma TBARS and AIMS scores correlated pretreatment but not after Vitamin E treatment. No relationship between neuroleptic dose and AIMS score.

Table 7.1. (continued)

Study and subjects	Study design	Vitamin E dose	Results and comments
Lohr (1993)			
n = 33 TD ?	DB PG	1600 IU/day for 8 weeks	AIMS scores ↓34%. ↓Severity of TD, if TD duration <5 years.
Dabiri et al. (1994)			
n = 11 6M; 5F 51 years (35–68) TD ?	DB nonCO	Week 1, 400 IU/day week 2, 800 IU/day weeks 3–12, 1200 IU/day	AIMS scores ↓36%. Neither age nor sex were predictors of improvement. Response independent of TD duration. Most improvement in buccolingual and limb dyskinesia.
Lam et al. (1994)			
n = 12 12Sz 62 ± 13 years TD ?	DB CO	Week 1, 400 IU/day; week 2, 800 IU/day; weeks 3–6, 1200 IU/day	Mean duration of illness, 20 years No significant change in AIMS scores. No changes in BPRS scores. Long duration of illness and possibly of TD may account for these findings.
Lohr and Caligiuri (1996)			
n = 35 33M; 2F TD ?	DB PG	1600 IU/day for 2 months	Modified AIMS scores ↓24%. (AIMS scores ↓35%, if TD duration <5 years, *versus* ↓11% if duration >5 years). Significant reduction in BPRS psychosis ratings in vitamin E group. No change in parkinsonism.
Dorevitch et al. (1997)			
n = 45 23M; 17F 64 years (32—80) TD >5 years (all except 1 patient)	DB CO	Week 1, 400 IU/day; week 2, 800 IU/day; week 3, 1200 IU/day weeks 4–8, 1600 IU/day	No significant change in AIMS scores. No change in BPRS ratings.
Adler et al. (1998)			
n = 40 (25 completed the entire trial)	DB PG	1600 IU/day for 36 weeks	↓AIMS score significant over the course of treatment. Treatment response significantly associated with shorter TD duration and lower antipsychotic dose. Study provides evidence for efficacy and safety of long-term treatment with Vitamin E for TD.

n, number of patients in the study; M, male; F, female; Sz, schizophrenic; Bp, bipolar; TD, tardive dyskinesia (mean duration); TDRS = Tardive Dyskinesia Rating Scale; IU, international units; DB, double-blind; CO, crossover; PG, parallel groups; OL(br), open-label, blind raters; AIMS, Abnormal Involuntary Movement Scale; BPRS, Brief Psychiatric Rating Scale; SANS, Scale for Assessment of Negative Symptoms; TBARS, Thiobarbituric acid reactive substances; ↑, increased; ↓, decreased.

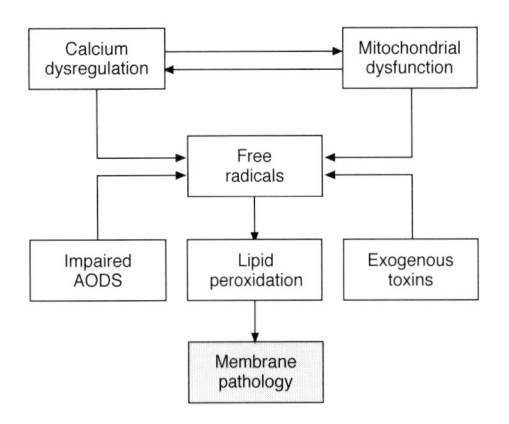

Figure 7.3. Simple schematic depiction of the multiple interactions between independent pathological processes that can lead to free radical generation and subsequent membrane pathology.

complex interactions between multiple factors converge to cause membrane pathology. In the absence of definite pathophysiological models, approaches to neuroprotection need to be rather broad and overinclusive. Since free radical pathology typically involves a cascade of events, each of the several steps contributing to an end result of neuronal membrane damage, the most effective strategies may involve interventions that reduce free radical generation as well as improve antioxidant efficiency.

ANTIOXIDANT TREATMENT IN SCHIZOPHRENIA

The use of antioxidants in schizophrenia has been almost exclusively limited to the use of vitamin E in the treatment of TD. Indirect, but persuasive evidence for a role of free radicals in TD comes from treatment studies with vitamin E (Reddy and Yao, 1996). Supranormal doses of vitamin E have been safely and effectively used to reduce the severity of TD. Several studies, albeit with relatively small sample sizes, have utilized double-blind random-assignment design, with and without crossover. Most of these studies, but not all, show that vitamin E treatment reduces TD severity (Table 7.1). A shorter duration of TD was associated with better therapeutic response. Most studies utilized a dose range of 1200–1600 IU/day. However, Peet et al. (1993) found a clinically significant response with 1200 IU/day, with the therapeutic effect maintained for 7–13 months after discontinuation of vitamin E. While most studies have been relatively brief (<12 weeks), Adler et al. (1998) conducted a 36-week study that showed robust effects of vitamin E in reducing dyskinesia severity. By contrast, the largest ($n = 158$) and longest (12 months) study to date (not yet published, but discussed by Lohr and Lavori, 1998) has shown reductions in dyskinesia severity in both treatment and placebo groups, but not significantly different between the two groups. In one study, significant decreases in psychiatric symptoms were found in schizophrenic patients following vitamin E treatment (Sram and Binkova, 1992). If indeed free radicals play a role in the development of TD, patients with inadequate AODS would be more likely to develop TD.

FUTURE DIRECTIONS

While it is tempting to begin treating all patients with some form of membrane-protective modality, such as antioxidants, it would be prudent to establish firm evidentiary foundations before doing so. There is a need to identify factors that modify, adversely or beneficially, the as yet unknown pathophysiology of schizophrenia.

For example, it would be important to know whether there are dietary factors that modify the illness, given that all of the antioxidants have to be consumed. High-calorie diets are associated with increased medical morbidity. By contrast, lower caloric intake in animals is associated with decreased oxidative stress and increased maximal life span (Sohal et al., 1994). It is interesting to note that lower total calories (as well as lower animal fats) was associated with better outcome in schizophrenic patients in developing countries (Christensen and Christensen, 1988); it is conceivable that lower caloric intake resulted in decreased free radical burden and decreased severity of membrane deficits. There may be other environmental and demographic factors that modify oxidative stress (Bridges et al., 1993), including cigarette smoking (Reddy et al., 1998), alcohol consumption (Nordmann et al., 1992), environmental pollutants (Papas, 1996), and comorbid medical conditions. These factors could interact with the pre-existing AODS abnormalities in schizophrenia to increase oxidative stress.

There remain significant gaps in the information necessary to develop sound intervention principles. With the exception of studies of vitamin E in the treatment of TD (Junker et al., 1992), no useful or recent antioxidant treatment trials exist for schizophrenia. Given the widespread use of multivitamin preparations and the availability everywhere of dietary antioxidants, it may be necessary to conduct clinical trials using pharmaceutical antioxidants, such as α-lipoic acid, that will increase the possibility of maximal between-group differences. Further, it is unclear whether any specific symptom complex or outcome variable would be a target for treatment with membrane-protective agents. It is possible that membrane-protective strategies may be most beneficial as nonspecific modifiers of the clinical course of the illness, increasing the likelihood of a favourable outcome. In particular, schizophrenic patients who have poor clinical outcome may benefit most from such interventions. It is possible to identify patients, early in the course of illness, who have general risk factors for poor outcome, such as an early age of onset, long pretreatment duration of psychosis, poor response to treatment, and so on. Such patients could be treated with a variety of membrane-protective methods to mitigate the possibility of poor outcome.

There is evidence of improved clinical state, albeit modest, with EFA supplementation in schizophrenia (reviewed in Mahadik and Evans, 1997). This strategy is based on the fairly consistent evidence that there are a variety of membrane deficits in schizophrenia, as discussed above and comprehensively reviewed elsewhere in this book. If indeed oxidative stress leads to these membrane deficits, then there may be merit in combining membrane-protective approaches, such as antioxidants, and EFA supplementation. The efficacy of a combined antioxidant and EFA supplementation strategy may be greater than either approach alone. Testing such a proposal is eminently feasible, utilizing a double-blind, random-assignment approach.

Independent of whether or not antioxidants or other membrane-protective strategies are utilized in future for the treatment of schizophrenia, there remains the task of untangling the complex relationships between oxidative stress, membrane deficits and pathophysiology in schizophrenia. In particular, relations between oxidative stress and membrane deficits need to be determined contemporaneously. With few exceptions, human studies have examined separately either the various indices of oxidative stress or measures of membrane pathology. Further, animal studies will need to be employed to clarify the cascade of events leading from free radical generation to membrane deficits. Findings from such investigations will determine the design and methodology of studies that will need to be conducted in patients. For example, longitudinal, within-subject, repeated-measures studies of first-episode and early-course schizophrenic patients will be necessary to examine relationships between oxidative stress, membrane deficits and clinical outcome. These studies will provide the quantitative clinical outcome measures that will help develop controlled treatment trials of membrane-protective agents. It is clear that the development of a rational approach to membrane-protective treatments will require systematic investigation and multidisciplinary collaborative effort.

ACKNOWLEDGEMENTS

This work was supported in part by the National Alliance for Research in Schizophrenia and Affective Disorders (NARSAD) Young Investigator Award (RR) and a Veterans Administration Merit Review grant (JKY).

REFERENCES

Abdalla DSP, Manteiro HP, Olivera JAC, Bechara CH. Activities of superoxide dismutase and glutathione peroxidase in schizophrenic and manic depressive patients. Clin Chem 1986; 32: 805–807.

Adler LA, Peselow E, Rotrosen J et al. Vitamin E treatment of tardive dyskinesia. Am J Psychiatry 1993; 150: 1405–1407.

Adler LA, Edson R, Lavori P et al. Long-term treatment effects of vitamin E for tardive dyskinesia. Biol Psychiatry 1998; 43: 868–872.

Akhtar S, Jajor TR, Kumar S. Vitamin E treatment of tardive dyskinesia. J Postgrad Med 1993; 39: 124–126.

Averback P. Structural lesions of the brain of young schizophrenics. Can J Neurol Sci 1981; 8: 73–76.

Ben-Schachar D, Zuk B, Glinka Y. Dopamine neurotoxicity: inhibition of mitochondrial respiration. J Neurochem 1995; 64: 718–723.

Beuttner GR. The pecking order of free radicals and antioxidants: lipid peroxidation, alpha-tocopherol, and ascorbate. Arch Biochem Biophys 1993; 300: 535–543.

Bridges AB, Scott NA, Parry GJ, Belch JJ. Age, sex, cigarette smoking and indices of free radical activity in healthy humans. Eur J Med 1993; 2: 205–208.

Brown K, Reid A, White T et al. Vitamin E, lipids, lipid peroxidation products and tardive dyskinesia. Biol Psychiatry 1998; 43: 863–867.

Buchsbaum MS, Neuchterlein KH, Haier RJ et al. Glucose metabolic rate in normals and schizophrenics during the continuous performance test assessed by positron emission tomography. Br J Psychiatry 1990; 156: 217–227.

Burton GW, Ingold KU. Vitamin E as an *in vitro* and *in vivo* oxidant. Ann N Y Acad Sci 1989; 570: 7–22.

Cadet JL, Kahler LA. Free radical mechanisms in schizophrenia and tardive dyskinesia. Neurosci Biobehav Rev 1994; 18: 457–467.

Cadet JL, Lohr JB. Possible involvement of free radicals in neuroleptic-induced movement disorders: evidence from treatment of tardive dyskinesia with vitamin E. Ann N Y Acad Sci 1989; 570: 176–185.

Cavelier L, Jazin EE, Eriksson I et al. Decreased cytochrome-c oxidase activity and lack of age-related accumulation of mitochondrial DNA deletions in the brains of schizophrenics. Genomics 1995; 29: 217–224.

Christensen O, Christensen E. Fat consumption and schizophrenia. Acta Psychiatr Scand 1988; 78: 587–591.

Cohen G. Enzymatic/nonenzymatic sources of oxyradicals and regulation of antioxidant defences. Ann N Y Acad Sci 1994; 738: 8–14.

Coyle JT, Puttfarcken P. Oxidative stress, glutamate, and neurodegenerative disorders. Science 1993; 262: 689–695.

Dabiri LM, Pasta D, Darby JK, Mosbacher D. Effectiveness of vitamin E for treatment of long-term tardive dyskinesia. Am J Psychiatry 1994; 151: 925–926.

Deicken RF, Merrin E, Calabrese G, Dillon W, Weiner MW, Fein G. ^{31}Phosphorus MRSI of the frontal and parietal lobes in schizophrenia. Biol Psychiatry 1993; 33: 46A.

Dorevitch A, Kalian M, Shlafman M, Lerner V. Treatment of long-term tardive dyskinesia with vitamin E. Biol Psychiatry 1997; 41: 114–116.

Egan MF, Hyde TM, Albers GW et al. Treatment of tardive dyskinesia with vitamin E. Am J Psychiatry 1992; 149: 773–777.

Elkashef AM, Ruskin PE, Bacher N, Barrett D. Vitamin E in the treatment of tardive dyskinesia. Am J Psychiatry 1990; 147: 505–506.

Floyd RA. Mitochondrial damage in neurodegenerative disease. In: Packer L, Hiramatsu M, Yoshikawa T, eds. Free radicals in brain physiology and disorders. Berlin: Academic Press, 1996: 313–329.

Fukuzako H, Takeuchi K, Fujimoto T et al. ^{31}P magnetic resonance spectroscopy of schizophrenic patients with neuroleptic resistant positive and negative symptoms. Biol Psychiatry 1992; 31: 204A–205A.

Fukuzako H, Fukuzako T, Takeuchi K et al. Phosphorus magnetic resonance spectroscopy in schizophrenia: correlation between membrane phospholipid metabolism in temporal lobe and positive symptoms. Prog Neuropsychopharmacol Biol Psychiatry 1996; 20: 629–640.

Glazov VA, Mamzev VP. Catalase in the blood and leucocytes in patients with nuclear schizophrenia. Zh Nevropatol Psikhiatr 1976; 4: 549–552.

Glen AIM, Glen EMT, Horrobin DF et al. A red cell membrane abnormality in a subgroup of schizophrenic patients: evidence for two diseases. Schizophr Res 1994; 12: 53–61.

Golse B, Debray-Ritzen P, Puget K, Michelson AM. Dosages de la superoxyde dismutases 1 plaquettaire dans les pychoses infantiles de développement. Nouv Pr Méd 1977; 6: 2449.

Golse B, Debray Q, Puget K, Michelson AM. Dosages érythrocytaires de la superoxyde dismutases 1 et de la glutathion peroxydase dans les schizophrénies de l'adulte. Nouv Pr Med 1978; 7: 2070–2071.

Guliaeva NV, Levshina IP, Obidin AM. Indices of lipid free-radical oxidation and the antiradical protection of the brain – the neurochemical correlates of the development of the general adaptation syndrome. Zh Vyssh Nerv Deiat 1988; 38: 731–737.

Hall ED. Antioxidant therapeutic strategies in CNS disorders. In: Connor A, ed. Metals and oxidative damage in neurological disorders. New York: Plenum Press, 1997: 325–339.

Hall ED, Yonkers PA, Andrus PK, Cox JW, Anderson DK. Biochemistry and pharmacology of lipid antioxidants in acute brain and spinal cord injury. J Neurotrauma 1992; 9 (Suppl): 425–442.

Hall ED, McCall JM, Means ED. Therapeutic potential of the lazaroids (21-aminosteroids) in CNS trauma, ischemia, and subarachinoid hemorrhage. Adv Pharmacol 1994; 28: 221–268.

Halliwell B. Reactive oxygen species and the central nervous system. J Neurochem 1992; 59: 1609–1623.

Halliwell B. Cigarette smoking and health: a radical view. J R Soc Health 1993; 113: 91–96.

Hoffer A, Osmond H, Smythies J. Schizophrenia: a new approach. J Ment Sci 1954; 100: 29–25.

Horrobin DF. Schizophrenia as a membrane lipid disorder which is expressed throughout the body. Prostagland Leukotr Essent Fatty Acids 1996; 55: 3–7.

Horrobin DF, Manku MS, Morse-Fisher N, Vaddadi KS. Essential fatty acids in plasma phospholipids in schizophrenics. Biol Psychiatry 1989; 25: 562–568.

Horrobin DF, Manku MS, Hillman S, Glen AIM. Fatty acid levels in brains of schizophrenics and normal controls. Biol Psychiatry 1991; 30: 795–805.

Horrobin DF, Glen AIM, Vaddadi K. The membrane hypothesis of schizophrenia. Schizophr Res 1994; 13: 195–207.

Iuliano L, Pedersen JZ, Pratico D, Rotilio G, Violi F. Role of hydroxyl radicals in the activation of human platelets. Eur J Biochem 1994; 221: 695–704.

Junker D, Steigleider P, Gattaz WF. Alpha-tocopherol in the treatment of tardive dyskinesia. Clin Neuropharmacol 1992; 15 (Suppl): 639B.

Kaiya H, Horrobin DF, Manku MS, Morse-Fisher N. Essential and other fatty acids in plasma in schizophrenics and normal individuals from Japan. Biol Psychiatry 1991; 30: 357–362.

Kalyanaraman B. Free radicals from catecholamine hormones, neuromelanins, and neurotoxins. In: Miquel J, Quintanilha AT, Weber H, eds. Handbook of free radicals and antioxidants in biomedicine. Vol I. Boca Raton: CRC Press, 1989: 147–159.

Katsuki H, Okuda S. Arachidonic acid as a neurotoxic and neurotrophic substance. Prog Neurobiol 1995; 46: 607–636.

Keshavan MS, Pettegrew JW. Magnetic resonance spectroscopy in schizophrenia and psychotic disorders. In: Krishnan KRR, Doraiswamy PM, eds. Brain imaging in clinical psychiatry. New York: Marcell-Dekker Inc., 1997: 381–400.

Keshavan MS, Pettegrew JW, Panchalingam K, Kaplan D, Bozik E. ^{31}P NMR spectroscopy detects altered brain metabolism before onset of schizophrenia. Arch Gen Psychiatry 1991; 48: 1112–1113.

Keshavan MS, Mallinger AG, Pettegrew JW, Dippold C. Erythrocyte membrane phospholipids in psychotic patients. Psychiatry Res 1993; 49: 89–95.

Khan NS, Das I. Oxidative stress and superoxide dismutase in schizophrenia. Biochem Soc Trans 1997; 25: 418S.

Kovaleva ES, Orlov ON, Tsutsul'kovskia MIA, Vladimirova TV, Beliaev TS. Lipid peroxidation processes in patients with schizophrenia. Zh Nevropatol Psikhiatr 1989; 89: 108–110.

Lam LCW, Chiu HFK, Hung SF. Vitamin E in the treatment of tardive dyskinesia: a replication study. J Nerv Ment Dis 1994; 182: 113–114.

Laugharne JDE, Mellor JE, Peet M. Fatty acids and schizophrenia. Lipids 1996; 31 (Suppl): S163–S165.

Lohr JB. Oxygen radicals and neuropsychiatric illness: some speculations. Arch Gen Psychiatry 1991; 48: 1097–1106.

Lohr JB. Vitamin E treatment of tardive dyskinesia. Presented at the Annual Meeting of the American Psychiatry Association. San Francisco, CA, USA, May 1993.

Lohr JB, Caligiuri MP. A double-blind placebo-controlled study of vitamin E in the treatment of tardive dyskinesia. J Clin Psychiatry 1996; 57: 167–173.

Lohr JB, Lavori P. Whither vitamin E and tardive dyskinesia? Biol Psychiatry 1998; 43: 861–862.

Lohr JB, Cadet JL, Lohr MA, Jeste DV, Wyatt RJ. Alpha-tocopherol in tardive dyskinesia. Lancet 1987; i: 913–914.

Lohr JB, Kuczenski R, Bracha HS, Moir M, Jeste DV. Increased indices of free radical activity in the cerebrospinal fluid of patients with tardive dyskinesia. Biol Psychiatry 1990; 28: 535–539.

Loven DP, James JF, Biggs L, Little K. Increased manganese-superoxide dismutase activity in postmortem brain from neuroleptic-treated psychotic patients. Biol Psychiatry 1996; 40: 230–232.

Mahadik SP, Evans DR. Essential fatty acids in the treatment of schizophrenia. Drugs Today 1997; 33: 5–17.

Mahadik SP, Mukherjee S, Correnti EE, Scheffer R. Plasma membrane phospholipid fatty acid composition of cultured skin fibroblasts from schizophrenic patients: comparison with bipolar and normal controls. Psychiatry Res 1996; 63: 133–142.

Mahadik SP, Mukherjee S, Scheffer R, Correnti EE, Mahadik JS. Elevated plasma lipid peroxides at the onset of nonaffective psychosis. Biol Psychiatry 1998; 43: 674–679.

McCreadie RG, MacDonald E, Wiles D, Campbell G, Paterson JR. The Nithsdale Schizophrenia Surveys. XIV. Plasma lipid peroxide and serum vitamin E levels in patients with and without tardive dyskinesia, and in normal subjects. Br J Psychiatry 1995; 167: 610–617.

Michel PP, Hefti F. Toxicity of 6-hydroxydopamine and dopamine for dopaminergic neurons in culture. J Neurosci Res 1990; 76: 428–435.

Michelson AM, Puget K, Durosay P, Bouneau JC. Clinical aspects of the dosage of erythrocuprein. In: Michelson AM, McCord JM, Fridovich I, eds. Superoxide and superoxide dismutase. London: Academic Press, 1977: 467–499.

Miyakawa T, Sumiyoshi S, Deshimaru M. Electron microscopic study on schizophrenia. Mechanism of pathological changes. Acta Neuropathol (Berl) 1972; 20: 67–77.

Mukherjee S, Mahadik SP, Correnti EE, Scheffer R, Kelkar H. Impaired antioxidant defense system at the onset of psychosis. Schizophr Res 1996; 19: 19–26.

Nordmann R, Ribiere C, Rouach H. Implication of free radical mechanisms in ethanol-induced cellular injury. Free Radic Biol Med 1992; 12: 219–240.

Packer L. Vitamin E is nature's master antioxidant. Sci Am Sci Med 1994; 1: 54–63.

Papas AM. Determinants of antioxidant status in humans. Lipids 1996; 31: S77–S82.

Patel M, Day BJ, Crapo JD, Fridovich I, McNamara JO. Requirement for superoxide in excitotoxic cell death. Neuron 1996; 16: 345–355.

Peet M, Laugharne J, Rangarajan N, Reynolds GP. Tardive dyskinesia, lipid peroxidation, and sustained amelioration with vitamin E treatment. Int Clin Psychopharmacol 1993; 8: 151–153.

Peet M, Laugharne JDE, Horrobin DF, Reynolds GP. Arachidonic acid: a common link in the biology of schizophrenia? Arch Gen Psychiatry 1994; 51: 665–666.

Peet M, Laugharne JDE, Mellor J, Ramchand CN. Essential fatty acid deficiency in eyrthrocyte membranes from chronic schizophrenic patients, and the clinical effects of dietary supplementation. Prostagland Leukotr Essent Fatty Acids 1996; 55: 71–75.

Pettegrew JW, Keshavan MS, Panchalingam K et al. Alterations in brain high-energy phosphate and membrane phospholipid metabolism in first-episode drug-naïve schizophrenics. A pilot study of the dorsal prefrontal cortex by in vivo phosphorus-31 nuclear magnetic resonance spectroscopy. Arch Gen Psychiatry 1991; 48: 563–568.

Pettegrew JW, Keshavan MS, Minshew NJ. [31]P nuclear magnetic resonance spectroscopy: neurodevelopment and schizophrenia. Schizophr Bull 1993; 19: 35–53.

Phillips M, Sabas M, Greenberg J. Increased pentane and carbon disulfide in the breath of patients with schizophrenia. J Clin Pathol 1993; 46: 861–864.

Prilipko LL. Activation of lipid peroxidation under stress and in schizophrenia. In: Kemali D, Morozov PV, Toffano G, eds. New research strategies in biological psychiatry. Biological psychiatry – new perspectives. Vol 3. London: John Libbey, 1984: 254–258.

Radi R, Castro L, Rodriguez M, Cassina A, Thomson L. Free radical damage to mitochondria. In: Beal MF, Howell N, Bodis-Wollner I, eds. Mitochondria and free radicals in neurodegenerative diseases. New York: Wiley-Liss, 1997: 57–89.

Ramchand CN, Das I, Ramchand R, Lee KH, Peet M. Biochemical alterations associated with membrane pathology in schizophrenia. A study using fibroblasts from schizophrenics. Schizophr Res 1997; 24: 66–67.

Reddy R, Yao JK. Free radical pathology in schizophrenia: a review. Prostagland Leukotr Essent Fatty Acids 1996; 55: 33–43.

Reddy R, Mahadik SP, Mukherjee S, Murthy JN. Enzymes of the antioxidant defense system in chronic schizophrenic patients. Biol Psychiatry 1991; 30: 409–412.

Reddy R, Kelkar H, Mahadik SP, Mukherjee S. Abnormal erythrocyte catalase activity in schizophrenic patients. Schizophr Res 1993; 9: 227.

Reddy R, van Kammen DP, Yao JK. Cigarette smoking and antioxidant status in schizophrenia. Biol Psychiatry 1998; 43: 112S–113S.

Rice-Evans CA. Formation of free radicals and mechanisms of action in normal biochemical processes and pathological states. In: Rice-Evans CA, Burdon RH, eds. Free radical damage and its control. Amsterdam: Elsevier, 1994: 131–153.

Roberts GW. Schizophrenia: a neuropathological perspective. Br J Psychiatry 1991; 158: 8–17.

Rotrosen J, Wolkin A. Phospholipid and prostaglandin hypotheses of schizophrenia. In: Meltzer H, ed. Psychopharmacology: the third generation of progress. New York: Raven Press, 1987: 759–764.

Schmidt M, Meister P, Baumann P. Treatment of tardive dyskinesia with vitamin E. Eur Psychiatry 1991; 6: 201–207.

Senitz D, Winkelmann E. Über morphologische Befunde in der orbitofrontalen Rinde bei Menschen mit schizophrenen Psychosen. Eine golgi-und eine elektonenoptische Studie. Psychiatr Neurol Med Psychol 1981; 33: 1–9.

Shriqui CL, Bradwejn J, Annable L, Jones BD. Vitamin E in the treatment of tardive dyskinesia: a double-blind placebo-controlled study. Am J Psychiatry 1992; 149: 391–393.

Sinet PM, Debray Q, Carmagnol F, Pelicier Y, Nicole A, Jerome H. Normal erythrocyte SOD values in two human diseases: schizophrenia and cystic fibrosis. In: Greenwald RA, Cohen G, eds. Oxy radicals and their scavenger systems. Vol. II: Cellular and medical aspects. New York: Elsevier, 1983: 302–304.

Sohal RS, Orr WC. Relationship between antioxidants, prooxidants, and the aging process. Ann N Y Acad Sci 1992; 663: 74–84.

Sohal RS, Ku HH, Agarwal S, Forster MJ, Lal H. Oxidative damage, mitochondrial oxidant generation and antioxidant defenses during aging and in response to food restriction in the mouse. Mech Ageing Dev 1994; 74: 121–133.

Sram RJ, Binkova B. Side-effects of psychotropic therapy. In: Packer L, Prilipko L, Christen Y, eds. Free radicals in the brain. Berlin: Spinger-Verlag, 1992: 153–166.

Stanley JA, Williamson PC, Drost DJ et al. An *in vivo* study of the prefrontal cortex of schizophrenic patients at different stages of illness *via* phosphorus magnetic resonance spectroscopy. Arch Gen Psychiatry 1995; 52: 399–406.

Stoklasova A, Zapletalek M, Kudrnova K, Randova Z. Glutathione peroxidase activity of blood in chronic schizophrenics. Sb Ved Pr Lek Fak Univerzity Hradci Kralove 1986; 29 (Suppl 1–2): 103–108.

Suboticanec K, Folnegovic-Smalc V, Korbar M, Mestrovic B, Buzina R. Vitamin C status in chronic schizophrenia. Biol Psychiatry 1990; 28: 959–966.

Therond P, Couturier M, Demelier JF, Lemonnier F. Hydroperoxides of erythrocyte phospholipid molecular species formed by lipoxygenase correlate with alpha-tocopherol levels. Lipids 1996; 31: 703–708.

Uyama O, Matsuyama T, Michishita H, Nakamura H, Sugita M. Protective effects of human recombinant superoxide dismutase on transient ischemic injury on CA1 neurons in gerbils. Stroke 1992; 23: 75–81.

Vaddadi KS, Courtney P, Gilleard CJ, Manku MS, Horrobin DF. A double-blind trial of essential fatty acid supplementation in patients with tardive dyskinesia. Psychiatry Res 1989; 27: 313–323.

Vaiva G, Thomas P, Leroux JM, Cottencin O, Dutoit D, Erb F. Erythrocyte superoxide dismutase (eSOD) determination in positive moments of psychosis. Thérapie 1994; 49: 343–348.

Wang H. An investigation on changes in blood CuZn-superoxide dismutase contents in type I, II schizophrenics. Chung Hua Shen Ching Ching Shen Ko Tsa Chih 1992; 25: 6–8.

Williamson PC, Drost D, Stanley J, Carr T, Morrison S, Merskey H. Localized phosphorus-31 magnetic resonance spectroscopy in chronic schizophrenic patients and normal controls. [Letter] Arch Gen Psychiatry 1991; 48: 578.

Wise CD, Baden MM, Stein L. Post-mortem measurement of enzymes in human brain: evidence of a central noradrenergic deficit in schizophrenia. J Psychiatr Res 1974; 11: 185–198.

Yamada K, Kanba S, Anamizu S et al. Low superoxide dismutase activity in schizophrenic patients with tardive dyskinesia. Psychol Med 1997; 27: 1223–1225.

Yao JK, van Kammen DP, Welker JA. Red blood cell membrane dynamics in schizophrenia. II. Fatty acid composition. Schizophr Res 1994; 13: 217–226.

Yao JK, Reddy R, McElhinny LG, van Kammen DP. Effect of haloperidol on antioxidant defense system enzymes in schizophrenia. J Psychiatr Res 1998a; 32: 385–391.

Yao JK, Reddy R, McElhinny LG, van Kammen DP. Reduced status of plasma total antioxidant capacity in schizophrenia. Schizophr Res 1998b; 32: 1–8.

Yao JK, Reddy R, van Kammen DP. Reduced level of plasma antioxidant uric acid in schizophrenia. Psychiatry Res 1998c; 80: 29–39.

Yao JK, Reddy R, van Kammen DP, Reddy R, Kelley ME. Superoxide dismutase and negative symptoms in schizophrenia. Biol Psychiatry 1998d; 43: 123S–124S.

Yao JK, Reddy R, van Kammen DP. Plasma specific glutathione peroxidase and symptom severity in schizophrenia. Biol Psychiatry 1999, in press.

Zhang F, Dryhurst G. Effects of l-cysteine on the oxidative chemistry of dopamine: new reaction pathways of potential relevance to idiopathic Parkinson's disease. J Med Chem 1994; 37: 1084–1098.

Zhang ZJ, Ramchand CN, Ramchand R, Milner E, Telang SD, Peet M. Glutathione peroxidase (GSHPx) activity in plasma and fibroblasts from schizophrenics and control. Biol Psychiatry 1998; 29: 103–104.

Membrane Abnormalities in Schizophrenia as Revealed by Tyrosine Transport

8

Lars Bjerkenstedt, Gunnar Edman and Frits-Axel Wiesel

INTRODUCTION

Before the introduction of neuroleptics, the only treatment effective in schizophrenia was insulin coma therapy, described 1935 in a monograph by Sakel entitled 'Neue Behandlingsmethode der Schizofreni'. The antipsychotic mechanism for this treatment has never been explained. However, one would expect that there should be a linkage between some of the insulin effects and pathophysiological findings in schizophrenic patients, and it has been suggested that this may be related to the fact that, in experimental animals, insulin treatment results in an excessive removal by the muscle of branched-chain amino acids from plasma (Fernstrom and Wurtman, 1972a,b; Munro et al., 1975). The passage of tyrosine, the precursor to dopamine, from plasma to brain is thereby facilitated. The corresponding process may, presumably, also take place in humans.

There are indications of disturbed monoamine metabolism in the brains of untreated schizophrenic patients. An alteration of dopaminergic transmission in the brains of schizophrenic patients has been postulated (Carlsson and Lindqvist, 1963; Randrup and Munkvad, 1965; van Rossum, 1966), and it has been suggested that the dopamine neurones projecting to the prefrontal cortex are involved in the pathogenesis of schizophrenia.

Dopamine is synthesized from the precursor amino acid, tyrosine. Recent experimental studies have also suggested that variations in brain tyrosine levels can significantly affect higher cortical functions subserved by the prefrontal cortex (Tam and Roth, 1997).

In a meta-analysis (Tuckwell and Koziol, 1993), the dopamine metabolite, homovanillic acid (HVA), has been shown to be significantly reduced in lumbar cerebrospinal fluid (CSF) in schizophrenics, compared to healthy controls. The HVA content in lumbar CSF has been shown to derive almost exclusively from the brain (Curzon et al., 1971; Post et al., 1973; Young et al., 1973; Gordon et al., 1975). Therefore, a reduced lumbar HVA level should, in all probability, reflect reduced central dopamine metabolism. The reason for reduced dopamine turnover is unknown. Quite recently, parkinsonism has also been observed in neuroleptic-naïve schizophrenic patients, suggesting that extrapyramidal motor signs may be part of schizophrenia (Caligiuri et al., 1993). These findings indicate reduced dopamine turnover in schizophrenia. In this chapter we will present results demonstrating that tyrosine transport in schizophrenia is disturbed, and that this may be due to cell membrane abnormalities affecting dopamine turnover.

AMINO ACIDS

Transport and brain levels

There are 23 amino acids (Table 8.1). Some of these can be synthesized in the body and are thus referred to as nonessential, while others, the essential amino acids, cannot be synthesized and must therefore be absorbed in the intestine from ingested food and distributed *via* the circulatory system.

In the human body, the amino acids have three main functions: they are the building blocks for protein synthesis; they act as transmitters; and they are precursors to the monoamines. It is in this latter role that the amino acids will mainly be referred to in the present chapter.

The precursor amino acid for dopamine and noradrenaline synthesis is tyrosine, and for serotonin synthesis tryptophan. Together with phenylalanine, these are called aromatic amino acids. Amino acids are polar molecules and cannot pass across membranes by passive diffusion but must be actively transported. In competition with three other large neutral amino acids (LNAAs), valine, isoleucine, and leucine (often referred to as branched-chain amino acids), the aromatic amino acids use a common transport system, the L-system

Table 8.1. Essential and nonessential amino acids and transport by the L-system.

Amino acid	L-system transport[a]
Essential	
Isoleucine	+
Leucine	+
Lysine	(+)
Methionine	(+)
Phenylalanine	+
Threonine	
Tryptophan	(+)
Valine	+
Nonessential	
Alanine	
α-Aminobutyrate	
Arginine	
Aspartate	
Aspargine	
Cysteine	
Glutamate	
Glutamine	
Glycine	
Histidine	(+)
Ornithine	
Proline	
Serine	
Taurine	
Tyrosine[b]	+

[a] + = L-system involved; (+) = L-system partly involved.
[b] Essential for the brain.

(where L is the abbreviation for 'large') (Pardridge and Oldendorf, 1977; Fernstrom and Faller, 1978). The L-system uses a so-far unidentified protein which is present in the membranes of all cells of the human body. Phorbol ester-induced membrane proteins, characterized in β-lymphocytes from chronic leukaemic patients, have quite recently been presented as candidate proteins for the L-system amino acid carrier (Woodlock et al., 1993). The L-system is specific for the six LNAAs, while other amino acids are transported by other systems. The transport from plasma to brain can be described as a passage facilitated by carrier molecules present in the endothelial cells lining brain capillaries, i.e., the blood-brain barrier.

In humans, the brain is the only organ for which amino acid transport is limited, so that competition occurs at physiological plasma concentrations (Pardridge and Oldendorf, 1977). For the brain, tyrosine and tryptophan are essential and must be absorbed by the intestine, i.e., transported over the intestinal mucosa (the first membrane passage), further transported over the capillary membrane (second membrane passage), and, finally, transported over the blood-brain barrier (third membrane passage) to the brain.

Accordingly, central monoamine turnover is partly regulated by the availability of tyrosine and tryptophan in plasma (Fernstrom and Wurtman, 1972a; Fernstrom and Faller, 1978). This has been demonstrated in experimental animals. Thus, a strong positive relationship has been found between the ratio of plasma tyrosine to plasma levels of the competing five amino acids (tryptophan, phenylalanine, valine, isoleucine, and leucine), and the brain levels of tyrosine (Fernstrom and Wurtman, 1972a). In other words, the pattern of LNAAs in the periphery may influence central monoamine metabolism. By studying the amino acid balance in plasma and the lumbar HVA levels simultaneously, an even more reliable measure of central dopamine metabolism can be achieved.

Influences on levels of LNAAs

The concentration of the LNAAs has been demonstrated to show a diurnal rhythm (Wurtman, et al., 1968; Eriksson et al., 1989). Besides affecting the concentrations of each LNAA, the diurnal rhythm will also influence their transport. Peak levels are observed in the afternoon and evening, and falling levels in the middle of the night period. Thus, when comparing levels of amino acids from different individuals, it is important to hold constant the time of day when blood samples are drawn.

Concentrations of alanine and glutamine are also dependent on muscle activity. Besides inborn errors of metabolism, latent alcoholism and starving could also influence amino acid levels. Finally, in females the concentrations of amino acids vary in accordance with the menstrual cycle phase, and with the intake of oral contraceptives (Möller, 1981).

Plasma levels and CSF monoamine metabolites

When the amino acids have reached the plasma pool, two membrane passages (that in the intestinal mucosa and that in the arterial capillaries) have taken place. So far, to our knowledge, no methods for studying the first passage have been applied. In the early 1980s our research group decided to study the third membrane passage, i.e., the relationship between plasma amino acids and CSF monoamine metabolites, in both schizophrenic patients and healthy controls.

One crucial question was the selection of the control group. Some earlier studies had, in that respect, used other patient groups, such as neurological patients; in other studies the controls were badly defined. We recruited healthy control subjects who had been thoroughly investigated, both clinically and biochemically, and who showed no clinically significant deviations from normal values in laboratory tests. The healthy volunteers were recruited from medical students, staff personnel and their friends. None had a history of mental illness. The healthy subjects all obtained ratings below 1.0 for all the items on the Comprehensive Psychopathological Rating Scale (CPRS) (Åsberg et al., 1978); such values are considered to be within the normal range for healthy subjects (Bjerkenstedt et al., 1978). The control group was treated, as far as possible, in the same way as the patients, i.e., they were admitted to the hospital, given an ordinary hospital diet, and instructed not to use alcohol or drugs in the 3 days before the investigation. In total, 65 (50 men and 15 women) healthy controls were recruited.

The patients ($n = 37$; 21 men and 16 women) all fulfilled the Research Diagnostic Criteria (RDC) (Spitzer et al., 1978) for schizophrenia, had been hospitalized for 3–14 days before the study, and had not taken any neuroleptic drugs during the preceding 2 weeks. Accordingly, the patients were in a psychotic state.

Samples of blood and lumbar CSF were taken between 08:00 and 09:00 after the subjects had been resting in bed for at least 8 h and fasting for 12 h. This is the definition of 'basal level'.

Compared to the healthy controls, the schizophrenic patients showed significant deviation in the basal levels of 10 amino acids in plasma (Table 8.2), among which four (phenylalanine, valine, leucine, and isoleucine) were elevated and transported by the L-system. In view

Table 8.2. Levels of amino acids (μmol/l) in the plasma of male and female healthy volunteers (HV) and schizophrenic patients (SP); means ± SD. Data from Bjerkenstedt et al. (1985).

Amino acid	Group	Men	Women	p
Alanine	HV	320 ± 87	346 ± 64	<0.001
	SP	392 ± 111	355 ± 113	
Glutamine	HV	632 ± 83	518 ± 89	<0.05
	SP	572 ± 116	517 ± 78	
Histidine	HV	90 ± 9	86 ± 9	<0.05
	SP	84 ± 11	64 ± 14	
Isoleucine	HV	68 ± 11	53 ± 7	<0.001
	SP	77 ± 14	64 ± 15	
Leucine	HV	159 ± 23	120 ± 11	<0.01
	SP	171 ± 30	141 ± 26	
Lysine	HV	189 ± 27	161 ± 21	<0.001
	SP	206 ± 29	186 ± 28	
Methionine	HV	25 ± 6	22 ± 4	<0.05
	SP	27 ± 7	26 ± 7	
Phenylalanine	HV	60 ± 7	52 ± 5	<0.01
	SP	64 ± 8	57 ± 8	
Taurine	HV	61 ± 17	42 ± 12	<0.001
	SP	67 ± 20	68 ± 14	
Valine	HV	257 ± 39	210 ± 19	<0.05
	SP	273 ± 45	232 ± 44	

Volunteers, 50 men and 15 women; schizophrenic patients, 21 men and 16 women.

Table 8.3. Levels of monoamine metabolites (pmol/ml) in the cerebrospinal fluid of male and female healthy volunteers (HV) and schizophrenic patients (SP); means ± SD. Data from Bjerkenstedt et al. (1985).

Monoamine metabolite	Group	Men	Women	p
HVA	HV	174 ± 75.2	202 ± 94.0	<0.01
	SP	110 ± 68.6	167 ± 74.5	
MHPG	HV	43.3 ± 7.2	42.1 ± 4.0	<0.05
	SP	44.6 ± 9.6	50.5 ± 7.4	
5-HIAA	HV	89.7 ± 34.2	94.7 ± 36.1	ns
	SP	75.8 ± 34.7	100.3 ± 27.1	

HVA = homovanillic acid; MHPG = 3-methoxy-4-hydroxy-phenylglycol; 5-HIAA = 5-hydroxyindole acetic acid. Volunteers, 50 men and 15 women; schizophrenic patients, 21 men and 16 women.

of the competition between LNAAs for transportation from plasma to the brain, it would be expected that tyrosine, the plasma precursor amino acid for dopamine, should be reduced in the brain, resulting in lower CSF levels of HVA. As can be seen from Table 8.3, this was also the case.

When correlating the plasma levels of the four elevated LNAAs with the levels of HVA, an interesting relationship was found. In the patient group, but not in the healthy subjects, there were significant and negative correlations between HVA and the plasma amino acid levels (Table 8.4). Thus, the higher the plasma levels of L-amino acids competing with tyrosine for transportation from plasma to brain, the lower the lumbar HVA levels. Apparently, a reduced transport of tyrosine can be assumed. It should be noted that six of the seven amino acids with elevated levels (all except taurine) in the schizophrenic patients are transported by the L-system. A change in the affinity of the L-system for its competing amino acids, or a decrease in its overall capacity, might be possible explanations for the observed deviations in plasma amino acids in schizophrenia. Disturbed amino acid transport may be a pathogenetic mechanism in the development of schizophrenia.

TYROSINE TRANSPORT

Transport in human cells

As has been emphasized above, all cell membranes of the human body contain transport systems for amino acids. In human genetics, fibroblasts have, for several years, been used for studying genetic traits (Gazzola et al., 1981). Thus, it should be possible to study the proposed transport defect using fibroblasts.

In a first *in vitro* study, skin biopsies were obtained from 10 male schizophrenic patients and compared with samples from seven healthy controls (Hagenfeldt et al., 1987). A significant isolated decrease in tyrosine transport velocity (V_{max}) was found in the schizophrenics (Table 8.5) but no significant difference in the value of the affinity constant (K_m). Furthermore, no difference in the overall capacity of the L-system was observed.

The finding of an isolated decrease in the value of V_{max} for tyrosine is not easily reconciled with present knowledge about amino acid transport mechanisms. The kinetic factors for other amino acids transported by the L-system or other systems were all unaffected. All attempts to explain the decreased transport capacity for tyrosine uptake in cells from schizophrenic patients in terms of amino acid transport has failed (Wiesel et al., 1994). Interestingly enough, a recent study by Ramchand and colleagues (Ramchand et al., 1996) has confirmed a reduced uptake of tyrosine across the membranes of fibroblasts in schizophrenics.

Of special interest is whether the changed V_{max} was receptor-mediated or not. Using the fibroblast technique, we therefore studied the effects of psychotropic drugs (Table 8.6) on tyrosine transport using the same cell lines (Wiesel et al., 1994). Tyrosine uptake was determined without drugs and also at three different concentrations of psychotropic drugs, and was found to be influenced only at very high drug concentrations. At therapeutic concentrations, no differences were found in tyrosine uptake in cell lines from schizophrenic patients and those from normal controls, and thus no support was provided for the view that receptor interaction might explain the

Table 8.4. Product-moment correlations between concentrations of MHPG, HVA and 5-HIAA in CSF and amino acids in the plasma of healthy volunteers (HV) and schizophrenic patients (SP). Data from Bjerkenstedt et al. (1985).

Amino acid	MHPG HV	MHPG SP	HVA HV	HVA SP	5-HIAA HV	5-HIAA SP
Alanine	+0.14	−0.24	+0.19	−0.11	+0.24	+0.04
α-Aminobutyrate	+0.21	−0.25	0.00	−0.27	+0.02	−0.29
Arginine	+0.26*	−0.18	+0.02	−0.15	+0.11	−0.08
Aspartate	+0.01	−0.12	+0.01	−0.21	+0.08	−0.24
Aspargine	+0.41†	+0.28	−0.01	−0.06	+0.12	−0.19
Cysteine	+0.23	−0.27	+0.13	+0.02	+0.19	+0.15
Glutamate	−0.05	−0.14	0.00	−0.09	+0.05	−0.02
Glutamine	+0.34**	−0.28	−0.08	−0.30	−0.02	−0.10
Glycine	+0.20	−0.11	+0.16	−0.14	+0.11	+0.04
Histidine	+0.21	−0.10	0.00	−0.17	+0.05	−0.06
Isoleucine	+0.35**	−0.10	−0.06	−0.44**	−0.04	−0.32*
Leucine	+0.36**	−0.24	−0.15	−0.51†	−0.07	−0.44**
Lysine	+0.25*	−0.12	−0.14	−0.33*	0.00	−0.27
Methionine	+0.33*	−0.12	+0.04	−0.36*	+0.06	−0.15
Ornithine	−0.02	−0.03	−0.18	−0.08	−0.12	0.00
Phenylalanine	+0.38**	−0.30	−0.07	−0.35*	+0.01	−0.42**
Proline	+0.32**	−0.12	+0.05	−0.15	+0.12	−0.05
Serine	+0.17	0.00	+0.06	−0.06	+0.05	+0.15
Taurine	+0.38**	+0.01	−0.03	+0.07	+0.02	+0.11
Threonine	+0.12	−0.39*	+0.13	−0.29	+0.21	−0.32*
Tryptophan	+0.33**	+0.01	0.00	+0.12	+0.11	+0.10
Tyrosine	+0.37**	−0.25	+0.06	−0.19	+0.16	−0.20
Valine	+0.33**	−0.09	−0.05	−0.36*	+0.02	−0.38**

$p <$: *0.05; **0.01; †0.001.

change in V_{max}. It appears likely that this finding reflects a more general alteration in plasma membrane function. Membrane abnormalities have, in earlier studies, been implicated in the aetiology of schizophrenia (Meltzer et al., 1980; Hitzemann, et al., 1984).

Transport across the blood–brain barrier

A change in membrane characteristics may have different functional effects, depending on the cell type. Neurones, and particularly dopaminergic neurones, may be more susceptible to disturbances in tyrosine transport, resulting in decreased dopamine synthesis in these cells and a change in dopaminergic transmission in schizophrenia. However, *in vitro* results are not immediately transferable to *in vivo* conditions. Therefore, a

Table 8.5. V_{max} values (nmol/min/mg protein) of amino acid transport in cultured fibroblasts from healthy volunteers (HV) and schizophrenic patients (SP); means ± SD. Data from Hagenfeldt et al. (1987).

Amino acid	SP	HV
Glycine	4.9 ± 2.7	3.9 ± 1.1
L-leucine	8.9 ± 1.0	8.0 ± 1.9
L-phenylalanine	4.8 ± 0.6	4.2 ± 1.1
L-tryptophan	4.6 ± 0.9	4.6 ± 1.1
L-tyrosine	4.5 ± 0.9**	7.8 ± 2.1

**In comparison with the corresponding value for healthy volunteers, $p < 0.01$ (Student's 2-tailed t test).

Table 8.6. Effect of incubation with different concentrations of psychiatric drugs on the uptake of L-tyrosine in fibroblasts from healthy volunteers (HV) and schizophrenic patients (SP). Data are presented as percentages of the uptake of L-[^{3}H]tyrosine in fibroblasts incubated without the psychiatric drug; the L-tyrosine concentration was 0.3 mmol/l. Data from Wiesel et al. (1994).

Drug	Group	n	10^{-6}	10^{-3}	1.0
Chlorpromazine	HV	1	86	68	2
	SP	1	82	61	0
Haloperidol	HV	3	96	83	0.2
	SP	1	117	94	2.0
Imipramine	HV	2	83	62	0
	SP	1	72	51	0
Insulin	HV	1	102	96	99
	SP	1	78	89	111
Isoproterenol	HV	2	98	100	102
	SP	4	104	108	118
Lithium	HV	1	76	73	61
	SP	3	86	91	70
D-propranolol	HV	1	86	77	59
	SP	1	100	101	30
L-propranolol	HV	1	87	90	0
	SP	1	83	96	0
Sulpiride	HV	4	77	80	75
	SP	2	77	72	70
Terbutaline	HV	1	83	111	123
	SP	1	75	102	119

Concentration (mmol/l)

study of the transport of tyrosine into the schizophrenic brain should be of the utmost interest.

In an *in vivo* study, the influx of tyrosine into the brains of five male neuroleptic-free schizophrenic patients and five male healthy controls was investigated using the positron emission tomography (PET) technique (Wiesel et al., 1991). The influx (I) is the product of the rate constant (K_1) of the in-transport and the tyrosine concentration in arterial plasma (C_a). The relationship between K_1, V_{max}, C_a and K_m is described in the following equation, implying that K_1 decreases with increasing concentrations of tyrosine:

$$K_1 = V_{max}/(C_a + K_m)$$

The PET investigation was performed in the morning (11:00) using L-[1-^{11}C]tyrosine. Fibroblasts were also taken by biopsy, and V_{max} was calculated for the tyrosine uptake.

The tyrosine influx into the brain was significantly reduced in the schizophrenics as compared to the healthy controls. No significant difference in K_1 was found (Wiesel et al., 1991). The most probable explanation of the reduced influx was the significantly lower concentration of tyrosine in plasma of the schizophrenic group. In the healthy subjects there appeared to be a relationship between an increase in the concentration of tyrosine and a corresponding reduction in the value of K_1, and *vice versa* (according to the equation). In the schizophrenic group, however, this relationship could not be analyzed because of the small range in tyrosine concentrations (Wiesel et al., 1991).

The existence of a disturbance in tyrosine transport

Table 8.7. The transport of tyrosine from plasma to the whole brain in healthy volunteers (HV) and schizophrenic patients (SP), according to a two-compartment model. Data from Wiesel et al. (1991).

Group	Tyrosine (nmol/ml)	K_1 (ml/g/min)	Influx rate ($K_1 \times C_a$) (nmol/g/min)
HV	44	0.080	3.50
	55	0.037	2.05
	60	0.058	3.47
	61	0.046	2.80
	78	0.039	3.02
Means	*60*	*0.052*	*2.97*
± SD	*± 12.3*	*± 0.018*	*± 0.59*
SP	41	0.047	1.91
	43	0.049	2.12
	43	0.035	1.49
	44	0.061	2.70
	45	0.034	1.52
Means	*43**	*0.045*	*1.95**
± SD	*± 1.5*	*± 0.011*	*± 0.50*

Whole brain was made up from the five highest slices; cerebellum, inferior temporal poles, gyri recti, and the vertex of the cortical surface were not included. Tyrosine kinetics were determined from data collected between 1 and 3.5 min after tracer injection. The patients had significantly lower tyrosine concentrations and influx rates than the healthy volunteers. The out-transport rate constant (k_2) values (min^{-1}) were 0.057 ± 0.051 in the healthy volunteers and 0.020 ± 0.035 in the schizophrenic patients (means ± SD). C_a = arterial concentration of tyrosine. *In comparison with the corresponding mean ± SD for healthy volunteers, $p < 0.05$ (Student's 2-tailed *t* test). The influx rates were decreased in all slice levels constituting the whole brain.

was further strengthened by the replication of a reduced V_{max} for tyrosine uptake in fibroblasts (Table 8.7) in this same patient group (Wiesel et al., 1994).

Accordingly, a disturbance of tyrosine transport has been demonstrated *in vitro* as well as *in vivo*. Together, the results support the hypothesis that schizophrenia is a systemic disorder with a primary disturbance in cell membrane function.

As mentioned above, the relationship between K_1 and C_a, as expressed in the formula, seemed to hold for healthy individuals but not for schizophrenics. In order to elucidate further the physiological mechanisms regulating tyrosine transport in schizophrenia compared to healthy controls, another PET study, including two PET investigations in the same day, i.e., before (at 09:00) and after (at 11:00) tyrosine loading, was performed in five patients and five healthy subjects (Wiesel et al., 1999). By this means, it should be possible to test the hypothesis that tyrosine concentrations in normals, but not in patients, influence the kinetics of transport. The reason for tyrosine loading was also to exclude the possibility that the LNAAs competing with tyrosine for transport might influence the results – which could have been the case in the PET study described above (Wiesel et al., 1991). The tyrosine loading should block the transportation of the other LNAAs from plasma to brain. The clinical condition of the patients had been stabilized with neuroleptic treatment before the participation in the study. The first PET investigation was done at 09:00, after which tyrosine was administered orally. The plasma tyrosine levels were increased by a factor of 3.0 after 2 h, when the second PET investigation was performed.

Comparing K_1 for the schizophrenics and the healthy controls, a significant reduction in the value of this parameter was found to have taken place in the healthy controls but not in the schizophrenics. The results are consistent with the prevailing notion that the brain's transport system for neutral amino acids works close to saturation in healthy subjects but probably not in schizophrenics. This finding of disturbed transport in schizophrenia is also suggestive of a cell membrane dysfunction.

TREATMENT OF SCHIZOPHRENIA WITH L-DOPA AND TYROSINE

As has been pointed out above, schizophrenia seems to involve a hypodopaminergic condition. An increase in central dopamine synthesis can be achieved by L-dopa or tyrosine treatment, and might be expected to have an alleviating effect on schizophrenia. However, the outcome of L-dopa treatment of schizophrenia is inconsistent between studies. The behavioural effects of L-dopa in schizophrenic patients were first studied about 25 years ago in a study by Angrist et al. (1973), who reported that a worsening of symptoms occurred in a majority of the patients. In two other studies (Gerlach and Lühdorf, 1975; Owens et al., 1990), the effect of L-dopa treatment in combination with conventional neuroleptics was partly successful. Without inducing or aggravating productive, accessory symptoms, L-dopa was effective against emotional withdrawal, blunted affect, tendency to isolation, and apathy. These studies, however, used a combination of L-dopa and neuroleptics. Accordingly, no definitive conclusions could be drawn regarding the effects of L-dopa treatment *per se*.

Low concentrations of serum tyrosine have been reported in neuroleptic-free patients whose schizophrenia was of early onset, suggesting a disturbance of the balance between tyrosine and phenylalanine (Wei et al., 1995). The consequence of this finding, in accordance with the results mentioned earlier regarding competition between amino acids for brain uptake, should be a reduced influx of tyrosine from plasma to brain (Bjerkenstedt et al., 1985; Wiesel et al., 1991). In a double-blind crossover (2 × 3 weeks) study in which schizophrenic patients received a combination of L-tyrosine (10 g/day) and neuroleptics, or placebo and neuroleptics (Deutsch et al., 1994), no significant improvement was conferred by L-tyrosine, in spite of significantly elevated plasma levels of tyrosine.

However, to our knowledge, the use of tyrosine *per se* to treat schizophrenia over a longer period of time has not been investigated, and an examination of the efficacy of such treatment would, therefore, be of great interest.

STUDIES OF MUSCLE CELLS IN SCHIZOPHRENIA

There are also other diseases in which membrane dysfunction occurs, e.g., myotonic dystrophy. This muscle disease is of special interest for schizophrenia research since it also affects the mental state of the patients, manifesting a personality disturbance during adolescence in addition to the muscle symptoms. Muscle biopsies from these patients are morphologically pathological.

Since the late 1960s, Meltzer and colleagues have reported elevated serum creatinine kinase activity in psychotic patients during acute phases (Meltzer, 1968, 1976). Moreover, the same group have found increased branching of subterminal motor nerves in psychotic patients (Meltzer and Crayton, 1974).

On the basis of this knowledge and the proposed membrane dysfunction in schizophrenia, we investigated muscle cells morphologically in eight untreated and eight neuroleptic-treated male schizophrenic patients (Borg et al., 1987). The main findings were a spectrum of pathological changes, including atrophic fibres, central nuclei, 'moth-eaten' fibres, 'ring' fibres, fibre splitting, and subsarcolemmal and intermyofibrillar glycogen droplets. The neuromuscular abnormalities could not be attributed to medication or drug abuse.

CONCLUSIONS

Disturbed tyrosine transport may be considered as marker for a membrane dysfunction in schizophrenia or as a pathophysiological mechanism behind the disease.

A related question is whether schizophrenia is one syndrome or a heterogeneous group of diseases. We assume that it is not a collection of separate and unrelated diseases but a single underlying entity with diverse expression. If it is one syndrome, the challenge is to identify the nature and function of the genes (Crow, 1995). It could also be hypothesized that virus infections and/or anoxia during the foetal period could result in membrane dysfunction.

Bearing in mind that disturbed tyrosine transport may be a marker of membrane dysfunction it is worth considering when and how it might appear. It could be a genetic phenomenon. It has, for example, been reported that skin fibroblasts from schizophrenic patients have an abnormal growth (Mukherjee et al., 1994), and this could indicate a coincidence between genetic factors regulating growth (protein synthesis/ neurodevelopment) and tyrosine uptake.

The importance of amino acid balance in the periphery (i.e., plasma) is demonstrated by a recent study of major depression, in which it was found that treatment with a tryptophan-free mixture of amino acids produced a relapse of depressive symptomatology within 7 h in recovered patients vulnerable to the disorder (Smith et al., 1997). It seems as though a continuous and balanced influx of essential amino acids, such as tyrosine and tryptophan, from plasma to brain, is a requisite for normal brain function.

Accordingly, in the near future our research group will start an open study in which schizophrenic patients will be treated with tyrosine alone; this study will encompass a longer period of time and will use the PET technique to evaluate biochemical effects.

REFERENCES

Angrist B, Sathananthan G, Gershon S. Behavioral effects of L-dopa in schizophrenic patients. Psychopharmacologia 1973; 31: 1–12.

Åsberg M, Perris C, Schalling D, Sedvall G. The CPRS – development and applications of a psychiatric rating scale. Acta Psychiatr Scand Suppl 1978; 271: 5–69.

Bjerkenstedt L, Härnryd C, Grimm V, Gullberg B, Sedvall G. A double-blind comparison of melperone and thiotixene in psychotic women using a new rating scale, the CPRS. Arch Psychiatrie Nervenkrank 1978; 226: 157–172.

Bjerkenstedt L, Edman G, Hagenfeldt L, Sedvall G, Wiesel FA. Plasma amino acids in relation to cerebrospinal fluid monoamine metabolites in schizophrenic patients and healthy controls. Br J Psychiatry 1985; 147: 276–282.

Borg J, Edström L, Bjerkenstedt L, Wiesel FA, Farde L, Hagenfeldt L. Muscle biopsy findings, conduction velocity and refractory period of single motor nerve fibres in schizophrenia. J Neurol Neurosurg Psychiatry 1987; 50: 1644–1655.

Caligiuri MP, Lohr JB, Jeste DV. Parkinsonism in neuroleptic-naïve schizophrenic patients. Am J Psychiatry 1993; 150: 1343–1348.

Carlsson A, Lindqvist M. Effect of chlorpromazine or haloperidol on formation of 3-methoxytyramine and normetanephrine in mouse brain. Acta Pharmacol Toxicol 1963; 20: 140–144.

Crow T. A continuum of psychosis, one human gene, and not much else – the case for homogeneity. Schizophr Res 1995; 17: 135–145.

Curzon G, Gumpert EJ, Sharpe DM. Amine metabolites in the lumbar cerebrospinal fluid of humans with restricted flow of cerebrospinal fluid. Nature 1971; 231: 189–191.

Deutsch S, Rosse RB, Schwartz BL, Banay-Schwartz M, McCarthy MF, Johri SK. L-Tyrosine pharmacotherapy of schizophrenia: preliminary data. Clin Neuropharmacol 1994; 17: 53–62.

Eriksson T, Voog L, Wålinder J, Eriksson TE. Diurnal rhythm in absolute and relative concentrations of large neutral amino acids in human plasma. J Psychiatry Res 1989; 23: 241–249.

Fernstrom JD, Faller DV. Neutral amino acids in the brain: changes in response to food ingestion. J Neurochem 1978; 30: 1531–1538.

Fernstrom JD, Wurtman RJ. Brain serotonin content: physiological regulation by plasma neutral amino acids. Science 1972a; 178: 414–416.

Fernstrom JD, Wurtman RJ. Elevation of plasma tryptophan by insulin in rat. Metabolism 1972b; 21: 337–342.

Gazzola GC, Dall'Asta V, Franchi-Gazzola R, White MF. The cluster-tray method for rapid measurement of solute fluxes in adherent cultured cells. Analyt Biochem 1981; 115: 368–374.

Gerlach J, Lühdorf K. The effect of L-dopa on young patients with simple schizophrenia, treated with neuroleptic drugs. A double-blind cross-over trial with Madopar and placebo. Psychopharmacologia 1975; 44: 105–110.

Gordon E, Perlow M, Oliver J, Ebert M, Kopin I. Origins of catecholamine metabolites in monkey cerebrospinal fluid. J Neurochem 1975; 25: 347–349.

Hagenfeldt L, Bjerkenstedt L, Venizelos N, Wiesel FA. Decreased tyrosine transport in schizophrenic patients. Life Sci 1987; 41: 2749–2757.

Hitzemann R, Hirschowitz J, Garver D. Membrane abnormalities in the psychoses and affective disorders. J Psychiatry Res 1984; 18: 319–326.

Meltzer HY. Creatine kinase and aldolase in serum: abnormality common to acute psychoses. Science 1968; 159: 1368–1370.

Meltzer HY. Neuromuscular dysfunction in schizophrenia. Schizophr Bull 1976; 2: 106–135.

Meltzer HY, Crayton JW. Subterminal motor nerve abnormalities in psychotic patients. Nature 1974; 249: 373–375.

Meltzer HY, Ross-Stanton J, Schlessinger S. Mean serum creatine kinase activity in patients with functional psychoses. Arch Gen Psychiatry 1980; 37: 650–655.

Möller SE. Effect of oral contraceptives on tryptophan and tyrosine availability: evidence for a possible contribution to mental depression. Neuropsychobiology 1981; 7: 192–200.

Mukherjee S, Mahadik SP, Schnur DB, Laev H, Reddy R. Abnormal growth of cultured skin fibroblasts associated with poor premorbid history in schizophrenic patients. Schizophr Res 1994; 13: 233–237.

Munro HN, Fernstrom JD, Wurtman RJ. Insulin, plasma amino acid imbalance, and hepatic coma. Lancet 1975; i: 722–724.

Owens DGC, Harrison-Read PE, Johnstone EC. L-dopa in very impaired schizophrenic patients. Clin Neuropharmacol 1990; 13 (Suppl 2): 174–175.

Pardridge WM, Oldendorf WH. Transport of metabolic substrates through the blood–brain barrier. J Neurochem 1977; 28: 5–12.

Post RM, Goodwin FK, Gordon E, Watkin DM. Amine metabolites in human cerebrospinal fluid: effect of cord transection and spinal fluid block. Science 1973; 179: 897–899.

Ramchand CN, Peet M, Clark AE, Gliddon AE, Hemmings GP. Decreased tyrosine transport in fibroblasts from schizophrenics: implications for membrane pathology. Prostagland Leukotr Essent Fatty Acids 1996; 55: 59–64.

Randrup A, Munkvad I. Special antagonism of amphetamine induced abnormal behaviour. Inhibition of stereotyped activity with increase of some normal activities. Psychopharmacologia 1965; 7: 416–422.

Smith KA, Fairburn CG, Cowen PJ. Relapse of depression after rapid depletion of tryptophan. Lancet 1997; 349: 915–919.

Spitzer RL, Endicott J, Robins E. Research diagnostic criteria. Arch Gen Psychiatry 1978; 35: 773–782.

Tam SY, Roth RH. Mesoprefrontal dopaminergic neurons: can tyrosine availability influence their functions? Biochem Pharmacol 1997; 53: 441–453.

Tuckwell HC, Koziol JA. A meta-analysis of homovanillic acid concentrations in schizophrenia. Int J Neuroscience 1993; 73: 109–114.

van Rossum JM. The significance of dopamine-receptor blockade for the action of neuroleptic drugs. Arch Int Pharmacodyn Ther 1966; 160: 492–494.

Wei J, Xu H, Ramchand CN, Hemmings GP. Low concentrations of serum tyrosine in neuroleptic-free schizophrenics with an early onset. Schizophr Res 1995; 14: 257–260.

Wiesel FA, Blomquist G, Halldin C et al. The transport of tyrosine into the human brain as determined with L-[1-^{11}C]tyrosine and PET. J Nucl Med 1991; 32: 2043–2049.

Wiesel FA, Venizelos N, Bjerkenstedt L, Hagenfeldt L. Tyrosine transport in schizophrenia. Schizophr Res 1994; 13: 255–258.

Wiesel FA, Andersson JLR, Westerberg G et al. Tyrosine transport is differently regulated in patients with schizophrenia. Submitted for publication, 1999.

Woodlock TJ, Young DA, Boal TR, Lichtman MA, Segel GB. Phorbol ester-induced membrane proteins in chronic leukemic β-lymphocytes. Candidate proteins for the L-system amino acid transporter? J Biol Chem 1993; 268: 16020–16027.

Wurtman RJ, Rose CM, Chou C, Larin FF. Daily rhythms in the concentration of various amino acids in human plasma. N Engl J Med 1968; 279: 171–175.

Young SN, Lal S, Martin JB, Ford RM, Sourkes TL. 5-hydroxyindoleacetic acid, homovanillic acid and tryptophan levels in CSF above and below a complete block of CSF. Psychiatry Neurol Neurochirurg 1973; 76: 439–444.

Membrane Peroxidation and the Neuropathology of Schizophrenia

9

Sahebarao P. Mahadik, Sandhya Sitasawad and Meena Mulchandani

INTRODUCTION

The biochemical basis of the aetiology of schizophrenia is unknown. However, substantial progress has been made to define its pathophysiology. Brain imaging and post-mortem analyses have provided evidence for a wide range of neuropathological changes. Several aetiopathological theories, including ones based on genetic, viral, autoimmune, nutritional, or neurotoxicity concepts, have been proposed to explain such a complex neuropathophysiology, which would contribute to a multitransmitter dysfunction. The degree of dysfunction in each transmitter system may vary among patients during the course of the illness. This has been the basis of current treatment strategies. Unfortunately, these treatments have shown a wide range of effectiveness in their ability to control the symptoms, and have often been associated with serious adverse effects. Alternative treatment strategies must therefore be sought that can improve the course and outcome of illness, and have fewer, and less marked, adverse effects.

Evidence has become increasingly available to support the view that some of these neuropathological changes in schizophrenia may be the result of increased free radical-mediated or reactive oxygen species (ROS) mediated neuronal injury (for reviews see Mahadik and Mukherjee, 1996; Reddy and Yao, 1996). This type of pathology was first considered to result from treatment with antipsychotic drugs (Cadet and Lohr, 1987), since treatment of animals with such drugs resulted in oxidative stress, i.e., a mismatch between the cellular generation of ROS and the antioxidant potential (see reviews by Mahadik and Mukherjee, 1996; Mahadik and Scheffer, 1996). ROS-mediated pathology has been also supported by the amelioration of some psychopathologies, and by the reduced lipid peroxidation, noted following treatment with antioxidants (see, e.g., Adler et al., 1993; Mahadik and Gowda, 1996; Mahadik and Scheffer, 1996; Reddy and Yao, 1996).

ROS-mediated neuronal injury (i.e., lipid peroxidation, and protein and DNA oxidation) occurs when oxidative stress exists. The brain is selectively susceptible to oxidative injury since it is generally under higher oxidative stress and is enriched in lipids that are selectively susceptible to oxidation. During development, the damaged neurones can drastically alter the brain structure and function and, if destroyed, cannot be replaced in the adult brain since they do not divide (Halliwell, 1992).

Neuronal membrane lipids are unique in terms of their quantity and quality (i.e., the type of fatty acid attached to them), and they are critical for brain development and differentiation, and neuronal function and survival (Simopoulos, 1991; Wainwright, 1992). The selective susceptibility of these lipids to peroxidation can affect the neurodevelopment, as well as the membrane receptor-mediated signal transduction, of neurotransmitters, hormones, and growth factors, and the transport of nutrients and ions. These effects may even lead to neuronal death and thus contribute to complex neuropathologies.

The primary objective of this chapter is to indicate that lipid peroxidation probably contributes to the neuropathophysiology of schizophrenia, and that prevention of lipid peroxidation may improve prognosis, probably by producing improvements in the structure, and thereby also in the functions, of neuronal membranes. The rationale and evidence will be discussed for the occurrence of lipid peroxidation due to oxidative stress in schizophrenia, and its implications for the neuropathophysiology of the disease. Possible neuroprotective strategies involving treatment with antioxidants and essential polyunsaturated fatty acids (EPUFAs) to prevent the neuronal lipid peroxidation and restore the membrane EPUFAs, will also be considered.

OXIDATIVE STRESS AND OXIDATIVE NEURONAL INJURY

Oxidative stress

Oxidative stress, a mismatch between cellular levels of ROS (also known as free radicals, e.g., $O_2^{\cdot-}$, $OH^{\cdot}$, $NO^{\cdot}$, $ONOO^-$) and antioxidant capacity, occurs under altered physiological situations, such as increased illness-related stress, caloric intake, alcohol consumption, smoking, infections, sedentary life style, and antipsychotic drug treatments. All these factors are relevant to schizophrenia (Mahadik and Gowda, 1996; see Figure 9.1). The increased oxidative stress will lead to oxidative cellular injury, i.e., peroxidative breakdown of lipids (Bielski et al., 1983; Gutteridge, 1988), proteins (Wolff and Dean, 1986; Stadtman, 1992) and DNA (Mellow-Filho and Meneghini, 1984; Ames et al., 1991). There is some evidence that membrane lipids suffer peroxidation before oxidation of proteins and DNA (Subbarao et al., 1990; Sohal et al., 1994). Effective prevention of membrane lipid peroxidation by antioxidants may allow restoration of the normal levels of lipids. However,

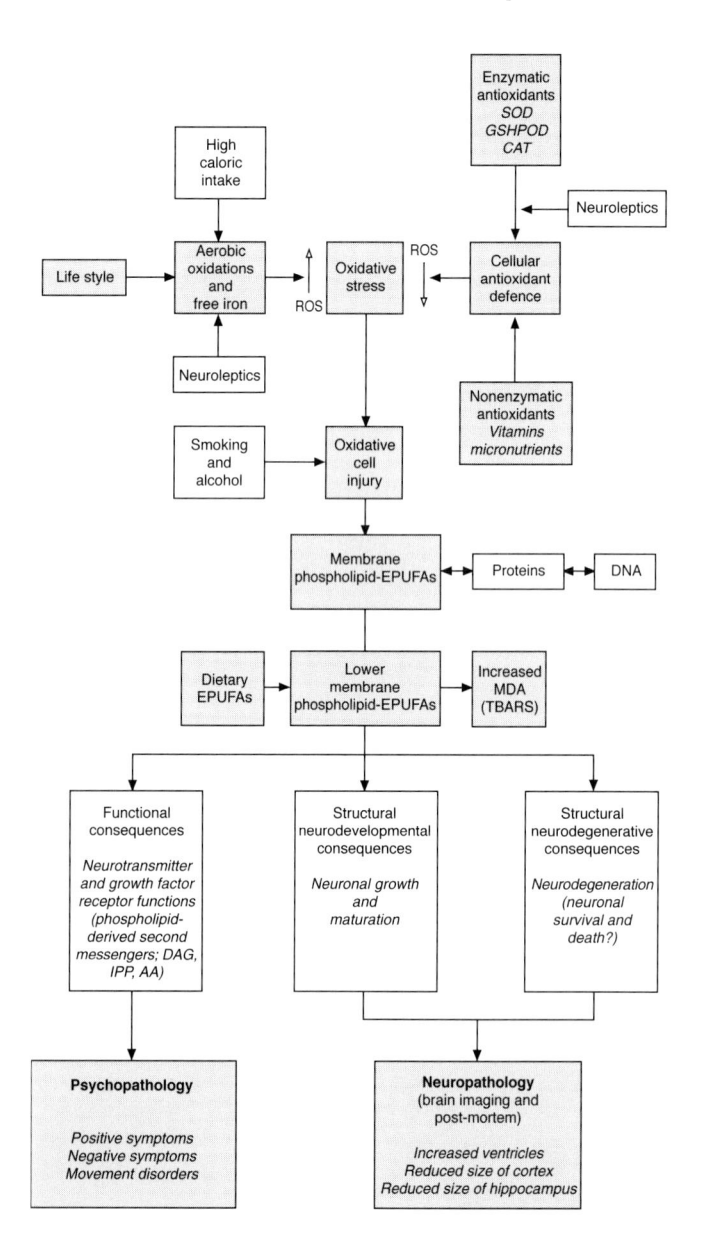

Figure 9.1. Mechanisms of oxidative stress and oxidative cell injury, and their neuropathological and psychopathological consequences. Oxidative stress is a mismatch between cellular levels of reactive oxygen species (ROS) and cellular antioxidant defence. ↑ and ↓ represent an increase and a decrease in ROS, respectively, the increase occurring by aerobic oxidation and in the presence of free iron, whilst the decrease occurs in response to cellular antioxidant defence. Also shown are factors such as caloric intake, administration of neuroleptics, smoking, and alcohol consumption, all of which may increase ROS and thereby contribute to oxidative stress. AA = arachidonic acid; DAG = diacylglycerol; DNA = deoxyribonucleic acid; EPUFAs = essential polyunsaturated fatty acids; IPP = inositol polyphosphate; MDA = malonyldialdehyde; TBARS = thiobarbituric acid reactive material. The arrows indicate the direction of the processes.

peroxidative breakdown of proteins and DNA may often lead to irreversible cellular injury.

Metabolism of ROS

The ROS generated during normal cellular metabolic processes, particularly by monoamine oxidases and errors in mitochondrial electron transport, are then converted into more potent species (Figure 9.2). Under normal physiological circumstances, the levels of ROS are controlled by a number of factors, including: the synergistic action of cellular antioxidant defence; superoxide dismutase (SOD), glutathione peroxidase (GSHPOD), catalase (CAT) and urate; and dietary antioxidants such as vitamins E and C, β–carotene, flavones and quinones. Figure 9.3 shows the synergistic actions of enzymatic and nonenzymatic antioxidants to protect against membrane lipid peroxidation, and against protein and DNA oxidation. SOD converts the oxyradical, $O_2^{\bar{\cdot}}$ to hydrogen peroxide, H_2O_2. CAT converts the H_2O_2 into H_2O and oxygen. If H_2O_2 is not removed by the catalase, it is converted into OH• in the presence of transition metals (e.g., free Fe^{2+}). OH• is a highly reactive species of oxyradical. Urate accounts for over 80% of the antioxidant potential in human plasma (Ames et al., 1981).

Preferential vulnerability of brain to oxidative injury

Brain is always under high oxidative stress since it uses 80% of the inhaled oxygen, and mitochondrial activity is very high to meet the energy demands for neuronal activity. This increases the chance of mitochondrial error, which is suggested to occur in schizophrenia (Marchbanks et al., 1995), and of the increased generation of oxyradicals. The brain is also enriched in lipids (see later) and proteins (enzymes and receptors with high disulphhydryl groups) that are more susceptible to peroxidation. In the adult brain, dead neurones, following DNA peroxidative breakdown, cannot be replaced since they do not divide. In addition, high levels of SOD, and generally low levels of CAT, keep the brain under high oxidative stress. All of these facts indicate that the increased oxidative stress and the preferential vulnerability of the brain to oxidative injury probably contribute to the associated neuropathophysiology, and thereby psychopathology, of schizophrenia.

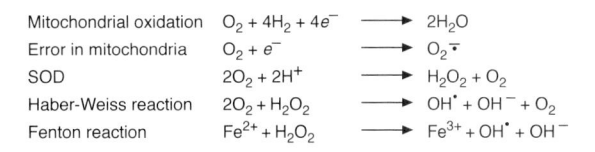

Mitochondrial oxidation	$O_2 + 4H_2 + 4e^-$	$\longrightarrow 2H_2O$
Error in mitochondria	$O_2 + e^-$	$\longrightarrow O_2^{\bar{\cdot}}$
SOD	$2O_2 + 2H^+$	$\longrightarrow H_2O_2 + O_2$
Haber-Weiss reaction	$2O_2 + H_2O_2$	$\longrightarrow OH^{\bullet} + OH^- + O_2$
Fenton reaction	$Fe^{2+} + H_2O_2$	$\longrightarrow Fe^{3+} + OH^{\bullet} + OH^-$

Figure 9.2. Mechanisms of oxygen metabolism and the generation of reactive oxygen species (ROS). H^+ = proton; e^- = electron; $O^{\bar{\cdot}}$ = oxyradical; $OH^{\bullet}$ = hydroxyl radical; H_2O_2 = hydrogen peroxide.

Neuronal membrane lipids and lipid peroxidation

Unlike plasma membranes of nonneuronal cells, neuronal plasma membranes, which contain 69.5% of the total lipids, constituting over 50% of the dry weight in human brain, are enriched in respect of four major phospholipids: phosphatidylcholine (PC); phosphatidylethanolamine (PE); phosphatidylserine (PS) and phosphatidylinositol (PI) (Suzuki, 1981). These phospholipids, particularly in the cortex, hippocampus

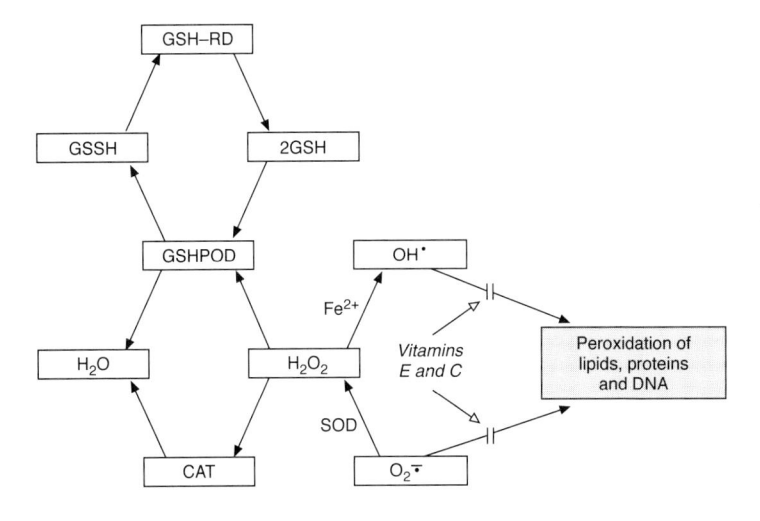

Figure 9.3. Mechanisms of cellular enzymatic and nonenzymatic antioxidant defence. $O^{\bar{\cdot}}$ = oxyradical; $OH^{\bullet}$ = hydroxyradical; H_2O_2 = hydrogen peroxide; CAT = catalase; GSH = glutathione; GSHPOD = glutathione peroxidase; GSSH = oxidized glutathione; SOD = superoxide dismutase. GSH-RD = glutathione reductase; The direction of the arrows indicates the direction of the reaction.

$$\text{Lipid–H} + \text{Oxyradical} \longrightarrow \text{Lipid}^\bullet + \text{Oxyradical–H}$$
$$\text{Lipid}^\bullet + O_2 \longrightarrow \text{Lipid–}O_2^\bullet$$
$$\text{Lipid }O_2^\bullet + \text{Lipid–H} \longrightarrow \text{Lipid–}O_2H + \text{Lipid}^\bullet$$

Figure 9.4. Mechanism of membrane lipid peroxidation chain-reaction. Lipid$^\bullet$ = lipid radical; Lipid-$O_2^\bullet$ = lipid peroxyl radical; Lipid-O_2H = lipid hydroperoxide. Notice that once Lipid$^\bullet$ is formed, it will continue producing lipid hydroperoxide in the presence of oxygen, i.e., a lipid peroxidation chain-reaction. This will not require any further oxyradicals.

and basal ganglia, are selectively enriched in EPUFAs, primarily arachidonic acid (AA) and docosahexaenoic acid (DHA) (O'Brien and Sampson, 1965; Carlson et al., 1986) that are selectively susceptible to lipid peroxidation due to the lowered bond dissociation energy of their allylic hydrogens. Hydrogen abstraction from their methylenic carbons can occur in the presence of ROS or drug radicals. Figure 9.4 shows the mechanisms of lipid peroxidation (Gutteridge, 1982; 1988; Bielski et al., 1983; Clemens and Waller, 1987).

Studies in erythrocytes indicate that lipid peroxidation may occur predominantly in the cell membrane (Clemens and Waller, 1987; Ramchand et al., 1996). It is also important to point out that, once the lipid peroxidation chain reaction starts, it continues without additional ROS. Therefore, membrane lipid peroxidation is predominantly affected during global oxidative stress and may profoundly and selectively affect neuronal membrane structure and function.

Analysis of lipid peroxides

Plasma malondialdehydes (MDA) and 4-hydroxyalkenals, well-defined byproducts of membrane phospholipid EFAs peroxidation, are generally measured by the assay procedure of Ohkawa et al. (1979) according to their reactivity with thiobarbituric acid (TBA). The levels of MDA are expressed as the TBA reactive substances (TBARS). However, this procedure is considered less selective for the lipid peroxides in biological materials (Janero, 1990). A high pressure liquid chromatography procedure with fluorescence detector that separates and measures the TBARS generated from lipid-bound EPUFAs has been considered more suitable (Young and Trimble, 1991). There is also a kit available for the selective determination of the lipid peroxidation byproducts (Bioxytech, Bonneuil/Marne, France).

Although there is sufficient evidence that plasma TBARS reflect the lipid peroxidation in the brain, concern has often been expressed regarding its relevance to brain lipid peroxidation. Support for the plasma TBARS as the preferred index for brain lipid peroxidation is based on the assumption that the lipid peroxidation, like the oxidative stress, is a global phenomenon, a view which is based partly on experimental evidence in animals (Kramer et al., 1987). There is also a suggestion that TBARS, like several other metabolites formed in the brain, enter the plasma *via* the cerebrospinal fluid (CSF). Also, since the brain is the predominant generator of TBARS under oxidative stress, the increased plasma levels probably reflect the oxidative lipid peroxides in the brain.

There have been some attempts to analyze the TBARS in the CSF from chronic schizophrenic patients (see later). Unfortunately, it is extremely difficult to collect CSF from drug-naïve first-episode patients, and the levels in the CSF from chronic patients may be confounded by the effects of years of treatment and illness. Post-mortem brain tissue is totally unsuitable for this purpose, since it yields highly variable values (unpublished data), probably due to variability in the procedures used to collect the tissues, and to patient heterogeneity. Breath alkanes have also been found to provide a useful index of *in situ* lipid peroxidation (van Gossum and Dekuyper, 1989).

Until ways are developed for determining the *in situ* brain levels of ROS and lipid peroxides, initial studies on the plasma TBARS and the effect of antioxidant treatments on the levels of TBARS, RBC membrane EPUFAs, and clinical outcome, may help to assess the role of membrane lipid peroxidation in the neuropsychopathophysiology of schizophrenia. Future studies then can address the molecular mechanisms underlying oxidative stress and lipid peroxidation.

Oxidative stress in schizophrenia

Evidence is increasing to support the hypothesis that oxidative stress exists in schizophrenia (Mahadik and Mukherjee, 1996; Reddy and Yao, 1996). There is no direct evidence for increased levels of ROS in schizophrenia, either with or without neuroleptic treatment. However, illness-related stress, high caloric intake, sedentary life style, smoking, alcohol consumption and antipsychotic drug treatments have been shown to increase ROS under experimental conditions (see e.g., Mahadik and Gowda, 1996); these are all very relevant to schizophrenia, and it is difficult to be certain whether oxidative stress is due to the disease itself or to the associated factors.

There is evidence for impaired enzymatic (Buckman et al., 1990; Reddy et al., 1991; Liday et al., 1995; Mukherjee et al., 1996; and for reviews see Mahadik and Mukherjee, 1996; Reddy and Yao, 1996) and nonenzymatic (Richardson-Andrews, 1990; Suboticanec et al., 1990; Brown, 1994; Liday et al., 1995) antioxidant defence systems. Although these indices of oxidative stress and oxidative injury are primarily derived from analyses of plasma and red blood cells, it is assumed that similar changes exist in the brain, since these enzymes are constitutively expressed in all tissues (Prohaska and Ganther, 1976; Kramer et al., 1987). Figure 9.1 shows the possible mechanisms that may be involved in increased oxidative stress, neuronal oxidative damage, and the neuropathophysiological consequences in schizophrenia.

The foregoing evidence also indicates that the oxidative stress probably predates the illness, since these changes are found in patients at the onset of psychosis, and may have a significant effect on brain development – and probably a continuing effect throughout life (Mukherjee et al., 1996; Mahadik et al., 1998). In addition, since treatment with typical neuroleptics increases oxidative stress and oxidative neuronal damage in animals (Heikkila et al., 1975; Murthy et al., 1989; Cadet and Perumal, 1990; Shivkumar and Ravindranath, 1993), neuroleptic treatment in schizophrenic patients is considered to be involved in the exacerbation of pre-existing oxidative stress (for reviews see, e.g., Cadet and Lohr, 1989; Mahadik and Mukherjee, 1996).

Both typical and atypical neuroleptics differ in their pro- and antioxidant properties (Jeding et al., 1995); thus, chlorpromazine has both pro- and antioxidant properties (Roy et al., 1984), whereas some atypical neuroleptics, e.g., clozapine, have pro-oxidant (Fisher, 1991; Liday et al., 1995) and others, e.g., olanzapine (unpublished results), probably antioxidant properties. Lower levels of MDA have been reported in schizophrenic patients treated with chlorpromazine (Bindoli et al., 1987). It is also possible that a neuroleptic drug may be an antioxidant by virtue of its ROS scavenger activity, but it may have pro-oxidant effects through its antipsychotic action and through acute increased catecholamine metabolism. In addition, heavy smoking, which is very common in schizophrenic patients, has been considered a major cause of oxidative damage (Morrow et al., 1995). It may therefore be suggested that the effects of neuroleptic drugs depend on their anti- or pro-oxidant properties and on the degree of the patient's oxidative stress, since together these may determine membrane lipid status.

MEMBRANE LIPID PEROXIDATION IN SCHIZOPHRENIA

Evidence for membrane lipid peroxidation in schizophrenia is based on increased TBARS in plasma and CSF, concomitant loss of membrane EPUFAs, increased pentane in the breath, and reduction of TBARS following treatment with antioxidants, with improvement in some aspects of the psychopathology of schizophrenia.

Membrane lipid peroxidation

Increased levels of lipid peroxides (e.g., TBARS) have been reported in plasma (Prilipko, 1984; Peet et al., 1993; McCreadie et al., 1995; Evans et al., 1996) and CSF (Pall et al., 1987; Lohr et al., 1989) from schizophrenic patients, with or without abnormal involuntary movements. Recently, we have reported increased plasma levels of lipid peroxides in drug-naïve patients at the onset of psychosis (Mahadik et al., 1998). Since the altered levels of indices of antioxidant defence, as well as of the lipid peroxides, exist at the onset of psychosis and correlate with poor premorbid function, it has been suggested that oxidative injury may predate the illness, possibly beginning during early brain development (Mahadik and Mukherjee, 1996; Mukherjee et al., 1996).

Altered membrane phospholipids and reduced esterified EPUFAs

There is now substantial evidence that both the quantity and quality of membrane phospholipids and esterified EPUFAs are altered in schizophrenia (for reviews see: Rotrosen and Wolkin, 1987; Horrobin et al., 1994; Horrobin, 1996; Mahadik et al., 1994; 1996a). However, it is not yet conclusively established that changes in schizophrenia result from increased peroxidation. It has been suggested that, in addition to increased peroxidation, the reduced dietary intake of both essential fatty acids (EFAs) and antioxidants, and possibly also the defective utilization of EFAs in the brain, may also play a critical role (Horrobin et al., 1994; Mahadik et al., 1996b). It will be important to investigate this further by within-patient measurements of lipid peroxides, levels of lipids and their esterified EPUFAs, and dietary intake of EPUFAs and antioxidants. However, there is substantial evidence that these membrane lipid constituents are altered in brain, blood, and even in cultured cells, from schizophrenic patients. There is also some indirect evidence for reduced levels of EFAs in erythrocyte membranes based on lower level of *in vitro* lipid peroxidation in erythrocytes from schizophrenic patients compared to normals, according to Ramchand et al. (1996), who have suggested that this lower level of lipid peroxidation is not due to neuroleptic treatment but is a result of illness.

Brain

Using ^{31}P-NMR spectroscopy, altered phospholipid metabolism, i.e., lower levels of phosphomonoesters (PME), indicative of reduced synthesis, and increased levels of phosphodiesters (PDE), indicative of increased degradation, have been found in the dorsal prefrontal cortex of first-episode, drug-naïve schizophrenic patients (Pettegrew et al., 1991). However, low levels of PME in chronic patients (Williamson et al., 1996) suggests that continued reduced phospholipid synthesis is probably due to the reduced availability of EPUFAs. Reduced levels of EPUFAs in phospholipids (PE and PI) have been reported in post-mortem frontal cortical tissue from schizophrenic patients (Horrobin et al., 1991). This is important, since several other pathophysiological processes have been found to be altered in frontal as well as in temporal cortices (Nasrallah, 1993). It will be important in future to establish the relationship between changes in CNS phospholipid metabolites and the peripheral membrane EPUFA status.

Blood

Studies on membrane phospholipids and their metabolites in plasma and erythrocytes have reported some inconsistencies (references for studies up to 1987 appear in a review by Rotrosen and Wolkin, 1987; Horrobin, 1992; Bates et al., 1992; Keshavan et al., 1993; Horrobin et al., 1994; Yao et al., 1994). These are probably due to confounding factors, since diet (Dougherty et al., 1987), neuroleptics (Maziere et al., 1988), hormonal state (Brenner, 1981), and defective utilization (Horrobin et al., 1994) can influence their levels. However, more consistent lower levels of phospholipid-EPUFAs, predominantly AA and DHA, have been reported in four separate studies (Vaddadi et al., 1989; Glen et al., 1994, Peet et al., 1994; Yao et al., 1994). The lower levels of AA and DHA have been implicated in negative symptoms in recent preliminary studies (Glen et al., 1994; Peet et al., 1994, 1995). It is important to establish firm clinical implications by using properly selected subgroups of schizophrenic patients and normal controls.

Cultured skin fibroblasts

We have now found lower levels of individual phospholipids (PS > PI > PE), primarily enriched in AA and DHA, in fibroblasts from chronic schizophrenic patients, as well as in first-episode, drug-naïve schizophrenic patients (Mahadik et al., 1994), which supports the altered distribution of their esterified EPUFAs (Mahadik et al., 1996a).

Increased breath pentane

Increased levels of pentane, a product of peroxidative breakdown of EFAs (van Gossum and Decuyper, 1989) have been reported in schizophrenic patients (Kovaleva et al., 1989; Phillips et al., 1995). This may be a very useful and suitable way of assessing the lipid peroxidation *in situ* under a variety of situations and stages of illness (Dodd, 1996), and may also help in monitoring the progress of the disease.

Antioxidant treatments and lipid peroxidation

There is only one study that has shown an effect of treatment which reduced lipid peroxidation, improved membrane levels of EFAs, and improved psychopathology (Peet et al., 1993). There are at least 12 published studies that have reported improved psychopathology, particularly tardive dyskinesia, after treatment with antioxidants, e.g., vitamin E (Adler et al., 1993; Mahadik and Gowda, 1996; Mahadik and Scheffer, 1996; Reddy and Yao, 1996). These studies have suggested that the effects of vitamin E are most likely to be exerted through the prevention of lipid peroxidation.

NEUROPATHOLOGICAL AND PSYCHOPATHOLOGICAL IMPLICATIONS

Since increased lipid peroxidation, and possibly associated altered membrane phospholipids, particularly lower levels of esterfied EPUFAs, are found in drug-naïve, first-episode psychotic patients as well as in chronic schizophrenic patients, this suggests that the lipid peroxidation probably predates the illness and continues throughout the life of the patient. This raises two questions. In the first place, was lipid peroxidation present during development, contributing to abnormal brain development? Secondly, does lipid peroxidation continue in adult life and contribute to the progression of neuropathophysiological changes and thereby the outcome of illness? The findings further suggest that lipid peroxidation probably contributes to structural brain pathology (organic) as well as neuronal plasma membrane pathology (functional), both of which may be correctable.

Lipid peroxidation and neurodevelopmental pathology

Again, there is no direct evidence that lipid peroxidation, and thereby altered lipids, contribute to neurodevelopmental pathology, particularly increased cerebral ventricular enlargement, neuronal disorganization, or altered size and shape of critical brain areas (e.g., frontal lobes, temporal cortex, hippocampus, thalamus), at the onset of psychosis in drug-naïve patients, or in the neuronal disorganization seen in post-mortem brain (for reviews see: Bloom, 1993; Nasrallah, 1993). These neurodevelopmental pathologies are the most replicated findings in schizophrenia. Down's syndrome may involve oxidative stress and possible lipid peroxidation during development, due to higher SOD, resulting from chromosome 21 trisomy (Sinet, 1982). Oxyradicals are considered to be needed for normal brain development and differentiation, but when produced in excess they can cause abnormal brain development (Allen and Balin, 1989; Allen, 1991).

We have found a low level of SOD in patients at the onset of psychosis in drug-naïve patients, suggesting that SOD may be lower during early development and may have contributed to neurodevelopmental pathology. Low SOD levels were correlated with poor premorbid performance (Mukherjee et al., 1996), and increased lipid peroxides were correlated with negative symptoms and lower GSHPOD activity in these patients (Mahadik et al., 1998).

Membrane EPUFAs and neurodevelopmental pathology

In the brain, the most serious consequence of lipid peroxidation during development may be through depletion of membrane EPUFAs. EPUFAs have been found to be critical for normal brain development in man and animals (Neuringer et al., 1986; Sinclair, 1990; Simopoulos, 1991; Crawford, 1992; Wainwright, 1992). Studies in animals have shown that the depletion of EFA, particularly ω-3 EFA, during development results in abnormal brain development and altered behavioural performance that are relevant to schizophrenia.

Lower levels of ω-3 EFA, particularly DHA, have been reported in drug-naïve patients at the onset of psychosis, indicating that these low levels probably contributed to the development of the illness and its associated neurodevelopmental pathology (Mahadik et al., 1996a; Peet et al., 1996). Recently, it has also been reported that schizophrenia was more prevalent in subjects who were formula-fed *versus* breastfed (for a full review and discussion, see Peet et al., 1999). Several baby formulas do not contain substantial amounts of ω-3 EFA, but mother's milk and even cord blood contain high quantities of ω-3 EFA, particularly DHA (Carlson et al., 1986). It will be very important to establish the causal relationship between membrane peroxidation, lower levels of membrane ω-3 EFA and psychopathology. These issues are raised because they are crucial in establishing the EPUFA status of membranes, and it should be possible to put them to empirical test.

Lipid peroxidation and neurodegenerative pathophysiology

Oxidative cellular injury has been implicated in several neurodegenerative diseases, such as Alzheimer's disease, Parkinson's disease, stroke, and amyotrophic lateral sclerosis (for reviews see: Fiskum, 1996; Simonian and Coyle, 1996). The occurrence of typical neurodegenerative neuropathology is still controversial in schizophrenia (Roberts and Crow, 1987; Hyde et al., 1991; Casanova et al., 1993; Freeman and Karson, 1993; Nasrallah, 1993). However, a few magnetic resonance imaging (MRI) studies have reported evidence for progressive ventricular enlargement in a subgroup of schizophrenic patients (Woods et al., 1990; Nair et al., 1997). Such changes have been suggested to be a result of progressive neurodegeneration, most probably due to oxidative damage (Garver, 1997). A negative correlation has been reported between the levels of GSHPOD, an enzyme crucial in preventing lipid peroxidation, and the degree of ventricular enlargement (Buckman et al., 1990).

There are several reports of the presence of diffuse pathology in the brain that may account for the loss of dendritic spines and synaptic contacts (Zipurski et al., 1992; Selemon et al., 1995). These changes suggest that oxidative injury may be restricted to membrane lipids, causing membrane pathology rather than significant breakdown of proteins and DNA that may lead to cell death. This may explain the reported absence of widespread gliosis indicative of neurodegeneration in the post-mortem brains (Casanova et al., 1990).

Lipid peroxidation, membrane pathology, and receptor-mediated signal transduction

Since lipid peroxidation can alter the quality and quantity of membrane phospholipids, this will contribute to the pathophysiology of schizophrenia by at least two mechanisms: (1) the altered distribution of phospholipids can change the physicochemical properties of membranes and this, in turn, can differentially influence the activities of membrane proteins (ion pumps and receptors); and (2) the altered distribution of phospholipids, with reduced levels of esterified AA, can result in reduced levels of neurotransmitter receptor-mediated generation of second messengers, e.g., AA, diacylglycerol (DAG) and inositol phosphate (IP) (Berridge, 1981; Agranoff, 1989; Axelrod, 1990; Rana and Hokin, 1990; Dennis et al., 1991; Farooqui et al., 1992). The levels of membrane phospholipids also play critical roles in membrane fluidity and in the function of several proteins (receptors, ion pumps and enzymes); their levels in plasma membranes thus represent the functional pool (Stubbs and Smith, 1990).

Lipid peroxidation has been shown to alter differentially the postsynaptic GABA receptor complex (Schwartz et al., 1988) as well as dopamine and GABA uptake in nerve terminals (Rafalowska et al., 1989). This may also explain the suggested abnormal differential multitransmitter neuronal signal transduction in schizophrenia (Essali et al., 1990; Hudson et al., 1993). Dopamine activation of the AA cascade has been shown to provide a basis for the D_1/D_2 dopamine receptor synergism (Piomelli et al., 1991) which is reported to be altered in schizophrenia (Seeman et al., 1989).

THERAPEUTIC STRATEGIES

Prevention of lipid peroxidation by antioxidants

Lipid peroxidation can be effectively prevented by antioxidants that may help to correct the active membrane pathology, e.g., membrane receptor-mediated signal transduction, which may then ameliorate some of the associated psychopathologies. However, such treatment will not restore the irreversible structural changes that occurred during development as well as during the course of illness and its treatment.

In schizophrenia, since the enzymatic antioxidant defence is altered, the use of exogenous nonenzymatic antioxidants has been a preferred choice, since they have been found to cross the blood–brain barrier and are effective in preventing oxidative injury in all areas of the brain in experimental systems. Fortunately, these are also available in pure form at reasonable cost.

Among the exogenous antioxidants; vitamins A, C and E, and β-carotene and quinones are the most common (Burton and Ingold, 1989; Rice-Evans and Diplock, 1993). These vitamin antioxidants fall into two categories: lipid soluble and water soluble. Vitamin E is a very potent antioxidant in the prevention of lipid peroxidation, being hydrophobic and able to remain in membranes for a long time. It occurs in high concentrations in vegetable oils, and wheat germ provides a particularly rich source. Its activity can be restored by vitamin C (Frei et al., 1989) which is present at high levels in all fruits and vegetables. However, schizophrenic patients, in general, do not eat these foodstuffs in sufficient quantities. Treatment with a combination of vitamins E and C may be even more effective in preventing lipid peroxidation (May et al., 1996). There are also several synthetic (pharmacological) antioxidants, such as retinol, retinyl esters and lazaroids, (21-aminosteroids that lack glucocorticoid activity and are potent against membrane lipid peroxidation) (Braughler et al., 1987).

Regular use of these antioxidants at pharmacological doses, i.e., vitamin A at <100 000 IU/day, vitamin E at <3200 mg/day and vitamin C at <4 g/day, has been considered to be quite safe, and no adverse effects have been reported with β-carotene, (however, there are some concerns about using vitamin C with iron supplements since iron can act as a pro-oxidant). The safety of their use is also assured, since these vitamins are metabolized without generating any known toxic intermediates (Meyers et al., 1996). This knowledge can help in choosing the appropriate antioxidant at a therapeutic dose level.

Control of oxidative stress may also be a useful strategy. High caloric intake has been shown to increase oxidative stress, leading to brain damage; food restriction can help to prevent this (Sohal et al., 1994). A large quantity of red meat in the diet substantially increases both the total caloric intake and the amount of iron that is ingested. It is difficult to advise patients to reduce red meat in the diet as well as to reduce the total calorie intake. There are, as yet, no clear guidelines as to how much red meat is safe and acceptable for those with an impaired antioxidant defence and with sedentary life style. The most difficult task is to persuade patients to reduce their caloric intake to a reasonable level: the degree of caloric restriction shown to decrease oxidative stress amounts to a daily intake of about 1600 calories, for those living a sedentary life. A dietary survey at our VA Medical Center revealed that most schizophrenic patients have a daily caloric intake of around 2600–3000/day. Smoking also increases oxidative stress and smoking cessation is usually the most difficult step of all. Regrettably, very little has been done to reduce the heavy smoking which is common amongst psychotic patients.

Present and future status of antioxidant treatment

A total of 14 studies have reported varying degrees (i.e., from no effect to a highly significant reduction) of efficacy of vitamin E in preventing the appearance of tardive dyskinesia in chronic schizophrenic patients (for reviews see: Mahadik and Scheffer, 1996; Mahadik and Gowda, 1996; Reddy and Yao, 1996). When poor responses have been obtained, this may have resulted from the inclusion of patients with pathology unrelated to lipid peroxidation, or with irreversible damage, or with the use of an inadequate dose of the antioxidant. In addition, none of the studies used a combination of membrane soluble and water soluble vitamins to provide a complete cellular antioxidant treatment.

It is also important to consider the supplementation of antioxidants with ω-3 EFAs, particularly eicosapentaenoic acid (EPA) and DHA, since lipid peroxidation may affect their levels, predominantly in the brain where they are enriched. The ω-6 EFAs are more widely distributed in the diet, whereas ω-3 EFAs are present only in certain diets (Simopoulos, 1991). The ω-3 EFAs have also been reported to be beneficial in the treatment of schizophrenic psychopathology (Peet et al., 1996).

Since the oxidative stress and lipid peroxidation probably predate the illness, it is very important that the efficacy of adjunctive use of antioxidants for the treatment of psychotic episodes should be tested right from the onset of illness. Antioxidants are known to work as neuroprotective agents through prevention of lipid peroxidation and may contribute to improved outcome of illness.

CONCLUSION

Lipid peroxidation may be a very important biochemical defect contributing to both neurodevelopmental and neurodegenerative pathology of schizophrenia. This may also explain the suggested multitransmitter dysfunction and the variable course of the illness (World Health Organization, 1979; Sartorius et al., 1986; Leff et al., 1992; Mahadik et al., 1999). Available treatment strategies involving the use of antipsychotic drugs are less than adequate, and may not be suitable to treat this neuropathology; such treatments are also very expensive due to the acquisition price of drugs, and the costs of clinical management and the control of comorbidities associated with the primary illness, as well as the costs involved in dealing with the adverse effects of drugs.

Alternative treatment strategies are badly needed. Prevention of lipid peroxidation is very effective with the use of commonly available and inexpensive dietary antioxidant supplements, and membrane lipid changes can be restored by supplementation with EPUFAs. This type of treatment can also be neuroprotective insofar as it prevents the oxidative injury before it becomes irreversible; neurodevelopmental pathologies may require intervention during early development. These treatments also may not have adverse effects and may help to improve some of the comorbidities, such as diabetes and hypertension, that appear to be associated with increased oxidative stress and lower EFAs.

REFERENCES

Adler LA, Peselow E, Rotrosen J et al. Vitamin E treatment of tardive dyskinesia. Am J Psychiatry 1993; 150: 1405–1407.

Agranoff B. Lipids. In: Siegel GJ, Albers RW, Agranoff BW, Katzman R, eds. Basic neurochemistry, 4th edn. Boston: Little, Brown and Company, 1989: 91–107.

Allen RG. Oxygen-reactive species and antioxidant responses during development: the metabolic paradox of cellular differentiation. Proc Soc Exp Biol Med 1991; 196: 117–129.

Allen RG, Balin AK. Oxidative influence on development and differentiation: an overview of a free radical theory of development. Free Radic Biol Med 1989; 6: 631–661.

Ames BN, Cathcart R, Schwier E, Hochstein P. Uric acid, an antioxidant in humans against oxidant- and radical-caused aging and cancer. A hypothesis. Proc Natl Acad Sci USA 1981; 78: 6858–6862.

Ames BA, Shingenaga MK, Park E-M. Oxyradicals and DNA damage. In: Davies KJA, ed. Oxidation damage and repair: chemical biological and medical aspects. Elmsford, NY: Pergamon Press, 1991: 181–187.

Axelrod J. Receptor-mediated activation of phospholipase A2 and arachidonic acid release in signal transduction. Biochem Soc Trans 1990; 18: 503–507.

Bates C, Horrobin DF, Ellis K. Fatty acids in plasma phospholipids and cholesterol esters from identical twins concordant and discordant for schizophrenia. Schizophr Res 1992; 6: 1–7.

Berridge MJ. Phosphatidylinositol hydrolysis: a multifunctional transducting mechanism. Mol Cell Endocrinol 1981; 24: 115–140.

Bielski BHJ, Arudi RL, Sutherland MW. A study of the reactivity of HO_2/O_2^- with unsaturated fatty acids. J Biol Chem 1983; 258: 4759–4761.

Bindoli A, Rigobello MP, Cavallini L, Libera AD, Galzigna I. Decrease of serum malondialdehyde in patients treated with chlorpromazine. Clin Chim Acta 1987; 169: 329–332.

Bloom F. Advancing neurodevelopmental origin for schizophrenia. Arch Gen Psychiatry 1993; 50: 224–227.

Braughler JM, Pregenzer JF, Chase RL et al. Novel 21-aminosteroids as potent inhibitors of iron-dependent lipid peroxidation. J Biol Chem 1987; 262: 10438–10440.

Brenner RR. Nutritional and hormonal factors influencing desaturation of essential fatty acids. Prog Lipid Res 1981; 20: 41–47.

Brown JS Jr. Role of selenium and other trace elements in the geography of schizophrenia. Schizophr Bull 1994; 20: 387–398.

Buckman TD, Kling AS, Sutphin MS, Steinberg A, Eiduson S. Platelet glutathione peroxidase and monoamine oxidase activity in schizophrenics with CT scan abnormalities: relation to psychosocial variables. Psychiatry Res 1990; 31: 1–14.

Burton GW, Ingold KU. Mechanisms of antioxidant action: preventive and chain breaking antioxidants. In: Migue J, Quintanilha AT, Weber H, eds. CRC Handbook of free radicals and antioxidants in biomedicine. Vol 2, Boca Raton: CRC Press, Inc., 1989: 29–43.

Cadet JL, Lohr JB. Free radicals and the developmental pathophysiology of schizophrenic burnout. Integr Psychiatry 1987; 5: 40–48.

Cadet JL, Lohr JB. Possible involvement of free radicals in neuroleptic-induced movement disorders: evidence from treatment of tardive dyskinesia with vitamin E. Ann N Y Acad Sci 1989; 570: 176–185.

Cadet JL, Perumal AS. Chronic treatment with prolixin causes oxidative stress in rat brain. Biol Psychiatry 1990; 28: 738–740.

Carlson SE, Rhodes PG, Ferguson MG. Docosahexaenoic acid status of preterm infants at birth and following feeding with human milk or formula 1-3. Am J Clin Nutr 1986; 44: 798–804.

Casanova MF, Stevens JR, Kleinman JE. Astrocytosis in the molecular layer of the dentate gyrus: a study in Alzheimer's disease and schizophrenia. Psychiatry Res: Neuroimaging 1990; 35: 149–166.

Casanova MF, Stevens JR, Kleinman JE. The neuropathology of schizophrenia: old and new findings. In: Weinberger DR, Kleinman JE, eds. New biological vistas of schizophrenia. New York: Brunner/Mazel Publishers, 1993: 82–109.

Clemens MR, Waller HD. Lipid peroxidation in erythrocytes. Chem Phys Lipids 1987; 45: 251–268.

Crawford MA. Essential fatty acids and neurodevelopmental disorder. In: Bazan NG, Toffano G, Horrobin DF et al., eds. Neurobiology of essential fatty acids. New York: Plenum Press, 1992: 307–314.

Dennis EA, Rhee SG, Billah MM, Hannun YA. Role of phospholipases in generating lipid second messengers in signal transduction. FASEB J 1991; 5: 2068–2077.

Dodd GH. The lipid membrane hypothesis of schizophrenia: implications for possible clinical breath tests. Prostagland Leukotr Essent Fatty Acids 1996; 55: 95–99.

Dougherty RM, Galli C, Ferro-Luzzi A. Lipid and phospholipid fatty acid composition of plasma, red blood cells, and platelets and how they are affected by dietary lipids: a study of normal subjects from Italy, Finland and the USA. Am J Clin Nutr 1987; 45: 443–455.

Essali MA, Das I, de Belleroche J, Hirsch SR. The platelet polyphosphoinositide system in schizophrenia: the effects of neuroleptic treatment. Biol Psychiatry 1990; 28: 475–487.

Evans DR, Puczkovski PY, Brandsma MJ, Mahadik JS, Mahadik SP. Elevated plasma lipid peroxides in schizophrenic patients without dementia. Biol Psychiatry 1996; 39: 588.

Farooqui AA, Hirashima Y, Horrocks LA. Brain phospholipases and their role in signal transduction. In: Baz·n NG, Murphy MG, Tofano G, eds. Neurobiology of essential fatty acids. New York: Plenum Press, 1992: 11–26.

Fisher AB. Possible role of free radical formation in clozapine (clozaril)-induced agranulocytosis. Mol Pharmacol 1991, 40: 846–853.

Fiskum G, ed. Neurodegenerative diseases: molecular and cellular mechanisms and therapeutic advances. George Washington University Medical Center, Department of Biochemistry and Molecular Biology Annual Spring Symposia. New York: Plenum Press, 1996.

Freeman T, Karson CN. The neuropathology of schizophrenia. Psychiatr Clin North Am 1993; 16: 281–293.

Frei B, England L, Ames BN. Ascorbate is an outstanding antioxidant in human blood plasma. Proc Natl Acad Sci USA 1989; 86: 6377–6381.

Garver DL. The etiologic heterogeneity of schizophrenia. Harward Rev Psychiatry 1997; 4: 1–11.

Glen AIM, Glen EMT, Horrobin DF et al. A red cell membrane abnormality in a subgroup of schizophrenic patients: evidence for two diseases. Schizophr Res 1994; 12: 53–61.

Gutteridge JMC. The role of superoxide and hydroxyl radicals in phospholipid peroxidation catalysed by iron salts. FEBS Lett 1982; 150: 454–458.

Gutteridge JMC. Lipid peroxidation: some problems and concepts. In: Halliwell B, ed. Oxygen radicals and tissue injury. Proc. Upjohn Symposium. Rockville, Bethesda, MD: FASEB Press, 1988: 9–19.

Halliwell B. Reactive oxygen species and the central nervous system. J Neurochem 1992; 59: 1609–1623.

Heikkila HS, Cohen G, Mannian AA. Reactivity of various phenothiazine derivatives with oxygen and oxygen radicals. Biochem Pharmacol 1975; 24: 363–368.

Horrobin DF. The relationship between schizophrenia and essential fatty acids and eicosanoid metabolism. Prostagland Leukotr Essent Fatty Acids 1992; 46: 71–77.

Horrobin DF. Schizophrenia as a membrane lipid disorder which is expressed throughout the body. Prostagland Leukotr Essent Fatty Acids 1996, 55: 3–7.

Horrobin DF, Manku MS, Hillman S, Glen AIM. Fatty acid levels in brains of schizophrenics and normal controls. Biol Psychiatry 1991; 30: 795–805.

Horrobin DF, Glen AIM, Vaddadi K. The membrane hypothesis of schizophrenia. Schizophr Res 1994; 13: 195–207.

Hudson CJ, Young LT, Li PP, Warsh JJ. CNS signal transduction in the pathophysiology and pharmacology of affective disorders and schizophrenia. Synapse 1993; 13: 278–293.

Hyde TM, Casanova MF, Kleinman JE, Weinberger DR. Neuroanatomical and neurochemical pathology in schizophrenia. In: Tasman A, Goldfinger SM, eds. Reviews of psychiatry. Washington DC: American Psychiatric Association Press, 1991; 10: 7–23.

Janero DR. Malondialdehyde and thiobarbituric acid-reactivity as diagnostic indices of lipid peroxidation and peroxidative tissue injury. Free Radic Biol Med 1990; 9: 515–540.

Jeding I, Evans PJ, Akanmu D et al. Characterization of the potential antioxidant and pro-oxidant actions of some neuroleptic drugs. Biochem Pharmacol 1995; 49: 359–365.

Keshavan MS, Mallinger AG, Pettegrew JW, Dippold C. Erythrocyte membrane phospholipids in psychotic patients. Psychiatry Res 1993; 49: 89–95.

Kovaleva ES, Orlov ON, Bogdanova ED et al. Study of the process of lipid peroxidation in patients with endogenous psychoses using gas chromatography. Zh Nevropatol Psikhiatr 1989; 89: 99–103.

Kramer K, Voss H-P, Grimberger JA, Timmerman H, Bast A. The effects of ischemia and recirculation, hypoxia and recovery on antioxidant factors and β-adrenoreceptor density: is the damage in erythrocytes a reflection of brain damage caused by complete cerebral ischemia and by hypoxia? Biochem Biophys Res Commun 1987; 149: 568–575.

Leff J, Sartorius N, Jablensky A, Korten A, Ernberg G. The international pilot study of schizophrenia: five-year follow-up findings. Psychol Med 1992; 22: 131–145.

Liday LA, Pippenger CE, Howard AA, Lieberman JA. Free radical scavenging enzyme activity and related trace metals in clozapine-induced agranulocytosis: a pilot study. J Clin Psychopharmacol 1995; 15: 353–360.

Lohr JB, Underhill S, Moir S, Jeste DV. Increased indices of free radical activity in the cerebrospinal fluid of patients with tardive dyskinesia. Biol Psychiatry 1989; 28: 535–539.

Mahadik SP, Gowda S. Antioxidants in the treatment of schizophrenia. Drugs Today 1996; 32: 1–13.

Mahadik SP, Mukherjee S. Free radical pathology and antioxidant defense in schizophrenia: a review. Schizophr Res 1996; 19: 1–17.

Mahadik SP, Scheffer RE. Oxidative injury and potential use of antioxidants in schizophrenia. Prostagland Leukotr Essent Fatty Acids 1996; 55: 45–54.

Mahadik SP, Mukherjee S, Correnti EE et al. Plasma membrane phospholipid and cholesterol distribution of skin fibroblasts from drug-naïve patients at the onset of psychosis. Schizophr Res 1994; 13: 239–247.

Mahadik SP, Mukherjee S, Correnti EE, Scheffer R. Plasma membrane phospholipid fatty acid composition of cultured skin fibroblasts from schizophrenic patients: comparison with bipolar and normal controls. Psychiatry Res 1996a; 63: 133–142.

Mahadik SP, Schendarkar NS, Scheffer R, Mukherjee S, Correnti EE. Utilization of precursor essential fatty acids in culture by skin fibroblasts from schizophrenic patients and normal controls. Prostagland Leukotr Essent Fatty Acids 1996b; 55: 65–70.

Mahadik SP, Mukherjee S, Scheffer R, Correnti EE, Mahadik JS. Elevated plasma lipid peroxides at the onset of nonaffective psychosis. Biol Psychiatry 1998; 43: 674–679.

Mahadik SP, Mulchandani M, Hegde MV, Ramjekar PK. Cultural and socio-economic differences in dietary intake of essential fatty acids and antioxidants: effects on the course and outcome of schizophrenia. In: Glen I, Peet M, Horrobin DF, eds. Phospholipid spectrum disorder in psychiatry. Carnforth: Marius Press, 1999: 167–179.

Marchbanks RM, Mulcrone J, Whatley SA. Aspects of oxidative metabolism in schizophrenia. Br J Psychiatry 1995; 167: 293–298.

May JM, Qu Z-C, Morrow JD. Interaction of ascorbate and α-tocopherol in resealed erythrocyte ghosts. J Biol Chem 1996; 271: 10577–10582.

Maziere C, Maziere J-C, Mora L, Auclair M, Polonovski J. Trifluoperazine increases fatty acid turnover in phospholipids in cultured human fibroblasts. Lipids 1988; 23: 419–423.

McCreadie RG, MacDonald E, Wiles D, Campbell G, Paterson JR. The Nithsdale Schizophrenia Surveys. XIV. Plasma lipid peroxide and serum vitamin E levels in patients with and without tardive dyskinesia, and in normal subjects. Br J Psychiatry 1995; 167: 610–617.

Mellow-Filho AC, Meneghini R. In vivo formation of single strand breaks in DNA by hydrogen peroxide is mediated by the Haber-Weiss reaction. Biochim Biophys Acta 1984; 781: 56–63.

Meyers DG, Maloley PA, Weeks D. Safety of antioxidant vitamins. Arch Intern Med 1996; 156: 925–935.

Morrow JD, Frei B, Longmire AW et al. Increase in circulating products of lipid peroxidation (F2-isoprostanes) in smokers: smoking as a cause of oxidative damage. N Engl J Med 1995; 332: 1198–1203.

Mukherjee S, Mahadik SP, Correnti EE, Scheffer R, Kelkar H. Impaired antioxidant defense system at the onset of psychosis. Schizophr Res 1996; 19: 19–26.

Murthy JN, Laev H, Karpiak S, Mahadik SP. Enzymes of oxyradical metabolism after haloperidol treatment of rat. Soc Neurosci 1989; 15: 139.

Nair TR, Christensen JD, Kingsbury SJ, Kumar NG, Terry WM, Garver DL. Progression of cerebroventricular enlargement and the subtyping of schizophrenia. Neuroimaging 1997; 74: 141–145.

Nasrallah HA. Neurodevelopmental pathogenesis of schizophrenia. Psychiatr Clin North Am 1993; 16: 269–280.

Neuringer M, Connor WE, Lin DS, Barstad L, Luck S. Biochemical and functional effect of prenatal and postnatal ω-3 fatty acid deficiency on retina and brain in rhesus monkeys. Proc Natl Acad Sci USA 1986; 83: 4021–4025.

O'Brien JS, Sampson EL. Lipid composition of the normal human brain: gray matter, white matter, and myelin. J Lipid Res 1965; 6: 537–544.

Ohkawa H, Ohishi N, Yagi K. Assay for lipid peroxides in animal tissues by thiobarbituric acid reaction. Analyt Biochem 1979; 95: 351–358.

Pall HS, Williams AC, Blake DR, Lunec J. Evidence of enhanced lipid peroxidation in the cerebrospinal fluid of patients taking phenothiazines. Lancet 1987; ii: 596–597.

Peet M, Laugharne J, Rangarajan N, Reynolds GP. Tardive dyskinesia, lipid peroxidation, and sustained amelioration with vitamin E treatment. Int Clin Psychopharmacol 1993; 8: 151–153.

Peet M, Laugharne J, Horrobin DF, Reynolds GP. Arachidonic acid: a common link in the biology of schizophrenia? Arch Gen Psychiatry 1994; 51: 665–666.

Peet M, Laugharne JDE, Rangarajan N, Horrobin DF, Reynolds G. Depleted red cell membrane essential fatty acids in drug-treated schizophrenic patients. J Psychiatr Res 1995; 29: 227–232.

Peet M, Laugharne JDE, Mellor J, Ramchand CN. Essential fatty acid deficiency in erythrocyte membranes from chronic schizophrenic patients, and the clinical effects of dietary supplementation. Prostagland Leukotr Essent Fatty Acids 1996; 55: 71–75.

Peet M, Poole J, Laugharne J. Breastfeeding, neurodevelopment and schizophrenia. In: Glen I, Peet M, Horrobin DF, eds. Phospholipid spectrum disorder in psychiatry. Carnforth: Marius Press, 1999: 159–166.

Pettegrew JW, Keshavan MS, Panchalingam K et al. Alterations in brain high-energy phosphate and membrane phospholipid metabolism in first-episode drug-naïve schizophrenics. A pilot study of the dorsal prefrontal cortex by *in vivo* phosphorus-31 nuclear magnetic resonance spectroscopy. Arch Gen Psychiatry 1991; 48: 563–568.

Phillips M, Erickson GA, Sabas M et al. Volatile organic compounds in the breath of patients with schizophrenia. J Clin Pathol 1995; 48: 861–864.

Piomelli D, Pilon C, Giros B, Sokoloff P, Martres M-P, Schwartz JC. Dopamine activation of the arachidonic acid cascade as a basis for D1/D2 receptor synergism. Nature 1991; 353: 164–167.

Prilipko LL. Activation of lipid peroxidation under stress and in schizophrenia. In: Kemali D, Morozov PV, Toffano G, eds. New research strategies in biological psychiatry. Biological psychiatry – new perspectives. Vol 3. London: John Libbey 1984: 254–258.

Prohaska JR, Ganther HE. Selenium and glutathione peroxidase in developing rat brain. J Neurochem 1976; 27: 1379–1387.

Rafalowska U, Liu G-J, Floyd RA. Peroxidation induced changes in synaptosomal transport of dopamine and gamma-aminobutyric acid. Free Radic Biol Med 1989; 6: 485–492.

Ramchand CN, Davies JI, Tresman RL, Griffins ICD, Peet M. Reduced susceptibility to oxidative damage of erythrocyte membranes from medicated schizophrenic patients. Prostagland Leukotr Essent Fatty Acids 1996; 55: 27–31.

Rana RS, Hokin LE. Role of phosphoinositols in transmembrane signaling. Physiol Rev 1990; 70: 115–164.

Reddy R, Yao J. Free radical pathology in schizophrenia: a review. Prostagland Leukotr Essent Fatty Acids 1996; 55: 33–43.

Reddy R, Mahadik SP, Mukherjee S, Murthy JN. Enzymes of the antioxidant defense system in chronic schizophrenic patients. Biol Psychiatry 1991; 30: 409–412.

Rice-Evans CA, Diplock AT. Current status of antioxidant therapy. Free Radic Biol Med 1993; 15: 77–96.

Richardson-Andrews RC. Unification of the findings in schizophrenia by reference to the effects of gestational zinc deficiency. Med Hypotheses 1990; 31: 141–153.

Roberts GW, Crow TJ. The neuropathology of schizophrenia – a progress report. Br Med Bull 1987; 43: 599–615.

Rotrosen J, Wolkin A. Phospholipid and prostaglandin hypotheses of schizophrenia. In: Meltzer HY, ed. Psychopharmacology: the third generation of progress. New York: Raven Press, 1987: 759–764.

Roy D, Pathak DN, Singh R. Effects of chlorpromazine on the activities of antioxidant enzymes and lipid peroxidation in the various regions of aging rat brain. J Neurochem 1984; 42: 628–633.

Sartorius N, Jablensky A, Korten A et al. Early manifestations and first-contact incidence of schizophrenia in different cultures. Psychol Med 1986; 16: 909–928.

Schwartz RD, Skolnick P, Paul SM. Regulation of γ-aminobutyric acid/barbiturate receptor gated chloride ion flux in brain vesicles by phospholipase A2: possible role of oxygen radicals. J Neurochem 1988; 50: 565–571.

Seeman P, Niznik HB, Guan H-C, Booth G, Ulpian C. Link between D1 and D2 dopamine receptors is reduced in schizophrenia and Huntington diseased brains. Proc Natl Acad Sci USA 1989; 86: 10156–10160.

Selemon LD, Rajkowska G, Goldman-Rakic PS. Abnormally high neuronal density in the schizophrenic cortex. Arch Gen Psychiatry 1995; 52: 805–818.

Shivkumar BR, Ravindranath V. Oxidative stress and thiol modifications induced by chronic administration of haloperidol. J Pharmacol Exp Ther 1993; 265: 1137–1141.

Simonian NA, Coyle JT. Oxidative stress in neurodegenerative diseases. Ann Rev Pharmacol Toxicol 1996; 36: 82–106.

Simopoulos AP. Omega-3 fatty acids in health and disease, and in growth and development. Am J Clin Nutr 1991; 54: 438–463.

Sinclair HM. History of essential fatty acids. In: Horrobin DF, ed. Omega-6 essential fatty acids: pathophysiological role in clinical medicine. New York: Alan R. Liss Inc., 1990: 1–19.

Sinet PM. Metabolism of oxygen derivatives in Down's syndrome. Ann N Y Acad Sci 1982; 396: 83–94.

Sohal RS, Ku H-H, Agarwal S, Forster MJ, Lal H. Oxidative damage, mitochondrial oxidant generation and antioxidant defenses during aging and in response to food restriction in the mouse. Mech Ageing Dev 1994; 74: 121–133.

Stadtman ER. Protein oxidation and aging. Science 1992; 257: 1220–1224.

Stubbs CD, Smith AD. Essential fatty acids in membrane: physical properties and function. Biochem Soc Trans 1990; 18: 779–781.

Subbarao KV, Richardson JS, Ang LC. Autopsy samples of Alzheimer's cortex show increased lipid peroxidation *in vitro*. J Neurochem 1990; 55: 342–345.

Suboticanec K, Folnegovic-Smalc V, Korbar M, Mestrovic B, Buzina R. Vitamin C status in chronic schizophrenia. Biol Psychiatry 1990; 28: 959–966.

Suzuki K. Chemistry and metabolism of brain lipids. In: Siegel GJ, Albers RW, Agranoff BW, Katzman R, eds. Basic neurochemistry, 3rd edn. Boston, MA: Little, Brown and Company, 1981: 355–370.

Vaddadi KS, Courtney P, Gilleard CJ, Manku MS, Horrobin DF. A double-blind trial of essential fatty acid supplementation in patients with tardive dyskinesia. Psychiatry Res 1989; 27: 313–323.

van Gossum A, Decuyper J. Breath alkanes as an index of lipid peroxidation. Eur Respir J 1989; 2: 787–791.

Wainwright PE. Do essential fatty acids play a role in brain and behavioural development? Neurosci Biobehav Rev 1992; 16: 193–205.

Williamson PC, Brauer M, Leonard S, Thomson T, Drost D. [31]P magnetic resonance spectroscopy studies in schizophrenia. Prostagland Leukotr Essent Fatty Acids 1996; 55: 115–118.

Wolff SP, Dean RT. Fragmentation of proteins by free radicals and its effect on their susceptibility to enzymic hydrolysis. Biochem J 1986; 234: 399–403.

Woods BT, Yurgelum-Todd D, Benes EM, Frankenburg FR, Pope HG Jr, McSparren J. Progressive ventricular enlargement in schizophrenia: comparison to bipolar affective disorder and correlation with clinical course. Biol Psychiatry 1990; 27: 341–352.

World Health Organization. Schizophrenia: an international follow-up study. New York: John Wiley and Sons, 1979.

Yao JK, van Kammen DP, Welker JA, Gurklis J. Red blood cell membrane dynamics in schizophrenia. III. Correlation of fatty acid abnormalities with clinical measures. Schizophr Res 1994; 13: 227–232.

Young IS, Trimble ER. Measurement of malondialdehyde in plasma by high performance liquid chromatography with fluorometric detection. Ann Clin Biochem 1991; 28: 504–508.

Zipursky RB, Lim KO, Sullivan EV, Brown BW, Pfefferbaum A. Widespread cerebral gray matter volume deficits in schizophrenia. Arch Gen Psychiatry 1992, 49: 195–205.

The Effects of Antipsychotic Drugs on Membrane Phospholipids: A Possible Novel Mechanism of Action of Clozapine

10

David F. Horrobin

INTRODUCTION

Conventional antipsychotics were introduced in the 1950s. Although the atypical antipsychotics were first discovered in the 1960s, the first of them, clozapine, did not become widely used until the 1990s. In the case of both groups, it is fair to say that the mechanisms of action remain to be firmly established.

The conventional antipsychotics have long been thought to act *via* blockade of dopamine receptors. Indeed, the consistency of the relationship between D_2 receptor blockade and drug potency has long been the strongest piece of evidence – some might say the only substantial piece of evidence – in favour of the dopamine theory of schizophrenia. Since D_2 receptor blockade always results in stimulation of prolactin secretion, this evidence is actually equally consistent with a prolactin deficiency theory of schizophrenia, and no-one has excluded the possibility that prolactin may contribute to antipsychotic efficacy. This serves to emphasize that any detailed inspection of the pharmacology of the conventional antipsychotics reveals that they have extraordinarily complex ranges of action. There are many other possible contenders for mechanisms which might contribute to their therapeutic effects.

Much the same is true of clozapine. Clozapine has very complex effects on many neurotransmitter systems, particularly dopaminergic and serotoninergic mechanisms. Many drugs have been synthesized which, to a greater or lesser degree, mimic the receptor interaction profile of clozapine. Several of these have been clinically tested and, indeed, have reached the market. However, a consensus is now emerging to the effect that while these novel atypical antipsychotics undoubtedly are different from the traditional drugs in their reduced risk of extrapyramidal effects, they are not equivalent to clozapine. Clozapine appears to have a quality of therapeutic effect in schizophrenia which is not shared by the newer atypical antipsychotic drugs. One possible conclusion is that clozapine has additional, hitherto unsuspected, mechanisms of action.

This book is devoted to the concept that disorders of membrane phospholipid metabolism may have a role to play in psychiatric disorders. There is substantial evidence, albeit of uneven quality, that conventional antipsychotics can have many different actions on membrane lipids. There are preliminary results, from two different sources, which suggest that clozapine also may have actions on lipid metabolism. This chapter briefly reviews some of the evidence.

CONVENTIONAL ANTIPSYCHOTICS

There are three main ways in which conventional antipsychotics may influence membrane lipid metabolism.

Indirect effects on cell signalling

Indirect effects on cell signalling may be produced by conventional antipsychotics, mediated through receptor blocking actions. Several receptors which are modulated by conventional antipsychotics interact with lipid-related cell signalling systems, such as the release of arachidonic acid by phospholipase A_2 or by phospholipase C in the course of the phosphatidyl–inositol cycle (Pacini et al., 1994).

Indirect effects on lipid metabolism

The conventional antipsychotics may produce indirect effects on lipid metabolism, mediated, for example, by the effect of prolactin on lipoprotein lipase (Hang and Rillema, 1997). All conventional antipsychotics stimulate prolactin secretion. Prolactin is a stimulator of lipoprotein lipase. As has been pointed out in several other chapters in this book, lipoprotein lipase is one of the key enzymes determining the rate of entry of fatty acids into the brain, and its activity is particularly high in the hippocampus (Eckel and Robbins, 1984; Shirai et al., 1986). It is therefore possible that some of the actions of conventional neuroleptics may, in part, be mediated by the effects of prolactin on lipoprotein lipase.

Direct effects on lipid metabolism

Large numbers of direct effects on lipid metabolism have been reported to be associated with conventional neuroleptics. There are, in fact, several hundred papers on the effects of conventional antipsychotics on lipid chemistry and metabolism, but most of them are very difficult to interpret in relation to their actions in schizophrenia. There are almost no published reports concerning the effects of antipsychotics on lipid metabolism in humans.

The proliferation of reports in this area relates to four major effects of conventional antipsychotics. First, they are lipophilic or amphiphilic compounds which readily insert themselves into the bilayer phospholipid membranes which constitute neuronal (and indeed all cell) outer membranes; the antipsychotics have thus been used extensively to probe the properties of such membranes. Second, they are compounds which can interfere with the effects of phospholipase A_2 and so have been used to explore the roles of this enzyme in a variety of situations. Third, they are compounds which have major effects on the phosphatidyl–inositol cycle and so have been used to investigate that system. Fourth, they bind to calmodulin and so have been used to investigate calcium-related cell signalling. Given this extraordinary range of nonreceptor-mediated effects, it is surprising that almost all the attention concerning their therapeutic mode of action has been directed at the single mechanism of dopamine blockade.

The real problem of relating these hundreds of publications to psychiatry is that most of the work has been done in cultured cells or cell-free membrane systems, and it is not at all clear how relevant these systems, and the drug concentrations used, are to clinical psychiatry. All that one can really say is that the lipid mechanisms deserve to receive much more attention when we are trying to understand the mechanisms of drug action.

Membrane structure and translocase proteins

Some sample papers on the effects of chlorpromazine on natural and synthetic membranes are those by Housley et al. (1986), Luxnat and Gall (1986), Hartmann and Glaser (1991), Anteneodo et al. (1995), and Chen and Huestis (1997). These studies demonstrate that, by reason of its chemistry, chlorpromazine has direct actions on membrane lipid structure. It may also have effects on translocase proteins which are able to flip phospholipids from one side of the membrane to the other.

Phospholipase A_2

There is also a substantial literature on the ability of phenothiazines and related compounds to inhibit the action of phospholipase A_2 (e.g., Holmsen et al., 1984; Ishigooka et al., 1985). This effect may well be related to the ability of these drugs to interact with calmodulin, which is one of the factors which regulate phospholipases (Rothenberg, 1987; Nakagawa and Waku, 1988).

The inositol cycle

There are many papers on the effects of conventional antipsychotics on the inositol cycle. The mechanisms are by no means certain, but the effects are a relatively consistent accumulation of phosphatidylinositol and certain inositol phosphates (Mullikin and Helmkamp, 1984; Leli et al., 1989; Essali et al., 1990; Wakatabe et al., 1991; Heiczman and Toth, 1995). These accumulations may be related to the *in vivo* phospholipid storage disorder seen with high doses of antipsychotics (Kodavanti et al., 1990). Given the importance of the inositol cycle in neuronal cell signalling, it is surprising that these effects have not received more attention from those trying to explain neuroleptic actions.

Other lipid-related effects

While the bulk of the papers relate to the above mechanisms, many other lipid-related effects of conventional antipsychotics have been reported. They include: pro-oxidant but, more consistently, also antioxidant actions (Jeding et al., 1995; Bindoli et al., 1988; Yamamoto et al., 1996); a shift of phospholipid synthesis from the formation of phosphatidylcholine and phosphatidylethanolamine to phosphatidylserine and phosphatidylinositol (Pelech and Vance, 1984; Leli and Hauser, 1987; Rabkin, 1989, 1994; Rhodes et al., 1993); activation of phospholipid acyltransferase and inhibition of cholesterol acyltransferase (Maziere et al., 1988); regulation of sphingomyelin metabolism (Albouz et al., 1986; Kolesnick and Herner, 1989; Hoshi and Fujino, 1992); and inhibition of phosphohydrolase (Holmsen and Dangelmaier, 1990).

How important any of these actions is in the management of psychiatric disorder is unknown. What is clear is that further investigation is required. At present, all that can be said is that conventional neuroleptic treatment does not appear to influence the levels of red cell fatty acids (Glen et al., 1994, 1996), but this certainly does not exclude the possibility of lipid-related actions being important in the brain.

CLOZAPINE

Most people agree that clozapine has both quantitatively and qualitatively atypical effects on schizophrenia. These are undoubtedly different from the conventional neuroleptics. However, it is now being recognized that clozapine also has effects which are different from the new generation of atypical neuroleptics. Some mechanism, additional to that of the known receptor blocking profile, is required to explain the effects. There are several possible hypotheses.

A possible prostaglandin E analogue

Clozapine behaves in some respects like a prostaglandin E analogue (Horrobin et al., 1978). Its structure is one which might theoretically interact with prostaglandin receptors. Its adverse effects of excess salivation and epilepsy are consistent with a prostaglandin E-like effect.

An antioxidant

Clozapine can exert antioxidant, anti-free radical effects (Joffe et al., 1998). Given the importance of membrane oxidation mechanisms in schizophrenia, discussed in several chapters in this volume, this mechanism may be relevant to clozapine's therapeutic effects.

A modifier of lipid metabolism

Clozapine may exert other, as yet undefined, effects on lipid metabolism as indicated by its actions on red cell membrane lipids.

When investigating the levels of the major unsaturated fatty acids in red cell phospholipids in several hundred schizophrenic patients, Glen and I noticed that those patients who were on clozapine appeared to have higher levels of these fatty acids than patients on other drugs. We wondered whether this might be an effect of clozapine, or whether it might be a characteristic of patients selected to receive clozapine (Glen et al., 1996; Horrobin et al., 1997). I therefore compared the levels of arachidonic acid and docosahexaenoic acid in 10 patients on starting clozapine and 8–12 weeks later. The results are shown in Figure 10.1. The administration of clozapine produced a substantial and significant elevation of these fatty acids. The mechanism at the

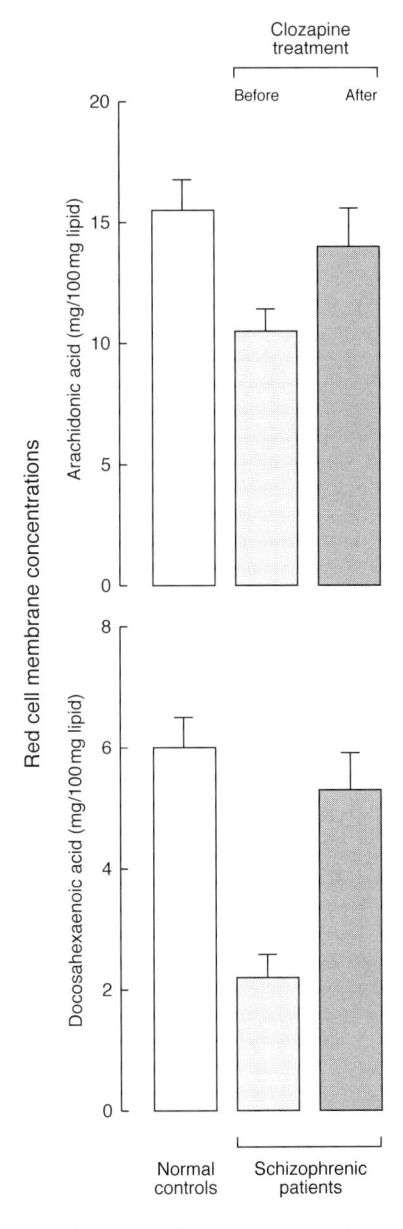

Figure 10.1. Red cell membrane arachdionic acid and docosahexaenoic acid levels before and after treatment with clozapine in schizophrenic patients ($n = 10$), compared with untreated normal controls.

moment is unknown. It may be explicable on the basis of the antioxidant/anti-free radical effects mentioned earlier, or may require other effects, such as inhibition of phospholipase A_2 or phospholipase C which remove these highly unsaturated fatty acids from cell membranes.

CONCLUSIONS

The possibility that some of the therapeutic effects of both typical and atypical neuroleptics may involve lipid-related actions has hardly been investigated. However, the evidence for the roles of membrane lipids in psychiatric disorders reviewed in this volume, and the evidence for lipid-related effects of these drugs, indicate that further study is required.

REFERENCES

Albouz S, Le Saux F, Wenger D, Hauw JJ, Baumann N. Modifications of spingomyeline and phosphatidylcholine metabolism by tricyclic antidepressants and phenothiazines. Life Sci 1986; 38: 357–363.

Anteneodo C, Bisch PM, Marques JF. Interaction of chlorpromazine with phospholipid membranes. An EPR study of membrane surface potential effects. Eur Biophys J 1995; 23: 447–452.

Bindoli A, Rigobello MP, Favel A, Galzigna L. Antioxidant action and photosensitizing effects of three different chlorpromazines. J Neurochem 1988; 50: 138–141.

Chen JY, Huestis WH. Role of membrane lipid distribution in chlorpromazine-induced shape change of human erythrocytes. Biochim Biophys Acta 1997; 1323: 299–309.

Eckel RH, Robbins RJ. Lipoprotein lipase is produced, regulated, and functional in rat brain. Proc Natl Acad Sci USA 1984; 81: 7604–7607.

Essali MA, Das I, de Belleroche J, Hirsch SR. The platelet polyphosphoinositide system in schizphrenia: the effects of neuroleptic treatment. Biol Psychiatry 1990; 28: 475–487.

Glen AIM, Glen EMT, Horrobin DF et al. A red cell membrane abnormality in a subgroup of schizophrenic patients: evidence for two diseases. Schizophr Res 1994; 12: 53–61.

Glen AIM, Copper SJ, Rybakowski J, Vaddadi K, Brayshaw N, Horrobin DF. Membrane fatty acids, niacin flushing and clinical parameters. Prostagland Leukotr Essent Fatty Acids 1996; 15: 9–15.

Hang J, Rillema JA. Prolactin's effects on lipoprotein lipase (LPL) activity and on LPL mRNA levels in cultured mouse mammary gland explants. Proc Soc Exp Biol Med 1997; 214: 161–166.

Hartmann J, Glaser R. The influence of chlorpromazine, on the potential-induced shape change of human erythrocyte. Biosci Rep 1991; 11: 213–221.

Heiczman A, Toth M. Effect of chlorpromazine on the synthesis of neutral lipids and phospholipids from [^{3}H]glycerol in the primordial human placenta. Placenta 1995; 16: 347–358.

Holmsen H, Dangelmaier CA. Trifluoperazine enhances accumulation and inhibits phosphohydrolysis of phosphatidate in thrombin-stimulated platelets. Thromb Haemost 1990; 64: 307–311.

Holmsen H, Daniel JL, Dangelmaier CA, Molish I, Rigmaiden M, Smith JB. Differential effects of trifluoperazone on arachidonate liberation, secretion and myosin phosphorylation in intact platelets. Thromb Res 1984; 36: 419–428.

Horrobin DF, Ally AI, Karnali RA, Karmazyn M, Manku MS, Morgan RO. Prostaglandins and schizophrenia: further discussion of the evidence. Psychol Med 1978; 8: 43–48.

Horrobin DF, Glen AIM, Cantrill RC. Clozapine: elevation of membrane unsaturated lipid levels as a new mechanism of action. Schizophr Res 1997; 24: 214.

Hoshi K, Fujino S. Difference between effects of chlorpromazine and perphenazone on microsomal phospholipids and enzyme activities in rat liver. J Toxicol Sci 1992; 17: 69–79.

Housley G, Born GV, Conroy DM, Belin J, Smith AD. Influence of dietary lipids on the effect of chlorpromazine on membrane properties of rabbit red cells. Proc R Soc Lond [Biol] 1986; 227: 43–51.

Ishigooka J, Shizu Y, Wakatabe H, Tanaka K, Miura S. Different effects of centrally acting drugs on rabbit platelet aggregation: with special reference to selective inhibitory effects of antipsychotics and antidepressants. Biol Psychiatry 1985; 20: 866–873.

Jeding I, Evans PJ, Akanmu D et al. Characterization of the potential antioxidant and pro-oxidant actions of some neuroleptic drugs. Biochem Pharmacol 1995; 49: 359–365.

Joffe G, Nyberg P, Gross A, Appelberg B. Is there an association between the effects of clozapine on the production of reactive oxygen metabolites by blood monocytes and clinical outcome in neuroleptic-resistant schizophrenia? Schizophr Res 1998; 29: 172.

Kodavanti UP, Lockard VG, Mehendale HM. In vivo toxicity and pulmonary effects of promazine and chlorpromazine in rats. J Biochem Toxicol 1990; 5: 245–251.

Kolesnick RN, Hemer MR. Trifluoperazine stimulates the coordinate degradation of spingomyelin and phosphatidylcholine in GH3 pituitary cells. J Biol Chem 1989; 264: 14057–14061.

Leli U, Hauser G. Modifications of phospholipid metabolism induced by chlorpromazine, desmethylimipramine and propranolol in C6 glioma cells. Biochem Pharmacol 1987; 36: 31–37.

Leli U, Ananth U, Hauser G. Accumulation of inositol phosphates induced by chlorpromazine in C6 glioma cells. J Neurochem 1989; 53: 1918–1924.

Luxnat M, Galla HJ. Partition of chlorpromazine into lipid bilayer membranes: the effect of membrane structure and composition. Biochim Biophys Acta 1986; 856: 274–282.

Maziere C, Maziere J-C, Mora L, Auclair M, Polonovski J. Trifluoperazine increases fatty acid turnover in phospholipids in cultured human fibroblasts. Lipids 1988; 23: 419–423.

Mullikin LJ, Helmkamp GM. Bovine brain phosphatidylinositol transfer protein. Selective inhibition by chlorpromazine and other amphiphilic amines. J Biol Chem 1984; 259: 2764–2768.

Nakagawa Y, Waku S. Selective inhibition of free arachidonic acid production in activated alveolar macrophages by calmodulin antagonists. Biochem Biophys Res Commun 1988; 156: 947–953.

Pacini L, Limatola C, Palma E, Spinedi A. Effects of perphenazine on the metabolism of inositol phospholipids in SK-N-BE(2) human neuroblastoma cells. Biochem Pharmacol 1994; 48: 1655–1657.

Pelech SL, Vance DE. Trifluoperazine and chlorpromazine inhibit phosphatidylcholine biosynthesis and CTP:phosphocholine cytidylyltransferase in HeLa cells. Biochim Biophys Acta 1984; 795: 441–446.

Rabkin SW. Effects of chlorpromazine and trifluoperazine on choline metabolism and phosphatidylcholine biosynthesis in cultured chick heart cells under normoxic and anoxic conditions. Biochem Pharmacol 1989; 38: 2349–2355.

Rabkin SW. Effect of hypoxia on choline metabolism and phosphatidylcholine biosynthesis in isolated adult rat ventricular myocytes: effects of trifluoperazine. Biochem Cell Biol 1994; 72: 289–296.

Rhodes PG, Hu ZY, Sun GY. Effects of chlorpromazine on phosphatidylserine biosynthesis in rat pup brain exposed to ethanol *in utero*. Neurochem Int 1993; 22: 75–80.

Rothenberg RJ. Effects of calmodulin inhibitors on rabbit synoviocyte phospholipase A_2. Prostaglandins Leukot Med 1987; 29: 61–69.

Shirai K, Saito Y, Yoshida S, Matsuoka N. Existence of lipoprotein lipase in rat brain microvessels. Tohoku J Exp Med 1986; 149: 449–450.

Wakatabe H, Tsukahara T, Ishigooka J, Miura S. Effects of chlorpromazine on phosphatidylinositol turnover following thrombin stimulation of human platelets. Biol Psychiatry 1991; 29: 965–978.

Yamamoto A, Itoh S, Hoshi K, Ichihara K. Chronic effect of phenobarbital, amitriptyline or chlorpromazine on lipid peroxidation in rat liver and brain. Res Commun Biol Psychol Psychiatry 1996; 21: 27–36.

Part IV

SCHIZOPHRENIA: RETINAL FUNCTION

Retinal Function in Schizophrenia

Fiona K. Skinner, Lois E. F. MacDonell and Iain Glen

INTRODUCTION

Dysfunctions of dopamine and other neurotransmitters are clearly important factors in schizophrenia but may not be primary causes (see Marchbanks et al., 1995). Evidence from recent studies suggests an alternative hypothesis based on the regulation of dopamine (DA) function by unsaturated fatty acids. A membrane hypothesis for schizophrenia has been proposed by Horrobin et al. (1994) which involves phospholipids. Essential fatty acids (EFAs) are very important in the development and function of both the cerebral cortex and the retina (Connor and Neuringer, 1988). These fatty acids are particularly concentrated where there is a need for rapid movement at a cellular level such as may be required in transport mechanisms at synaptic junctions. Prostaglandins, which are EFA derivatives, modulate nerve conduction, velocity, neurotransmitter release and postsynaptic transmitter action (Crawford, 1983).

The study of visual information processing can help an understanding of vision as well as suggesting how other systems in the brain may respond to stimulation. Abnormalities in the visual system, e.g., hallucinations, have been observed in schizophrenia and there are indications that some, e.g., eye movement disorder, may be relatively specific to schizophrenic patients.

The brain is the most difficult part of the body to study because of its structural, biochemical and physiological complexity, and because of the problem of access to obtain information. The vertebrate retina is a part of the central nervous system and originates embryologically from the primitive forebrain. It possesses many of the characteristics of the brain. It is a simpler system than the brain and can serve as an alternative site for the study of transmitter function and general neural systems. The retina is also easily accessible and contains relatively few neurones – only six basic types arranged in an orderly fashion (Dowling, 1970). Despite this simplicity, much information processing does occur in the retina.

If similar neuronal systems are present in both brain and visual system, a dysfunction of a particular type of neurone may be studied more easily in man from an examination of visual responses; also, a study of drug effects on retinal level may lead us to a better understanding of the action of those drugs on neural function. Thus it is possible that studies of the retina and higher levels of the visual system in schizophrenic patients may improve our understanding of the nature of the disorder and/or improve our ability to monitor changes in the disorder.

This chapter will first summarize some of the main research findings on vision in patients with schizophrenia, and will then illustrate the important role of EFAs in vision; finally, studies in which the role of EFAs in vision has been particularly investigated in schizophrenia will be examined.

VISUAL ABNORMALITIES IN SCHIZOPHRENIA

Visual perceptual abnormalities

Kraepelin (1896) and Bleuler (1911) did not regard abnormal perception as particularly important when examining schizophrenic psychopathology. Until the 1950s, abnormal perception was not considered as a candidate for a role in delusions. However, the importance of perception began to be realized in the 1950s and 1960s when psychiatrists obtained detailed accounts of altered perception from the early stages of the illness in their schizophrenic patients (e.g., Chapman, 1966).

Since that time, several reports have referred to the percentages of patients experiencing abnormal perceptions at the onset of their illness (e.g., Phillipson and Harris, 1985; Cutting and Dunne, 1986). Overall, visual distortions appear to be present in no less than 60% of any sample of schizophrenic patients. Cutting and

Dunne (1986) emphasized the need for psychiatrists to appreciate how large a proportion of schizophrenic patients experience these perceptual changes at this stage. Bracha et al. (1989) reviewed chart notes from discharged schizophrenic patients, and found that 32% had documented evidence of visual hallucinations, but, when a prospective assessment was carried out, 56% admitted to experiencing visual hallucinations at some time. It was felt that clinicians do not ask specifically about visual hallucinations as often as they should, since this type of hallucination is taught as being more typical of drug-induced or organic psychoses. This assumption is likely to have been based on the findings of a major study in the 1960s which reported only 18% of schizophrenic patients experiencing visual hallucinations (Goldberg et al., 1965).

The investigation of visual hallucination can also help predict other areas of concern in the illness. Mueser et al. (1990) found that the global severity of illness was related to the presence of visual hallucinations and not to other types (auditory, tactile and olfactory). Recognition of the early signs of schizophrenia can help an early diagnosis to be established and appropriate treatment to be given early, with consequent improvement in prognosis. Phillipson and Harris (1985) emphasized the importance of early detection of abnormal perceptions which may later develop into the more recognizable features of schizophrenia i.e., delusions and hallucinations.

Various higher-level theories have been put forward to explain the presence of these abnormal perceptions. These include a disorder of attention (McGhie and Chapman, 1961) or a breakdown in gestalt (Cutting and Dunne, 1986). The membrane lipid hypothesis for schizophrenia proposes that deficiency of certain EFAs causes upregulation of DA which, in turn, may be responsible for the visual distortion. Whatever the cause, the effect in schizophrenia may well be a contribution to the content of hallucinations and delusions and to the patient's lack of communication.

Visual function abnormalities

Eye movement disorder

In 1908, Diefendorf and Dodge reported abnormal smooth pursuit eye movements (SPEM) in schizophrenic patients and this was rediscovered by Holzman and co-workers in 1973. Since the latter report was published, a number of studies have been conducted on possible links between schizophrenia and abnormalities in oculomotor function. The results suggest that eye movement dysfunction (EMD), which includes specifically SPEM, seems to be a trait in schizophrenia that is stable over time and independent of clinical state. Clementz and Sweeney (1990) reviewed studies on EMD in schizophrenic patients and their first-degree relatives and suggested that EMD was a potential biological marker for schizophrenia. EMD appears to be one of the most consistent biological findings in schizophrenia, with 51–57% of schizophrenic patients exhibiting the dysfunction, compared to a base rate of about 8% in the normal population. Approximately 45% of the first-degree relatives exhibited SPEM abnormalities. It has consequently been suggested that SPEM dysfunction may be a phenotypic expression of factors associated with genetic vulnerability to schizophrenia (Holzman et al., 1988).

Visual evoked potentials

Analysis of flash visual evoked potentials (VEPs) has shown that they are delayed by a decrease in DA levels (Bodis-Wollner et al., 1982) and can be differentially influenced by the type of schizophrenic symptoms (Connolly et al., 1983) as well as by the stage of the illness, i.e., by whether the condition is acute or chronic (Landau et al., 1975). It is generally found that larger amplitudes and reduced wave shape variability in the first 100 ms after stimulus onset are present in schizophrenic patients who are chronic and have more positive 'psychotic' symptoms. VEP latencies are negatively correlated with positive symptoms and positively correlated with negative symptoms. Therefore, the shorter latencies associated with positive symptoms may relate to the findings of Bodis-Wollner et al. (1982), who noted that higher levels of DA, which have been shown to be associated with positive symptoms (Crow et al., 1986), would induce a shorter latency.

Forward and backward masking

In visual backward masking, an informational target stimulus is presented, followed, after an interstimulus interval, by a masking stimulus that interferes with, or interrupts, the target identification. In visual forward masking, the mask precedes the target. Using these techniques, researchers have demonstrated a visual information processing deficit in individuals with schizophrenia, i.e., they require a longer interval between target and mask to be able to identify the target. The deficits have been found to be more prominent in those with negative symptoms (Slaghuis and Bakker, 1995) and not to be a product of neuroleptic medication, since neuroleptics have been shown to increase speed of processing rather than to reduce it (Braff and

Saccuzzo, 1982). However, it appears that the deficits are not entirely specific to the symptoms or to schizophrenia for backward masking. Similar deficits were found in chronic manic inpatients (Green et al., 1994) as well as in attention-deficit/hyperactivity disorder (Rund et al., 1996). Green and colleagues (1997) also showed that unaffected siblings of schizophrenics demonstrated problems on this test, but interestingly these siblings showed only problems associated with the early sensory–perceptual processes rather than the later processes which are susceptible to attention problems. The deficit found in schizophrenia has been subject to various interpretations based on the two components: the early one reflecting sensory–perceptual processes which is based on two types of visual channels – transient and sustained; and the later one reflecting two neuropsychological processes of integration and interference which are susceptible to attention problems.

Electroretinography

In response to a flash of light, the electroretinogram (ERG) measures a negative potential called the a-wave (associated with retinal photoreceptors), and a positive b-wave (associated with the inner nuclear layer neurones). The ERG b-wave components have been shown to be sensitive to levels of DA and the a-wave components to levels of EFAs. There have been conflicting results from studies of ERG responses in schizophrenia. A fuller discussion of the electroretinographic findings is given by Warner and Peet (1999).

Visual aftereffects

The perception of a contour of a visual stimulus can influence contours of a subsequent visual stimulus so that the second stimulus is perceived to be different from its appearance when not so preceded. If the first (adapting) stimulus is presented and then removed before the second (test) stimulus is presented, what the observer perceives is an aftereffect (e.g., Magnussen and Kurtenbach, 1980). More specifically, Harris and Calvert and their co-workers have demonstrated that the use of the tilt aftereffect (TAE) may be of benefit when investigating the effects of DA on the visual system (Harris et al., 1986; Calvert at al., 1990). The TAE test may allow DA abnormalities to be assessed in schizophrenia in a noninvasive manner, and it has been found to be abnormal in patients with schizophrenia, as well as in patients suffering from Parkinson's disease (Calvert et al., 1991, 1992; Skinner, 1994), with the size of the TAE corresponding positively to the levels of dopaminergic activity. However, there have been inconsistent results for the motion aftereffect test and Harris (1994) has proposed that clinical status and medication appear to be the main causes of these inconsistencies.

EFAs AND VISION

A general overview of retinal anatomy, function and terminology may be useful before the specific effects of EFAs on the visual system are discussed. By detailed electron microscopy, Dowling (1970) established how the different classes of neurone connect synaptically. Figure 11.1 summarizes these findings. This general description is applicable to most mammalian species, including man. However, the anatomy of the retina is not the same in all species. Light energy is transformed into electrical energy by the photoreceptors *via* phototransduction. The photoreceptors contain photopigments, the main function of which is to absorb light. Stimulation causes the membranes to hyperpolarise, which is the opposite to what normally occurs in receptor membranes. This appears to release other neurones in the visual pathway from inhibition. The photoreceptor pigments induce signals in the bipolar and horizontal neurones by electrical current flow across the synaptic gaps *via* chemical transmitters. The signal is transmitted from photoreceptor to bipolar to ganglion cell but also spreads laterally through networks of horizontal and amacrine cells. Interplexiform cells can spread the signal laterally in the inner plexiform layer, but also feed it back to the outer plexiform layer to influence incoming signals. As well as the chemical synapses, gap junctions have been detected between those cells which spread signals laterally. Gap junctions are low-resistance channels bridging the gap between coupled cells and they have been shown to mediate electrical conduction (S-potential spread). The ganglion cells are the final stage before the signal leaves the retina, and their electrical responses are characterized by the formation of propagated spike potentials. The electrical responses recorded from photoreceptor, horizontal and bipolar cells are all graded, nonpropagated potentials.

Within the visual system, as well as in the brain, there is a wide range of neurotransmitters and it is well documented that DA can influence the visual system (for reviews see: Daw et al., 1982; Ehinger, 1983). Horizontal cells in the retina are electrically coupled *via* gap junctions and can be uncoupled by DA (Lasater and Dowling, 1985) or by arachidonic acid (AA) metabolites (Miyachi et al., 1994), which in turn can influence visual sensitivity. Miyachi et al. (1994) showed that it is the lipoxygenase metabolites of AA, rather than the acid itself, that modify the gap junctions. These findings

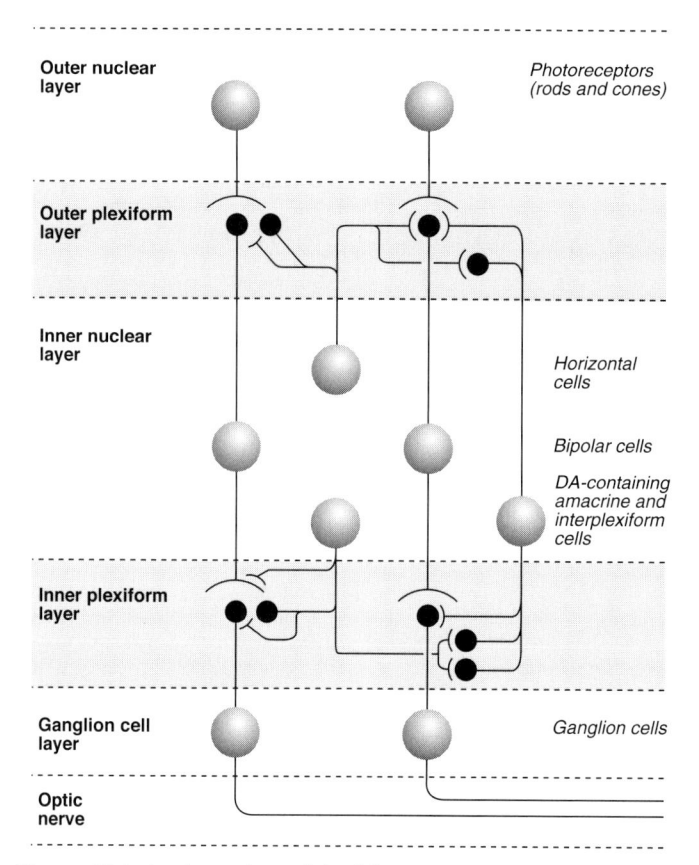

Figure 11.1. A schematic model of the retina (see text for explanation). After Hadjiconstantinou and Neff (1984).

suggest that associations might be found between visual sensitivity in human subjects and levels of AA, or its lipoxygenase products.

One of the long-chain fatty acids, docosahexaenoic acid (DHA), is also important in visual function. DHA-rich phospholipids are tightly bound to rhodopsin, the photosensitive pigment of rod photoreceptors, and are a major component of the outer segment disc membrane in which rhodopsin rests (reviewed by Fliesler and Anderson, 1983; Bazán et al., 1986).

Deficiencies of EFAs have been found to affect visual acuity and the size of the 'a' wave amplitude of the ERG (Connor and Neuringer, 1988).

The importance of EFAs in the visual system, and the fact that EFA supplementation can change visual function, has been investigated in preterm and term infants by many research workers. For example, Uauy-Dagach and colleagues (1994) stated that their studies provide clear evidence of an effect of dietary ω-3-EFA deficiency on eye and brain function of preterm infants as shown by the results of ERG and cortical VEP measurements and behavioural testing of visual acuity. They concluded that the maturation of visual and brain function is influenced by the levels of EFAs in the early diet.

Stordy (1995) also demonstrated the importance of EFAs in the visual system when she found that individuals who suffer from dyslexia improved their night vision, as measured by dark adaptation, after EFA supplementation.

Retinitis pigmentosa involves the loss of rod photoreceptor cells, beginning with impairments in the outer cell segments. Because the photoreceptor cells contain such large quantities of DHA, an alteration in the metabolism or supply of this fatty acid could affect the functional properties of visual cells. Indeed, red blood cell (RBC) and plasma DHA content has been reported as being depressed in patients with retinitis pigmentosa, for autosomal dominant forms only (Simonelli et al., 1996).

There is evidence then that EFAs can modify the absolute sensitivity of the visual system through their modulation of rhodopsin activity, and also modify its spatial resolution by possibly modulating the function of horizontal cells.

STUDIES INVESTIGATING THE EFFECTS OF EFAs ON VISUAL FUNCTION

Contrast sensitivity

The aim of the first study which was part of a larger investigation (Skinner, 1994) to examine the functional relationship between DA, EFAs and visual function in schizophrenia, was to explore the relationship between EFAs and visual spatial sensitivity.

The contrast sensitivity (CS) test allows information to be obtained about vision over a wide range of spatial frequencies (SFs) from coarse to fine detail, i.e., from low to high SF. DA and AA acid metabolites have been found to alter the horizontal cell receptive field size by closing the gap junctions which causes the receptor field surround of bipolar cells to become weaker; this, in turn, affects the first stage in detection of spatial contrast by effectively increasingly the overall signal. This, therefore, alters the contrast and improves visual acuity.

It was hypothesized that the level of unsaturated fatty acids would be negatively correlated with CS for fine lines, i.e., high SFs, since DA has been shown to be down-regulated by EFAs and a positive correlation had been reported by others (Domenici et al., 1985; Bodis-Wollner et al., 1987; Harris et al., 1990) between DA and CS at high SFs.

Subjects

Forty-five schizophrenic patients (with a DSM-III-R diagnosis) recruited from Craig Dunain Hospital, Inverness, outpatient clinics and the community were seen, but it was possible to assess only 29 on the CS test as the others had significant impairments of sustained attention (Skinner, 1994). Of the 29 tested, fatty acid data existed for 18. All the patients on treatment were receiving only antipsychotic medication, an important consideration since other drugs can influence levels of DA and vision (e.g., Seggie, 1988; Kahn et al., 1990; Bowers et al., 1991). The 18 patients comprised one drug-naïve, one drug-free, nine on oral antipsychotic medication and seven receiving the drug by depot. The mean (± SD) chlorpromazine equivalent (CPZ100) for the 16 patients receiving antipsychotic medication was 393.2 ± 627.3; range 50–2500 mg/day.

Twenty-two normal controls, recruited mainly from staff at the hospital (sampling from all the different occupations), were also assessed on the CS test. The control participants had no known psychiatric illness, were receiving no medication, and had normal or corrected vision.

The mean age for the schizophrenic group was 34.6 years (SD 12.96) and for the controls 29.8 years (SD 9.91). There was no significant difference between the two groups for age.

Method

Contrast sensitivity. In order to obtain a CS function, the experimenter determined the contrast required just to detect the grating, i.e., the threshold for spatial frequencies of 0.5 , 1, 2, 3, 4, 5, 6, 8 and 10 cycles per degree (c/deg) . To measure CS, the lowest frequency grating was first set at the lowest physical contrast, i.e., the highest attenuation (measured in decibels), so that the grating could not be seen. Contrast was then slowly increased until the subject reported that he or she could just detect the lines; this was taken as the threshold. This procedure was completed for each SF. The process was repeated three times, the median score being taken if any discrepancies emerged.

Essential fatty acid estimation. Levels of fatty acids were estimated from 10 ml blood samples. Each blood sample was taken into two 5 ml EDTA tubes to prevent clotting, and centrifuged within 1 h at 5000 g for 20 min. The separated plasma and RBCs were pipetted into Sarstedt tubes and deep frozen (−70°C) under code before being flown to the Efamol Research Institute, Nova Scotia, for analysis by gas-liquid chromatography (see Manku et al., 1982). Freezing the samples is an acceptable procedure (Stanford et al., 1991).

Results

Table 11.1 shows the values and significance levels of Pearson product-moment correlation coefficients between CS threshold, as measured by relative contrast attenuation (db) at SFs of 0.5–10 c/deg, and (a) the unsaturation index and (b) the AA levels for RBC total phospholipid for 18 schizophrenic patients and 22 normal controls. High numbers for the unsaturation index indicate that the RBC membranes have more unsaturated EFAs, including AA and DHA, than saturates; high numbers for the CS indicates that the individual did not require a lot of contrast to be able to detect the lines of the grating and therefore showed high sensitivity. All the correlations for normal controls were negative, whereas

Table 11.1. Correlations (Pearson product-moment correlation coefficients) between the contrast sensitivity threshold and the EFA unsaturation index, and between the contrast sensitivity threshold and the levels of arachidonic acid in red blood cells, for contrast sensitivity thresholds at spatial frequencies 0.5–10 c/deg.

Contrast sensivity threshold (c/deg)	Schizophrenic patients	Controls
EFA unsaturation index		
0.5	+0.237	−0.394§
1	−0.027	−0.501*
2	+0.001	−0.617***
3	+0.350	−0.620***
4	+0.301	−0.498*
5	+0.398	−0.500*
6	+0.512*	−0.661†
8	+0.565*	−0.449*
10	+0.597**	−0.404§
AA levels in RBC		
0.5	+0.160	−0.397§
1	−0.042	−0.519*
2	+0.006	−0.643†
3	+0.285	−0.632***
4	+0.270	−0.500*
5	+0.340	−0.506*
6	+0.435§	−0.655†
8	+0.471*	−0.440*
10	+0.480*	−0.412§

§$0.1 > p > 0.05$ (borderline significance); $p <$: *0.05; **0.01; ***0.005; †0.001.

those for the schizophrenic group were mainly positive. No significant correlations were found for either group for plasma unsaturated EFAs. No significant correlations were found between age and the RBC longer-chain EFAs. No significant differences were found between the two groups for the longer-chain unsaturated EFAs, e.g., AA and DHA, in RBC membranes.

Discussion

The results support the hypothesis for the group of normal controls but not for the schizophrenic patients, i.e., a negative correlation was found for the controls between the RBC unsaturated EFA index and CS measures at high spatial frequencies; a positive correlation was, however, found for the schizophrenic patients. The levels of RBC unsaturated EFAs were not significantly different between the two groups.

Previous studies have shown that increased DA as well as AA metabolites are associated with increased visual acuity or CS at high SFs (e.g., 4–10 c/deg), whereas low DA is associated with reduced visual acuity or CS at low SFs (e.g., 0.5 c/deg) (Domenici et al., 1985; Bodis-Wollner et al., 1987; Harris et al., 1990; Miyachi et al., 1994). This would suggest that a positive correlation would be expected between EFAs (in particular AA) and CS, which was found for the schizophrenic patients. The increasing sensitivity of the visual system to the higher SFs with higher levels of unsaturated EFAs might indicate that some modulation of the intensity process is involved. This could be explained by the findings of Miyachi et al. (1994) that AA metabolites modified the gap junctions of horizontal cells, since this is one of the important neural features governing lateral interaction at a retinal level. Another explanation might be that, since Myachi's study was *in vitro* and it is not possible to determine what equivalent level of AA metabolites would be required *in vivo* for the same result, then it could be that a U-shaped curve is involved, but it is unclear which part of the curve this *in vivo* study might be dealing with. It is obviously not yet clear exactly what is happening in the visual system of schizophrenic patients.

In the light of findings from EFA studies, it seems possible that metabolism of AA *via* the lipoxygenase pathway or *via* the cyclo-oxygenase system may be dysfunctional in schizophrenia. This would be in keeping with recent reports on clinical studies of the cyclo-oxygenase pathway using the technique of niacin-induced prostaglandin D2-mediated skin flushing (described in detail by Ward and Glen, 1999). This might account for our finding of the opposite direction of the correlations between unsaturation and visual acuity between patients and controls, while the mean values for fatty acids are not significantly different between the two groups.

Dark adaptation

This study, which is still in progress, is part of a research project concerned principally with measuring dark adaptation in adults with dyslexic-type problems, as compared with controls. Carroll et al. (1994) found that 12 out of 41 dyslexic readers had abnormally poor dark adaptation. Since Stordy (1995) demonstrated impaired dark adaptation and significant improvements following supplementation with DHA, it has been suggested by her that dyslexics are characterized both by dark adaptation and by DHA deficiency. Richardson et al. (1997) have demonstrated, with functional magnetic resonance spectroscopy imaging, raised phosphomonoester levels in a dyslexic group, compared with controls, suggesting reduced incorporation or problems with biosynthesis in membrane phospholipids (see also Puri and Richardson, 1999).

We are currently examining the effectiveness of measuring DHA deficiencies by means of both dark adaptation testing and taking blood samples for EFA estimation. Horrobin et al. (1995) postulate a relationship, based on phospholipid abnormalities and genetic interactions, between schizophrenia and dyslexia noting that there is evidence for reduced incorporation of DHA and AA into cell membranes in dyslexia, while in schizophrenic patients the rate of loss of DHA and AA from membranes appears to be increased because of enhanced phospholipase A_2 activity.

Thus it is hypothesized that schizophrenics may also show impairment of dark adaptation and it was decided to incorporate a sample of schizophrenics into the dark adaptation study design. Preliminary findings reported here are for the schizophrenic sample, compared with controls.

Subjects and procedure

Ten schizophrenic patients were recruited in the same way as for the CS test, and eight control subjects were recruited from within the Hospital and from Inverness College. A Snellen eye chart was used to determine the dominant eye. The non-dominant eye was then occluded before 10 min exposure to 600–800 lux. Immediately afterwards, and in total darkness, there was exposure to a series of dim flashes of light on a Friedmann Visual Field Analyser to establish levels of dark adaptation over 25 min.

The Wilkins Sustained Attention Test (Wilkins et al., 1987) was also administered, to the schizophrenic patients only, in order to try to ascertain whether or not they had sufficiently good attention and thus to ensure beyond reasonable doubt that poor performance on the dark adaptation test was not due to inability to attend to the task. In the test, short tones were generated by a computer; the subject had to listen to the tones, count the number heard and, when the last tone was emitted, tell the experimenter how many had been counted. The tones were presented in five series of 12 presentations (the first two of the 12 counted as a practice and were not scored), at 1, 2, 3, 5 and 7 Hz. If an individual reported a number greater or less than the correct number of beeps presented, or was unable to give an answer, this was counted as an error. More than two errors out of 10 presentations at 2 Hz was regarded as inability to attend satisfactorily: Skinner (1994) reported that 90% of schizophrenics who were able to complete a simple visual test (tilt aftereffect), and 80% who could not complete this test, were correctly categorized.

Blood samples were taken under code for RBC and plasma fatty acid analysis.

Results

Two schizophrenic patients were untestable on the dark adaptation test and also failed the attention test; one because of a high error rate and the other because of inability to complete the test. A third schizophrenic failed the attention test and had very poor dark adaptation. One schizophrenic has not yet done the attention test. The remaining six completed both tests. The resulting schizophrenic group of seven patients (six male, one female) had a mean age of 42.6 ± 12.2 years and the eight controls (four male, four female) had a mean age of 35.8 ± 9.6 years. The difference in ages was not significant.

Figure 11.2 shows the control group values as a 95% confidence interval band around the mean, and the individual results from the schizophrenics, which are mainly outwith this band, demonstrating poorer dark adaptation. All subjects in the schizophrenic group were outwith the control band when 'area under curve' (AUC, i.e., average of time points 20 to 26 mins) was calculated. The difference between the schizophrenic and controls group for AUC was statistically significant ($p < 0.005$).

Significant differences between the groups for the eighteen RBC phospholipids were found in only two fatty acids: 16:0 ($p < 0.05$) and 18:3n-3 ($p < 0.005$), and for the plasma phospholipids (values for seven controls only) in three: 18:1n-9 ($p < 0.005$), 18:3n-6 ($p < 0.01$) and 22:4n-6 ($p < 0.005$).

Discussion

It is to be expected, and it is well documented (Cornblatt et al., 1985), that schizophrenic patients will have poor attention. In a review of biological markers in schizophrenia Szymanski et al. (1991) concluded that a major candidate for such a role might be the ability to maintain sustained focused attention. Results from tests purporting to measure variables other than attention must therefore be regarded with caution until an attention component has been ruled out. We have attempted in our studies to control for attention, but an exploration of the reasons for lack of attention is beyond the remit of this chapter. Having reasonably reliable results for seven of the 10 original schizophrenics is not ideal.

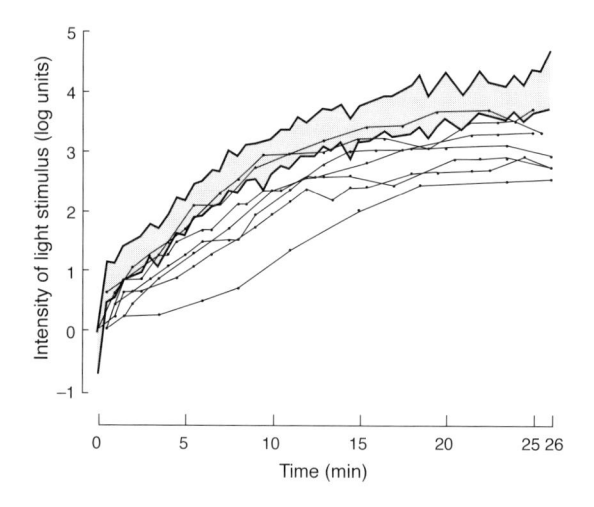

Figure 11.2. Dark adaptation curves for control subjects (shown as confidence intervals ± 2 SEM) and schizophrenic patients (individual curves illustrated).

Also, bearing in mind that the schizophrenics were taking a variety of medications, it might be expected that such a high degree of uncontrolled variance inherent in such data would result in the group not being cohesive enough for any difference to emerge between it and any other diagnostic group. The fact that statistically significant differences have emerged between the very small schizophrenic group and the control group is remarkable, and it indicates that the effect of schizophrenia must be a robust one to show up so clearly. Thus it seems that schizophrenics really do have poor dark adaptation. This evidence supports the theory of poor dark adaptation in schizophrenics, but the evidence from fatty acid estimations is less convincing. Numbers are at present extremely small. However, results from plasma fatty acid estimations probably reflect dietary differences between the groups, since hospital diets, and the diets of those living alone after discharge from hospital, are notoriously lacking in fresh and healthy produce. The RBC fatty acid results do pose interesting possibilities: either the method of estimating the acids does not truly reflect levels in the retina which are being assessed by the dark adaptation test or indeed there is no connection between EFA levels, particularly DHA, and dark adaptation. These are preliminary results and it is too early to draw any definite conclusion about this relationship, but the fact that dark adaptation improved in dyslexics supplemented with DHA in the study by Stordy (1995) should perhaps still be borne in mind.

GENERAL DISCUSSION

It was suggested at the beginning of this chapter that the study of individuals who have abnormalities in vision can provide more information about the visual system and the illness (e.g., schizophrenia) from which the individual suffers. Has this been shown to be the case?

It has been shown that schizophrenics not only suffer from visual hallucinations but that abnormal visual perception early on in the illness might help with early diagnosis, which is beneficial to the individual if it results in appropriate treatment being given.

When specific visual functions are assessed in groups of schizophrenics, a variety of important observations are made. First the eye movement disorder appears to be an important potential biological marker for the illness, with its features of stability over time and independence of clinical state being rare among measures used to date. Second, like so many other measures, visual function can be sensitive to psychiatric symptoms and to levels of DA, e.g., VEPs seem dependent on whether the schizophrenic symptoms are positive or negative, and upon the levels of DA; the latter also influences visual aftereffects. However, visual masking studies, especially those involving the backward type of masking, have found that these deficits, although initially shown to be influenced by symptoms, might not be specific to schizophrenia, since similar deficits were found in manic inpatients, as well as in attention-deficit/hyperactivity disorder. The third interesting observation is clearly demonstrated in the masking studies. When individuals suffering from schizophrenic illness have specific visual functions assessed, the importance of the visual systems involved and the role of attention should be considered. Overall, there is increasing evidence that the transient visual system, i.e., low spatial frequencies (thick lines) and high temporal frequencies (faster presentation), may be more sensitive than the sustained system, i.e., high spatial frequencies (fine detail) and low temporal frequencies (slower presentation). It is well documented that schizophrenic patients have poor attention, with the ability to sustain attention being suggested as another potential trait marker. Interestingly, the ability to sustain attention has been shown to improve if neuroleptics are given (e.g., Nestor et al., 1991). Matthyse (1978) discussed in detail how DA may affect attention, proposing that involuntary shifts in the focus of attention, and the way in which it is coupled to stimuli and internal states, may be at least partly under dopaminergic control. Cornblatt et al. (1985) found that positive symptoms and distractibility were related, whereas negative symptoms were related to lowered cognitive processing capacity. Neuchterlein et al. (1986) showed that deficits on measures of sustained attention were consistently associated with negative symptoms.

Finally, the link between EFAs and vision has been established (e.g., Fliesler and Anderson, 1983) and the specific role of EFAs in the visual system in schizophrenia is now emerging, although the precise mechanism remains unclear. The retina contains the highest levels of DHA of any organ in the body and the largest amounts are found in the outer segments of rod photoreceptor cells. The constant renewal of disc membranes requires a sustained supply of DHA. However, retinal cells have a limited ability to synthesize DHA, and therefore DHA synthesis by the liver, with its arrival to the eye from plasma and its retrieval from phagosomal lipids back to photoreceptors, is an important contribution to the acquisition and preservation of this essential component of disc membrane phospholipids (Bazán et al., 1993). Rhodopsin has as its prosthetic group a derivative of vitamin A, called retinal; this molecule is the primary visual pigment of the retina. When retinal absorbs light energy it undergoes a conformational change from the 11-cis to the all-trans configuration, thereby inducing a conformational change in the rhodopsin molecule of which it is part. This rhodopsin molecule then catalytically activates the heterotrimeric G-protein, transducin. Litman and Mitchell (1996) proposed a role for DHA in modulating the G-protein signalling system in visual transduction. It may be that since DHA and cis-retinal molecules take up a lot of space in the membranes, then if the levels of DHA decrease and are replaced by straighter saturated fatty acids, the space available for cis-retinal will be reduced, thus impairing the function of the rod cells for visual function. This could account for the impairment found in dark adaptation and electroretinography studies. With regard to the inner retina, it appears that unsaturated fatty acids may regulate visual function, possibly in part by the effects of their hydroxy metabolites controlling the gap junctions of the horizontal cells and thus influencing visual acuity.

ACKNOWLEDGEMENT

The studies investigating the effects of EFAs on visual function were supported by the Scottish Hospital Endowment Research Trust (grant No. 904) and by Scotia Pharmaceuticals.

REFERENCES

Bazán NG, Reddy TS, Bazan HEP, Birkle DL. Metabolism of arachidonic and docosahexaoic acids in the retina. Prog Lipid Res 1986; 25: 595–606.

Bazán NG, Rodriguez de Turco EB, Gordon WC. Pathways for the uptake and conversation of docosahexaenoic acid in photoreceptors and synapses: biochemical and autoradiographic studies. Can J Physiol Pharmacol 1993; 71: 690–698.

Blueler EP. Dementia praecox or the group of schizophrenias. Translated by Zinkin J, New York: International Universities Press, 1950; 1911.

Bodis-Wollner I, Yahr MD, Mylin L, Thornton J. Dopaminergic deficiency and delayed visual evoked potentials in humans. Ann Neurol 1982; 11: 478–483.

Bodis-Wollner I, Marx MS, Mitra S, Bobak P, Mylin L, Yahr M. Visual dysfunction in Parkinson's disease: loss in spatiotemporal contrast sensitivity. Brain 1987; 110: 1675–1698.

Bowers MB, Hoffman FJ, Morton JB. Diazepam and haloperidol: effect on regional brain homovanillic acid levels. Neuropsychopharmacology 1991; 5: 65–69.

Bracha HS, Wolkowitz OM, Lohr JB, Karson CN, Bigelow LB. High prevalence of visual hallucinations in research subjects with chronic schizophrenia. Am J Psychiatry 1989; 146: 526–528.

Braff DL, Saccuzzo DP. Effect of antipsychotic medication on speed of information processing in schizophrenic patients. Am J Psychiatry 1982; 139: 1127–1130.

Calvert JE, Harris JP, Phillipson OT. Effects of L-Dopa on the tilt aftereffect with differing stimulus contrast and test duration. Clin Vis Sci 1990; 5: 87–93.

Calvert JE, Harris JP, Phillipson OT. Tilt aftereffect reveals early visual processing deficits in Parkinson's disease and in chronic schizophrenic patients on depot neuroleptic. Psychopathology 1991; 24: 375–380.

Calvert JE, Harris JP, Phillipson OT. Probing the visual system of Parkinson's disease and chronic schizophrenic patients on depot neuroleptic using the tilt aftereffect. Clin Vis Sci 1992; 7: 119–127.

Carroll TA, Mullaney P, Eustace P. Dark adaptation in disabled readers screened for scotopic sensitivity syndrome. Percept Mot Skill 1994; 78: 131–141.

Chapman J. The early symptoms of schizophrenia. Br J Psychiatry 1966; 112: 225–251.

Clementz BA, Sweeney JA. Is eye movement dysfunction a biological marker for schizophrenia? A methodological review. Psychol Bull 1990; 108: 77–92.

Connolly JF, Gruzelier JH, Manchanda R, Hirsch SR. Visual evoked potentials in schizophrenia: intensity effects and hemispheric asymmetry. Br J Psychiatry 1983; 142: 152–155.

Connor WE, Neuringer M. The effects of n-3 fatty acid deficiency and repletion upon the fatty acid composition and function of the brain and retina. Prog Clin Biol Res 1988; 282: 275–294.

Cornblatt BA, Lensenweger MF, Dworkin RH, Erlenmeyer-Kimling L. Positive and negative schizophrenic symptoms, attention and information processing. Schizophr Bull 1985; 11: 397–408.

Crawford MA. Background to essential fatty acids and their prostanoid derivatives. Br Med Bull 1983; 39: 210–213.

Crow TJ, Ferrier IN, Johnstone EC. The two-syndrome concept and neuroendocrinology of schizophrenia. Psychiatr Clin North Am 1986; 9: 99–113.

Cutting J, Dunne F. The nature of the abnormal perceptual experiences at the onset of schizophrenia. Psychopathology 1986; 19: 347–352.

Daw NW, Ariel M, Caldwell JH. Function of neurotransmitters in the retina. Retina 1982; 2: 322–331.

Diefendorf AR, Dodge R. An experimental study of the ocular reactions of the insane from photographic records. Brain 1908; 31: 451–489.

Domenici L, Trimarchi C, Piccolino M et al. Dopaminergic drugs improve human visual contrast sensitivity. Hum Neurobiol 1985; 4: 195–197.

Dowling JE. Organisation of vertebrate retinas. Invest Opthalmol 1970; 9: 655–680.

Ehinger B. Functional role of dopamine in the retina. Prog Retinal Res 1983; 2: 213–232.

Fliesler SJ, Anderson RE. Chemistry and metabolism of lipids in the vertebrate retina. Prog Lipid Res 1983; 22: 79–131.

Goldberg SC, Klerman GL, Cole JO. Changes in schizophrenic psychopathology and ward behaviour as a function of phenothiazine treatment. Br J Psychiatry 1965; 111: 120–133.

Green MF, Nuechterlein KH, Mintz J. Backward masking in schizophrenia and mania. II: Specifying the visual channels. Arch Gen Psychiatry 1994; 51: 945–951.

Green MF, Nuechterlein KH, Breitmeyer B. Backward masking performance in unaffected siblings of schizophrenic patients. Arch Gen Psychiatry 1997; 54: 465–472.

Hadjiconstantinou M, Neff NH. Catecholamine systems of retina: a model for studying synaptic mechanisms. Life Sci 1984; 35: 1135–1147.

Harris JP. The duration of the movement aftereffect as an index of psychiatric illness. Perception 1994; 23: 1145–1153.

Harris JP, Gelbtuch MH, Phillipson OT. Effects of haloperidol and nomifensine on the visual aftereffects of tilt and movement. Psychopharmacology 1986; 89: 177–182.

Harris JP, Calvert JE, Leendertz, JA, Phillipson OT. The influence of dopamine on spatial vision. Eye 1990; 4: 806–812.

Holzman PS, Proctor LR, Hughes DW. Eye-tracking patterns in schizophrenia. Science 1973; 181: 179–180.

Holzman PS, Kringlen E, Matthysse S et al. A single dominant gene can account for eye tracking dysfunctions and schizophrenia in offspring of discordant twins. Arch Gen Psychiatry 1988; 45: 641–647.

Horrobin DF, Glen AIM, Vaddadi K. The membrane hypothesis of schizophrenia. Schizophr Res 1994; 13: 195–207.

Horrobin DF, Glen AIM, Hudson CJ. Possible relevance of phospholipid abnormalities and genetic interactions in psychiatric disorders: the relationship between dyslexia and schizophrenia. Med Hypotheses 1995; 45: 605–613.

Kahn EM, Schulz SC, Perel JM, Alexander JE. Change in haloperidol level due to carbamazepine – a complicating factor in combined medication for schizophrenia. J Clin Psychopharmacol 1990; 10: 54–57.

Kraeplin E. Psychiatrie; Leipzig: Barth, 1896.

Landau SG, Buchsbaum MS, Carpenter W, Strauss I, Sacks M. Schizophrenia and stimulus intensity control. Arch Gen Psychiatry 1975; 10: 1239–1245.

Lasater EM, Dowling JE. Dopamine decreases conductance of the electrical junctions between cultured retinal horizontal cells. Proc Natl Acad Sci USA 1985; 82: 3025–3029.

Litman BJ, Mitchell DC. A role for phospholipid polyunsaturation in modulating membrane protein function. Lipids 1996; 31 (Suppl): S193–S197.

Magnussen S, Kurtenbach W. Linear summation of tilt illusion and tilt aftereffect. Vision Res 1980; 20: 39–42.

Manku MS, Horrobin DF, Morse N et al. Reduced levels of prostaglandin precursors in the blood of atopic patients. Defective delta-6 desaturase functions as a biochemical basis for atopy. Prostagland Leukotr Med 1982; 9: 615–628.

Marchbanks RM, Mulcrone J, Whatley SA. Aspects of oxidative metabolism in schizophrenia. Br J Psychiatry 1995; 167: 293–298.

Matthyse S. A theory of the relation between dopamine and attention. J Psychiatry Res 1978; 14: 241–248.

McGhie A, Chapman J. Disorders of attention and perception in early schizophrenia. Br J Med Psychol 1961; 34: 103–116.

Miyachi E, Kato C, Nakaki T. Arachidonic acid blocks gap junctions between retinal horizontal cells. NeuroReport 1994; 5: 485–488.

Mueser KT, Bellack AS, Brady EU. Hallucinations in schizophrenia. Acta Psychiatr Scand 1990; 82: 26–29.

Nestor PG, Faux SF, McCarley RW, Sands SF, Horvath TB. Neuroleptic improve sustained attention in schizophrenia: a study using signal detection theory. Neuropsychopharmacology 1991; 4: 145–149.

Neuchterlein KH, Edell WS, Norris M, Dawson ME. Attentional vulnerability indicators, thought disorder, and negative symptoms. Schizophr Bull 1986; 12: 408–426.

Phillipson OT, Harris JP. Perceptual changes in schizophrenia: a questionnaire survey. Psychol Med 1985; 15: 859–866.

Puri BK, Richardson AJ. Brain phospholipid metabolism in dyslexia assessed by magnetic resonance spectroscopy. In: Glen I, Peet M, Horrobin DF, eds. Phospholipid spectrum disorder in psychiatry. Carnforth: Marius Press, 1999: 234–249.

Richardson AJ, Cox IJ, Sargentoni J, Puri BK. Abnormal cerebral phospholipid metabolism in dyslexia indicated by phosphorus-31 magnetic resonance spectroscopy. NMR Biomed 1997; 10: 309–314.

Rund BR, Oie M, Sundet K. Backward-masking deficit in adolescents with schizophrenia disorders or attention deficit hyperactivity disorder. Am J Psychiatry 1996; 153: 1154–1157.

Seggie J. Lithium and the retina. Prog Neuropsychopharmacol Biol Psychiatry 1988; 12: 241–253.

Simonelli F, Manna C, Romano N, Nunziata G, Voto O, Rinaldi E. Evaluation of fatty acids in membrane phospholipids of erythrocytes in retinitis pigmentosa patients. Ophthalmic Res 1996; 28: 93–98.

Skinner FK. Dopamine and visual function in schizophrenia: a psychophysical investigation using the tilt aftereffect and contrast sensitivity tests. PhD Thesis, University of Aberdeen, Aberdeen, Scotland, 1994.

Slaghuis WL, Bakker VJ. Forward and backward visual masking of contour by light in positive- and negative-symptom schizophrenia. J Abnorm Psychol 1995; 104: 41–54.

Stanford JL, King I, Kristal AR. Long-term storage of red blood cells and correlations between red cell and dietary fatty acids: results from a pilot study. Nutr Cancer 1991; 16: 183–188.

Stordy BJ. Benefit of docosahexaenoic acid supplements to dark adaptation in dyslexics. Lancet 1995; 346: 385.

Szymanski S, Kane JM, Lieberman JA. A selective review of biological markers in schizophrenia. Schizophr Bull 1991; 17: 99–111.

Uauy-Dagach R, Birch EE, Birch DG, Hoffman DR. Significance of ω3 fatty acids for retinal and brain development of preterm and term infants. World Rev Nutr Diet 1994; 75: 52–62.

Ward PE, Glen I. Oral and topical niacin flush testing in schizophrenia. In: Glen I, Peet M, Horrobin DF, eds. Phospholipid spectrum disorder in psychiatry. Carnforth: Marius Press, 1999: 139–144.

Warner RW, Peet M. Essential fatty acids and the electroretinogram in schizophrenia. In: Glen I, Peet M, Horrobin DF, eds. Phospholipid spectrum disorder in psychiatry. Carnforth: Marius Press, 1999: 133–136.

Wilkins AJ, Shallice T, McCarthy R. Frontal lesions and sustained attention. Neuropsychologia 1987; 25: 359–365.

Essential Fatty Acids and the Electroretinogram in Schizophrenia

12

R. W. Warner and Malcolm Peet

THE ELECTRORETINOGRAM AND RETINAL FUNCTION

The electroretinogram (ERG) (Figure 12.1) is a recording of the mass electrical potential from the corneal surface of the eye. The eyes are exposed to stimuli of moderate or intense light flashes of standardized length and intensity, and measurements are made under standard conditions (International Standardisation Committee, 1989). When evoked by a flash of light, an initial, corneally negative potential is produced, called the a-wave, which has been associated with the electrical activity of retinal photoreceptors (Hood and Birch, 1990). The a-wave is followed by a cornea positive b-wave, which is thought to reflect depolarisation of Muller cells, a result of stimulated retinal neurones in the nuclear layer. These latter are represented by a series of small, fast components superimposed on the b-wave – the oscillatory potentials (Heynen et al., 1985).

In the dark-adapted eye, dim flashes of light evoke responses dominated by rod photoreceptors and their subsequent neurone pathway. As the flashes become brighter, a cone receptor component is added. The cone receptor response may be isolated by exposing the eye to high levels of background light to suppress rod receptor activity, or by presenting a rapidly flickering light stimulus which cannot be distinguished by the less sensitive rod receptor.

Reduction in ERG amplitude can result from changes in a number of aspects of retinal function (Hood and Birch, 1990), including: reduced numbers of photoreceptors; reduced length of the outer segments of photoreceptors; reduced density of visual pigment; or altered transmission from photoreceptors to deeper retinal layers. These usually have secondary effects on the b-wave. Changes in the a-wave are throught to arise from alterations in photoreceptor function. Changes in b-wave amplitude in the absence of a-wave changes reflect changes in transmission in the inner layers of the retina and are more difficult to localize. Changes in the temporal pattern of the ERG (e.g., the time from stimulus to maximum b-wave response) are not easy to localize, but appear to occur in diffuse retinal disease, such as retinitis pigmentosa (Birch and Fish, 1987).

FATTY ACIDS, THE RETINA AND THE ERG

The outer segments of photoreceptors in the retina are rich in n-3 fatty acids, particularly docosahexaenoic acid (22: 6n-3; DHA) (Neuringer et al., 1994). A decrease in ERG amplitude has been demonstrated in rats deficient in essential fatty acids, specifically n-3 fatty acids (Benolken et al., 1973). Dietary deficiency of n-3 essential fatty acids in infant rhesus monkeys has been associated with reduced ERG amplitudes and delayed temporal responses which may be irreversible (Neuringer et al., 1986). In most studies, the effect of DHA depletion has been primarily on the a-wave, suggesting a relationship with photoreceptor function. There does not seem to be an associated reduction in photoreceptor number or length of outer segments,

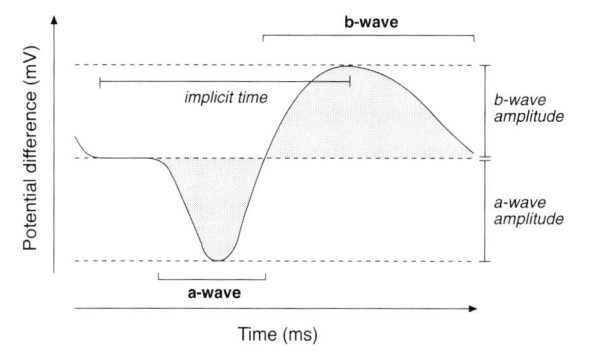

Figure 12.1. A diagrammatic representation of an electroretinogram.

suggesting that DHA may be important in affecting the function, rather than the structure of the photoreceptors (Neuringer, 1992). More recent studies on the effects of DHA levels on the ERG of the guinea pig, suggests that DHA concentrations account for up to 35% of the variability in ERG responses (Weisinger et al., 1996).

THE ERG AND DOPAMINE

Dopamine, along with other neurotransmitters, is important in the vertebrate retina, particularly in the inner and outer plexiform layers. It appears to modulate retinal function (see review by Daw et al., 1982). Dopamine has been implicated in various functional roles in the retina, including cell growth, photomechanical movement, horizontal cell synaptic transmission and light/dark adaptation (see review by Witkovsky and Dearry, 1991).

Blockade of dopamine receptors has a variable effect on the ERG in animals. Depending on the drug used and the dose, both increases and decreases in b-wave amplitude, and increases in b-wave implicit time, have been demonstrated (Jagadeesh et al., 1980; Sato et al., 1987; Schneider and Zrenner, 1987; Bodis-Wollner et al., 1989; Wioland et al., 1990); implicit time is a measure of the time latency from stimulus to the peak of the b-wave, and changes in this value occur in pathological conditions involving diffuse retinal damage, such as retinitis pigmentosa. In humans, selective blockade of D_1 and D_2 receptors reduces the amplitude of b-wave responses in the ERG (Holopigian et al., 1994). There is no effect on b-wave implicit times. Reduced ERG b-wave amplitudes have been found shortly after drug withdrawal in cocaine addicts (Roy et al., 1997), who are likely to have decreased D_3 receptor availability, and in patients with untreated Parkinson's disease (Ellis et al., 1987).

THE ERG IN SCHIZOPHRENIA

Three studies of ERG responses in schizophrenic patients have been reported. Marmor et al. (1988) looked at the ERGs of 12 unmedicated male schizophrenic patients and nine control subjects. As abnormalities in dopaminergic transmission had been postulated to have aetiological significance in schizophrenia, the investigators were interested in electrophysiological correlates of dopamine function, and therefore in measuring changes in oscillatory potentials of the ERG, as these reflect the activity of retinal neurones in the inner nuclear layers. They found no differences between schizophrenics and controls in oscillatory potential, peak amplitude, or latency. They also reported no differences in a-wave and b-wave forms, but gave no details of the parameters measured.

Raese et al. (1982) examined the variance in amplitude of oscillatory potentials in a group of 11 men with schizophrenia and 11 control subjects. Patients with schizophrenia had been medication-free for 2 weeks. Although subjects with schizophrenia appeared to have a higher variance of amplitude of oscillatory potentials, this difference was not statistically significant, due to the heterogeneity of the control group. Interestingly, the authors were able to demonstrate that administration of oral amphetamines (15 mg) to subjects significant increased the amplitude of oscillatory potentials.

Gerbaldo et al. (1992) reported ERG findings in nine patients with schizophrenia (DSM-III-R criteria) compared with 13 controls. They reported only measurements of b-wave amplitude and implicit time, which did not differ significantly between the schizophrenics and controls, despite seven of the schizophrenic subjects being on regular doses of haloperidol 5–30 mg/day. However, six of the nine subjects defined as demonstrating photophilic behaviour (sun-gazing or light-seeking) had significantly lower b-wave amplitudes than observed in controls in light-adapted conditions (isolated cone response). The investigators postulated that there is a subgroup of schizophrenics who have an abnormality in information processing at the retinal level, as reflected by the ERG responsiveness, and that this may be related to dysfunction of the dopaminergic system in the retina. The clinical significance of this particular proposed subgroup of schizophrenics is not clear.

If the reduced levels of n-3 essential fatty acids found in patients with schizophrenia (Peet et al., 1995) are reflected in reduced levels in neuronal cell membranes it would be expected that reduced ERG photoreceptor amplitudes (a-wave) would be particularly marked in patients with schizophrenia as compared with normal controls. We have conducted a study comparing ERGs in nine patients with schizophrenia (DSM-IV criteria) and nine age- and sex-matched controls. The schizophrenic subjects were found to have significantly lower mean a-wave and b-wave amplitudes in the dark-adapted ERG than were shown by the controls. However, the light-adapted ERG findings showed a differential group effect on a-wave amplitude alone and no differences in the b-wave responses (Table 12.1). There were no significant correlations between medication dose, in terms of chlorpromazine equivalents, and any of the ERG

Table 12.1. Results of ERG recordings in schizophrenic ($n = 9$) and control ($n = 9$) subjects; means ± SD.

ERG	Controls	Schizophrenics
Dark adapted		
Rod ERG		
b-wave amplitude (μV)	214.2 ± 63.2	157.7 ± 55.0§
Maximal ERG		
a-wave latency (ms)	21.7 ± 1.1	21.6 ± 1.0
a-wave amplitude (μV)	305.1 ± 55.5	215.1 ± 49.7**
b-wave amplitude (μV)	586.6 ± 115.9	459.5 ± 97.5*
Light adapted		
Single-flash cone ERG		
a-wave latency (ms)	16.2 ± 0.5	15.7 ± 0.50§
a-wave amplitude (μV)	56.6 ± 8.8	40.4 ± 9.9***
b-wave amplitude (μV)	196.0 ± 44.6	194.8 ± 65.2

In comparison with the corresponding value for control subjects, $p <$: *0.05; **0.01; ***$p < 0.005$; §$0.1 > p > 0.05$ (borderline significance); other differences were statistically nonsignificant (Student's t test).

recorded measurements. One subject in the schizophrenic group had been medication-free for over 6 months and in this particular subject the light-adapted b-wave responses corresponded to those of controls rather than to those of the other schizophrenic subjects. However, this was not the case for the a-wave amplitude, which was in accord with the mean values for schizophrenic subjects.

CONCLUSION

Investigation of ERG responses in schizophrenic patients has produced conflicting results. The amplitudes of a-waves, reflecting the activities of photoreceptors, have not been routinely measured in ERG studies, as investigators have concentrated on dopaminergic activity in the retina. Changes in a-wave amplitude attributable to alterations in the photoreceptors may be related to low levels of n-3 fatty acids, which have been demonstrated to be associated with a-wave changes in animals. There is thus some initial support from ERG investigations for the hypothesis that abnormalities in n-3 series fatty acid metabolism are associated with schizophrenia. Further research needs to be conducted to investigate the relationship between abnormal ERG findings, cell fatty acid composition and neuroleptic medication, and particularly to establish whether fatty acid supplementation can reverse the effects on the ERG.

REFERENCES

Benolken RN, Anderson RE, Wheeler TG. Membrane fatty acids associated with the electrical response in visual excitation. Sciences 1973; 182: 1253–1256.

Birch DG, Fish GE. ERGs in retinitis pigmentosa and cone rod degeneration. Invest Ophthalmol Vis Sci 1987; 28: 140–147.

Bodis-Wollner I, Marx MS, Guilardi F. Systemic haloperidol administration increases the amplitude of light and dark adapted flash ERG in monkeys. Clin Vis Sci 1989; 4: 19–26.

Daw N, Ariel M, Caldwell JH. Functions of neurotransmitters in the retina. Retina 1982; 2: 322–331.

Ellis CJK, Allen TGJ, Marsden CD, Ikeda H. Electroretinographic abnormalities in idiopathic Parkinson's disease and the effects of L-dopa administration. Clin Vis Sci 1987; 1: 347–355.

Gerbaldo H, Thaker G, Tittel PG, Vane-Gedge J, Moran M, Demisch L. Abnormal electroretinography in schizophrenic patients with a history of sun gazing. Neuropsychobiology 1992; 25: 99–101.

Heynen H, Wachtmerester L, van Norrend D. Origin of the oscillatory potentials in the primate retina. Vis Res 1985; 25: 1365–1367.

Holopigian K, Clewner L, Seiple W, Kupersmith MJ. The effects of dopamine blockade on the human flash electroretinogram. Doc Ophthalmol 1994; 86: 1–10.

Hood DC, Birch GB. The a-wave of the human electroretinogram and rod receptor function. Invest Opthalmol Vis Sci 1990; 31: 2070–2081.

International Standardisation Committee. Standard for clinical electroretinography. Arch Ophthalmol 1989; 107: 816–819.

Jagadeesh JM, Leigh HC, Salazer Bookaman M. Influence of chlorpromazine on the rabbit ERG. Invest Ophthalmol Vis Sci 1980; 19: 1449–1456.

Marmor MF, Hock P, Schechter G, Pfefferbaum A, Berger PA, Maurice R. Oscillatory potentials as marker for dopaminergic disease. Doc Ophthalmol 1988; 69: 255–261.

Neuringer M. The relationship of fatty acid composition to function in the retina and visual system. In: Dobbing J, Benson JD, eds. Lipids, learning and the brain. Report of the 103rd Ross Conference on Paediatric Research. Columbus, OH: Ross, 1992: 134–163.

Neuringer M, Connor WE, Lin DS, Barstad L, Luck S. Biochemical and functional effects of prenatal and postnatal ω-3 fatty acid deficiency on retina and brain in rhesus monkeys. Proc Natl Acad Sci USA 1986; 83: 4021–4025.

Neuringer M, Reisbeck S, Janowsky J. The role of n3 fatty acids in visual and cognitive developments: current evidence and methods of assessment. J Paediatr 1994; 125: S39–S47.

Peet M, Laugharne JDE, Rangarnjan N, Horrobin DF, Reynolds G. Depleted red cell membrane essential fatty acids in drug-treated schizophrenic patients. J Psychiatr Res 1995; 29: 227–232.

Raese D, King RJ, Barnes D et al. Retinal oscillatory potential in schizohrenia: implications for the assessment of dopamine transmission in man. Psychopharmacol Bull 1982; 18: 72–77.

Roy M, Roy A, Williams J, Weinberger L, Smelson D. Reduced blue cone ERG in cocaine withdrawn patients. Arch Gen Psychiatry 1997; 54: 152–156.

Sato T, Yaneyama T, Kim HK, Susuki TA. The effect of dopamine and haloperidol on the b-wave and light peak of light-induced retinal responses in the chick eye. Doc Ophthalmol 1987; 65: 359–371.

Schneider T, Zrenner E. The effect of fluphenazine on rod-mediated retinal responses. Doc Ophthalmol 1987; 65: 287–296.

Weisinger HS, Vingys AJ, Sinclair AJ. The effect of docosahexaenoic acid on the electroretinogram of the guinea pig. Lipids 1996; 31: 65–70.

Wioland N, Rudolph G, Bonadventure N. Electroretinographic study in the chicken after dopamine and haloperidol. Doc Ophthalmol 1990; 75: 175–180.

Witkovsky P, Dearry A. Functional roles of dopamine in the vertebrate retina. Progr Retinal Res 1991; 11: 247–292.

Part V

SCHIZOPHRENIA: NIACIN FLUSH TEST

Oral and Topical Niacin Flush Testing in Schizophrenia

13

Pauline E. Ward and Iain Glen

INTRODUCTION

Niacin, as nicotinic acid, in an adequate oral dose (>2 mg/kg), produces marked flushing of the face and upper body (e.g., Miller and Hayes, 1982). This response had been described prior to this, but the actual mechanism was not known until Eklund et al. (1979) demonstrated an association between niacin-induced flushing and increased formation of prostaglandins. Absence or diminution of the flush in response to large doses of oral niacin amongst individuals with schizophrenia was first noted by Hoffer (1962); Horrobin (1980) extended that observation and suggested that clinical improvement might be associated with the restoration of normal flushing. Attempts to quantify the flush response in schizophrenics by measuring skin temperature change and/or change in blood flow resulted in no differences being detected between schizophrenia sufferers and normal controls in two studies (Fiedler et al., 1986; Wilson and Douglass, 1986). Rybakowski and Weterle (1991) elaborated on these results by making similar observations on temperature increase, i.e., that there were no differences between controls and schizophrenics; however, they also made the observation that a significant number of the schizophrenics failed to flush in response to oral niacin, a failure that was not noted among the controls, nor among severely depressed individuals. Hudson et al. (1996) reported that about one-third of schizophrenic individuals failed to flush normally in response to 200 mg nicotinic acid, whereas all normal individuals flushed and all those with a bipolar disorder flushed either normally or excessively. In a multicentre study of patients selected for a predominance of negative symptoms, more than half of the schizophrenics failed to flush following 200 mg oral nicotinic acid (Glen et al., 1996). Both flushers and non-flushers were receiving similar antipsychotic drugs at similar doses, so the absence of flushing was not related to drug treatment.

Although it was known that the flushing seen following ingestion of niacin in large doses was due to the release of prostaglandin D2, the realization that the release was within the skin, and probably from skin macrophages, came in 1996 after one of us pursued an understanding of the flush mechanism and came upon the work of Morrow et al. (1992). This prompted the development of a skin test which is semi-quantitative and clearly shows that schizophrenics differ greatly in their flushing response to topically applied niacin compared to normal individuals (Ward et al., 1998).

The upper body skin flushing induced by an oral dose of nicotinic acid can be uncomfortable, even unpleasant, and is not readily quantifiable. The skin test which is widely used in research in dermatology and in the development of nonsteroidal anti-inflammatory drugs (NSAIDs) is quick, easily repeated and semi-quantitative. It is also acceptable to individuals with schizophrenia, more so when they can see that their response differs from that of the tester. It enables them to accept that their condition has a biochemical basis which may have the potential to be amended.

The relationship between a flushing response to niacin and abnormalities of essential fatty acid metabolism will have become apparent in other chapters of this book. In order to have a flush response to niacin there must be available sufficient of the precursor of prostaglandin D2, arachidonic acid. Elsewhere in this book the deficiency or unavailability of arachidonic acid in schizophrenia, and possible causes thereof, are discussed.

BACKGROUND

The prostaglandin deficiency hypothesis for schizophrenia, first postulated by Horrobin (1977), is substantiated to some extent by the observation that some schizophrenics fail to flush following ingestion of a large dose of niacin (Hoffer, 1962; Horrobin, 1980;

Rybakowski and Weterle, 1991; Hudson et al., 1996). Kunin (1976) suggested that niacin flushing might be due to increased prostaglandin formation because it could be blocked by drugs which inhibit prostaglandin synthesis. This was confirmed by Eklund and colleagues (1979) who demonstrated that niacin flushing was associated with a rise in prostaglandin E blood levels, thus adding strength to the hypothesis that schizophrenia may be linked to a prostaglandin deficiency. Later workers have established an association between niacin flushing and prostaglandin D2 blood levels (Morrow et al., 1989, 1992). Both prostaglandin D2 and E2 are involved in the vasodilatation seen in the inflammatory response. They both result from the mobilization of arachidonate from membrane phospholipids. Recent work (Glen et al., 1994; Peet et al., 1994) has shown the erythrocyte membranes of schizophrenics to be somewhat depleted in arachidonic acid. Morrow et al. (1992) demonstrated that the flush seen following niacin ingestion is almost entirely due to the release of prostaglandin D2 in the skin, and most probably from skin macrophage cells. Could it be that the failure to flush in some schizophrenics is due to the depletion of arachidonic acid in macrophage membrane phospholipid, or does the problem lie elsewhere in the arachidonate pathway (Figure 13.1)?

Until very recently all studies in this area used the response to oral niacin in an attempt to tease out differences in schizophrenics to find a biochemically homogeneous group which may offer a route for fruitful exploration. Some of these studies have found no difference in the responses of schizophrenics from those of nonschizophrenics. Very recently, a study using a topical application of niacin has reported differences between schizophrenics and healthy controls. An overview of these studies is given below.

STUDIES USING THE ORAL NIACIN TEST IN SCHIZOPHRENIA

The first published studies in the area reported no differences between schizophrenics and healthy controls. Wilson and Douglass (1986) gave 16 drug-free schizophrenics and 18 healthy matched controls an oral dose of 3 mg/kg of nicotinic acid and assessed the skin response by measuring blood flow using a photoplethysmograph attached to the left ear lobe. This was based on the assumption that a flush response would necessarily be accompanied by an increase in blood flow, whilst a lack of response would show no change in blood flow. They reported no differences between schizophrenics and controls in their study.

Fiedler and his colleagues (1986) also failed to detect any differences between schizophrenics ($n = 9$) and normal controls ($n = 8$) when individuals were given 25 mg of sodium nicotinate intravenously over a period of 2 min. They measured malar temperature change and converted it to a malar thermal circulation index (Wilkin, 1982).

Rybakowski and Weterle (1991) employed a method similar to that of Wilson and Douglass (1986) by administering 200 mg of nicotinic acid (2.5–4 mg/kg) orally. They used a larger number of schizophrenics ($n = 33$) and compared them with a psychiatrically ill control group which comprised 18 people with endogenous depression. In this study, the method of Fiedler et al. (1986) was used to assess temperature change and, in addition, individuals were classified into flushers and nonflushers, depending on the appearance of sudden facial erythema during the 3 h following ingestion of the niacin. The data (Table 13.1) led to three groups being identified: flushing schizophrenics ($n = 25$); nonflushing schizophrenics ($n = 8$); and flushing depressives ($n = 18$). There were significant differences between the flushing schizophrenia group and the other groups in the temperature increase, though all three groups demonstrated a rise in temperature. There was also a longer time to maximum temperature in the nonflushing schizophrenia group, the difference from other groups in this respect being statistically significant.

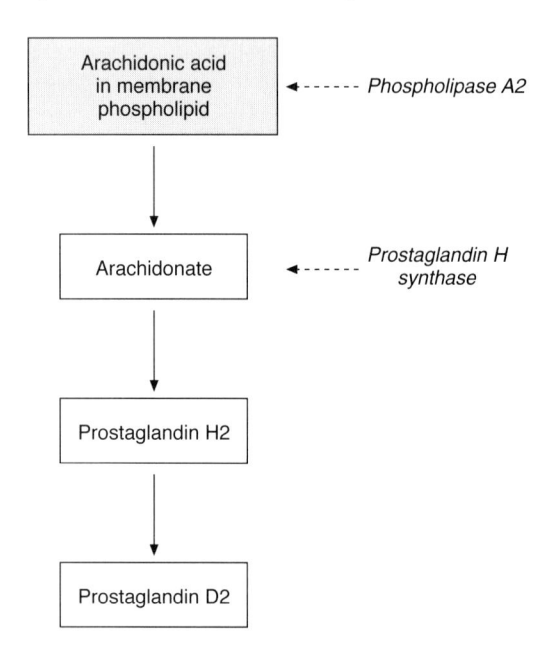

Figure 13.1. Pathway of production of arachidonate and prostaglandins H2 and D2 from arachidonic acid.

The use of the plethysmograph to measure response by change in blood flow may have led to the recording of blood flow increases in rather deeper layers of the skin, i.e., the blood flow which gives rise to an increase in temperature but not necessarily to erythema; erythema is caused by dilatation of microvessels in the surface layers of the skin. The earlier studies, then, may have relied too heavily on temperature change as an indicator of response, or they may have used too small a sample size either to detect differences or to identify a subgroup of schizophrenics.

In the course of a double-blind trial of n-6 fatty acid supplementation in schizophrenics with predominantly negative symptoms, Glen and colleagues (1996) took measures of erythrocyte fatty acids and the niacin flush response. The data shown in Table 13.2 suggests an association between red blood cell membrane fatty acid levels and response to a niacin challenge.

By this time the niacin challenge test was being standardized to some extent among researchers as the presence or absence of facial flush within 1 h of ingesting 200 mg of niacin. Hudson and his colleagues (1996) used the test to define a group who were participating in a genetic study which had as its focus the promoter region of the gene for cytosolic phospholipase A_2 (PLA_2), this being one of the enzymes which selectively cleaves arachidonic

Table 13.1. Malar temperature changes in schizophrenic and depressed patients following oral administration of 200 mg nicotinic acid; means ± SEM. Data from Rybakowski and Weterle (1986).

Patient group	n	Baseline temperature (°C)	Time to maximum temperature (h)	Maximum rise in temperature (°C)
Depressed	18	30.6 ± 0.5	1.3 ± 0.1*	3.5 ± 0.5
Schizophrenic	33	30.5 ± 0.4	1.4 ± 0.2	4.1 ± 0.3
Flushing	25	30.5 ± 0.4	1.2 ± 0.1*	4.5 ± 0.3*
Nonflushing	8	30.4 ± 0.5	1.7 ± 0.2	3.4 ± 0.4

*In comparison with the corresponding value for nonflushing schizophrenic patients, $p < 0.05$ (Mann-Whitney U test).

Table 13.2. Red cell membrane essential fatty acids and related parameters in responders and nonresponders to oral administration of 200 mg nicotinic acid. Fatty acids were measured in mg/100 ml total phospholipid; means ± SD (number of patients in parentheses).

EFA	Responders	Nonresponders
Individual EFAs		
18:0	13.42 ± 3.37 (44)**	15.09 ± 3.14 (41)
20:3n-6	1.13 ± 0.54 (44)*	0.81 ± 0.44 (41)
20:4n-6	8.86 ± 4.68 (44)***	5.79 ± 4.23 (41)
22:6n-3	2.73 ± 1.83 (40)**	1.83 ± 1.80 (30)
Ratios		
DGLA/AA	0.14 ± 0.05 (44)*	0.17 ± 0.06 (41)
LA/AA	1.56 ± 1.05 (44)†	2.42 ± 1.58 (41)
n-6/n-3	11.16 ± 15.23 (42)*	22.29 ± 26.82 (36)

AA = arachidonic acid; DGLA = dihomo-γ-linolenic acid; LA = linoleic acid. In comparison with the corresponding value for nonresponders, $p <$: *0.05; **0.01; ***0.005; †0.001. During this trial, significant increase occurred in the erythrocyte arachidonic acid level in subjects who changed in the course of the study from nonresponder to responder. Data from Glen et al. (1996).

acid from the Sn2 position of the phospholipid. Excess activity of PLA_2 (Gattaz et al., 1995) could account for the depletion of arachidonic acid seen in some schizophrenics, which could, in turn, account for the reduced niacin-induced vasodilatation. Hudson et al. (1996) found a significant relationship between the flush response to niacin and the lengths of the alleles in the promoter region of this gene, the non-flushers having significantly greater representation in the longer alleles.

In 1980, Horrobin proposed this test as a possible independent method of monitoring status or improvement in schizophrenia, rather as the dexamethasone suppression test was used in endogenous depression. This could be fraught with difficulties. Very often when individuals with schizophrenia are unwell they can have little trust in anyone and may be suspicious when asked to swallow 'vitamin tablets' to assess their possible response to them. Clinicians may be in a quandary when considering the benefits to be gained from subjecting their patients to a test which may or may not have an effect, and which may have an effect which can be extremely uncomfortable and unsettling. It is also time-consuming and can only be properly administered when the patient is fasted.

These difficulties, and an incident involving a control subject, married to one of our researchers, where he 'over reacted', becoming flushed very quickly and experiencing palpitations and faintness, led us to search for more information on the mechanism involved with the flush reaction. This search uncovered a wealth of literature in dermatology journals describing the use of topical niacin in the monitoring of skin penetration kinetics and efficacy of NSAIDs which block the cyclooxygenase pathway. This led the way to the study which is described next.

STUDY USING THE SKIN TEST

The first published study (Ward et al., 1998) using a topical application of niacin was designed to ascertain the feasibility of using such a method. Four concentrations of aqueous methyl nicotinate (AMN), i.e., 10^{-1} M, 10^{-2} M, 10^{-3} M and 10^{-4} M, were applied topically to the forearm skin in 38 patients with schizophrenia (DSM-III-R criteria) and 22 control subjects with no history of mental illness. Four gauze patches were soaked in the AMN solutions, one patch per concentration, and applied to a subject's forearm for 5 min by means of a plastic strip: in this way, each subject received all four concentrations simultaneously. Following removal of the strip and patches, the redness produced by any resulting vasodilatation was rated on a four-point scale from 0 (no redness relative to the background skin) through 1 (slight redness), and 2 (moderate redness) to 3 (maximal redness). Assessments were made at 5, 10, 15, 20 and 25 min following initial application of the patches.

At all concentrations of AMN, the responses produced in the schizophrenic patients were highly significantly different from those in the controls. One concentration (10^{-2} M) gave the greatest degree of differentiation between schizophrenic patients and controls, and this was sustained over the full 25 min period of the study.

Figure 13.2 shows the dose–response curves for the two groups immediately after 5 min exposure to the concentrations of AMN. At this concentration at 5 min,

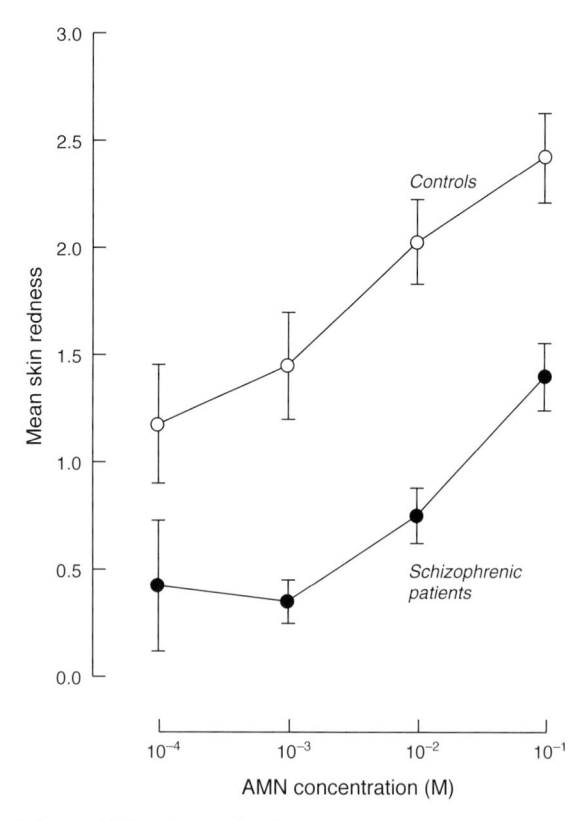

Figure 13.2. Relationship between mean redness score in the flushing response to the niacin skin test and the dose of aqueous methyl nicotinate (AMN) administered topically to the forearm skin in schizophrenic patients ($n = 38$) and normal controls ($n = 22$). Amongst the schizophrenic patients, 38 received 0.1 M AMN and 35 also received other concentrations; amongst the controls, 17 received 0.0001 M AMN and all 22 received other concentrations. Error bars are ± SEM. Data from Ward et al. (1998).

83% of schizophrenics, but only 23% of controls, had a zero or minimal response to AMN: these early data therefore suggest a sensitivity of 83% and a specificity of 77% at certain strengths (Figure 13.3).

Studies using the skin test as a semi-quantitative method of assessing prostaglandin D2 availability/activity are now proliferating. Results from these studies have yet to be reported. We have as yet unpublished data relating to mania and depression which suggest that schizophrenia sufferers are singular in having an impaired response to niacin, although sufferers from depression seem to have a slower than normal response. This and other studies are now being carried out in several centres looking at skin response in relation to diagnosis and to movement disorders.

DISCUSSION

Schizophrenia is diagnosed at present using clinical criteria which are useful but perhaps not robust enough to define the biological mechanism of schizophrenia which would lead to genetically determined vulnerability in metabolic pathways. The niacin skin test may prove to be a useful diagnostic aid and a potential biological marker, perhaps being one of a number of such tests which may be developed.

The early data on the skin test suggest a sensitivity (the proportion of true positives correctly identified by the test) of 83%, and a specificity (the proportion of true negatives correctly identified) of 77% (Altman and Bland, 1994). When a larger data set has been gathered, the predictive value of the test can be addressed. The likely way forward with the skin test is for it to be administered by clinical staff as part of a battery of tests which will outline an abnormal metabolic pathway.

We are reporting here on the niacin skin test at a very early stage in its development. There remains much work to be done. Yao and van Kammen (1994) found that membrane fluidity was predictive of relapse in schizophrenia. Yao et al. (1994) correlated membrane fluidity to fatty acid unsaturation index, a large part of which was due to a change in the arachidonic acid level. Given that response to oral niacin can be associated with levels of polyunsaturated fatty acids in the membrane (Glen et al., 1996) then we could anticipate that perhaps a poor skin response would be predictive of relapse. There may be a role in the monitoring of people with schizophrenia. The whole area of state-dependence over the course of a schizophrenic illness must also be examined, there being a possibility that the response to the niacin skin test may vary in some

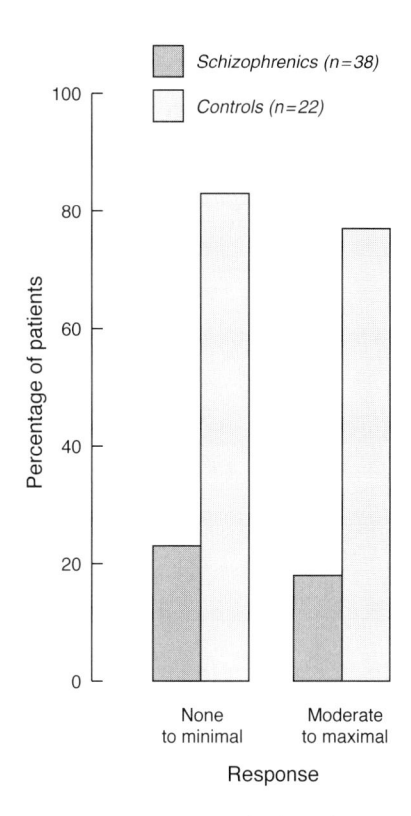

Figure 13.3. Proportions of schizophrenic and normal control patients in the study by Ward et al. (1998) who showed either no (or minimal) response or a moderate-to-maximal response, to the niacin flush test, assessed 5 min after topical administration of 0.01 M AMN.

schizophrenic individuals in accordance with variations in their illness (either illness severity or symptom profile).

Other areas which must also be considered are variations in response over a 24-h period due to fluctuations either in availability of prostaglandin or in skin penetration. The applicability and validity of such a test in individuals with pigmented skin will also have to be examined.

There can be little doubt that this test is a major progression in the field of defining a biochemically distinct group in schizophrenia. It will assist in persuading those involved in the field of schizophrenia research that there is an abnormality of basic fatty acid metabolism which they can easily assess in a semi-quantitative fashion and that this alternative hypothesis for schizophrenia is as acceptable as any other, and perhaps even more so. Its test may herald a paradigm shift in our view of the cause of schizophrenia.

REFERENCES

Altman DG, Bland JM. Diagnostic tests. 1: Sensitivity and specificity. Br Med J 1994; 308: 1552.

Eklund B, Kaijser L, Nowack J, Wennmalm A. Prostaglandins contribute to the vasodilatation induced by nicotinic acid. Prostaglandins 1979; 17: 821–830.

Fiedler P, Wolkin A, Rotrosen J. Niacin-induced flush as a measure of prostaglandin activity in alcoholics and schizophrenics. Biol Psychiatry 1986; 21: 1347–1350.

Gattaz WF, Schmitt A, Maras AM. Increased platelet phospholipase A_2 activity in schizophrenia. Schizophr Res 1995; 16: 1–6.

Glen AIM, Glen EMT, Horrobin DF et al. A red cell membrane abnormality in a subgroup of schizophrenic patients: evidence for two diseases. Schizophr Res 1994; 12: 53–61.

Glen AIM, Cooper SJ, Rybakowski J, Vaddadi K, Brayshaw N, Horrobin DF. Membrane fatty acids, niacin flushing and clinical parameters. Prostagland Leukotr Essent Fatty Acids 1996; 55: 9–15.

Hoffer A. Niacin therapy in psychiatry. Springfield: C.C. Thomas, 1962.

Horrobin DF. Schizophrenia as a prostaglandin deficiency disease. Lancet 1977; i: 936–937.

Horrobin DF. Niacin flushing, prostaglandin E and evening primrose oil. A possible objective test for monitoring therapy in schizophrenia. J Orthomolec Psychiatry 1980; 9: 33–34.

Hudson CJ, Kennedy JL, Gotowiec A et al. Genetic variant near cytosolic phospholipase A_2 associated with schizophrenia. Schizophr Res 1996; 21: 111–116.

Kunin RA. The action of aspirin in preventing the niacin flush and its relevance to the anti-schizophrenic action of megadose niacin. J Orthomolec Psychiatry 1976; 5: 89–100.

Miller DR, Hayes KC. Vitamin excess and toxicity. In: Hathcock JN, ed. Nutritional toxicology. Vol. 1. New York: Academic Press, 1982: 81–133.

Morrow JD, Parsons W, Roberts L. Release of markedly increased quantities of prostaglandin D_2 in vivo in humans following the administration of nicotinic acid. Prostaglandins 1989; 38: 263–274.

Morrow JD, Awad JA, Oates JA, Roberts LJ. Identification of skin as a major site of prostaglandin D2 release following oral administration of niacin in humans. J Invest Dermatol 1992; 98: 813–815.

Peet M, Laugharne JDE, Horrobin DF, Reynolds GP. Arachidonic acid: a common link in the biology of schizophrenia? Arch Gen Psychiatry 1994; 51: 665–666.

Rybakowski J, Weterle R. Niacin test in schizophrenia and affective illness. Biol Psychiatry 1991; 29: 834–836.

Ward PE, Sutherland J, Glen EMT, Glen AIM. Niacin skin flush in schizophrenia: a preliminary report. Schizophr Res 1998; 29: 269–274.

Wilkin JK. Chlorpropamide-alcohol flushing, malar thermal circulation index and baseline malar temperature. Metabolism 1982; 31: 948–954.

Wilson DWS, Douglass AB. Niacin skin test is not diagnostic of schizophrenia. Biol Psychiatry 1986; 21: 974–977.

Yao JK, van Kammen DP. Red blood cell membrane dynamics in schizophrenia. I. Membrane fluidity. Schizophr Res 1994; 11: 209–216.

Yao JK, van Kammen DP, Welker JA. Red blood cell membrane dynamics in schizophrenia. II. Fatty acid composition. Schizophr Res 1994; 13: 217–226.

Family Studies in Schizophrenia

14

Iain Glen

INTRODUCTION

The idea that a spectrum of phospholipid abnormalities may underlie the major psychiatric disorders may provide a framework for understanding the close relationship between manic-depressive illness and schizophrenia. Such a model may also explain the association between some causes of borderline handicap and schizophrenia, because of the influence of lipids on brain development. Since alcohol has profound effects on phospholipid metabolism, the link between alcoholic psychosis and schizophrenia may similarly become understandable; Bleuler (1924) was well aware of this latter association when he suggested that 'alcoholic hallucinosis could...be a mere syndrome of schizophrenia induced by alcohol'. Finally, and rather more recently, studies of the cannabinoid receptors seem to explain the significantly increased risk of cannabis psychosis in individuals with a family history of schizophrenia, since anandamide occupies the cannabis receptor and is derived from the arachidonic metabolic pathway (Di Marzo et al., 1994; McGuire et al., 1995).

Our findings of bimodality in certain essential fatty acids (EFAs) in the red blood cell (RBC) membranes of schizophrenic patients (Glen et al., 1994) reinforced the concept of a spectrum of phospholipid abnormalities. We were able to test these findings further in an investigation of the families of schizophrenic probands in the north of Scotland, a study carried out jointly with the University of Aberdeen and funded by the Chief Scientist Office of the Scottish Office. The purpose of this chapter is to place this large family study of phospholipids in schizophrenia in the context of our own previous work and that of others; and also to review the evidence for the occurrence of a spectrum of disorders – manic-depressive illness, borderline handicap, alcoholism – in the families of schizophrenic probands.

MEMBRANE ABNORMALITIES IN PSYCHIATRIC DISORDERS

Psychiatry has been blessed (or bedevilled) by serendipitous discoveries. Thus the discovery that an anti-tuberculosis drug, isoniazid, had mood-elevating properties, associated with amine oxidase inhibition, led to the early view that amine neurotransmitters were causally implicated in manic-depressive illness. Similarly, the development of chlorpromazine in the 1950s from antihistamine-like compounds, which had useful temperature-lowering properties for certain types of surgery, was followed by the observation that it possessed calming properties in psychiatric illness: the serendipitous discovery of the tranquillizer had been made, and the findings were also to be interpreted in terms of the blockade of the newly discovered neurotransmitters as a primary abnormality in the major psychoses. The Research Councils understandably began to fund receptor studies in manic-depressive illness and schizophrenia. Only recently has it become clear that chlorpromazine may have other important actions, including, for example, effects on phospholipase A_2 (PLA_2) and on membranes (Leli and Hauser, 1987).

The earlier work in the 1920s and 1930s on cholesterol and lipid metabolism in manic-depressive illness received little attention (Brice, 1935; Randall and Cohen, 1939), perhaps because these studies were interrupted by the Second World War, and also because the technology for detecting the structure of fatty acids by gas chromatography had not been invented. After the war, the emphasis was on neurotransmitters, largely to the exclusion of investigation of membrane lipids, at least in clinical practice. The new tranquillizers had remarkable therapeutic effects compared to the existing treatments for schizophrenia – morphine, bromide and paraldehyde. The positive symptoms of schizophrenia – hallucinations, delusions and paranoia – were for the first time effectively treated, as were manic symptoms of elation and hyperactivity. Prior to the introduction of chlorpromazine, prolonged catatonic stupor or excitement in schizophrenia was not uncommon, but following the introduction of the phenothiazines these symptoms were seldom seen. However, the lack of effects of classical neuroleptics on negative symptoms and on the course of the illness prompted some investigators to look closely at receptor function and membrane systems for alternative aetiological solutions.

The accidental discovery of the clinical action of lithium in manic-depressive illness by Cade could not be readily fitted to the amine hypothesis for depression, mania and schizophrenia and was initially disregarded (Cade, 1949, 1978). Such a discovery by a little-known clinical psychiatrist in Australia seemed, in the face of the power of basic scientific and clinical research in amine transmitters, to be of doubtful significance; subsequent studies, however, confirmed the prophylactic effect of lithium in manic-depressive illness (see Schou, 1978). This action of lithium seemed more likely to be a receptor or membrane effect than the result of any direct action on neurotransmitter synthesis, and provided support for our own early studies on membrane transport deficits in manic-depressive illness (Glen et al., 1968, 1969). Coppen and his colleagues had carried out studies of the distribution of sodium between cells and the extracellular space, suggesting a disorder of aldosterone in manic-depressive illness (Coppen et al., 1966). These isotope studies were difficult to carry out and we devised a simple technique for measuring Na^+ transport across membranes using saliva (Glen et al., 1968, 1969). Further studies of the effect of lithium also pointed to a membrane transport dysfunction (Glen et al., 1972). These studies were followed by evidence that the transport systems in cell membranes, i.e., ATPases, were abnormal in manic-depressive illness (Hesketh et al., 1978). The effect of lithium on these ATPase systems and on calcium binding established a strong case for a primary abnormality in membranes in manic-depressive illness (Glen, 1985).

At about the same time, the amine hypothesis was beginning to run into further difficulties because post-mortem brain studies were bedevilled by the pre-mortem effect of the tranquillizers on receptors, and the separation of the drug effect from the illness proved difficult. Then the studies of amine metabolites in CSF proved inconclusive: there was no difference between dopamine, 5HT and noradrenaline metabolites taken from patients during the acute phase of the illness and those taken from normal control subjects. We suggested that the amine hypothesis might be replaced by a modified amine hypothesis (Ashcroft et al., 1972), introducing the concept of receptors being modified by membrane effects.

Although membrane dysfunction, e.g., altered membrane fluidity, was seen at the time to lead to potential receptor functional changes, this was not considered in terms of specific effects of fatty acids. Clinically, lithium did not have any major effect in schizophrenia. However, publication of the studies on membranes in manic-depressive illness led to an exchange of ideas with David Horrobin, then working on prostaglandins in Montreal, and an understanding of his view of the potential importance of prostaglandins and the precursor fatty acids, especially arachidonic acid (AA), in schizophrenia as well as manic-depressive illness (Horrobin, 1977). It is clear now, that minimal alterations in the composition of fatty acids alter receptor function and carrier systems across membranes: these observations are discussed by Horrobin elsewhere in this book. The changes in ATPases in manic-depressive illness, which we and others found, do not appear to be present to the same extent in schizophrenia, although this has not been so well researched. Peet, in this volume, and others, have described fatty acid abnormalities in depression.

Can a spectrum of illnesses be attributed entirely to abnormalities in membrane phospholipids? The studies of gene expression of PLA_2, and the concept of variable gene expression, are at only an early stage, and clarification of the linkages to lipid peroxidation and to the cyclooxygenase system are not yet well understood. In this chapter, we examine the range of disorders found in sporadic schizophrenics and in the families of schizophrenic probands, in terms of variable phospholipid dysfunction.

BACKGROUND TO THE FAMILY STUDY

In previous studies of fatty acids in phospholipids we had identified a general increase in saturates and a decrease in unsaturates in plasma and in brain of schizophrenic patients compared with controls (Horrobin et al., 1989; 1991). These studies were of great interest, although the changes were small, leading us to consider whether they might be secondary, i.e., associated with lifestyle changes and poor nutrition, or possible side effects of neuroleptic treatment. In a multicentre study, we examined the effects of drugs on fatty acids in RBCs using covariance analysis, and found no effect attributable to drugs (Glen et al., 1996). However, in view of the undoubted fact that the deficits of fatty acids were small, and because we had still not evaluated a possible effect of impaired nutrition, we remained uncertain of the significance of the findings. From a careful assessment of diet, Laugharne et al. (1996) concluded that nutritional effects were not a primary cause of the fatty acid deficits. In a further study (Glen et al., 1992), we identified a subgroup of schizophrenic patients who had markedly reduced levels of AA and docosahexaenoic acid (DHA) in RBC membranes, and another larger group with normal levels of AA and DHA; the patients with low AA and DHA were clinically severely impaired and many of them showed marked negative symptoms and borderline handicap with schizophrenia. This preliminary study led us to see whether we could find bimodality in a wider study of unselected schizophrenic patients and controls from a number of centres (Glen et al., 1994). We found clear evidence of a subgroup of about one-third of schizophrenic patients with very low levels of AA and DHA in RBC membranes and another, larger, group comprising the remaining two-thirds who had normal levels of fatty acids and were indistinguishable from a control population. The plasma levels of fatty acids in all the patients were normal. This finding of discontinuity in fatty acid levels seemed unlikely to be associated with dietary stress alone, and suggested instead a genetic influence in an as yet unidentified pathway.

We again examined for confounding factors to account for the subgroup of schizophrenic patients with the low AA and DHA. We could find no drug effect to account for the differences between the two subgroups of schizophrenic patients. On the face of it, the two populations appeared to have been treated in the same institutions and would have received the same diet, but we still could not entirely exclude a nutritional cause accounting for the differences. However, since the plasma levels showed no abnormality, we postulated that the low levels of fatty acids resulted from either an incorporation defect or an increased breakdown through increased release from membranes with increased peroxidation. The latter seemed the likelier since Gattaz et al. (1987, 1990, 1995) had reported increased levels of PLA_2, and Peet and others had also observed increased levels of lipid peroxidation in schizophrenia (e.g., Peet et al., 1995). Our findings of abnormalities in the RBC fatty acids in phospholipids were soon replicated by Peet et al. (1994) and by Yao et al. (1994). Further evidence for increased breakdown of membranes came from nuclear magnetic resonance spectroscopy, also reported elsewhere in this volume.

THE FAMILY STUDY

Structure of the study

The North of Scotland is uniquely suited to family studies of psychotic illness. While emigration has taken its toll, the remaining population is still cohesive and has been indigenous for many generations. More importantly, these Highland families are supportive of psychiatric research through a still well-integrated Health Service. We are indebted to them for their contribution to this study and to our psychiatric colleagues for their assistance. The same applies to the North-east – the Grampian catchment area: the families are identifiable through the Health Service contacts and are also most co-operative. In both Highland and Grampian regions, consultant colleagues in the psychiatric service have a geographically-based service which is a further aid to family research.

The families were selected on the basis that, in addition to the presenting proband with schizophrenia, there was at least one other psychotic (schizophrenic, schizoaffective, or manic-depressive) first-degree relative. The primary purpose of the family study was to see whether the fatty acid abnormalities were present equally in the proband schizophrenics and in their families. The secondary purpose was to determine the degree to which nutritional factors and drug exposure might contribute to any fatty acid abnormalities. We argued that, if there were a fatty acid abnormality, this would then be present to a greater extent in the affected than in the unaffected members of the family. The family study also presented the opportunity to begin to test the hypothesis that there is a spectrum of illness associated with phospholipid disorder.

A first analysis of the fatty acid studies in terms of bimodality of distribution has been completed, although much information remains to be evaluated (Glen et al., 1997. The fatty acid laboratory analysis was undertaken in the University of Stirling in the Unit of Aquatic Biochemistry in the Department of Biological and Molecular Science. Our initial analysis of the data was designed to answer the following questions: (1) are the findings of low AA and DHA in membrane phospholipids replicated; (2) are similar abnormalities found in individuals with a familial disorder; and (3) are they found in relatives without a psychotic illness?

We argued that, if we could replicate our previous findings of bimodality of distribution of AA and DHA, we could assess the subjects in the groups with 'low' and 'high' fatty acids with regard to diet, smoking, drug and alcohol consumption, and thus see whether the 'low' group was differentiated from the 'high' group by a significantly poorer diet, heavier smoking, increased alcohol consumption or increased exposure to neuroleptics.

The families

Eighty-four families were recruited from Grampian and the Highlands and Islands of Scotland. Inclusion in the study required that there be in the family an individual (proband) fulfilling DSM-IV criteria for the diagnosis of schizophrenia, a first-degree relative who had, or had had, a psychotic illness, i.e., schizophrenia or manic-depressive illness, also fulfilling DSM-IV criteria (affected relative), and another first-degree relative over the age of 40 years and without such an illness (unaffected relative). All individuals involved gave written consent, or where this was not possible, an uninvolved consultant psychiatrist and/or next of kin gave such consent.

The controls

Healthy subjects were recruited from the general population. All were drug-free with no personal or family history of mental illness.

Fatty acids

Blood samples were processed within an hour of venepuncture. Where necessary, the sample was kept on ice until centrifugation for 20 min at $5000 \times g$. Plasma and erythrocytes were separated and stored at −20°C for up to a month prior to transfer to −70°C. Samples taken in the Outer Hebrides were stored at −40°C prior to storage at −70°C. The erythrocyte pellet was thawed at room temperature and 1 ml was mixed with 5 ml chloroform/BHT in two stages and then centrifuged at $2000 \times g$. Fatty acid methyl esters (FAME) were prepared by acid-catalysed transmethylation and the extracts were evaporated under nitrogen. FAMEs were separated by gas liquid chromatography, and individual esters identified by comparison with known standards. The absolute amount of each fatty acid (using internal standards) was calculated relative to the total membrane phospholipid content (Bell and Tocher, 1989; Wilson and Tocher, 1991).

The potential confounders

Neuroleptic drug exposure. This was recorded for schizophrenic probands and their affected relatives and expressed as daily chlorpromazine equivalent (Foster, 1989).

Alcohol use. This was assessed as part of the MONICA dietary questionnaire in terms of weekly alcohol consumption.

Tobacco use. Subjects were asked to disclose their typical daily tobacco use as number of cigarettes smoked (or equivalent tobacco consumption as number of cigarettes smoked).

Dietary intake. Subjects completed a 10-page dietary questionnaire, extracted from *Monitoring Trends and Determinants in Cardiovascular Disease* (MONICA) (World Health Organization, 1988), with assistance from the interviewer where necessary. Conversion of the raw data to dietary values was carried out in the University of Dundee, Department of Cardiovascular Epidemiology.

Statistical analysis

A test for bimodality in frequency distributions was carried out. A mixture of two normal distributions was fitted to the AA (20:4n-6) and DHA (22:6n-3) fractions of probands ($n = 84$) by a direct function minimisation method described by Venables and Ripley (1994). In each case, a Likelihood Ratio Test (LRT) of bimodality *versus* unimodality was computed. In addition, the Wilk-Shapiro W test was also performed as a comparison (Mendell et al., 1991). The parameters of the mixture distributions were estimated by the method of maximum likelihood.

Results

Bimodality

Our previous findings were confirmed. There were 12 schizophrenic probands of the 84 families recruited (14%) that formed a 'low fatty acid' subgroup. This was a smaller number than in the previous study of sporadically occurring schizophrenia, but nevertheless, a highly significant bimodal distribution emerged using the LRT ($p < 0.0001$), and the Wilcoxon matched-pairs test ($p < 0.0001$). Values for fatty acids were expressed as mg/100 mg total phospholipid in the RBC membranes; for AA the value (mean ± SD) for distribution 1 was 4.075 ± 1.566 and for distribution 2, 11.961 ± 1.131; for DHA the values were 0.832 ± 0.395 and 4.029 ± 0.863, respectively.

We next considered the numbers in each of the four population groups that comprised the subjects with low AA; 12./84 (14%) of probands had low AA, compared with 4/59 (6.7%) of affected relatives, 6/64 (9.3%) of unaffected relatives, and 1/68 (1.4%) of controls.

The potential confounders

We next examined the possibility that the 'low' subgroup of patients showed low levels of AA and DHA because of poor diet (low intake of precursors or of unsaturated fatty acids or low intake of antioxidants). We argued that a comparison of confounders in the low and high fatty acid groups should reveal differences if that were the case. All the potential confounders (diet, alcohol, smoking and neuroleptic exposure) were examined for differences between the two groups.

There was no significant difference in age structure between the low AA and high AA groups: the mean age for the low group was 44.8 ± 16 (mean ± SD) years ($n = 12$) and for the high group 44.3 ± 14 years ($n = 72$) ($t = 0.91$).

Neuroleptic drug exposure. There was no significant difference ($t = 0.57$) between the low AA group (630 ± 603, $n = 12$) and the high AA group (529 ± 561, $n = 72$) (means ± SD) for chlorpromazine equivalence, the commonly used method for comparing neuroleptic intake.

Alcohol use. The mean daily consumption of alcohol was calculated as g/day. A problem arose, in that the number in the low AA group of schizophrenics was too small for statistical analysis: of the 12 probands, only three consumed alcohol. We therefore referred to the complete data for all probands (Table 14.1). The probands consumed less alcohol (mean 10.4 g/day) than the controls (mean 14.3 g/day). Furthermore, the affected relatives had a lower consumption (3.2 g/day) than the unaffected relatives (9.9 g/day). In each group there were high standard deviations. We could not interpret the findings in terms of an effect of alcohol accounting for the fatty acid deficits.

Tobacco use. We compared the number of cigarettes smoked daily in the low AA group ($n = 12$) and the high AA group ($n = 67$). The mean number of cigarettes smoked was 17 in the low group and 12 in the high group. We examined the significance using Levene's test for the equality of variances and found $F = 0.032$, which was not significant. We also carried out a t test and found no significant difference between the means. We concluded there was no evidence of an effect of smoking on level of AA, i.e., tobacco use did not affect the bimodality.

Dietary intake. The numbers were too small to allow direct comparison of the low and high AA groups. We therefore compared all the probands with all the affected

Table 14.1. Daily intake of alcohol and a variety of nutrient dietary factors for probands, affected relatives, unaffected relatives, and control subjects. Data are presented as means ± SD, with the number of subjects in parentheses.

Intake factor	Probands	Affected relatives	Unaffected relatives	Controls
Alcohol (g)	10.4 ± 21.6 (54)	3.2 ± 6.4 (44)	9.9 ± 22.2 (33)	14.3 ± 17.0 (51)
β-Carotene (μg)	2891.1 ± 2057.5 (29)	4026.2 ± 2510.7 (38)	4888.4 ± 2085.0 (29)	3989.2 ± 2509.1 (51)
α-Tocopherol (mg)	10.5 ± 7.4 (27)	9.9 ± 7.4 (35)	10.2 ± 8.0 (22)	8.1 ± 3.7 (51)
Vitamin C (mg)	60.2 ± 33.4 (57)	74.8 ± 34.4 (46)	80.4 ± 37.0 (35)	86.5 ± 35.2 (51)
Retinol (μg)	572.4 ± 318.7 (29)	661.0 ± 642.1 (35)	620.6 ± 394.3 (26)	417.5 ± 362.8 (51)
Iron (mg)	14.1 ± 8.0 (44)	5.6 ± 14.6 (39)	15.8 ± 6.7 (29)	14.2 ± 5.3 (51)
Fat (g)	94.2 ± 34.6 (28)	97.2 ± 41.2 (36)	84.9 ± 25.2 (26)	70.0 ± 30.6 (51)
Cholesterol (mg)	330.7 ± 121.7 (29)	379.7 ± 207.4 (35)	370.4 ± 158.2 (26)	258.0 ± 134.9 (51)
Polyunsaturates (g)	14.4 ± 7.7 (25)	13.9 ± 7.0 (36)	12.7 ± 6.6 (26)	11.0 ± 4.9 (51)
Saturates (g)	37.5 ± 14.9 (25)	40.5 ± 18.8 (36)	35.1 ± 11.2 (26)	27.9 ± 12.4 (51)
Carbohydrate (g)	322.0 ± 131.1 (54)	300.9 ± 113.9 (44)	309.1 ± 110.7 (33)	265.2 ± 76.4 (51)
Starch (g)	164.8 ± 88.0 (56)	163.9 ± 76.4 (46)	173.8 ± 76.2 (35)	150.6 ± 47.9 (51)
Sugar (g)	151.6 ± 68.5 (56)	133.3 ± 52.3 (45)	139.2 ± 55.0 (35)	114.5 ± 37.0 (51)
Kilocalories	2530.9 ± 907.8 (28)	2467.0 ± 842.5 (35)	2353.9 ± 592.1 (26)	2106.9 ± 704.8 (51)
Protein (g)	83.9 ± 32.5 (57)	88.0 ± 30.8 (46)	90.3 ± 24.9 (35)	85.2 ± 27.0 (51)
Linoleic acid (g)	12.2 ± 7.1 (27)	11.4 ± 6.4 (35)	11.1 ± 6.7 (22)	9.1 ± 4.4 (51)

and unaffected relatives and controls. For the range of antioxidants and pro-oxidants, lipids and cholesterol, no clear pattern emerged, e.g., for α-tocopherol the mean value for probands (10.5 mg/day) was higher than that found in controls (8.1 mg/day) but similar to that in unaffected relatives (10.2 mg/day) and close to that in affected relatives (9.9 mg/day). However, the vitamin C value for probands was 60.2 mg/day, which was significantly lower than in any of the other groups, and there was a highly significant difference between the groups using a χ^2 test ($p < 0.0002$). There was also a significant difference between the groups for β-carotene ($p < 0.001$).

The polyunsaturate intake had a mean of 14.4 g for probands, 13.9 g for affected relatives, 12.7 g for unaffected relatives and 11.1 g for controls, and the standard deviations were similar. In the instance of total saturates, the mean value for probands was 37.5 g, for affected relatives 40.5 g, for unaffected relatives 35.1 g and for controls 27.9 g. The total calorific intake was marginally higher in the probands and affected relatives than in the unaffected relatives and controls.

Membrane fatty acids

When the four population groups were examined as a whole for the levels of fatty acids in red cell membranes (Table 14.2), there was a gradation of values from probands to normal controls. For example, AA level (mg/100 ml phospholipid) in probands was 10.8; in affected relatives, 11.54; in unaffected relatives, 11.60; and in controls, 11.99. The same gradation held for DHA (22:6n-3) – the mean in probands was 3.59 mg/100 ml phospholipid; in affected relatives, 4.26; in unaffected relatives, 4.06; and in controls 4.39.

Discussion of the fatty acid data

The most striking observations are the bimodality data, the evidence for the bimodal distribution for AA and DHA confirming our previous observations among sporadic schizophrenic subjects from a number of different centres. Because of the bimodal distribution, the mean values of the fatty acids, although grading in the expected direction from schizophrenic proband to normal control, are not so strikingly different from each other. How can we account for the bimodality in distribution of the fatty acids and these low levels of AA and other acids?

In preliminary studies, Sargent and his colleagues in Stirling established that these low levels of AA are associated with remarkably reduced levels of phosphatidylethanolamine (PE) and in these studies it appears that the decrease was offset by an increase in partially peroxidised fatty acids (Sargent, personal communication). The low level of AA could then be accounted for by either (a) peroxidation of the unsaturates in PE *in situ*, followed by removal of, or (b) hydrolysis of, the fatty acids in PE by an overactive PLA$_2$, followed by peroxidation. There is a third possibility: it could be an *in vitro* artifact, whereby blood from those patients with unsaturated fatty acids in red cell membranes genetically more susceptible to peroxidation or hydrolysis by PLA$_2$ is degraded during storage or thawing. Whatever the cause, there remains a striking difference between the process in normal control subjects, schizophrenic probands and their relatives. This must mean that the process is not primarily an *in vitro* effect but a manifestation of a biological difference between these population groups. Although the differences in polyunsaturated fatty acids between probands, affected relatives and controls did

Table 14.2. Levels of fatty acids in RBC membranes in for probands, affected relatives, unaffected relatives, and control subjects. Data are presented as means ± SD.

Fatty acid	Probands	Affected relatives	Unaffected relatives	Controls
18: 2n-6	7.64 ± 1.60	8.01 ± 1.27	8.51 ± 1.59	8.50 ± 1.09
18: 4n-3	0.18 ± 0.06	0.19 ± 0.06	0.18 ± 0.06	0.16 ± 0.04
20: 2n-6	0.26 ± 0.07	0.27 ± 0.05	0.27 ± 0.05	0.26 ± 0.04
20: 3n-6	1.34 ± 0.44	1.39 ± 0.37	1.30 ± 0.29	1.31 ± 0.32
20: 4n-6	10.83 ± 3.03	11.54 ± 1.97	11.60 ± 1.93	11.99 ± 1.52
22: 5n-6	0.26 ± 0.11	0.29 ± 0.09	0.24 ± 0.08	0.28 ± 0.10
22: 5n-3	2.07 ± 0.69	2.19 ± 0.46	2.26 ± 0.47	2.21 ± 0.41
22: 6n-3	3.59 ± 1.82	4.26 ± 1.32	4.06 ± 1.14	4.39 ± 1.01

not support a dietary stress in patients (the controls had a lower intake of polyunsaturates) there were some significantly lower intakes of some antioxidants in the patients (vitamin C and β-carotene)

The spectrum of illness in the families

In this analysis we have classified the groups within the families of probands as affected or unaffected. We have not as yet carried out a detailed analysis of the diagnostic subgroups. In an initial analysis of the families in the Highlands and Islands only, we examined the proportion of borderline handicap occurring in association with schizophrenia. Turner (1989) found three times more schizophrenic patients than expected among mentally retarded subjects. Many family studies of schizophrenic probands have concentrated on so-called typical schizophrenics and have excluded those families with other diagnostic categories, for example with coexisting psychosis and/or learning difficulty. In this study, all that mattered was that the proband was clearly schizophrenic. Patients with schizophrenia and coexisting borderline handicap, according to DSM-III-R, were allocated to Code 317 if the IQ level was 50–70, and to Code V 40 if the IQ level fell into the 71–84 range based on the Quick Test score. Patients were also assessed on the National Adult Reading Test (NART) for premorbid IQ and on the Quick Test for current IQ. NART is well established in a wide range of diagnoses for assessing premorbid levels of intellectual functioning (e.g., Crawford et al., 1992). The Quick Test measures current IQ by means of perceptual verbal performance and has a strong correlation with other measures, i.e., WAIS and WAIS-R, especially for below-average IQs (e.g., Traub and Spruill, 1982). Of 22 families with complete data for proband and affected relatives, the age structure is shown in Table 14.3. Table 14.4 shows the number of individuals with and without learning difficulties among the probands and affected relatives. IQ results are presented in Table 14.5.

In this preliminary sample from the Highland Health Board area, we found that approximately 25% of the probands and their affected relatives had evidence of learning difficulty. This is a much higher incidence than would be expected in the general population. The question arises whether this can be explained on the basis of an association with schizophrenia or with some cause such as Down's Syndrome or Fragile X. These two latter syndromes were excluded on clinical grounds but we have not carried out a chromosomal analysis at this time.

The presence of manic-depressive illness in the families of schizophrenic probands has been extensively described (Tsuang, 1994). The question arises, and has been the subject of much discussion, as to whether or not manic-depressive illness and schizophrenia lie on a continuum or are separate and distinct phenomena. In terms of the phospholipid hypothesis and in epidemiological terms we see evidence for a continuum with discontinuities. In other studies (Glen et al., 1996; Ward et al., 1998) we have examined the cyclooxygenase pathway through the niacin skin patch test. Here we find impaired flushing (reduced activity in the pathway) in schizophrenia but normal or excessive flushing in manic-depressive illness, indicating a normally func-

Table 14.3. Age structure of subjects entered into the family study.

Group	n	Mean	SD	Minimum	Maximum
All families					
All probands	32	49.2	15.06	17	83
Male	18	48.9	16.94	17	83
Female	14	49.6	12.86	29	72
Selected families					
All probands	22	49.6	15.03	27	83
Male	12	50.5	16.72	27	83
Female	10	48.7	13.55	29	72
All affected relatives	22	46.0	17.29	19	76
Male	10	37.7	16.72	19	66
Female	12	52.9	15.09	30	76

Table 14.4. The number of individuals with and without learning difficulties, as assessed by the premorbid IQ on the National Adult Reading Test (NART), the current IQ on the Quick Test, and clinical evidence contained in the case notes. The percentages of individuals with learning difficulties as determined by each of the assessment methods are shown in parentheses.

	NART (Premorbid IQ)			Quick Test (Current IQ)			
Group	Normal (>84)	Mild to borderline (50–84)	Not testable[a]	Normal (>84)	Mild to borderline (50–84)	Not testable	Clinical case notes
Probands without affected relatives ($n = 32$)	20	3 (9%)	9	16	9 (28%)	7	8 (25%)
Probands with affected relatives ($n = 22$)	14	1 (5%)	7	12	3 (14%)	7	4 (18%)
Affected relatives ($n = 22$)	20	0 (0%)	2	12	7 (32%)	3	6 (27%)

[a] Includes problems due to symptoms, attention, noncooperation, illiteracy, or indistinct speech.

Table 14.5. Premorbid and current IQ for probands and affected relatives, with and without learning difficulties; frequencies, with percentages in parentheses.

	Premorbid IQ[a]			Current IQ[b]		
Group	>84[c]	50–84[d]	Not testable	>84	50–84	Not testable
Learning difficulty[e]						
8/all 32 probands	1 (12.5)	3 (37.5)	4 (50.0)	0 (0.0)	6 (75.0)	2 (25.0)
12/22 probands	1 (8.3)	1 (8.3)	2 (16.7)	0 (0.0)	2 (16.7)	2 (16.7)
6/22 AR[f]	5 (83.3)	0 (0.0)	1 (16.7)	0 (0.0)	5 (83.3)	1 (16.7)
No learning difficulty[e]						
24/all 32 probands	19 (79.2)	0 (0.0)	5 (20.8)	16 (66.7)	3 (12.5)	5 (20.8)
18/22 probands	13 (72.2)	0 (0.0)	5 (27.8)	12 (66.7)	1 (16.7)	5 (27.8)
16/22 AR	15 (93.8)	0 (0.0)	1 (6.3)	12 (75.0)	2 (12.5)	2 (12.5)

[a] Measured using the National Adult Reading Test (NART); [b] measured using the Quick test; [c] normal; [d] mild/borderline; [e] established from clinical evidence in the case notes; [f] affected relatives.

tioning or even overactive pathway. Table 14.6 shows niacin skin patch test results in bipolar manic-depressive subjects, in unipolar depressive patients and in schizophrenia. The index of measurement (area under the curve, AUC) is measured at four concentrations of niacin on the skin (AUCp1-AUCp4) representing concentrations of 0.1 M, 0.01 M, 0.001 M, 0.0001 M. AUCt5, AUCt10 and AUCt15 represent the area under the curve for 0–5 min (AUCt5), for 5–10 min (AUCt10) and 10–15 min (AUCt15). The bipolar manic-depressive patients were, on the whole, not significantly different from controls and only on one measure (AUCp4) was there a significant increase over the control value, i.e., a more sensitive response. The schizophrenic patients were all significantly lower, i.e., less sensitive than the control response, apart from AUCp4 which was not significantly different. The unipolar depressive patients were less responsive than control

Table 14.6. Results of the niacin skin patch test of the cyclooxygenase pathway in patients with bipolar affective disorder ($n = 15$), unipolar depression ($n = 24$), and schizophrenia ($n = 35$), compared with control subjects ($n = 48$). The index of measurement (area under the curve) is shown for four different concentrations of niacin, and three different time intervals (see text for further explanation).

Index	Bipolars	Unipolars	Schizophrenics	Controls
Concentrations				
AUCp1 (0.1 M)	32.17 ± 6.54	27.19 ± 11.19*	22.86 ± 9.87†††	32.74 ± 7.57
AUCp2 (0.01 M)	21.83 ± 12.48	17.19 ± 12.47†††	14.31 ± 9.95†††	29.94 ± 8.92
AUCp3 (0.001 M)	12.67 ± 12.69*	7.50 ± 6.84	5.26 ± 7.89***	11.77 ± 10.52
AUCp4 (0.0001 M)	10.00 ± 11.99	3.65 ± 4.60	2.59 ± 7.27	1.59 ± 3.39
Time intervals				
AUCt5 (0–5 min)	3.40 ± 2.51	1.77 ± 1.62†††	1.33 ± 1.78†††	3.84 ± 1.85
AUCt10 (5–10 min)	4.87 ± 2.79	3.90 ± 2.55*	3.16 ± 2.00††	5.18 ± 1.73
AUCt15 (10–15 min)	5.70 ± 2.53	4.71 ± 2.53	4.26 ± 2.13*	5.50 ± 1.88

In comparison with the corresponding value for the control subjects, $p <$: *0.05; ***0.005; ††0.0005; †††0.0001; all other comparisons were statistically nonsignificant.

patients but the mean response was intermediate between controls and schizophrenics.

PLA$_2$ has not been studied in manic-depressive illness, but we have carried out preliminary observations of the PLA$_2$ expressor site on Chromosome 1 and find an association between the number of poly-adenosine repeats and schizophrenia (over 50 repeats being associated only with schizophrenia, accounting for 40% of subjects, whereas the manic-depressive patients were not distinguishable from controls in this respect). Interestingly the schizoaffective patients were not so different in this regard from the schizophrenic patients (Ward, personal communication).

DISCUSSION

Evidence has been presented in this chapter in support of the concept of a spectrum of phospholipid disorders. Our early studies in manic-depressive illness indicated a disorder of transport across membranes. We could not explain the abnormalities in the ATPase systems which were found, not only by our group, but also by Naylor et al. (1976). These ATPase abnormalities were found in the non-nucleate RBC and the explanation seemed to lead us to some steroid, or as yet unknown hypothalamic control system, possibly a neuropeptide. In the event, the abnormalities in ATPase transport systems can be clearly explained by alterations in the membrane fatty acids.

In our earlier studies of fatty acids in phospholipids in schizophrenia the findings were unimpressive and it was only when we found a bimodality and discontinuity in these fatty acid changes that the highly significant differences within the schizophrenic population became clear and suggested genetic control. The observation of bimodality needed to be replicated, although it had been confirmed by Peet et al. (1994) and Yao et al. (1994). The findings might still have been explained by confounders, such as abnormalities of diet, smoking, etc., within the population, but we believe that the family study has excluded this possibility. This view is further supported by recent evidence confirming a reduction in polyunsaturated fatty acids in frontal lobe of postmortem brain of schizophrenic subjects (Yao et al., 1999) There is also further evidence for increased PLA$_2$ activity in brain, confirming early reports of increased PLA$_2$ in peripheral blood cells (Ross et al., 1999)

The question arises of the reason for a spectrum of illness within families. Perhaps the likeliest explanation lies in a multiple gene hypothesis where gene expression in one field is influenced by the interaction of a neighbouring gene. In this case, the interaction of phospholipase and cyclooxygenase seems a likely possibility, although there are other potential candidate gene interactions. It is our intention to study the identified families in the north of Scotland displaying a spectrum of illness, in order to elucidate this matter further. A number of routes of investigation have been envisaged. Individuals with coexisting borderline handicap and psychosis or, indeed, individuals with borderline handicap in the absence of psychiatric illness, do occur in these families and investigation so far has not revealed any other genetic or chromosomal abnormality to account for the impairment. We know of one such individual, for whom there is a family history of schizophrenia in both parents, who presented in late childhood with borderline handicap and a schizophrenia-like psychosis. He had very low levels of AA and DHA in his RBC membranes. It seems possible that a major lipid deficit of early onset would have a profound effect on brain development. It is our intention to pursue the investigation of borderline handicap associated with schizophrenia in terms of early effects produced by maximal gene expression.

Turning to schizophrenia itself, others have investigated the possibility that 'positivity' or 'negativity' of symptoms would be found predominantly within the same families. No evidence for the predominance of one or other group of symptoms in one family has been found, and our own preliminary findings (not shown here) confirm this. Thus, in families with more than one schizophrenic individual, one sibling may have positive symptoms and another sibling may have negative symptoms. It may be that the possession of negative symptomology indicates earlier onset, and a more severe problem of gene expression, and indeed the data we have would suggest that chronic severe negative symptoms are associated with more severe lipid abnormality. Patients with positive symptoms seem more closely related to individuals with manic-depressive illness, and this has been pointed out in clinical studies previously (Tsuang, 1994). It may be that while there is increased breakdown of phospholipids in those with both negative and positive symptoms, patients with positive symptoms are more able to synthesise new fatty acids and phospholipids and so have a high turnover. Clearly, this is open to investigation using such techniques as ^{13}C labelling of fatty acids.

The role of lipid peroxidation needs to be considered. Several studies discussed above have described increased lipid peroxidation in schizophrenia. We are currently developing a new technique for measuring volatile products of lipid peroxidation in breath. Previous studies (reviewed by Dodd, 1996) indicate that these peroxidation products are increased as breath volatiles in schizophrenia, but not in manic-depressive illness. We have here, therefore, another avenue for exploring the differences in the phospholipid spectrum between manic-depression and schizophrenia.

We have discussed above the findings from the niacin skin test that measure the cyclooxygenase pathway and show that our manic-depressive patients appear to have normal or increased functioning of these enzymes.

Schizoaffective illness, from the clinical aspect, would seem to be placed somewhere between schizophrenia and manic-depressive illness, but the results from our skin testing so far indicate that the cyclooxygenase pathway is as impaired in schizoaffective illness as it is in schizophrenia, unlike manic-depressive illness, where we have, if anything, an overactive cyclooxygenase pathway, as judged by skin test results.

In earlier studies we found marked abnormalities in the ATPase systems, both in manic-depressive illness and in depression. In severe depressive illness, we find an impairment in the cyclooxygenase pathway, as measured by the skin test, although the time course of the response is different, i.e., patients with schizophrenia tend to have a prolonged and impaired response, whereas depressive patients, although less responsive than controls, lie somewhat between schizophrenia and controls.

An important clinical differentiation between manic-depressive illness and schizophrenia is made by evaluating the degree to which manic-depressive illness is periodic whereas schizophrenia is persistent. This periodicity may well be mediated by the anandamide system (Gravatt et al., 1995). Animal work suggests that periodic occurrences, such as wakefulness and sleep, are functionally controlled by this system. Thus it is interesting that, while schizophrenia appears to be a more serious and chronic illness, there is no sleep impairment, whereas the periodic illnesses of depression and mania are accompanied by profound sleep disorder. It is, however, of interest, given the increased incidence of cannabis psychosis in individuals with a family history of schizophrenia, that the cannabis receptor is an anandamide (an amide of AA). The anandamide system is clearly an important area for investigation.

In this chapter, the early history has been reviewed of linkages between transport systems in membranes and membrane dysfunction with the discovery that fatty acids can profoundly affect these systems. We have presented further data to show that bimodality or discontinuity in lipid abnormalities in membranes are unlikely to be caused by confounding agents such as heavy smoking and bad diet, although such factors may play some part in determining absolute levels of fatty acids.

We have described some of the features of the spectrum of illness which we find in the families of schizophrenic probands, and we have outlined current approaches to investigating the nature of this phospholipid spectrum abnormality. The treatment prospects are described elsewhere. These, together with the new approaches to objective diagnosis, present prospects for testable hypotheses using measurable parameters in a way which we have not seen before in psychiatry.

ACKNOWLEDGEMENTS

The family study was supported by a grant from the Chief Scientist of the Scottish Office jointly to the Department of Mental Health, University of Aberdeen (Professor L.J. Whalley) and the Highland Psychiatric Research Group (Dr I. Glen). Fatty acid measurements were carried out in the Department of Biological and Molecular Science at the University of Stirling by Professor John Sargent and Dr Douglas Tocher. The Highland Psychiatric Research Group received support from the Highland Communities NHS Trust, Laxdale Ltd, and Scotia Pharmaceuticals. I am grateful for contributions to this chapter from my colleagues, Dr Joanne Sutherland, Dr Evelyne Glen and Pauline Ward, and to our research secretaries, Alison Obern and James Miller.

REFERENCES

Ashcroft GW, Eccleston D, Murray LG et al. Modified amine hypothesis for aetiology of affective illness. Lancet 1972; ii: 573–577.

Bell MV, Tocher DR. Molecular species composition of the major phospholipids in brain and retina from rainbow trout. Biochem J 1989; 264: 909–915.

Bleuler EP. Textbook of psychiatry (trans. AA Brill). NY: Dover Publications, 1924.

Brice AT. The blood fats in schizophrenia. J Nerv Ment Dis 1935; 81: 613–632.

Cade JFJ. Lithium salts in the treatment of psychotic excitement. Med J Aust 1949; 2: 349–352.

Cade JFJ. Lithium – past, present and future. In: Johnson FN, Johnson S, eds. Lithium in medical practice. Lancaster: MTP Press, 1978: 5–16.

Coppen A, Shaw DM, Malleson A, Costain R. Mineral metabolism in mania. Br Med J 1966; 1: 71–75.

Crawford JR, Moore JW, Cameron IM. Verbal fluency: a NART-based equation for the estimation of premorbid performance. Br J Clin Psychol 1992; 31: 327–329.

Di Marzo V, Fontana A, Cadas H et al. Formation and inactivation of endogenous cannabinoid anandamide in central neurons. Nature 1994; 372: 686–691.

Dodd GH. The lipid membrane hypothesis of schizophrenia: implications for possible clinical breath tests. Prostagland Leukotr Essent Fatty Acids 1996; 55: 95–99.

Foster P. Neuroleptic equivalence. Pharmaceut J 1989; 30: 431–432.

Gattaz WF, Köllisch M, Thuren T, Virtanen JA, Kinnunen PKJ. Increased plasma phospholipase-A_2 activity in schizophrenic patients: reduction after neuroleptic therapy. Biol Psychiatry 1987; 22: 421–426.

Gattaz WF, Hübner CK, Nevalainen TJ, Thuren T, Kinnunen PKJ. Increased serum phospholipase A_2 activity in schizophrenia: a replication study. Biol Psychiatry 1990; 28: 495–501.

Gattaz WF, Steudle A, Maras A. Increased platelet phospholipase A_2 activity in schizophrenia. Schizophr Res 1995; 16: 1–6.

Glen AIM. Measurement of change. The importance of brain compartments: CSF, glial, extracellular, subcellular, with special reference to lithium. Presentation, 9th CINP Meeting, Paris, 1974.

Glen AIM. Lithium prophylaxis of recurrent affective disorders. J Affective Disord 1985; 8: 259–265.

Glen AIM, Ongley CG, Robinson, K. Diminished membrane transport in manic-depressive psychosis and recurrent depression. Lancet 1968; ii: 241–243.

Glen AIM, Ongley GC, Robinson K. Effect of a sensory stimulus on an impaired membrane transport system in man. Nature 1969; 221: 565–566.

Glen AIM, Bradbury MWB, Wilson J. Stimulation of the sodium pump in the red blood cell by lithium and potassium. Nature 1972; 239: 399–401.

Glen AIM, Glen EMT, Horrobin DF et al. Essential fatty acids in schizophrenic patients with borderline mental handicap. Presentation, Schizophrenia 1992 Conference, Vancouver, Canada, 19–22 July, 1992.

Glen AIM, Glen EMT, Horrobin DF et al. A red cell membrane abnormality in a subgroup of schizophrenic patients: evidence for two diseases. Schizophr Res 1994; 12: 53–61.

Glen AIM, Cooper SJ, Rybakowski J, Vaddadi K, Brayshaw N, Horrobin DF. Membrane fatty acids, niacin flushing and clinical parameters. Prostagland Leukotr Essent Fatty Acids 1996; 55: 9–15.

Glen AIM, Ward P, Fox H, Tocher D, Sargent J, Whalley LJ. Confirmation of bimodality of arachidonic acid and docosahexaenoic acid in schizophrenia. Prostagland Leukotr Essent Fatty Acids 1997; 57: 266.

Gravatt BF, Prospero-Garcia O, Siuzdak G et al. Chemical characterization of a family of brain lipids that induce sleep. Science 1995; 268: 1506–1511.

Hesketh JE, Loudon JB, Reading HW, Glen AIM. The effect of lithium treatment on erythrocyte membrane ATPase activities and erythrocyte ion content. Br J Clin Pharmacol 1978; 5: 323–329.

Horrobin DF. Schizophrenia as a prostaglandin deficiency disease. Lancet 1977; i: 936–937.

Horrobin DF, Manku MS, Morse-Fisher N, Vaddadi KS. Essential fatty acids in plasma phospholipids in schizophrenics. Biol Psychiatry 1989; 25: 562–568.

Horrobin DF, Manku MS, Hillman S, Glen AIM. Fatty acid levels in the brains of schizophrenics and normal controls. Biol Psychiatry 1991; 30: 795–805.

Laugharne JDE, Mellor JE, Peet M. Fatty acids and schizophrenia. Lipids 1996; 31 (Suppl): S163–S165.

Leli U, Hauser G. Modifications of phospholipid metabolism induced by chlorpromazine, dimethylimipramine and propranolol in C6 glioma cells. Biochem Pharmacol 1987; 36: 31–37.

McGuire PK, Jones P, Harvey I, Williams M, McGuffin P, Murray RM. Morbid risk of schizophrenia for relatives of patients with cannabis-associated psychosis. Schizophr Res 1995; 15: 277–281.

Mendell NR, Thide HC, Finch SJ. The likelihood ratio test for the two component normal mixture problem: power and sample size analysis. Biometrics 1991; 47: 1143–1148.

Naylor GJ, Dick DAT, Dick EG et al. Erythrocyte membrane carrier in mania. Psychol Med 1976; 6: 659–663.

Peet M, Laugharne JDE, Horrobin DF, Reynolds GP. Arachidonic acid: a common link in the biology of schizophrenia? Arch Gen Psychiatry 1994; 51: 665–666.

Peet M, Laugharne JDE, Rangarajan N, Horrobin DF, Reynolds G. Depleted red cell membrane essential fatty acids in drug-treated schizophrenic patients. J Psychiatr Res 1995; 29: 227–232.

Randall LO, Cohen LH. The serum lipids in schizophrenia. Psychiatr Q 1939; 13: 441–448.

Ross BM, Turenne S, Moszczynska A et al. Differential alteration of phospholipase A(z) activities in brain of patients with schizophrenia. Brain Res 1999; 821: 407–413.

Schou M. The range of clinical uses of lithium. In: Johnson FN, Johnson S, eds. Lithium in medical practice. Lancaster: MTP Press, 1978: 21–39.

Traub GS, Spruill J. Correlations between the Quick Test and Wechsler Adult Intelligence Scale – Revised. Psychol Rep 1982; 51: 309–310.

Tsuang MT. Genetics, epidemiology, and the search for causes of schizophrenia. Am J Psychiatry 1994; 151: 3–6.

Turner TH. Schizophrenia and mental handicap: an historical review, with implications for further research. Psychol Med 1989; 19: 301–314.

Venables WN, Ripley BD. Distribution and data summaries. In: Venables WN, ed. Modern applied statistics with S-plus. Berlin: Springer-Verlag, 1994: 163–190.

Ward P, Sutherland J, Glen E, Glen A. The response of the niacin skin test in the functional psychoses. Presented at the 21st CINP Congress, Glasgow, Scotland, 12–16 July, 1998.

Wilson R, Tocher DR. Lipid and fatty acid composition is altered in plaque tissue from multiple sclerosis brain compared with normal brain white matter. Lipids 1991; 26: 9–12.

World Health Organization. MONICA Project Principal Investigators (prepared by Tunstall-Pedoe H). The World Health Organization MONICA Project. J Clin Epidemiol 1988; 44: 105–111.

Yao JK, Leonard S, Reddy RD. Membrane phospholipid abnormalities in postmortem brains from schizophrenic patients. 1999, submitted.

Yao JK, van Kammen DP, Welker JA. Red blood cell membrane dynamics in schizophrenia. II. Fatty acid composition. Schizophr Res 1994; 13: 217–226.

Part VI

SCHIZOPHRENIA: DIETARY INFLUENCES AND TREATMENT

Breastfeeding, Neurodevelopment, and Schizophrenia

15

Malcolm Peet, Jacqui Poole and Jonathon D. E. Laugharne

INTRODUCTION

The human brain has a growth spurt during the last trimester of pregnancy and the first few months postnatally (Dobbing and Sands, 1970). This brain growth is not uniform, and growth spurts occur in different brain regions at different times. Neurones multiply, dendrites and synaptic connections develop between neurones, and myelination occurs. This requires an abundant supply of polyunsaturated fatty acids (PUFAs). Nerve tissue contains around 50% of lipid on a dry weight basis and 10% wet weight (Sastry, 1985). There is a particularly high concentration of arachidonic acid (AA) and docosahexaenoic acid (DHA) in neuronal membranes, so that an adequate supply of these PUFAs must be assured (Crawford et al., 1997). In the uterus, supply of these PUFAs depends upon maternal sources and thus ultimately on maternal nutrition. After birth, adequate amounts of AA and DHA must be provided in feeds, because human infants, especially those who are premature, cannot adequately convert dietary linoleic acid (LA) and α-linolenic acid (ALA) into other PUFAs (Koletzko, 1992).

The normal western diet is relatively deficient in n-3 PUFAs (Taylor et al., 1979; Rice, 1984). During pregnancy, the placenta appears to extract DHA and AA preferentially, so that these PUFAs are present in significantly greater concentrations in cord blood than in the maternal circulation (Crawford et al., 1997). In the final trimester of pregnancy, circulating levels of maternal DHA diminish (Holman et al., 1991). Supplementing the diet of pregnant women with sardines and fish oil leads to substantially increased DHA levels in erythrocytes and plasma of newborn infants (Connor et al., 1996). There is evidence that long-chain PUFA status at birth affects postnatal PUFA levels independently of postnatal diet (Foreman-Van Drongelen et al., 1995). Thus, maternal nutrition may affect PUFA status not only in the foetus but also subsequently.

INFANT FEEDING AND PUFA

It is well established that preterm and term infants fed on formula feeds have lower plasma and erythrocyte levels of DHA and AA than breast-fed infants. Formula feeds for preterm infants need to be supplemented with DHA and AA.

Boehm et al. (1996) studied 41 very low birth-weight infants fed with breast milk, standard formula or formula supplemented with DHA and AA in proportions similar to human milk. DHA and AA levels declined in plasma phospholipids and erythrocyte membranes of formula-fed infants during the first few weeks of life, whereas these levels remained constant in the breast-fed and supplemented formula-fed infants. This is further evidence that premature infants cannot adequately synthesize DHA and AA from ALA and LA in standard formula.

Koletzko et al. (1996) gave either human milk or formula to healthy infants in a study of AA metabolism. AA in plasma phospholipids was significantly lower in the formula-fed than in the breast-fed infants at 1 week, and at 1 and 2 months. Four neonates with phenylketonuria were fed with corn oil, and the synthesis of AA was estimated by measuring the conversion of natural ^{13}C enrichment from the corn oil into plasma AA. It was estimated that full-term infants can endogenously synthesize only about 23% of plasma AA by day 4, so that supplementation is necessary. Salem et al. (1996) also demonstrated that AA and DHA can be synthesized from 18-carbon fatty acid precursors by human infants at term, but the quantities synthesized may not match those available to breast-fed infants.

Ghebremeskel et al. (1995) showed that incorporation of DHA into formula feed led to increased plasma and erythrocyte levels of DHA, but reduced the conversion of LA to AA. This further indicates the need to provide a proper balance of n-3 and n-6 PUFAs in formula feeds. It seems clear that preterm infants require formula feeds to be supplemented with both DHA and AA. Term infants have more capacity to synthesize these long-chain PUFAs from their 18-carbon precursors, but are still likely to benefit from supplementation.

Studies in both animals and humans have investigated the effects of infant feeding on brain accumulation of DHA and AA. Early studies in rats focused on investigating the biological effects of marked depletion of brain n-3 PUFAs produced by dietary deprivation over several generations. Recently, more subtle approaches have been used. For example, Jumpsen et al. (1997) fed nursing dams from parturition, and pups from weaning, on diets with varying levels and ratios of n-6 and n-3 PUFAs, within the range proposed for infant formulas. They found that brain phosphatidylethanolamine and phosphatidylcholine PUFA composition in the frontal region, cerebellum and hippocampus reflected the composition of the diet and varied between brain regions and cell types. In the rhesus monkey, new born infants have low concentrations of n-3 PUFAs in plasma, erythrocytes and brain when their mothers have been deprived of dietary n-3 during pregnancy (Connor et al., 1991). DHA is particularly low. Levels of n-3 PUFAs fall even more when dietary deficiency is continued postnatally.

In the human infant, two important studies have investigated brain PUFA levels in relation to infant feeding. In a study of human infants who died of cot death, the phospholipid composition of cerebral cortex grey matter was compared between those breast-fed and those formula-fed (Farquharson et al., 1992). Formula-fed infants had significantly less DHA in brain phospholipid, but the overall percentage of long-chain PUFAs was similar in the two groups because of increased incorporation of n-6 fatty acids in brain phospholipid in the formula-fed group. Makrides et al. (1994) also compared brain, retina and erythrocyte fatty acids in infants who had suffered sudden death. Again, breast-fed infants had a significantly greater proportion of DHA in both erythrocytes and brain cortex relative to formula-fed infants. Brain cortex DHA concentration showed a significant positive correlation with duration of breastfeeding.

It is plain from these studies that the PUFA content of brain phospholipid is sensitive to dietary changes, both during pregnancy and postnatally. Use of formula feeds leads to reduced tissue levels of DHA and AA relative to infants who are breast-fed, and this is reflected in brain PUFA levels, particularly DHA.

PUFA AND BRAIN AND COGNITIVE DEVELOPMENT

There have been many studies in animals, and several in humans, investigating the effect of PUFA depletion during pregnancy and infancy on subsequent brain development and function. Levels of AA and DHA in cord blood at birth have been shown to be positively correlated with head circumference (Crawford et al., 1993). Maternal diet is important in determining foetal development. Badart-Smook et al. (1997) analyzed maternal diet and found that maternal intake of n-3 PUFAs plus AA correlated positively with foetal growth.

Studies in rodents

Most studies of the behavioural effects of PUFA depletion during pregnancy and lactation have been conducted on animals, particularly rodents. Data from rodents are difficult to extrapolate to humans, partly because brain growth patterns differ. Also, many of the earlier experiments involved PUFA deprivation over several generations, because the rodent brain is relatively resistant to dietary deprivation of DHA. There are many studies showing impaired learning ability using a variety of models, in rats deficient in n-3 PUFAs during pregnancy and infancy. However, it has been pointed out that PUFA have been shown to affect pain tolerance and retinal function, both of which could affect apparent performance in some learning tasks (Wainwright, 1992).

Studies in monkeys

In monkeys, brain development more closely parallels that in humans, and so primate studies are perhaps more pertinent. Rhesus monkeys whose mothers were fed a low n-3 fatty acid diet during pregnancy, and who continued on a low n-3 diet after birth, showed very low n-3 fatty acid levels in plasma, erythrocytes, brain and retina at birth and subsequently. The visual acuity of n-3-deficient monkeys was reduced by half at 8 and 12 weeks of age, and was associated with abnormalities of the electroretinogram (ERG). The visual effects were associated with decreased DHA levels in retinal membranes (Neuringer et al., 1986). Addition of fish oil to the diet of these monkeys did not reverse the ERG changes, even though tissue levels of n-3 fatty acids were normalized (Connor et al., 1990). Monkeys deficient in n-3 fatty acids also developed polydipsia (Reisbick et al., 1990). In the longer term, it was shown that monkeys chronically deficient in n-3 fatty acids showed more stereotyped behaviour, and a higher level of whole body locomotion, than seen in normal control monkeys.

These effects were considered typical of rhesus monkeys raised under conditions of partial social isolation, or those whose surroundings had been disrupted (Reisbick et al., 1994).

Studies in humans

In the human, there is increasing evidence that PUFA depletion in infancy has physiological and behavioural consequences. Work has mostly focused on comparing breast-fed with formula-fed infants. In an early study, Rodgers (1978) followed up a cohort of children born during one week in 1946 in Great Britain. Those who were breast-fed were compared with those who were formula-fed, which at that time was done with diluted cow's milk and added sugar. Family, social and economic variables were controlled for. It was found that, at 8 years of age, breast-fed children scored better on picture intelligence. At the age of 15 years, children who had been breast-fed scored better than those who had been bottle-fed, on tests of nonverbal ability, sentence completion and mathematics.

Morrow-Tlucak et al. (1988) found that breast-fed infants scored better than those bottle-fed, on the mental development index of the Bayley Scales (Bayley, 1969) at age 1 and 2 years, but not at 6 months. The effect persisted after controlling for potential confounding variables, including measures of maternal intelligence, authoritarian ideology and home environment.

Rogan and Gladen (1993) studied a cohort of 855 babies through school age. Breast-fed infants showed significantly higher scores on the Bayley index of mental development and the McCarthy Scale between 2 and 5 years of age. Breast-fed children also had higher English grades on school report cards. These effects were still seen after multivariate statistical analysis controlling for potential confounding variables.

Morley et al. (1988) investigated the effects on child development of breast milk *versus* formula feeding for low birth-weight, premature infants. Assessment of developmental status at 18 months showed significantly higher scores on the Bayley index of mental development in breast-fed infants, and this persisted after adjusting for relevant demographic and perinatal factors. The same cohort was found to have an 8.3 point advantage in mean IQ at the age of 8 years, after adjustment for differences between groups in maternal education and social class (Lucas et al., 1992). This difference was shown on both verbal and performance scales of the Wechsler Intelligence Scale for Children. This advantage was unaffected by whether children had been given breast milk entirely by nasogastric feed or whether they had been put to the breast. This indicates a pharmacological effect of breast milk rather than a psychological effect. Jacobson and Jacobson (1992), however, sounded a note of caution regarding the interpretation of such studies. They found that IQ was significantly higher in breast-fed than in bottle-fed infants and that this difference remained statistically significant after including education and social class as covariates; however, including maternal IQ and parenting score (derived by direct observation of parent–child interaction) reduced the difference to nonsignificant levels.

Temboury et al. (1994) conducted a prospective study of 229 healthy term infants and found that lower results on the Bayley index of mental development were associated with bottle-feeding, lower social class, elementary education of the mother, temper tantrums, and having siblings. Johnson et al. (1996) investigated 204 3-year-old children of normal birth-weight, controlling for environmental variables and maternal intelligence. It was found that breast-fed infants had, on average, a 4.6 point higher intelligence.

Riva et al. (1996) retrospectively compared IQ scores of 26 school age phenylketonuric children who were either breast-fed or formula-fed before phenylketonuria was diagnosed. Breast-fed children had an IQ advantage of 14 points relative to those formula-fed. This IQ advantage persisted after adjusting for social status and maternal education.

Lanting et al. (1994) investigated minor neurological dysfunction in 9-year-old children given breast milk or formula milk as babies. A standardized neurological examination was carried out and children were classified as normal, having minor neurological dysfunction, or abnormal. Minor neurological dysfunction included such abnormalities as mild hypotonia, dyskinesia, coordination difficulties or dyspraxia. Breastfeeding showed an advantage in neurological status at 9 years after correcting for obstetric, perinatal, neonatal, neurological and social differences.

Carlson et al. (1993) gave standard formula or marine oil-supplemented formula to healthy preterm infants and found that their visual acuity was better, at 2 and 4 months, in the n-3 supplemented group. Visual acuity correlated with erythrocyte DHA levels. Werkman and Carlson (1996), in a randomized double-blind trial, found that preterm infants whose formula feed was supplemented with DHA until they were 9 months of age, showed improved visual attention (more discrete looks at both novel and familiar stimuli) and shorter look duration, which indicates more rapid information processing. Furthermore, DHA supplementation until 2 months post-term produced similar benefits at 12 months, indicating lasting benefit from short-term supplementation (Carlson and Werkman, 1996).

Faldella et al. (1996) measured flash visual evoked potentials, flash electroretinography and brain stem acoustic evoked potentials in 58 healthy preterm infants at 52 weeks postgestational age. The infants were fed with either standard preterm formula, PUFA-supplemented formula, or breast milk. Those fed standard formula showed abnormal wave morphology and longer wave latencies in the visual evoked potential relative to those fed breast milk or supplemented formulas. Erythrocyte DHA levels were significantly higher in the breast-fed and supplemented groups.

Innis et al. (1996) tested preferential looking acuity and novelty preference in healthy full-term infants at 9 months of age, and related this to whether the infants had been breast-fed or formula-fed, though this was not at random. No significant differences were found. It was concluded that formulas containing adequate LA and ALA, but no AA or DHA, provided adequate PUFA nutrition to healthy term infants, as measured by visual development.

Overall, the data suggest that breast milk, or formula feeds with additional PUFA supplements, have significant advantages over standard formula feeds, with respect to neurocognitive development. Effects are seen more strongly in preterm than in full-term infants.

INFANT FEEDING AND NEUROLOGICAL AND PSYCHIATRIC DISORDERS

Several studies have attempted to relate infant feeding practice to more major psychiatric and neurological disorders. In an early study, Menkes (1977) found that only 13.8% of children with learning disorders had been breast-fed, compared to 47.2% of a control group with neurological disorders other than learning disabilities.

Tanoue and Oda (1989) investigated infant feeding practices in children with autism, a disorder characterized by markedly abnormal social interaction and communication and a limited range of activities and interests, and which has features in common with schizophrenia. They found that 24.8% of patients, but only 7.5% of normal controls, were weaned by the end of 1 week, a significant difference. Early weaning was more commonly because of the mother's condition in the patient group relative to the controls. However, this study did not control for other variables, including socioeconomic status.

Pisacane et al. (1994) investigated the relationship between breastfeeding and multiple sclerosis, using a case-control methodology. Controls were patients in the same department, during the same period, matched for age and sex. Duration of breastfeeding was 8.4 months for cases and 12.5 months for controls, a significant difference. Statistical correction for other variables, including social class, birth-weight and type of delivery, did not affect this finding.

Thus, there is evidence that PUFA effects on neuropsychological development may lead to subsequent neurological and psychiatric disorders.

SCHIZOPHRENIA AS A NEURODEVELOPMENTAL DISORDER

There is growing evidence that functional neurodevelopment is abnormal in infants and children who later become schizophrenic. Several studies have found that schizophrenic patients have reduced head circumference at birth (Kanugi et al., 1995). Schizophrenic patients also generally have low birth-weight and this predicts poor premorbid social adjustment and cognitive impairment in schizophrenic men (Rifkin et al., 1994). All of these characteristics are associated with lower AA and DHA levels in cord blood, as well as an increased requirement for AA and DHA in feeds (Crawford et al., 1997).

In a large birth cohort followed up by Jones et al. (1994), it was found that those who became schizophrenic had delayed milestones of motor development, particularly walking, which was delayed by an average of 1.2 months. By age 2 years, a higher proportion of schizophrenic cases than controls had not attained all the milestones of talking, or sitting, standing and walking alone. Speech problems were more common in cases up to age 15 years. Educational test scores were lower at ages 8, 11 and 15 years, with particular deficits in verbal, nonverbal and mathematical skills, but less impairment of vocabulary and reading. Cases also showed solitary play preference at ages 4 and 6 years, were less socially confident as children and, at age 15 years, both anxiety and IQ were independent predictors of future schizophrenia. Aylward et al. (1984) also showed a premorbid IQ deficit in a meta-analysis of early studies of schizophrenic patients.

Walker et al. (1994, 1996) examined the neuromotor development of patients using childhood home movies and showed significant deficits in preschizophrenic children compared to controls. These were mostly postural and movement abnormalities of the upper limbs, particularly during the first 2 years of life.

Data on visual function are not available from schizophrenic patients as infants, but our group has shown abnormal ERG recordings in adult schizophrenics which echo those shown in bottle-fed infants.

Thus, the IQ deficits and minor neurological dysfunction described in preschizophrenic children mirror the deficits described earlier in formula-fed infants, particularly those born preterm. Poor premorbid childhood adjustment has been linked to structural brain abnormalities, as shown by CT and MRI scans in chronic schizophrenic patients (Weinberger et al., 1980; Walker et al., 1996).

PUFAs and schizophrenia

Direct evidence for an abnormality of membrane PUFA composition in adult schizophrenic patients has been described in detail elsewhere in this book. The evidence points strongly to a deficit, particularly of AA and DHA, which may be related to increased activity of phospholipase A_2 which may be genetic in origin. We have seen that PUFA, particularly AA and DHA, are essential to brain development, and that a relative lack of these PUFA results in cognitive and neurological deficits similar to those seen in bottle-fed preterm infants. Any such predisposition would be exacerbated by a poor dietary supply of these PUFA, whether during pregnancy, early feeding, or later adult nutrition.

There is increasing evidence that PUFA intake, particularly n-3 PUFAs, is related to the course and outcome of established schizophrenia. However, much less attention has been paid to issues of maternal and infant nutrition as possible determinants of future schizophrenia. Butler et al. (1994) have reviewed evidence relating to nutritional deprivation during pregnancy as a possible risk factor in schizophrenia, but without specific reference to PUFA. Susser and Lin (1992) showed a significantly increased risk of schizophrenia in the offspring of women pregnant during the Dutch Famine, though the women suffered multiple dietary deficiencies and not just a deficiency of PUFAs.

Breastfeeding and schizophrenia

It is clear from the data discussed so far that relative deprivation of AA and DHA during early infant feeding, resulting from bottle-feeding rather than breastfeeding, would be expected to compound any genetically determined pre-existing deficiency of these PUFA, which would further compromise neurodevelopment and lead to increased risk of schizophrenia. We therefore decided to investigate feeding practices amongst schizophrenic patients during infancy, and to compare these with a matched control group.

We identified 55 schizophrenic patients meeting DSM-IV diagnostic criteria. They were taken from a larger group of patients being screened for inclusion in a double-blind trial of n-3 supplementation. Only those with mothers who were alive and available for interview, either in person or by telephone, were included. Patients were matched for age, sex and parental socioeconomic status (ascertained from the mother) with 55 control subjects recruited from outpatients attending a Fracture Clinic, and from administrative staff. Medical and paramedical staff were not used, so as to avoid possible bias. The selection process ensured that the two groups were closely matched, each comprising 47 males and eight females, with a mean age of 34 years. The mother of each patient and each control subject was interviewed in regard to how the subject had been fed as an infant. In the patient group, 33 (60%) had been breast-fed, compared with 43 (78%) in the control group. Significance levels were assessed using the McNemar Test. There were six pairs with only the schizophrenic patient breast-fed but 16 pairs with only the control breast-fed ($\chi^2 = 4.45$; $p = 0.033$). With regard to breastfeeding for more than 4 weeks, this occurred in 44% of patients and 67% of controls. There were nine pairs of subjects with only the schizophrenic patient having 4 weeks or more of breastfeeding, but 22 pairs with only the control having 4 weeks or more ($\chi^2 = 5.45$; $p = 0.020$). When asked the reasons for failing to breastfeed, three mothers of control subjects cited behavioural problems in the baby, whilst only one schizophrenic patient's mother suggested similar difficulties.

In another study, McCreadie (1997) asked the mothers of 45 schizophrenic patients to complete a questionnaire about breastfeeding, which was defined as having been put to the breast at least once, and they were also questioned to determine the prevalence of breastfeeding at various ages. Patients were compared with their siblings and with data from national surveys of breastfeeding. It was found that the overall incidence of breastfeeding was 29% in patients and 38% in their siblings. At 4 weeks of age, 22% of patients and 34% of siblings were still being breast-fed; at 8 weeks only 18% of patients, but 30% of their siblings, were being breast-fed. Though there is a clear trend for a lower rate of breastfeeding amongst patients than amongst their unaffected siblings, these findings do not reach statistical significance. This study did not include a matched control group, but the figures on breastfeeding were compared with population surveys of breastfeeding in the UK and Scotland in the 1940s and 1950s. The Scottish breastfeeding figures were substantially lower than those for the whole of the UK: only 51% of infants were breast-fed, and 43% were still breastfeeding by 8 weeks, in a 1958 survey. The rate of breastfeeding in the patients included in the study of McCreadie (1997) was significantly lower than that in the Scottish survey data. Patients not breast-fed had significantly lower IQ than those who were breast-fed. There were no significant differences in personality traits and social adjustment between breast-fed patients and their normal siblings, but within the patient group those who had not been breast-fed had significantly more schizoid and schizotypical traits and poorer social adjustment at ages 5–11 and ages 12–16 years. The authors suggested that lack of breast milk may be a risk factor in the neurodevelopmental form of schizophrenia.

DISCUSSION AND CONCLUSIONS

A reduced rate of breastfeeding in infants who later became schizophrenic has been demonstrated in two independent studies in different populations, one using case control methodology and the other using whole population comparisons. However, there are difficulties of interpretation of these data which will now be considered.

Both studies of breastfeeding in schizophrenia used retrospective maternal accounts of breastfeeding and the reliability of this could be questioned. However, van den Bogaard et al. (1991) showed 97% accuracy in retrospective accounts of mothers regarding breastfeeding 10–19 years after the event, when checked against medical notes held at the Child Health Clinic.

The data from these two studies are consistent with the hypothesis that lack of breastfeeding is a risk factor for schizophrenia. However, other interpretations are possible. Bauchner et al. (1986) summarized the methodological problems in breastfeeding studies under the headings: avoidance of detection bias; adjustments for potential confounding variables; definition of the outcome event; and definition of breastfeeding. Detection bias occurs when the outcome event is detected more readily in one group than in another. This is particularly pertinent to the study of the effect of breastfeeding on the prevalence of childhood infections. In the case of schizophrenia, however, distinction between those affected with the disorder and unaffected controls posed no problem in our case-control study. With regard to confounding variables, the main variable affecting breastfeeding is socioeconomic status. This was controlled for in our case-control study. The study of McCreadie (1997) did not specifically control for socioeconomic status, but the author argued that there was no significant difference in this variable between the general population and their subpopulation of schizophrenic patients. Important issues are parent–child interaction and home environment, which may differ between schizophrenic and nonschizophrenic populations as infants, and which may also affect breastfeeding. Jones et al. (1994) showed, using health visitors' ratings, that significantly more mothers of schizophrenic cases than mothers of controls had worse than average general understanding and management of their children, even though none was mentally ill. Adjusting for home environment tends to reduce the differences in cognitive development between children breast-fed and those bottle-fed, and Jacobson and Jacobson (1992) found that including a parenting score, derived by direct observation of parent–child interaction, as a covariate, reduced the difference in childhood IQ consequent upon breastfeeding or bottle-feeding to a statistically nonsignificant level. Thus, it is possible that deficient mothering skills led to both failure to breastfeed and also to schizophrenia. The finding of McCreadie (1997) of a strong, though statistically nonsignificant, trend for infants of the schizophrenic group to have less frequent and less prolonged breastfeeding than their unaffected siblings, provides some argument against such an effect. However, maternal factors cannot be definitely excluded in either study. It could also be suggested that people with the neurodevelopmental form of schizophrenia could show abnormalities as babies which would mitigate against breastfeeding. However, a problem with the baby was cited more often by parents of control subjects than by parents of schizophrenics as reasons for failure to breastfeed. With regard to definition of the outcome event, both studies used clear diagnostic criteria, which again causes fewer problems than occur in studies of the effects of breastfeeding on infections and other diseases in children. With regard to the definition of breastfeeding, both studies define this as having been put to the breast and both recorded the duration of breastfeeding. The distinction was thus made between those who had received breast milk and those who had received only formula feed. There was no separate category for those who were breast-fed but also supplemented with formula, and inclusion of these subjects in the breast-fed group would tend to reduce apparent differences between bottle-feeding and breastfeeding.

If the relationship between failure to breastfeed and schizophrenia is causal, then factors other than PUFA content should be considered. These include nucleotides, immunoglobulins, digestive enzymes and other potentially relevant constituents of human milk (Hamosh, 1997). However, the wealth of evidence reviewed in this chapter relating PUFAs to neurodevelopment must make these the most likely factor relating breastfeeding to subsequent schizophrenia.

SUMMARY

The foetal and infant brain requires substantial quantities of AA and DHA for normal development. Babies, particularly those born preterm, show neurodevelopmental abnormalities if their diet is not supplemented with AA and DHA. Schizophrenia is now widely regarded as a neurodevelopmental disorder, and there is good evidence of abnormal PUFA metabolism, which may be of genetic origin, in adult schizophrenic patients. Any predisposition to depletion of AA or DHA would be aggravated or ameliorated by adjustments to the dietary intake of these PUFAs, and this would be especially critical during early brain development. Two studies have now shown that schizophrenic patients are less likely than nonschizophrenic individuals to have been breast-fed as infants. Whilst other explanations cannot be ruled out, the data are consistent with the hypothesis that alterations of cell membrane PUFA composition are of aetiological importance in schizophrenia.

REFERENCES

Aylward E, Walker E, Bettes B. Intelligence in schizophrenia: a meta-analysis. Schizophr Bull 1984; 10: 430–459.

Badart-Smook A, van Houwelingen AC, Al MD, Kester AD, Hornstra G. Fetal growth is associated positively with maternal intake of riboflavin and negatively with maternal intake of linoleic acid. J Am Diet Assoc 1997; 77: 867–870.

Bauchner H, Leventhal JM, Shapiro ED. Studies of breast-feeding and infections: how good is the evidence? JAMA 1986; 256: 887–892.

Bayley N. Bayley scales of infant development. New York: The Psychological Corporation, 1969.

Boehm G, Borte M, Bohles HJ, Muller H, Kohn G, Moro G. Docosahexaenoic and arachidonic acid content of serum and red blood cell membrane phospholipids of preterm infants fed breast milk, standard formula or formula supplemented with n-3 and n-6 long-chain polyunsaturated fatty acids. Eur J Paediatr 1996; 155: 410–416.

Butler PD, Susser ES, Brown AS, Kaufmann CA, Gorman JM. Prenatal nutritional deprivation as a risk factor in schizophrenia: preclinical evidence. Neuropsychopharmacology 1994; 11: 227–235.

Carlson SE, Werkman SH. A randomised trial of preterm infants fed docosahexaenoic acid until two months. Lipids 1996; 31: 85–90.

Carlson SE, Werkman SH, Rhodes PG, Tolley EA. Visual acuity development in healthy preterm infants: effect of marine-oil supplementation. Am J Clin Nutr 1993; 58: 35–42.

Connor WE, Neuringer M, Lin DS. Dietary effects upon brain fatty acid composition: the reversibility of n-3 fatty acid deficiency and turnover of docosahexaenoic acid in the brain, erythrocytes and plasma of Rhesus monkeys. J Lipid Res 1990; 31: 237–248.

Connor WE, Neuringer M, Reisbick S. Essentiality of n-3 fatty acids: evidence from the primate model and implications for human nutrition. In: Simopoulos AP, Kifer RR, Martin RE, Barlow SM, eds. Health effects of n-3 polyunsaturated fatty acids in seafoods. World Rev Nutr Diet 1991; 66: 118–132.

Connor WE, Lowensohn R, Hatcher L. Increased docosahexaenoic acid levels in human newborn infants by administration of sardines and fish oil during pregnancy. Lipids 1996; 31 (Suppl 31): S183–S187.

Crawford MA, Doyle W, Leaf A, Leighfield M, Ghebremeskel K, Phylactos A. Nutrition and neurodevelopmental disorders. Nutr Health 1993; 9: 81–97.

Crawford MA, Costeloe K, Ghebremeskel K, Phylactos A, Skirvin L, Stacey F. Are deficits of arachidonic and docosahexaenoic acids responsible for the neural and vascular complications of preterm babies? Am J Clin Nutr 1997; 66 (Suppl): 1032S–1041S.

Dobbing J, Sands J. Timing of neuroblast multiplication in the developing human brain. Nature 1970; 226: 639–640.

Faldella G, Govoni M, Alessandroni R et al. Visual evoked potentials and dietary long chain polyunsaturated fatty acids in preterm infants. Arch Dis Child; Fetal Neonatal Edn 1996; 75: F108–F112.

Farquharson J, Cockburn F, Patrick WA, Jamieson EC, Logan RW. Infant cerebral cortex phospholipid fatty acid composition and diet. Lancet 1992; 340: 810–813.

Foreman-van Drongelen MMFP, van Houwelingen AC, Kester ADM, Hasaart THM, Blanco CE, Hornstra G. Long chain polyunsaturated fatty acids in preterm infants: status at birth and its influence on postnatal levels. J Paediatr 1995; 126: 611–618.

Ghebremeskel K, Leighfield M, Leaf A, Costeloe K, Crawford M. Fatty acid composition of plasma and red cell phospholipids of preterm babies fed on breast milk and formulae. Eur J Paediatr 1995; 154: 46–52.

Hamosh M. Should infant formulas be supplemented with bioactive components and conditionally essential nutrients present in human milk? J Nutr 1997; 127 (Suppl 5): 971S–974S.

Holman RT, Johnson SB, Ogburn PL. Deficiency of essential fatty acids and membrane fluidity during pregnancy and lactation. Proc Natl Acad Sci USA 1991; 88: 4835–4839.

Innis SM, Nelson CM, Lwanga D, Rioux FM, Waslen P. Feeding formula without arachidonic acid and docosahexaenoic acid has no effect on preferential looking acuity or recognition memory in healthy full-term infants at 9 months of age. Am J Clin Nutr 1996; 64: 40–46.

Jacobson SW, Jacobson JL. Breast feeding and intelligence. Lancet 1992; 926: 339.

Johnson DL, Swank PR, Howie VM, Baldwin CD, Owen M. Breast-feeding and children's intelligence. Psychol Rep 1996; 79: 1179–1185.

Jones P, Rodgers B, Murray R, Marmot M. Child developmental risk factors for adult schizophrenia in the British 1946 birth cohort. Lancet 1994; 344: 1398–1402.

Jumpsen J, Lien EL, Goh YK, Clandinin MT. Small changes of dietary (n-6) and (n-3) fatty acid content ratio alter phosphatidylethanolamine and phosphatidylcholine fatty acid composition during development of neuronal and glial cells in rats. J Nutr 1997 ; 127: 724–31.

Kanugi H, Nanko S, Takei N, Saito K, Murray RM, Kazamatsuri H. Small head circumference at birth in schizophrenia. Schizophr Res 1995; 15: 192–193.

Koletzko B. Fats for brains. Eur J Clin Nutr 1992; 46 (Suppl 1): S51–S62.

Koletzko B, Decsi T, Demmelmair H. Arachidonic acid supply and metabolism in human infants born at full term. Lipids 1996; 31: 79–83.

Lanting CI, Fidler V, Huisman M, Tonwen BC, Boersma ER. Neurological differences between 9-year-old children fed breast milk or formula milk as babies. Lancet 1994; 344: 1319–1322.

Lucas A, Morley R, Cole TJ, Lister G, Leeson-Payne C. Breast milk and subsequent intelligence quotient in children born preterm. Lancet 1992; 339: 261–264.

Makrides M, Neumann MA, Byard RW, Simmer K, Gibson RA. Fatty acid composition of brain, retina and erythrocytes in breast-fed and formula-fed infants. Am J Clin Nutr 1994; 60: 180–194.

McCreadie RG. The Nithsdale Schizophrenia Surveys. 16. Breast-feeding and schizophrenia: preliminary results and hypotheses. Br J Psychiatry 1997; 170: 334–337.

Menkes JH. Early feeding of children with learning disorders. Devel Med Child Neurol 1977; 19: 169–171.

Morley R, Cole TJ, Powell R, Lucas A. Mothers choice to provide breast milk and developmental outcome. Arch Dis Child 1988; 63: 1382–1385.

Morrow-Tlucak M, Haude RH, Ernhart CB. Breastfeeding and cognitive development in the first 2 years of life. Soc Sci Med 1988; 26: 635–639.

Neuringer MD, Connor WE, Lin DS, Barstad L, Luck S. Biochemical and functional effects of prenatal and postnatal ω-3 fatty acid deficiency on retina and brain in rhesus monkeys. Proc Natl Acad Sci USA 1986; 83: 4021–4025.

Pisacane A, Impagliazzo N, Russo M et al. Breast feeding and multiple sclerosis. Br Med J 1994; 308: 1411–1412.

Reisbick S, Neuringer M, Hasnain R, Connor WE. Polydipsia in rhesus monkeys deficient in omega-3 fatty acids. Physiol Behav 1990; 47: 315–323.

Reisbick S, Neuringer M, Hasnain R, Connor WE. Home cage behaviour of rhesus monkeys with long-term deficiency of omega-3 fatty acids. Physiol Behav 1994; 55: 231–239.

Rice RD. The effects of low doses of MaxEPA for long periods. Br J Clin Pract 1984; 38 (Suppl): 85–88.

Rifkin L, Lewis S, Jones P, Toone B, Murray R. Low birth weight and schizophrenia. Br J Psychiatry 1994; 165: 357–362.

Riva E, Agostini C, Biasucci G et al. Early breastfeeding is linked to higher intelligence quotient scores in dietary treated phenylketonuric children. Acta Paediatr 1996; 85: 56–58.

Rodgers B. Feeding in infancy and later ability and attainment: a longitudinal study. Devel Med Child Neurol 1978; 20: 421–426.

Rogan WJ, Gladen RC. Breast feeding and cognitive development. Early Hum Devel 1993; 31: 181–193.

Salem N, Wegher B, Mena P, Uauy R. Arachidonic and docosahexaenoic acids are biosynthesised from their 18-carbon precursors in human infants. Proc Natl Acad Sci USA 1996; 93: 49–54.

Sastry PS. Lipids of the nervous tissues: composition and metabolism. Prog Lipid Res 1985; 24: 169–176.

Susser ES, Lin SP. Schizophrenia after prenatal exposure to the Dutch Hunger Winter of 1944–1945. Arch Gen Psychiatry 1992; 49: 983–988.

Tanoue Y, Oda S. Weaning time of children with infantile autism. J Autism Devel Disord 1989; 19: 425–434.

Taylor TG, Gibney MJ, Morgan JB. Homeostatic function and polyunsaturated fatty acids. Lancet 1979; ii: 1378.

Tembury MC, Otero A, Polanco I, Arribas E. Influence of breastfeeding on the infant's intellectual development. J Paediatr Gastroenterol Nutr 1994; 18: 32–36.

van den Bogaard C, Van den Hoogen HJ, Huygen FJ, van Weel C. The relationship between breast-feeding and early childhood morbidity in a general population. Fam Med 1991; 23: 510–515.

Wainwright PE. Do essential fatty acids play a role in brain and behavioural development? Neurosci Biobehav Rev 1992; 16 : 193–205.

Walker EF, Savoie T, Davis D. Neuromotor precursors of schizophrenia. Schizophr Bull 1994; 20: 441–451.

Walker EF, Lewine RRJ, Neumann C. Childhood behavioural characteristics and adult brain morphology in schizophrenia. Schizophr Res 1996; 22: 93–101.

Weinberger D, Cannon-Spoor E, Potkin S, Wyatt R. Poor premorbid adjustment and CT scan abnormalities in chronic schizophrenia. Am J Psychiatry 1980; 137: 1410–1413.

Werkman SH, Carlson SE. A randomised trial of visual attention of preterm infants fed docosahexaenoic acid until nine months. Lipids 1996; 31: 91–97.

Cultural and Socioeconomic Differences in Dietary Intake of Essential Fatty Acids and Antioxidants: Effects on the Course and Outcome of Schizophrenia

Sahebarao P. Mahadik, Meena Mulchandani, Mahabaleshwar V. Hegde and Prabhakar K. Ranjekar

INTRODUCTION

Diet and life style have long been considered to cause as well as to cure many diseases, including major psychiatric diseases such as schizophrenia. Both diet and life style are unique and essential aspects of each culture and socioeconomic class. There is now increasing evidence that these factors can at least affect the course and outcome of schizophrenia. Multinational studies coordinated by the World Health Organization (WHO) have found that the incidence, prevalence, and manifestations of schizophrenia are similar across different countries and cultures, but that the course and outcome vary widely, the outcome being generally mild in the developing countries but tending to be serious and chronic in the developed countries (World Health Organization, 1973; Sartorius et al., 1986; Jablensky, 1987; Jablensky et al., 1991). This has led to the notion of a 'universality' of schizophrenia with a variability in outcome. It has also been reported that, within a culture, the outcome of schizophrenia may be related to the socioeconomic class; thus, patients from higher social and economic classes had poor outcome in developing countries (see Nandi et al., 1980 and studies reported therein), but had better outcome in the USA (Eaton, 1985). Several variables, such as the degree of stigma associated with schizophrenia, family support, type of treatment, and family history examined in the WHO studies, and several other factors examined in other independent studies (Hopper, 1991; Karno and Jenkins, 1993; Edgerton and Cohen, 1994; Craig et al., 1997), could not satisfactorily account for this cross-national/cross-cultural variability in outcome. These findings suggest that differences in diet and life style probably contribute to the variable course and outcome of schizophrenia.

Christensen and Christensen (1988) first narrowed this down to the variation in the intake of dietary fat. They observed that 98% of the variation in the course of schizophrenia could be explained by variations in fat intake; developing countries with a low fat content diet and major dietary fat being derived from vegetables and sea-food (low saturated fatty acid and high essential polyunsaturated fatty acid [EPUFA] contents) had a better course of the disease as compared to the developed countries with a high fat content diet and the major dietary fat content coming from land animals and birds (high saturated fatty acids and low EPUFA contents). Several studies have also reported variable changes in membrane phospholipids (for reviews see Rotrosen and Wolkin, 1987; Horrobin et al., 1994) and their esterified EPUFAs (e.g., Glen et al., 1994; Horrobin, 1996; Mahadik and Evans, 1997) in schizophrenic patients, particularly those with poor outcome. These reports strongly suggest that the variable course and outcome of schizophrenia in patients from different cultures and socioeconomic status may be related to the differences among these patients in the intake of EPUFAs, particularly ω-3 EFAs, and of the antioxidants that prevent cell membrane EPUFA breakdown.

ω-3 EFAs are consistently found to be critical for brain development and differentiation, and for neuronal function and survival (Simopoulos, 1991; Wainwright, 1992). Antioxidants protect EFAs from breakdown by free radicals, also known as reactive oxygen species (ROS). This protection occurs at many levels: in the food during storage and cooking, in the gut, and in the neuronal membranes. The dietary intake of EPUFAs, particularly ω-3 EFAs, varies greatly among populations from different cultures, socioeconomic classes and geographical locations (Simopoulos, 1989, 1991; World Health Organization Study Group on Diet, Nutrition and Prevention of Noncommunicable Diseases, 1990; Food and Agriculture Organization of the United Nations/World Health Organization, 1994), and their intake is reflected in their erythrocyte membrane levels (Farquhar and Ahrens, 1963; Iacono et al., 1974; Dougherty et al., 1987). The changes in erythrocyte membrane levels of ω-3 EFAs in response to diet are considered to be relevant to changes in the brain since the percentage change in erythrocyte membranes parallels that in the brain (Connor et al., 1990). Sudden crosscultural migration and/or change in socioeconomic status may both affect the intake of EPUFAs and antioxidants. In addition, the stress related to crosscultural and socioeconomic differences (life style) and illness may increase the oxidative stress that may then, in its turn, exacerbate the loss of neuronal membrane EPUFAs by oxidative breakdown.

This chapter will present the unitary hypothesis that the differences in the intake of primarily ω-3 EFAs and antioxidants in different cultures and socioeconomic classes may be associated with the variable course and outcome of schizophrenia. We will also discuss the possible effects of family history and size, prenatal and neonatal factors, seasonality of birth, birth order, sex, and migration (e.g., rural to urban, developing to developed country, and tropical to cold) on the intake of EPUFAs and antioxidants, and on the incidence, course and outcome of schizophrenia. This is a refutable hypothesis; if supported by the evidence, it will have a major impact on our understanding of the possible aetiopathology of schizophrenia, and on its treatment and management.

CULTURES, SOCIOECONOMIC CLASSES, AND DIET

An interesting editorial by Murphy (1984) addressed the issue of diseases of civilization. It was suggested that diseases such as general peresis, peptic ulcer, and schizophrenia could be caused as well as cured by civilization. Civilization is conceived as a process, rather than as a state, that combines single human individuals into one great unity (Freud, 1961). Torrey (1980) has suggested a close correlation between the prevalence of schizophrenia and the degree of civilization; he favoured a viral theory of schizophrenia. Others have blamed the diet for the diseases of civilization. It has also been suggested that the pathogenic factors that cause these diseases may be incidental, rather than essential, aspects of civilization, but evidence is increasing to indicate that the dietary patterns, and the existence of specific types of viruses, are, in fact, essential aspects of each civilization.

The role played by the dietary patterns of cultures and socioeconomic classes in determining the diseases of civilization, such as schizophrenia, is a complex issue. However, the discussion will focus here on the relevant specific ingredients in the diet, primarily EPUFAs and antioxidants, differences in their intake between cultures and socioeconomic classes, effects on the course and outcome of schizophrenia, possible underlying mechanisms, and future perspectives, in view of the worldwide rapid cultural and socioeconomic changes that are currently taking place.

Diet: EPUFAs and antioxidants

Dietary fat from animals and vegetables contains primarily cholesterol, nonessential fatty acids (can be made in the body), and essential fatty acids (EFAs) (cannot be made in the body). The requirement for EFAs, which are primarily present in vegetables, was first established by Burr and Burr (1929, 1930). Much is now known about the food sources, metabolism, and requirements for EFAs, as well as their involvement in both communicable and noncommunicable diseases, and their worldwide consumption (Sinclair, 1958, 1990; Bang et al., 1980; Food and Agriculture Organization, 1980; Simopoulos, 1989; Gunstone et al., 1994; Food and Agriculture Organization of the United Nations/World Health Organization, 1994). EFAs are of two types, n-6 (ω-6) series, starting with linoleic acid (C18:2n-6), and the n-3 (ω-3) series, starting with α-linolenic acid (C18:3n-3). It has now been well established that ω-6 EFAs are more widely distributed than ω-3 EFAs, and are often excessively consumed from both animal and vegetable diets; ω-3 EFAs are primarily available from a diet rich in vegetables and natural habitat fish (for reviews see Simopoulos, 1991; Mahadik and Evans, 1997).

EPUFAs are broken down by ROS (e.g., Bielski et al., 1983; for a review see Mahadik and Gowda, 1996). Under normal circumstances, adequate dietary intake of antioxidants, such as β-carotene, and vitamins E, A and C, can prevent the breakdown of these EFAs in the brain. Environmental stressors (e.g., socioeconomic and emotional stress, temperature, environmental pollutants) and high caloric intake, that increase oxidative stress, can also increase the breakdown of EPUFAs.

EPUFAs are used to synthesize cellular membrane phospholipids. Two of these EPUFAs are arachidonic acid (AA; C20:4n-6) and docosahexaenoic acid (DHA; C22:6n-3); DHA, in particular, is highly enriched in the brain and is critical for brain and behavioural development (Simopoulos, 1991; Wainwright, 1992). This suggests that the selective intake of EPUFAs and antioxidants in various cultures and socioeconomic classes may be related to the differences in course and outcome of schizophrenia.

EPUFAs, antioxidants, and pathophysiology of schizophrenia

There is now sufficient evidence to indicate that in schizophrenia there is abnormal cell membrane phospholipid metabolism (for reviews see Rotrosen and Wolkin, 1987; Horrobin et al., 1994; Horrobin, 1996; Mahadik and Evans, 1997). These phospholipid changes are considered to be a result of lower membrane levels of EPUFAs, particularly AA and DHA (Horrobin, 1996; Mahadik et al., 1996a), as have been reported in some schizophrenic patients (Horrobin et al., 1991; Glen et al., 1994; Yao et al., 1994; Mahadik et al., 1996b; Peet et al., 1996). The lower levels of EPUFAs are thought to be due to lower dietary intake, defective utilization and/or excessive peroxidative breakdown (Mahadik and Scheffer, 1996; Mahadik et al., 1996b; Reddy and Yao, 1996). A possible lower intake of ω-3 PUFAs is also supported by the observation of clinical improvement following their dietary supplementation (e.g., Mahadik and Evans, 1997; Peet et al., 1996).

Evidence is also accumulating that lower levels of membrane EPUFAs result from their increased ROS-mediated peroxidative breakdown, since increased lipid peroxidation products have been reported in the plasma as well as in cerebrospinal fluid (Lohr et al., 1989; Peet et al., 1993; McCreadie et al., 1995; Mahadik et al., 1998). The ROS-mediated peroxidative breakdown of EPUFAs is probably a result of oxidative stress (i.e., a mismatch between the cellular generation of ROS and the antioxidant defense) in schizophrenia, even at the onset of psychosis (Mahadik and Mukherjee, 1996; Mukherjee et al., 1996; Reddy and Yao, 1996; Mahadik et al., 1998). Support for this view is provided by improvements in the clinical status of patients, concomitant with improved plasma lipid peroxide levels, which result from treatment with antioxidants (e.g., Adler et al., 1993; Peet et al., 1993; Mahadik and Gowda, 1996).

These studies suggest that the intake of ω-3 PUFAs and antioxidants may crucially determine the aetiology, course and outcome of schizophrenia.

THE INTAKE OF EPUFAs AND ANTIOXIDANTS, AND THE COURSE AND OUTCOME OF SCHIZOPHRENIA

Cultural and socioeconomic differences in the intake of EPUFAs and antioxidants

Before industrialization

Each civilization (culture) evolved where plentiful food and water, and other suitable environmental features, were available. The population had to adapt to seasonal variability in the environment, and in the quantity and quality of food; those who could not adapt did not survive. Social and economic classes probably evolved on the basis of the individual's abilities. Generally, an upper social class has been also an upper economic class in most cultures, except in India where there are four distinct classes based on social and economic differences: an upper social class subdivided into those with higher or lower economic status, and a lower social class also with higher or lower economic status subdivisions. However, 75 years ago, the lower social class did not have a subgroup with higher economic status, and at present the urban population is divided only into upper and lower economic status. There is also a complex caste system which was originally primarily based, for reasons that are unclear, on the expected type of job in society and also on birth.

The dietary patterns of populations from different cultures varied widely, primarily due to the various geographical factors that determined food availability. In addition to these factors, behavioural consequences within the context of psychosocial influences also play a critical role in food choices (Nestle et al., 1998). Understanding these factors will be very important in the future development of dietary recommendations, nutritional programmes, and educational messages that will assist the population in choosing a healthy diet, and in promoting dietary changes. There are no published data on the precise intake of specific quantities of EPUFAs and antioxidants in different cultures or socioeconomic classes. However, the intake of fat, a primary source of EPUFAs, probably remained stable until the beginning of industrialization when it began to increase rapidly (Simopoulos, 1991). During the hunter-gatherer period, man consumed primarily meat (probably containing EPUFAs) from herbivorous animals, supplementing this with fruits and vegetables. This diet probably provided adequate quantities of EPUFAs and antioxidants. With the establishment of organized agriculture, increasing quantities of fruits and vegetables became available, whilst the quality and quantity of fat, EPUFAs and antioxidants remained more or less constant. Cultures closer to permanent water resources probably supplemented their diet with fish, which are rich in ω-3 EPUFAs; Greenland and Alaska Eskimo cultures consumed primarily sea-food, rich in ω-3 PUFAs, all year round (Bang et al., 1980). Winter and summer were probably associated with changes in the intake of EPUFAs and antioxidants, due to seasonal changes in the availability of fruits and vegetables. Upper social and economic classes probably had the same type of food as the rest of the population, though they probably had access to greater quantities, whilst doing less physical work.

During industrialization

For the last 75 years, the changes that have occurred as a consequence of western industrialization have had a major impact on the dietary intake of EPUFAs and antioxidants. This is largely due to an increased availability of foods that are poor in EPUFAs and antioxidants (Simopoulos, 1991) as well as to changes in the socioeconomic structure of society and in the environment. These changes have also divided the world into two major groups: the developed and developing regions. Furthermore, industrialization has led to extensive migration, creating multicultural societies; it has also reduced urban–rural differences, and has permitted sudden changes to occur in the economic status of an individual or group. These changes have been accompanied by changes in dietary patterns and thereby in the EPUFA status (i.e., cell membrane levels of EPUFAs) of some populations (Keys, 1970; Lands et al., 1990). However, the dietary patterns and life styles in most of the rural populations in developing countries, such as India and Nigeria, have remained largely unchanged.

In the USA in the last 30 years, emphasis has been placed on the problems of the overconsumption of food, particularly fat (Kennedy and Powell, 1996; Lichtenstein et al., 1998). Fat consumption in the general population has been steadily increasing in spite of US national recommendations that total fat intake should be 30% or less of total energy requirements, and that saturated fat intake should be less than 10% of total energy requirements, for all individuals over the age of 2 years. It is not clear whether the percentage or the absolute amount of fat in the diet is the more important, nor do the recommendations address the issue of the quality of fat being consumed, i.e., the levels of ω-6 and ω-3 EFAs. The fat actually consumed is primarily from farm animals and is generally low in ω-3 EFAs.

Recently, Holman (1998) has indicated that, in different human populations, a wide range of proportions of dietary ω-3 and ω-6 EFA proportions occur e.g., high ω-3 and low ω-6 content to low ω-3 and high ω-6 content. The populations in Nigeria and in Kerala, India, consume very high amounts of ω-3 EFAs and very low amounts of ω-6 EFAs, whilst American infants and control populations in Minnesota show a high consumption of ω-6 EFAs but have a low intake of ω-3 EFAs. It has been suggested that the relatively low dietary ω-3 EFA levels of the American population are of nutritional origin, since, in modern times, the major food sources of ω-3 EFAs have been exchanged for ω-6-rich EFAs and ω-3-poor EFA sources to increase the shelf-life of food products.

There are also several indirect consequences of industrialization on the EPUFA status. A sudden cross-cultural change, as well as a sudden shift in social or economic status, can increase the stress that is involved in adapting to a new environment (e.g., temperature, pathogenic viruses and microbes, social rules and regulations, and life style); these stressors can increase the oxidative breakdown of EPUFAs, as noted previously. The adaptive changes take time and involve the activation of new sets of genes in response to changes in environment and diet in order to cope with these changes. Sudden change may therefore affect the health of an individual, possibly irreversibly. Animal studies have shown that sudden changes in environment and diet, particularly in the intake of ω-3 PUFAs, can affect the development of brain and behaviour (Simopoulos, 1991; Carlson and Salem, 1991; Wainwright, 1992). All of these factors are now considered to be involved in the clinical course and outcome of schizophrenia.

Relation between intake of EPUFAs and antioxidants, and the incidence, course and outcome of schizophrenia

Methodological issues in studies on incidence, course and outcome

Any theory regarding the biological basis of schizophrenia must be able to account for its various clinical definitions. It has, for example, been conceptualized as a syndrome that can be divided into subtypes, each of which may have distinct aetiological origins, but it has also been seen as an illness with a symptom complex where each symptom varies in its severity during the course of the illness (van der Velde, 1976; Kety, 1980; Jeste et al., 1982). It has also been suggested that mental disorders represent a continuum of brain dysfunction, with schizophrenia situated at one extreme. These different interpretations probably result from a variety of methodological approaches and from the use of different diagnostic scales to define schizophrenia. The scales used for these studies, particularly the International Classification of Diseases (ICD-9) and revised ICD-10 in Europe, and DSM-III, DSM-III-R and, most recently, DSM-IV in the USA, differ significantly in their diagnostic criteria and this can affect quantitative descriptions of the incidence, course and outcome of the illness. In spite of these differences, schizophrenia in its early stages seems to be very similar in different cultures around the world.

In addition to broad cultural and socioeconomic differences, there are several other factors (e.g., prenatal and postnatal factors, seasonality of birth, birth order, family size, sex, smoking, alcohol consumption, family history, and geographical migration) that are essential aspects of culture and socioeconomic status which can affect the availability, intake or the metabolism of EPUFAs, and thereby contribute to the altered course and outcome of schizophrenia.

Cross-cultural differences

A consistent finding across the WHO studies, such as the International Pilot Study of Schizophrenia (IPSS) and the Determinants of Outcome of Severe Mental Disorders (DOSMD) study, was that clinical and social outcomes were far better for schizophrenic patients in developing countries, such as India and Nigeria, than for their counterparts in developed industrialized countries, such as the USA, UK, and Denmark (World Health Organization, 1973, 1979; Sartorius et al., 1977; Jablensky, 1987; Jablensky et al., 1991; Leff et al., 1992). The classification of 'developing' *versus* 'developed' was based arbitrarily on prevailing socioeconomic conditions. A greater proportion of schizophrenic patients in developing countries experienced complete recovery and sustained remission from psychosis during the follow-up period than did their counterparts in developed countries. The relatively high frequency of complete recovery (approximately every fourth patient in developing countries, and every seventh in developed countries) after a psychotic episode qualifying for a diagnosis of schizophrenia was mentioned as one of the most important findings of these studies. Variables examined in the WHO studies could not satisfactorily account for this cross-national variability in outcome. In summarizing the findings of the DOSMD study, Jablensky and his colleagues (1991) remarked on the clear and consistant differences in the prognosis of schizophrenia between the centres in developed countries and the centres in developing countries.

In the WHO studies, the initial diagnosis of schizophrenia was based on the ICD-9 criteria, which did not include a temporal criterion of 6 months duration of symptoms as did the DSM-III or DSM-III-R. It was therefore not established that the occurrence of schizophrenia, as defined by DSM-III-R or DSM-IV criteria, is similar in different countries. However, Kulhara and Chandiramani (1988), after 18–30 months follow-up of 112 patients suffering from schizophrenia, defined according to ICD-9 using five diagnostic systems (e.g., CATEGO, Research Diagnostic Criteria, Feighner's Criteria, DSM-II, and Schneider's First Rank Symptoms), have reported that the course and outcome of the disorder did not reveal significant variability.

A multicentre study in India has found that the outcome of schizophrenia was better in patients from rural areas than in those from urban areas (Verghese et al., 1989). The investigators used the St Louis criteria (Feighner et al., 1972), but modified the temporal criterion to 3 months to avoid the exclusion of acute schizophrenic patients. Inclusion was limited to patients within 2 years of their onset of psychosis. They found the percentage of patients with good outcome (66.3%) to be identical to that reported for patients at Agra, India, in the IPSS (66%). A similar outcome (67%) has also been reported more recently with a 10-year follow-up (Thara et al., 1994).

It was first reported by Christensen and Christensen (1988) that there was a highly significant correlation between a favourable rating of course and outcome of schizophrenia in patients from different countries (cultures) and a low percentage of dietary total fat ($r = 0.8$–0.9; $p < 0.05$) and fat from land animals and birds (composed mainly of saturated fat) ($r = 0.91$–0.95; $p < 0.01$). They observed that 98% of the variation in the course of schizophrenia could be explained by variations in fat intake (Food and Agricultural Organization, 1980); patients in developing countries where the major dietary fat is obtained from vegetables and sea-food (enriched in ω-PUFAs) had a better course of the disease than seen in patients in the developed countries where a high fat diet is common and major dietary fat comes from land animals and birds (poor in ω-PUFAs).

Based on the availability of edible fats and oil, there are now two global trends of fat consumption (Food and Agriculture Organization of the United Nations/World Health Organization, 1994). The total *per capita* fat consumption, based on the statistics related to production, trade, stock and non-food use, is much more in developed than in developing countries (128 *versus* 50 g/person/day). However, the intake of animal fat is greater than that of vegetable fat (70 *versus* 58 g/person/day) in developed countries, whereas the intake of vegetable fat was greater than that of animal fat (32 *versus* 18 g/person/day) in developing countries. This favours the higher intake of ω-PUFAs in developing countries.

In developing countries, such as India and Nigeria, which have the best outcome of schizophrenia, the diet consists primarily of fruits and vegetables that are generally rich in ω-3 PUFAs and antioxidants, such as vitamins E, A and C, and β-carotene, flavones and quinones. However, in developed countries, such as the USA, with worst outcome, only one in 10 people get an adequate daily supply of antioxidants (Packer, 1984), and the intake of ω-PUFAs is steadily declining (Simopoulos, 1991). In addition, the caloric intake of patients from India is very low (1400–1600 calories/day) compared to that in patients from the USA (>2600 calories/day, not counting snacks). Such high caloric intake and a sedentary life style may also increase the peroxidative loss of EPUFAs since caloric restriction in animals has been found to reduce the loss of EPUFAs, predominantly in the brain. Also, increased socioeconomic stress in developed countries as compared to developing countries such as India, where the environmental situation has been stable for several hundred years, may increase the stress-mediated peroxidative loss of ω-3 PUFAs. A better outcome of schizophrenia has been reported in stable, traditional rural societies (Murphy and Taumoepeau, 1980).

The conclusions of the WHO studies on the epidemiology of schizophrenia have been questioned by some (e.g., Stevens, 1987; Stevens and Wyatt, 1987; Torrey, 1987a; 1987b; Edgerton and Cohen, 1994; Mason et al., 1997). It has, for example, been suggested that the equal incidence and prevalence of schizophrenia in developing and developed countries, and the better outcome in developing countries might arise from the inclusion in the category of schizophrenia of brief, remitting psychoses which might occur at a higher rate in developing countries. In support of this, Stevens (1987) reported that, of patients admitted with a diagnosis of schizophrenia at mental hospitals in Harare, Zimbabwe, only 10–15% met DSM-III criteria for schizophrenia. Most appeared to have a brief reactive psychosis. Studies by Susser et al. (1995) have suggested a separate class of syndrome, an acute transient psychosis that is different from schizophrenia of brief duration and from atypical affective psychosis.

This is an important issue. If, in the WHO studies, there was a greater proportion of patients in developing than in developed countries who had a brief reactive or schizophreniform psychosis that was classified as schizophrenia, the incidence and prevalence of schizophrenia in developing countries, such as in India, is not the same as in developed countries. If, on the other hand, patients in developing and developed countries do have the same disorder (schizophrenia), the better outcome in the former requires an explanation. Since factors such as stigma, family history, family support, type of treatment, and some environmental factors (e.g., viruses) did not explain the outcome differences, such differences may be related to the intake of EPUFAs and antioxidants.

Socioeconomic differences in course and outcome

Studies in industrialized and urbanized Western countries have typically found an excess of schizophrenia in lower socioeconomic groups, or they have failed to show a class effect (Faris and Dunham, 1939; Hollingshead and Redlich , 1958; Goldberg and Morrison, 1963; Eaton, 1985), whereas studies in India have consistently found a higher prevalence of schizophrenia amongst members of the upper social classes, particularly among those more educated and urbanized (Dhunjibhoy, 1930; Rao, 1966; Dube, 1970; Elnagar et al., 1971; Dube and Kumar, 1972; Saxena et al., 1972; Nandi et al., 1979; 1980). This issue is not addressed in reviews of the epidemiology of schizophrenia (Eaton, 1986; Häffner, 1987; Gottesman, 1991), except by one author (Torrey, 1980a; 1987).

Faris and Dunham (1939) found that first-admission rates for schizophrenia diminished progressively, from 102 per 100 000 for those living in the slums of central Chicago, to 25 per 100 000 in affluent neighbourhoods on the periphery of the city. Similar findings were reported by Eaton (1985), who used the Maryland psychiatric case register and found the rates of first hospitalization for schizophrenia to be twice as high in central city areas than in other urban or rural areas. By using occupational status rather than social class as a predictor, he found that male blue-collar workers had a rate of first hospitalization for schizophrenia that was five times higher than that observed for professional and technical workers. Goldberg and Morrison (1963) demonstrated that the social class effect could be explained by a 'downward social drift' of affected individuals, rather than a greater propensity of individuals in lower socioeconomic classes to develop the disorder. It was also suggested that increased rates of schizophrenia in urban areas may be a result of migration of affected individuals from rural areas. However, it is also true that urban poor people, and particularly schizophrenic patients, may suffer more from a reduced dietary availability of EPUFAs and antioxidants, due to a lack of fish or fresh fruits and vegetables.

A number of studies in India have found schizophrenia to be more prevalent in the upper social classes. These comprise surveys of the social class of patients admitted at mental hospitals, including a study of first admissions, as well as door-to-door surveys of populations of towns and villages. In an early comment on dementia praecox, Dhunjibhoy (1930), a British trained psychiatrist, recorded his experience that the condition was more common in those Indian communities that had most embraced Western civilization and culture.

These impressions were later echoed by others in studies of social class backgrounds of patients at mental hospitals (Rao, 1966). These increased rates of chronic illness can be related to the altered EPUFA status and life style in the affluent population.

It has been found that *per capita* total fat consumption rises very rapidly with increase in income (Food and Agriculture Organization of the United Nations/World Health Organization, 1994). However, the patterns of quality of fat show even larger differences. Vegetable fat consumption is higher than that of animal fat (26 *versus* 10 g/day) in low economic classes and is reversed (44 *versus* 90 g/day) in very high economic classes. Urbanization has also been found to increase the fat consumption eight-fold (Hassan and Ahmed, 1992). It is also important to point out that the edible oils used by members of the urban population are often processed in a way that alters the quality of EPUFAs (Food and Agriculture Organization of the United Nations/World Health Organization, 1994) and probably also the amount of antioxidants present in the natural source, whereas oils in rural areas are generally freshly collected. The urban higher socioeconomic class may thus have a reduced intake of EPUFAs and antioxidants, which, when combined with high caloric intake and a more sedentary life style, may seriously affect the EPUFA status. Schizophrenic patients may be at even greater risk of not having adequate EPUFAs and antioxidants.

In developed countries, economic status is now much more variable within and between generations, and there are no significant urban–rural differences. During the early period of industrialization, patients from urban slums did show poor outcome in the USA. Over the last 25 years, the upper economic classes in the developed world have become more aware of dietary and health issues. They are reducing their intake of red meat and increasing the vegetable content of their diet, reducing caloric intake, and doing more exercise. On the other hand, the lower economic classes remain at risk and suffer from socioeconomic stress. These situations may result in better EPUFA-status and better outcome in the upper economic class than in the lower economic class in the developed countries such as the USA.

Effects of factors that affect the intake and metabolism of EPUFAs and antioxidants on the course and outcome of schizophrenia

Seasonality of birth

Several studies have reported that, in both nothern and southern hemispheres, schizophrenic patients are more likely to have been born in the winter than in the summer (e.g., Bradbury and Miller, 1985; Dalen, 1990; O'Callahan et al., 1991; McGrath et al., 1995). It has also been reported that enlarged ventricles, indicative of abnormal neurodevelopment, were present predominantly in these patients (Reveley et al., 1984; Zipursky and Schulz, 1987), and that, surprisingly, these patients also had low genetic risk (Kinney and Jacobsen, 1978; Shur, 1982; O'Callahan et al., 1991). These reports are important, particularly in terms of intake of EPUFAs and antioxidants. Populations living in winter zones can suffer from the nonavailability of fresh fruits and vegetables, and can be subjected to winter weather stress which can increase oxidative stress. Since DHA is critical for fertility and for the normal growth of the foetus (Carlson and Salem, 1991), a lack of this substance might also affect brain development. There are some indications that this season-of-birth effect in schizophrenia is disappearing, probably due to economic factors that help to protect individuals from the harmful effects of poor diet. This trend is more in evidence amongst females than amongst males (Eagles et al., 1995); this is very important, since the female EFA status is much more protected than males (see later). In tropical areas and in developing countries there are no significant seasonal food variations. This issue must be investigated systematically.

Prenatal and postnatal factors

Several prenatal and neonatal factors, such as nutrition (famine), maternal stress, smoking, drugs of abuse, alcohol consumption, obstetric complications such as neonatal hypoxia, and breast feeding, have been associated with schizophrenia (Geddes and Lawrie, 1995; McNeil, 1995; Mahadik and Gowda, 1996; Glover, 1997; Hultman et al., 1997). These factors have in common the potential to affect cellular membrane EPUFA status. Undernutrition, as well as malnutrition, may primarily affect neurodevelopment, due more to the reduced intake of ω-3 PUFAs and antioxidants than to the reduced intake of protein and carbohydrate. The effects of lower protein intake may be compensated during postnatal development. Hypoxia may also affect brain development through oxidation of EFAs. Low birth weight, which is associated with DHA deficiency, is associated with poor premorbid function and later schizophrenia (Foerster et al., 1991).

Several factors, such as maternal stress, use of alcohol and drugs of abuse, and smoking, can affect the intake of EPUFAs and antioxidants as well as increasing their peroxidative breakdown. In the developed countries these factors are a major concern; so far, in the rural part of the developing countries they are far less evident.

Recently, it has been reported that fewer schizophrenics than nonschizophrenic patients had been breast fed (McCreadie, 1997). It is well known that the milk of all mammals contains high concentrations of ω-3 EFAs, particularly DHA, and is needed for the normal growth and development of infants (Carlson et al., 1986; Carlson and Salem, 1991). The DHA concentration of milk varies with the mother's dietary intake and stress (Finley et al., 1985; Koletzko et al., 1992; Chulei et al., 1995). None of the formula milk products has contained these EFAs, until very recently, and breast-fed children have been found to have higher developmental scores and higher IQ (Lucas et al., 1992) than seen in formula-fed children. This is a very important factor between developing countries and developed countries as well as between rural *versus* urban populations. In rural parts of the developing countries, 100% of women breast feed their children, often over a year or more, whereas in urban women the practice is rapidly decreasing. However, in developed countries, the incidence of breast feeding is substantially below 50% and declining further. Since DHA contributes to brain and behavioural development, and milk also contains growth hormones and factors, breast feeding by women with adequate intake of EPUFAs and antioxidants may be an important factor in the better outcome of schizophrenia.

It has been suggested that the better outcome of schizophrenia in developing countries may be related to the increased child mortality of those who suffered prenatal insults and who, had they survived, would later have developed schizophrenia. This possibility needs to be systematically investigated.

Sex differences

Many studies have reported that female schizophrenic patients show better premorbid functioning, and a later onset and more benign course of their illness (Lewine, 1988; Hambrecht et al., 1992; Castle et al., 1995). Among the several hypotheses tested, oestrogen appears to play a critical role in this sex difference (Haffner et al., 1998). The desaturases, enzymes involved in the synthesis of PUFAs, are known to be regulated by oestrogen (Brenner, 1981). Animal studies have shown that female rat pups maintain brain ω-EFA status much better than male rat pups during periods of ω-EFA deficiency (Yamamoto et al., 1987). In addition, in developing countries women have traditionally less demanding social and family responsibilities, other than taking care of children. This is, however, changing in urban and developed countries and is reflected in a reduced sex difference in the clinical course and outcome of schizophrenia.

Family history, family size and birth order

Increased incidence, prevalence and poor outcome of schizophrenia seem to be associated with a family history of the illness, suggesting genetic transmission (Kety, 1980; Gottesman, 1991). However, debate continues as to what is transmitted and whether this relates to prenatal and postnatal maternal environment (e.g., nutrition, virus, autoantibodies, defective adaptive mechanisms for increased stress) or to a specific gene (Davis et al., 1995). It is most likely that an interaction between genetic and environmental factors determines the incidence and outcome of schizophrenia. EPUFAs, particularly ω-3 PUFAs, as well as antioxidants, have been found to play critical roles in the expression of several genes involved in adaptive and survival mechanisms (e.g., Fernandes et al., 1996; Palmer and Paulson, 1997).

In the developing countries, such as India, the average family size is four to six children in the rural areas but less than three in the urban upper socioeconomic class, the latter being similar to the developed countries. In a family of large size, it is generally the first and second position siblings that are reported to be at risk for psychotic disorders (Rao, 1964; Sunderaj and Rao, 1966). This is attributed to the socioeconomic pressures put on the older children to provide for the needs of younger siblings and family. This can disrupt the education and also affect the available quantity and quality of food (and thereby the EPUFA status) of the older children. However, with decreasing family size and with increasing child-bearing age of women, the role of this factor may need to be reexamined.

Migration

Migration is going to be a very important factor in coming years due to world-wide industrialization and the establishment of a global economy. Populations from stable, low-stress cultures from developing countries are migrating to fast-changing, high-stress cultures in developed countries, and rural populations are migrating to urban centres to take advantage of economic opportunities and social assistance. All such changes will have dramatic effects on the intake of EPUFAs and antioxidants, as well as on life style. There are already several reports which suggest that there is an increased risk for these migrant populations for diseases that are generally associated with EPUFAs, e.g., hypertension, cardiovascular disease, diabetes, cancer, immune disease, and some neurodegenerative diseases (Bang et al., 1980;

Kromhout, 1989; Gupta et al., 1995; Calder, 1998). There are very few studies yet published to indicate the impact of migration on the outcome of schizophrenia. A study in Manchester, England, found readmission rates for psychosis to be higher among African-Caribbeans and Asian Indians than amongst patients of European origin (Thomas et al., 1993). The higher rates of psychosis reported for African-Caribbeans in Britain are not related to pregnancy and birth complication (Hutchinson et al., 1997). Several hypotheses have been tested to explain the higher rates of schizophrenia in migrants (Cochrane and Bal, 1987); some role for stress related to socioeconomic differences, was suggested. The major factors may, however, be the alterations in dietary intake and life style which migration entails.

MECHANISMS BY WHICH DIETARY EPUFAs AND ANTIOXIDANTS MAY AFFECT OUTCOME IN SCHIZOPHRENIA

Theoretically, the intake of EPUFAs and antioxidants may play a critical role in determining the outcome of schizophrenia in one of two ways: by an effect upon neurodevelopment; and by altering receptor signal transduction. Since a major role of antioxidants is probably to protect the EPUFAs, these two possible roles of EPUFAs will be discussed.

EPUFAs and abnormal neurodevelopment

There is overwhelming support for the role of EPUFAs in brain and behavioural development (Sinclair, 1990; Simopoulos, 1991; Crawford, 1992; Wainwright, 1992). Brain imaging studies have reported a wide range of neurodevelopmental abnormalities even in first-episode drug-naïve young schizophrenic patients (see reviews by Bloom, 1993; Nasrallah, 1993; Murray, 1994). Also, as indicated earlier, lower levels of membrane EPUFAs are reported in schizophrenic patients than in nonschizophrenic controls (Horrobin, 1994; Peet et al., 1996; Mahadik and Evans, 1997). The membrane levels of EPUFAs have also been found to correlate with psychopathology, i.e., higher DHA levels were associated with better outcome (Peet et al., 1996). This indicates that the increased intake of EPUFAs during prenatal and postnatal development may ameliorate abnormal neurodevelopment. Unfortunately, studies have not yet been published which show a direct relationship between the intake of EPUFAs and either improved neurodevelopment or a better outcome to schizophrenia.

The exact mechanisms underlying the role of DHA in brain development are not yet fully understood. However, DHA deficiency predominantly affects brain development (Neuringer et al., 1986), and lower levels are found in preterm than in term infants (Carlson et al., 1986; Farquharson et al., 1992). It has been suggested that DHA is needed to maintain the rapid rate of neuronal plasma membrane synthesis, since these membranes are selectively enriched with very high levels of DHA (O'Brien and Samson, 1965). DHA is also critical for maintaining the high membrane fluidity that may help promote growth and membrane receptor function (Stubbs and Smith, 1990).

EPUFAs and membrane receptor signal transduction

EPUFAs are crucial in determining the quantity and quality of neuronal membrane phospholipids (Horrocks et al., 1982; Thomson, 1992). These phospholipids probably maintain the membrane fluidity appropriate for membrane receptors, and specific phospholipids are hydrolyzed by receptor-mediated processes generating intermediates that act as second messengers, e.g., diacylglycerol, inositol polyphosphates, arachidonic acid, prostaglandins, and cytokines (Berridge, 1981; Axelrod, 1990; Rana and Hokin, 1990; Horrobin et al., 1994). In particular, dopamine receptor activation of the AA cascade seems to be the basis for D_1/D_2 receptor synergism (Piomelli et al., 1991). Altered membrane receptor-mediated signal transduction of several neurotransmitters (and also probably of growth factors), has been considered in schizophrenia (Hudson et al., 1993). This is probably a result of common second messengers derived from altered membrane phospholipids.

CONCLUSIONS

Evidence is increasing to support the view that the outcome of schizophrenia may be related to the intake and metabolism of EPUFAs, primarily ω-3 PUFAs, and antioxidants. Cultural and socioeconomic differences in the intake of EPUFAs and antioxidants probably affect the course and outcome of schizophrenia. Life style also plays a critical role in EPUFA status by directly affecting EPUFA intake as well as metabolism, since life style is influenced by environmental and socioeconomic factors that act as stressors. Migration of populations, due to global industrial growth and emerging economic opportunities, is also going to have a major impact on the dietary intake of EPUFAs. EPUFAs and antioxidants probably play a critical role in both the amelioration of abnormal neurodevelopment and in the alteration of membrane receptor-mediated signal transduction of several neurotransmitters, and possibly growth factors, that are generally considered as being of importance in schizophrenia. Dietary supplementation of EPUFAs and antioxidants may be a preferred choice for improving the course and outcome of schizophrenia, since it is difficult to advise on voluntary changes in dietary intake and life style.

REFERENCES

Adler LA, Peselow E, Rotrosen J et al. Vitamin E treatment of tardive dyskinesia. Am J Psychiatry 1993; 150: 1405–1407.

Axelrod J. Receptor-mediated activation of phospholipase A_2 and arachidonic acid release in signal transduction. Biochem Soc Trans 1990; 18: 503–507.

Bang HO, Dyerberg J, Sinclair HM. The composition of the Eskimo food in north western Greenland. Am J Clin Nutr 1980; 33: 2657–2661.

Berridge MJ. Phosphatidylinositol hydrolysis: a multifunctional transducting mechanism. Mol Cell Endocrinol 1981; 24: 115–140.

Bielski BHJ, Arudi RL, Sutherland MW. A study of the reactivity of $HO_2^·/O_2^{-·}$ with unsaturated fatty acids. J Biol Chem 1983; 258: 4759–4761.

Bloom F. Advancing neurodevelopmental origin for schizophrenia. Arch Gen Psychiatry 1993; 50: 224–227.

Bradbury TN, Miller GA. Season of birth in schizophrenia: a review of evidence, methodology and etiology. Psychol Bull 1985; 98: 569–594.

Brenner RR. Nutritional and hormonal factors influencing desaturation of essential fatty acids. Prog Lipid Res 1981; 20: 41–47.

Burr GO, Burr MM. A new deficiency disease produced by the rigid exclusion of fat from the diet. J Biol Chem 1929; 82: 345–367.

Burr GO, Burr MM. On the nature and role of the fatty acids essential in nutrition. J Biol Chem 1930; 85: 587–621.

Calder PC. Dietary fatty acids and the immune system. Nutr Rev 1998; 56: S70–S83.

Carlson SE, Salem N, Jr. Essentiality of ω-3 fatty acids in growth and development in infants. In: Simopoulos AP, Kifer RR, Martin RE, Barlow SM, eds. Health effects of ω-3 pulyunsaturated fatty acids in seafood. World Rev Nutr Diet 1991: 66: 74–86.

Carlson SE, Rhodes PG, Ferguson MG. Docosahexaenoic acid status of preterm infants at birth and following feeding with human milk or formula 1-3. Am J Clin Nutr 1986; 44: 798–804.

Castle DJ, Abel K, Takei N, Muray RM. Gender differences in schizophrenia: hormonal effects or subtypes? Schizophr Bull 1995; 21: 1–12.

Christensen O, Christensen E. Fat consumption and schizophrenia. Acta Psychiatr Scand 1988; 78: 587–591.

Chulei R, Xiaofang L, Hongsheng M et al. Milk composition in women from five different regions of China: the great diversity of milk fatty acids. J Nutr 1995; 125: 2993–2998.

Cochrane R, Bal SS. Migration and schizophrenia: an examination of five hypotheses. Soc Psychiatry 1987; 22: 181–191.

Connor WE, Neuringer M, Lin DS. Dietary effects upon brain fatty acid composition: the reversibility of n-3 fatty acid deficiency and turnover of docosahexaenoic acid in the brain, erythrocytes and plasma of Rhesus monkeys. J Lipid Res 1990; 31: 237–248.

Craig TJ, Siegel C, Hopper K, Lin S, Sartorius N. Outcome in schizophrenia and related disorders compared between developing and developed countries. Br J Psychiatry 1997; 170: 229–233.

Crawford MA. Essential fatty acids and neurodevelopmental disorder. In: Bazan NG, Toffano G, Horrobin DF et al., eds. Neurobiology of essential fatty acids. New York: Plenum Press, 1992: 307–314.

Dalen P. Does age incidence explain all season-to-birth effects in the literature? Schizophr Bull 1990; 16: 11–12.

Davis JO, Phelps JA, Bracha HS. Prenatal development of monozygotic twins and concordance for schizophrenia. Schizophr Bull 1995; 21: 357–366.

Dhunjibhoy JE. A brief résumé of the types of insanity commonly met within India, with a full description of 'Indian hemp insanity' peculiar to the country. J Ment Sci 1930; 40: 254–264.

Dougherty RM, Galli C, Ferro-Luzzi A. Lipid and phospholipid fatty acid composition of plasma, red blood cells, and platelets and how they are affected by dietary lipids: a study of normal subjects from Italy, Finland and the USA. Am J Clin Nutr 1987; 45: 443–455.

Dube KC. A study of prevalence of biosocial variables in mental illness in a rural and an urban community in Uttar Pradesh, India. Acta Psychiatr Scand 1970; 46: 327–359.

Dube KC, Kumar N. An epidemiological study of schizophrenia. J Biosoc Sci 1972; 4: 187–195.

Eagles JM, Hunter D, Geddes JR. Gender-specific changes since 1900 in the season-of-birth effects in schizophrenia. Br J Psychiatry 1995; 167: 469–472.

Eaton WW. Epidemiology of schizophrenia. Epidemiol Cal Rev 1985; 7: 105–126.

Eaton WW. The epidemiology of schizophrenia. In: Burrows GD, Norman TC, Rubinstein G, eds. Handbook of studies on schizophrenia. Part 1: Epidemiology, etiology, and clinical features. Amsterdam: Elsevier, 1986: 11–33.

Edgerton RB, Cohen A. Culture and schizophrenia: the DOSMD challenge. Br J Psychiatry 1994; 164: 222–231.

Elnagar MN, Maitra P, Rao MN. Mental health in an Indian rural community. Br J Psychiatry 1971; 118: 499–503.

Faris REL, Dunham HW. Mental disorders in urban areas. Chicago: Chicago of University Press, 1939.

Farquhar JW, Ahrens EH. Effects of dietary fats on human erythrocyte fatty acid patterns. J Clin Invest 1963; 42: 675–685.

Farquharson J, Cockburn F, Patrick WA, Jamieson EC, Logan RW. Infant cerebral cortex phospholipid fatty acid composition and diet. Lancet 1992; 340: 810–813.

Feighner JP, Robins E, Guze SB, Woodruff RA, Winokur G, Munoz R. Diagnostic criteria for use in psychiatric research. Arch Gen Psychiatry 1972; 26: 57–63.

Fernandes G, Chandrasekar B, Luan X, Troyer DA. Modulation of antioxidant enzymes and programmed cell death by n-3 fatty acids. Lipids 1996; 31: S91–S96.

Finley DA, Lonnerdal B, Dewey KG, Grivetti LE. Breast milk composition: fat content and fatty acid composition in vegetarians and non-vegetarians. Am J Clin Nutr 1985; 41: 787–800.

Foerster A, Lewis SW, Owen MJ, Murray RM. Low birth weight and a family history of schizophrenia predict poor premorbid functioning in psychosis. Schizophr Res 1991; 5: 13–20.

Food and Agriculture Organization. Food balance sheets 1975–1977. Average and *per capita* food supplies, 1961–1965; average 1967 to 1977. Rome: Food and Agriculture Organization, 1980.

Food and Agriculture Organization of the United Nations/World Health Organization. Global trends in the availability of edible fats and oils. Reports on fats and oils in human nutrition. 1994: 25–32.

Freud S. Civilization and its discontents. In: Strachey J, ed. The standard edition of the complete psychological work of Sugmund Freud. Vol. 21. London: Hogarth, 1961: 59–145.

Geddes JR, Lawrie SM. Obstetric complications and schizophrenia: a meta-analysis. Br J Psychiatry 1995; 167: 786–793.

Glen AIM, Glen EMT, Horrobin DF et al. A red cell membrane abnormality in a subgroup of schizophrenic patients: evidence for two diseases. Schizophr Res 1994; 12: 53–61.

Glover V. Maternal stress or anxiety in pregnancy and emotional development of the child. Br J Psychiatry 1997; 171: 105–106.

Goldberg EM, Morrison SL. Schizophrenia and social class. Br J Psychiatry 1963; 109: 785–802.

Gottesman II. Schizophrenia genesis: the origins of madness. New York: WH Freeman and Co., 1991.

Gunstone F, Harwood JL, Padley FB, eds. The lipid handbook. 2nd edn. London: Chapman and Hall, 1994.

Gupta S, Belder A, de Hughes LO. Avoiding premature coronary deaths in Asians in Britain. Br Med J 1995; 311: 1035–1036.

Häffner H. Epidemiology of schizophrenia. In: Häffner H, Gattaz WF, Janzarik W, eds. Search for the causes of schizophrenia. Berlin: Springer-Verlag, 1987: 47–74.

Häffner H, an der Heiden W, Behrens S et al. Causes and consequences of the gender differences in age at the onset of schizophrenia. Schizophr Bull 1998; 24: 99–113.

Hambrecht M, Maurer K, Haffner H, Sartorius N. Transnational stability of gender differences in schizophrenia. Eur Arch Psychiatry Neurol Sci 1992; 242: 6–12.

Hassan N, Ahmed KU. Studies on food and nutrient intake by urban population of Bangladesh: comparison between intakes of 1962–64 and 1985–86. Ecol Food Nutr 1992; 28: 131–148.

Hollingshead AB, Redlich FC. Social class and mental illness. New York: Riley, 1958.

Holman RT. The slow discovery of the importance of ω3 essential fatty acids in human health. J Nutr 1998; 128: 427S–433S.

Hopper K. Some old questions for the new cross-cultural psychiatry. Med Anthropol Q 1991; 5: 299–329.

Horrobin DF. Schizophrenia as a membrane lipid disorder which is expressed throughout the body. Prostagland Leukotr Essent Fatty Acids 1996; 55: 3–7.

Horrobin DF, Manku MS, Hillman S, Glen AIM. Fatty acid levels in brains of schizophrenics and normal controls. Biol Psychiatry 1991; 30: 795–805.

Horrobin DF, Glen AIM, Vaddadi K. The membrane hypothesis of schizophrenia. Schizophr Res 1994; 13: 195–207.

Horrocks LA, Ansell GB, Porcellati G, eds. Phospholipids in the nervous system. Vol. 1, Metabolism. New York: Raven Press, 1982.

Hudson CJ, Young LT, Li PP, Warsh JJ. CNS signal transduction in the pathophysiology and pharmacology of affective disorders and schizophrenia. Synapse 1993; 13: 278–293.

Hultman CM, Ohman A, Cnattingius S, Wieselgren I-M, Lindstrom LH. Prenatal and neonatal risk factors for schizophrenia. Br J Psychiatry 1997; 170: 128–133.

Hutchinson G, Takei N, Bhugoa D et al. Increased rate of psychosis among African-Caribbeans in Britain is not due to an excess of pregnancy and birth complications. Br J Psychiatry 1997; 171: 145–147.

Iacono JM, Zellner DC, Paoletti R, Ishikawa T, Frigeni V, Fumagalli R. Comparison of blood platelet and erythrocyte lipids in man in three age groups from three regions: Milan, Cincinnati and Sicily. Haemostasis 1974; 2: 141–162.

Jablensky A. Multicultural studies and the nature of schizophrenia: a review. J R Soc Med 1987; 80: 162–167.

Jablensky A, Sartorius N, Ernberg G et al. Schizophrenia: manifestations, incidence and course in different cultures. Psychol Med Monogr Suppl 1991; 20: 1–97.

Jeste DV, Kleinman JE, Potkin SG, Luchins DJ, Weinberger DR. Ex uno multi: subtyping the schizophrenic syndrome. Biol Psychiatry 1982; 17: 199–222.

Karno M, Jenkins JH. Cross-cultural issues in the course and treatment of schizophrenia. Psychiatr Clin North Am 1993; 16: 339–350.

Kennedy E, Powell R. Changing eating patterns of American children: a view from 1996. J Am Coll Nutr 1997; 16: 524–529.

Kety SS. The syndrome of schizophrenia: unresolved questions and opportunities for research. Br J Psychiatry 1980; 136: 421–436.

Keys A, ed. Coronary heart disease in seven countries. Circulation 1970; 4 (Suppl 1): 1–238.

Kinney DK, Jacobson B. Environmental factors in schizophrenia: new adoption study evidence. In: Wynn LC, Cromwell RL, Matthysse S, eds. The nature of schizophrenia: new approaches to research and treatment. New York: John Wiley and Sons, 1978: 38–51.

Koletzko B, Thiel J, Abiodum PO. The fatty acid composition of human milk in Europe and Africa. J Pediatr 1992; 120: S62–S70.

Kromhout D. n-3 fatty acids and coronary heart disease: epidemiology from Eskimos to Western populations. J Int Med 1989; 225: 47–51.

Kulhara P, Chandiramani K. Outcome of schizophrenia in India using various diagnostic systems. Schizophr Res 1988; 1: 339–349.

Lands WEM, Hamazaki T, Yamazaki K et al. Changing dietary patterns. Am J Clin Nutr 1990; 51: 991–993.

Leff J, Sartorius N, Jablensky A, Korten A, Ernberg G. The international pilot study of schizophrenia: five-year follow-up findings. Psychol Med 1992; 22: 131–145.

Lewine RRL. Gender and schizophrenia. In: Nasrallah HA, ed. Handbook of schizophrenia, Vol. 3. Amsterdam: Elsevier, 1988: 379–397.

Lichtenstein AH, Kennedy E, Barrier P et al. Dietary fat consumption and health. Nutr Rev 1998; 56: S3–S28.

Lohr JB, Underhill S, Moir S, Jeste DV. Increased indices of free radical activity in the cerebrospinal fluid of patients with tardive dyskinesia. Biol Psychiatry 1989; 28: 535–539.

Lucas A, Morley R, Cole TJ, Lister G, Leeson-Payne C. Breast milk and subsequent intelligence quotient in children born pre-term. Lancet 1992; 339: 261–264.

Mahadik SP, Evans DR. Essential fatty acids in the treatment of schizophrenia. Drugs Today 1997; 33: 5–17.

Mahadik SP, Gowda S. Antioxidants in the treatment of schizophrenia. Drugs Today 1996; 32: 1–13.

Mahadik SP, Mukherjee S. Free radical pathology and antioxidant defense in schizophrenia: a review. Schizophr Res 1996; 19: 1–17.

Mahadik SP, Scheffer RE. Oxidative injury and potential use of antioxidants in schizophrenia. Prostagland Leukotr Essent Fatty Acids 1996; 55: 45–54.

Mahadik SP, Mukherjee S, Correnti EE, Scheffer R. Plasma membrane phospholipid fatty acid composition of cultured skin fibroblasts from schizophrenic patients: comparison with bipolar and normal controls. Psychiatry Res 1996a; 63: 133–142.

Mahadik SP, Schendarkar NS, Scheffer R, Mukherjee S, Correnti EE. Utilization of precursor essential fatty acids in culture by skin fibroblasts from schizophrenic patients and normal controls. Prostagland Leukotr Essent Fatty Acids 1996b; 55: 65–70.

Mahadik SP, Mukherjee S, Scheffer R, Correnti EE, Mahadik JS. Elevated plasma lipid peroxides at the onset of nonaffective psychosis. Biol Psychiatry 1998; 43: 674–679.

Mason P, Harrison G, Croundance T, Glazebrook C, Medley I. The predictive validity of a diagnosis of schizophrenia. Br J Psychiatry 1997; 170: 321–327.

McCreadie RG. The Nithsdale Schizophrenia Surveys. 16. Breast-feeding and schizophrenia: preliminary results and hypotheses. Br J Psychiatry 1997; 170: 334–337.

McCreadie RG, MacDonald E, Wiles D, Campbell G, Paterson JR. The Nithsdale Schizophrenia Surveys. XIV. Plasma lipid peroxide and serum vitamin E levels in patients with and without tardive dyskinesia and in normal subjects. Br J Psychiatry 1995; 167: 610–617.

McGrath J, Welham J, Pemberton M. Month of birth, hemispere of birth and schizophrenia. Br J Psychiatry 1995; 167: 783–785.

McNeil TF. Perinatal risk factors and schizophrenia: selective review and methodological concepts. Epidemiol Rev 1995; 17: 107–112.

Mukherjee S, Mahadik SP, Correnti EE, Scheffer R, Kelkar H. Impaired antioxidant defense system at the onset of psychosis. Schizophr Res 1996; 19: 19–26.

Murphy HBM. Diseases of civilization? Psychol Med 1984; 14: 487–490.

Murphy HBM, Taumoepeau BM. Traditional and mental heath in the South Pacific: a re-examination of an old hypothesis. Psychol Med 1980; 10: 471–482.

Murray RM. Neurodevelopmental schizophrenia: the rediscovery of dementia precox. Br J Psychiatry 1994; 165 (Suppl 25): 6–12.

Nandi DN, Banerjee G, Boral GC et al. Socio-economic status and prevalence of mental disorders in certain rural communities in India. Acta Psychiatr Scand 1979; 59: 276–293.

Nandi DN, Mukherjee SP, Boral GC et al. Socio-economic status and mental morbidity in certain tribes and castes in India – a cross-cultural study. Br J Psychiatry 1980; 136: 73–85.

Nasrallah HA. Neurodevelopmental pathogenesis of schizophrenia. Psychiatr Clin North Am 1993; 16: 269–280.

Nestle M, Wing R, Birch L et al. Behavioral and social influences on food choice. Nutr Rev 1998; 56: S50–S74.

Neuringer M, Connor WE, Lin DS, Barstad L, Luck S. Biochemical and functional effects of prenatal and postnatal ω-3 fatty acid deficiency on retina and brain in rhesus monkeys. Proc Natl Acad Sci USA 1986; 83: 4021–4025.

O'Brien JS, Samson EL Lipid composition of the normal human brain: gray matter, white matter, and myelin. J Lipid Res 1965; 6: 537–544.

O'Callahan E, Gibson T, Colohan HA et al. Season of birth in schizophrenia: evidence for confinement of an excess of winter births to patients without a family history of mental disorder. Br J Psychiatry 1991; 158: 764–769.

Packer L, ed. Oxygen radicals in biological systems. Methods Enzymol Vol. 105. New York: Academic Press, 1984.

Palmer HJ, Paulson KR. Reactive oxygen species and antioxidants in signal transduction and gene expression. Nutr Rev 1997; 55: 353–361.

Peet M, Laugharne J, Rangarajan N, Reynolds GP. Tardive dyskinesia, lipid peroxidation, and sustained amelioration with vitamin E treatment. Int Clin Psychopharmacol 1993; 8: 151–153.

Peet M, Laugharne JDE, Mellor J, Ramchand CN. Essential fatty acid deficiency in erythrocyte membranes from chronic schizophrenic patients, and the clinical effects of dietary supplementation. Prostagland Leukotr Essent Fatty Acids 1996; 55: 71–75.

Piomelli D, Pilon C, Giros B, Sokoloff P, Martres M-P, Schwartz JC. Dopamine activation of the arachidonic acid cascade as a basis for D1/D2 receptor synergism. Nature 1991; 353: 164–167.

Rana RS, Hokin LE. Role of phosphoinositols in transmembrane signaling. Physiol Rev 1990; 70: 115–164.

Rao S. Birth order and schizophrenia. J Nerv Ment Dis 1964; 138: 87–89.

Rao S. Caste and mental disorders in Bihar. Am J Psychiatry 1966; 122: 1045–1055.

Reddy R, Yao J. Free radical pathology in schizophrenia: a review. Prostagland Leukotr Essent Fatty Acids 1996; 55: 33–43.

Reveley AM, Revley MA, Murray RM. Cerebral ventricular enlargement in non-genetic schizophrenia: a controlled twin study. Br J Psychiatry 1984; 144: 89–93.

Rotrosen J, Wolkin A. Phospholipid and prostaglandin hypotheses of schizophrenia. In: Meltzer HY, ed. Psychopharmacology: the third generation of progress. New York: Raven Press, 1987: 759–764.

Sartorius N, Jablensky A, Shapiro R. Two-year follow-up study of the patients included in the WHO International Pilot Study of Schizophrenia: preliminary communication. Psychol Med 1977; 7: 529–541.

Sartorius N, Jablensky A, Korten A et al. Early manifestations and first-contact incidence of schizophrenia in different cultures. Psychol Med 1986; 16: 909–928.

Saxena BM, Bhaskaran K, Ananth JV. Social class and schizophrenia: a study based on the caste system in India. Transcult Psychiatr Res Rev 1972; 9: 130–133.

Shur E. Season of birth in high and low genetic risk schizophrenics. Br J Psychiatry 1982; 140: 410–415.

Simopoulos AP. Summary of the NATO advanced research workshop on dietary ω-3 and ω-6 fatty acids: biological effects and nutritional essentiality. J Nutr 1989; 119: 521–528.

Simopoulos AP. Omega-3 fatty acids in health and disease growth and development. Am J Clin Nutr 1991; 54: 438–463.

Sinclair HM, ed. The essential fatty acids. London: Butterworths, 1958.

Sinclair HM. History of essential fatty acids. In: Horrobin DF, ed. Omega-6 essential fatty acids: pathophysiological role in clinical medicine. New York: Alan R. Liss Inc., 1990: 1–19.

Stevens JR. Brief psychoses: do they contribute to the good prognosis and equal prevalence of schizophrenia in developing countries? Br J Psychiatry 1987; 151: 393–396.

Stevens JR, Wyatt RJ. Similar incidence worldwide of schizophrenia: case not proven. Br J Psychiatry 1987; 151: 131–132.

Stubbs CD, Smith AD. Essential fatty acids in membrane: physical properties and function. Biochem Soc Trans 1990; 18: 779–781.

Sunderaraj N, Rao SR. Order of birth and schizophrenia. Br J Psychiatry 1966; 112: 1127–1129.

Susser E, Verma VK, Malhotra S, Conover S, Amador XF. Delineation of acute transient psychotic disorders in developing country setting. Br J Psychiatry 1995; 167: 216–219.

Thara R, Henrietta M, Joseph A, Rajkumar S, Eaton WW. Ten-year course of schizophrenia – the Madras longitudinal study. Acta Psychiatr Scand 1994; 90: 329–336.

Thomas CS, Stone K, Osborn M, Thomas PF, Fisher M. Psychiatric morbidity and compulsory admission among UK-born Europeans, Afro-Caribbeans, and Asians in Central Manchester. Br J Psychiatry 1993; 163: 91–99.

Thomson GA, ed. The regulation of membrane lipid metabolism. 2nd edn. Boca Raton: CRC Press, 1992.

Torrey EF. Schizophrenia and civilization. New York: Jason Aronson, 1980.

Torrey EF. Prevalence studies in schizophrenia. Br J Psychiatry 1987a; 150: 598–608.

Torrey EF. Similar incidence worldwide of schizophrenia: case not proven. Br J Psychiatry 1987b; 151: 132–133.

van der Velde CD. Variability in schizophrenia. Arch Gen Psychiatry 1976; 33: 489–496.

Verghese A, John JK, Rajkumar S, Richard J, Sethi BB, Trivedi JK. Factors associated with the course and outcome of schizophrenia in India: results of a two-year multicentre follow-up study. Br J Psychiatry 1989; 154: 499–503.

Wainwright PE. Do essential fatty acids play a role in brain and behavioural development? Neurosci Biobehav Rev 1992; 16: 193–205.

World Health Organization. The international pilot study of schizophrenia. Vol. 1. Geneva: World Health Organization, 1973.

World Health Organization. Schizophrenia: an international follow-up study. New York: John Wiley and Sons, 1979.

World Health Organization. Study group on diet, nutrition, and prevention of non-communicable diseases. Diet, nutrition and the prevention of chronic diseases: report of WHO study group. World Health Organization technical report series; 797. Geneva: World Health Organization, 1990.

Yamamoto N, Saitoh M, Moriuchi A, Nomura M, Okuyama H. Effect of dietary α-linolenate/linoleate balance on brain lipid compositions and learning ability of rats. J Lipid Res 1987; 28: 144–151.

Yao JK, van Kammen DP, Welker JA, Gurklis JA. Red blood cell membrane dynamics in schizophrenia. III. Correlation of fatty acid abnormalities with clinical measures. Schizophr Res 1994a; 13: 227–232.

Zipursky RB, Schulz SC. Seasonality of birth and CT findings in schizophrenia. Biol Psychiatry 1987; 22: 1288–1297.

Sustained Remission of Symptoms Following Treatment with Eicosapentaenoic Acid in a Case of Schizophrenia with Dyslexia

Alexandra J. Richardson and Basant K. Puri

INTRODUCTION

Double-blind trials have shown that treatment with ω-3 fatty acids, particularly eicosapentaenoic acid (EPA), can be of benefit in reducing schizophrenic symptoms in medicated patients (Mellor et al., 1996; Peet et al., 1996, 1997). In these studies, improvements were particularly apparent for positive symptoms. Here results are presented from a single case, open study of treatment with ω-3 fatty acids in an otherwise unmedicated patient with schizophrenia. The initial dramatic improvement in both positive and negative symptoms of schizophrenia has already been reported (Puri and Richardson, 1998), but treatment has been continued at the request of the patient and further details of this case are provided here. Follow-up has now been going on for more than 15 months and the remission of psychiatric symptoms has been sustained during this time.

An additional interesting feature of this case is that the patient had previously been identified as dyslexic. Additional psychological assessments relevant to this condition were therefore carried out before and after treatment. Results from these are presented, showing that treatment with ω-3 fatty acids was also associated with improvement across a range of dyslexic symptomatology.

The rationale for fatty acid treatment in schizophrenia

Horrobin's membrane phospholipid hypothesis of schizophrenia (Horrobin, 1977, 1996, 1998) provides an underlying explanation not only for those aspects of schizophrenia traditionally explained by the dopamine hypothesis, but also for other clinical features. These include: the inverse relationship between schizophrenia and some inflammatory disorders; the high resistance to pain shown by some patients; the dramatic remission of symptoms that may occur with pyrexia; the increased risk associated with exposure to viral infections or maternal malnutrition during foetal development; and the difference in severity and prognosis in different countries (Horrobin et al., 1994). Consistent with this hypothesis, findings from biochemistry, cerebral magnetic resonance spectroscopy (MRS) and molecular genetics suggest that schizophrenia is related to a deficiency in cell membranes of arachidonic acid (AA) and docosahexaenoic acid (DHA), arising from excess activity of one or other of the phospholipase A_2 (PLA_2) group of enzymes, as discussed elsewhere in this book (and see Pettegrew et al., 1991; Glen et al., 1994; Horrobin, 1996, 1998; Hudson et al., 1996). Whilst there is thus increasing evidence to support the membrane phospholipid hypothesis, a very important question is whether this hypothesis has any useful implications for treatment.

Atypical antipsychotics, such as clozapine, represent a considerable improvement over standard (typical) neuroleptics. However, the mechanism of action of clozapine has not adequately been explained on the basis of neurotransmitter actions, and in this regard it is interesting that two decades ago Horrobin suggested that the structure and pharmacological actions of clozapine are consistent with its being a prostaglandin E analogue. E prostaglandins are potent stimulators of cyclic AMP formation, and cyclic AMP inhibits PLA_2 (Horrobin et al., 1978). Furthermore, pharmacotherapy with clozapine has also been shown to be associated with a dramatic rise in erythrocyte membrane concentrations of certain polyunsaturated fatty acids (Glen et al., 1996). These findings raise the possibility that the pharmacotherapeutic value of clozapine in schizophrenia may be a function of its action on membrane phospholipid composition (Horrobin, 1996, 1997).

The membrane phospholipid hypothesis leads to the prediction that treatment with PLA_2 inhibitors should result in clinical improvement in schizophrenia (Horrobin, 1996). As EPA is a PLA_2 inhibitor (Finnen and Lovell, 1991), and also a constituent of brain phospholipids and a precursor of DHA, then it follows from the hypothesis that treatment with an essential fatty acid (EFA) such as EPA should be of clinical value in schizophrenia.

Schizophrenia and dyslexia

The subject of the case study reported here suffered from both dyslexia and schizophrenia. There are a number of similarities between these conditions, suggesting that there may be common elements at the level of biological predisposition. Shared features at the level of phenomenology include a vulnerability to perceptual distortions and associated unusual beliefs, such that dyslexic individuals score highly on measures of schizotypal personality traits (Richardson, 1994, 1997). Other clinical similarities include disordered language, poor visuomotor coordination and attentional problems, while at the neurobiological level, both dyslexia and schizophrenia are associated with reduced cerebral lateralization, and with specific abnormalities of visual perception implicating the fast magnocellular stream of visual processing.

Epidemiological and genetic evidence also supports an association between dyslexia and schizophrenia. Reading problems at school, as well as an excess of non-right-handedness, characterized those children in a large-scale, random population study who went on to develop schizophrenia (Crow et al., 1995). Most compelling, however, is the fact that an unusually high incidence of dyslexia has repeatedly been found in the children of schizophrenic parents (Marcus, 1974; Rieder and Nichols, 1979; Erlenmeyer-Kimling et al., 1984; Fish, 1987). This is consistent with a genetic component to dyslexia that is carried by those with schizophrenia.

There is already substantial evidence for abnormal phospholipid metabolism in schizophrenia, as is amply discussed elsewhere in this book. With respect to dyslexia, Stordy (1995) found that visual dysfunction in dyslexic adults was corrected following treatment with ω-3 fatty acids. This would suggest a phospholipid abnormality in dyslexia also, and there is other evidence to support this. Horrobin and colleagues (1995) therefore proposed a model whereby genetic interactions in this domain could explain the aggregation of schizophrenia, dyslexia and other disorders within families. Specifically, they suggested two separate, but interactive, abnormalities, one involving excessive phospholipid breakdown (probably *via* PLA$_2$ overactivity), as appears to characterize schizophrenia, and the other involving problems in the synthesis or incorporation of membrane phospholipids, which they suggested may be the case in dyslexia. The results of an initial ^{31}P MRS study of dyslexia were consistent with this proposal (Richardson et al., 1997).

FATTY ACID TREATMENT IN A CASE OF SCHIZOPHRENIA WITH DYSLEXIA

Background to the case

The subject was a man aged 30 years at the start of this study, who first came to the attention of the psychiatric services at the age of 28 years when he was diagnosed as suffering from schizophrenia by DSM-IV criteria (American Psychiatric Association, 1994). His symptoms included daily auditory hallucinations and a complex delusional system, both of which had started in his early teenage years. His profile had always been predominantly one of unremitting positive symptoms, although more recently he had also begun to suffer from negative symptoms, including anhedonia, social anxiety and social withdrawal. At the time of diagnosis he was prescribed sulpiride, but owing to a severe extrapyramidal reaction he rejected this after a single dose, and refused medication thereafter. However, in the attempt to understand (and rid himself of) his symptoms he was very keen to participate in research studies, so his case had been extremely well documented over the 2 years preceding this study. Over this period his symptoms had not changed.

The patient volunteered that he had previously been identified as dyslexic, having been assessed for this both at primary school and again during adolescence. This was confirmed by his performance on standardized measures of reading and spelling relative to his general ability, as well as the particular deficits he showed in tasks involving auditory sequential memory and phonological skills. Having heard that double-blind trials of EFA treatment in dyslexia were being set up, he expressed an interest in taking part in these, although this was precluded by the co-diagnosis of schizophrenia. Instead, he gave full informed consent to enter into an open, single-case study of treatment with a high-EPA emulsion (Kirunal, 30 ml/day, supplying 2 g EPA), as used in some double-blind studies of schizophrenia.

The treatment study

Psychiatric ratings were carried out before treatment commenced, and then at monthly intervals for 12 months, using the Schedules for the Assessment of Positive (SAPS) and Negative Symptoms (SANS) (Andreasen, 1984a,b). Additional psychological, experimental, biochemical and other measures were also used. These included interview and questionnaire ratings of dyslexia and features associated with this condition, psychometric assessments of reading and related skills, psychophysical measures of visual and auditory function, blood biochemical measures, and cerebral MRS and imaging.

A minimal set of such assessments was carried out monthly, and the others at 3-month intervals, for 12 months from the initiation of EPA treatment. Treatment and follow-up has since continued at the subject's request, with a reduced set of measures conducted at 3-month intervals. It is now more than 15 months since EPA treatment commenced. No adverse effects from this treatment have been experienced.

Results

Clinical impressions

At the first monthly follow-up there was a clear improvement in the patient's appearance, and notably in the condition of his skin and hair, but subjectively he reported feeling that nothing had changed. Experimental measures, psychiatric ratings and his own daily and weekly records largely seemed to support that picture. He was somewhat sceptical about the treatment, although his compliance with it, record-keeping, and motivation during testing continued to be model.

After the second month of treatment, his appearance was still much healthier, and at this visit he also seemed more calm and focused. He was still maintaining that he himself had noticed little change. Nonetheless, his conversation was much more lucid and coherent; his usual anxiety and agitation were minimal; and it emerged that he had not heard any hallucinatory voices for over a month.

By the 3-month follow-up the improvements were even more pronounced, and the patient himself admitted that he felt much better. He was still free of auditory hallucinations, and the content and clarity of his thought and speech were very much improved from baseline. He also volunteered that he now felt very embarrassed at some of the 'rubbish' (i.e., accounts of his bizarre experiences and his interpretations of these) that he had written in his study record book during the first month. He appeared more positive and outgoing, and seemed to be coping with much more interaction with the world.

Further improvements followed, and these have now been sustained for well over a year. The patient has now resumed studying for a degree and is coping well with the course, whereas his previous attempts to do this had been disrupted by his symptoms to such an extent that neither further education nor employment had been an option.

Psychiatric ratings

Psychiatric rating scores (SAPS and SANS) over a period of 15 months from the initiation of EPA treatment are shown in Figure 17.1. These scores fell dramatically after two months, and this improvement has been sustained, such that the subject is now virtually symptom-free. These changes are particularly impressive, considering that his symptom profile had remained constant over the 2 years preceding this study.

Dyslexia symptom ratings

As the patient had a history of dyslexia, interview checklist ratings of a range of associated symptoms were also carried out. These included visual symptoms experienced when reading, auditory language confusions, expressive language problems, and motor coordination difficulties. Ratings were taken at baseline and then at 3-month intervals for 12 months. As shown in Figure 17.2, improvements were reported across all domains, but as his initial symptoms predominantly involved auditory language and spoken language problems this was the domain for which the reductions were most apparent.

Reading and spelling measures

The patient's reading and spelling performance also improved following treatment (see Figure 17.3). Results are shown in this figure for the first 3 months only, as although there were further improvements beyond this point, repetition of the same materials may have been a factor. However, the passage reading test used, i.e., the Gray Oral Reading Test, 3rd Edition (Wiederholt and Bryant, 1992), involves a series of up to 13 passages which are graded in difficulty. Two alternative forms of the test are available, one of which was used at baseline and the other after 3 months. On this standardized test of oral passage reading his performance rose from below-average to above-average levels, with improvements in reading speed, accuracy, overall fluency and comprehension. Single word reading performance remained unchanged, which might be expected in view of the strong influence of vocabulary on this kind of measure, but his spelling, while remaining below average, also showed some improvement.

Essential fatty acid deficiency signs

Ratings of clinical signs associated with EFA deficiency (Stevens et al., 1995) were taken at baseline and at

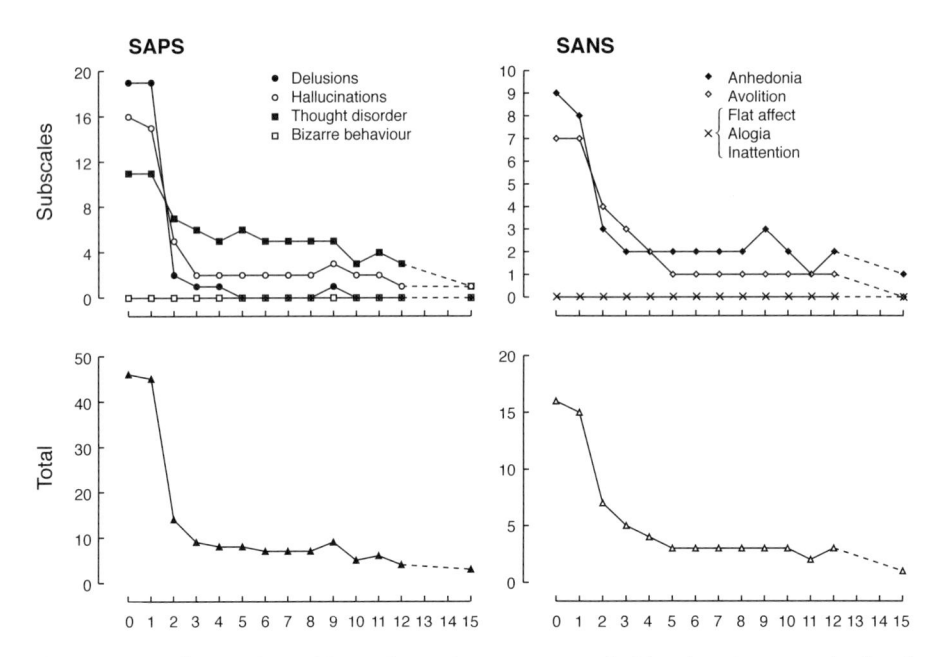

Figure 17.1. Reduction in positive and negative symptoms of schizophrenia, assessed using the SAPS and SANS ratings, respectively, in a patient treated with EPA over a 15-month period. Ratings for individual symptoms and total ratings are shown. Note that for the SANS ratings flat affect, alogia and inattention were all zero from pretreatment baseline and thereafter throughout treatment and so are represented by a single symbol in the graph.

3-month intervals for 12 months. This scale includes the assessment of seven items (excessive thirst, frequent urination, dry skin, dry hair, brittle nails, dandruff and follicular keratosis) on a four-point ordinal scale. Although each of these symptoms can have other causes, scores on this scale have been found to relate to blood biochemical measures of EFA deficiency (Stevens et al., 1995). The results for this patient are shown with reference to mean values for adult dyslexic and control groups from trials involving the use of fatty acids to treat dyslexia (Richardson et al., 1999b) (see Figure 17.4). EFA deficiency signs were initially high, at a level slightly above the mean for the dyslexic group which were, in their turn, significantly higher than those of controls. This initial high score was mainly attributable to the patient's strong endorsement of the items concerning excessive thirst, dry skin and hair, and brittle nails.

Following treatment EFA deficiency signs were reduced, as might be expected, and in this the patient's self-reports were consistent with clinical impressions of improvement in the quality of his skin, hair and nails. Within 3 months his total score for EFA deficiency signs had normalized, and from then on his scores remained below the mean for adult controls.

Visual motion sensitivity

Experimental assessments included thresholds for detecting coherent motion in random dot patterns, an index of magnocellular visual function. Impaired motion sensitivity is associated with dyslexia (Cornelissen et al., 1995) and has also been found in unmedicated patients with schizophrenia (Richardson et al., 1996). Motion sensitivity was therefore assessed at baseline and at 3-month intervals for 12 months.

The test used was the same as in the study of dyslexia by Cornelissen and colleagues (1995). Results for this patient are therefore shown with reference to mean values for the adult dyslexic and control groups from this study (see Figure 17.5). Initially, the patient showed an elevated threshold, comparable with the mean for dyslexic subjects, but over the course of 12 months his performance improved steadily, with thresholds falling to a level below the control group mean.

Laterality

One very interesting accompaniment to symptom remission following EPA treatment was an apparent shift in the patient's handedness (Richardson et al., 1999a).

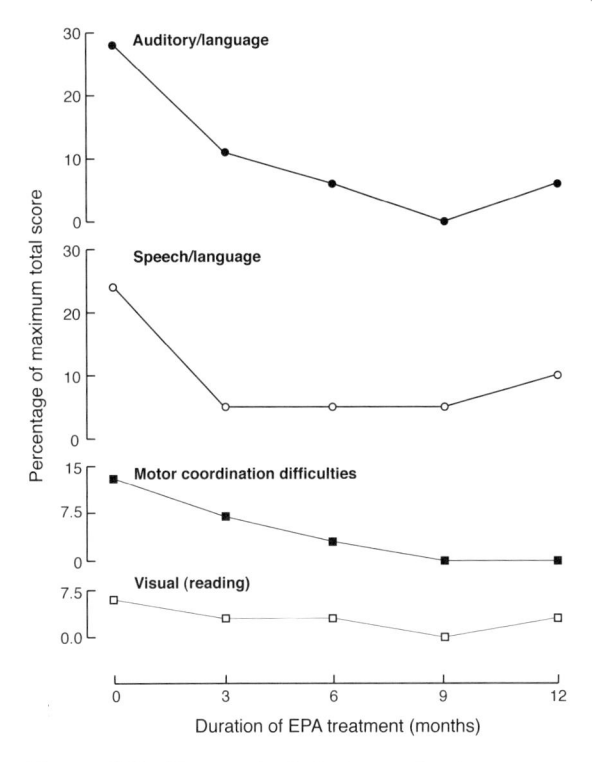

Figure 17.2. Changes in dyslexia-associated symptoms over a period of 12 months treatment with EPA in a single patient showing symptoms of both schizophrenia and dyslexia.

Initially he showed a strong right-hand advantage on a pegboard task (Annett, 1985), consistent with his reported hand preference. However, after 3 months his performance on this task had become much more symmetrical, owing to a marked improvement in his left-hand scores (see Figure 17.6). On retest at 6, 9 and 12 months this reduction in asymmetry was maintained. The fact that the patient's handedness on this measure had not changed in the year preceding EPA treatment also adds to our confidence in the veracity of this result.

DISCUSSION

This report concerns a unique case study of an individual with both schizophrenia and dyslexia who was treated with EPA in the absence of any other medication. Treatment was followed within 2 months by a dramatic reduction in both positive and negative symptoms of schizophrenia (Puri and Richardson, 1998), and this remission continues to be sustained at the time of writing, more than 15 months since treatment was started. It is unlikely that this improvement represented either a spontaneous remission or a placebo response. The patient's clinical profile had remained essentially unchanged over the two previous years, and prior to this there is no evidence of spontaneous remission or an episodic quality to the illness. Furthermore, other research studies incorporating a nonpharmacological treatment element had yielded no benefit, and it is

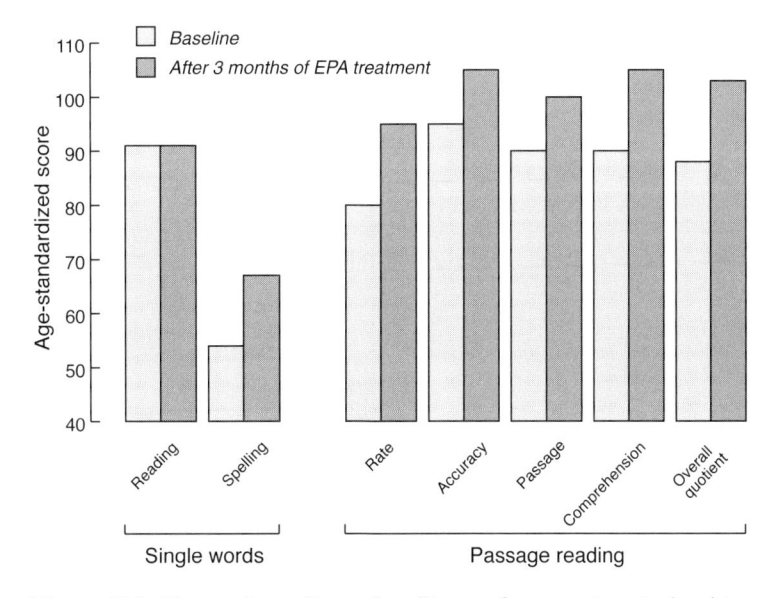

Figure 17.3. Changes in reading and spelling performance in a single schizophrenic/dyslexic patient before and 3 months after treatment with EPA.

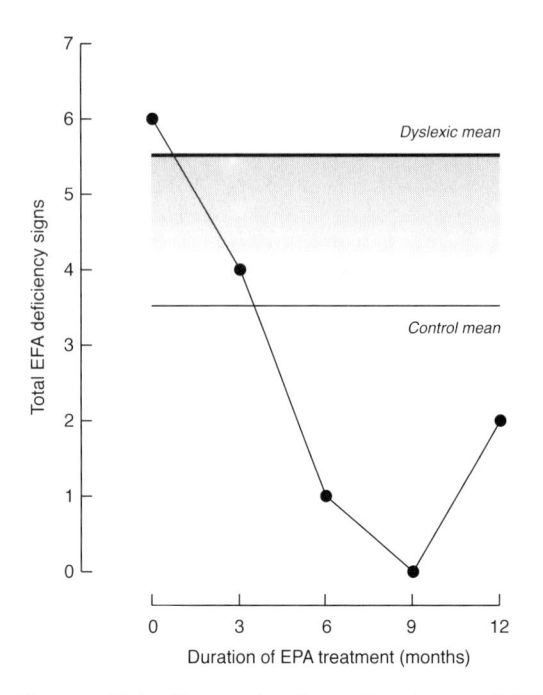

Figure 17.4. Change in the rating for total EFA deficiency signs in a single schizophrenic/dyslexic patient over a period of 12 months of treatment with EPA. Means for dyslexic and control subjects taken from earlier trials are shown for comparison.

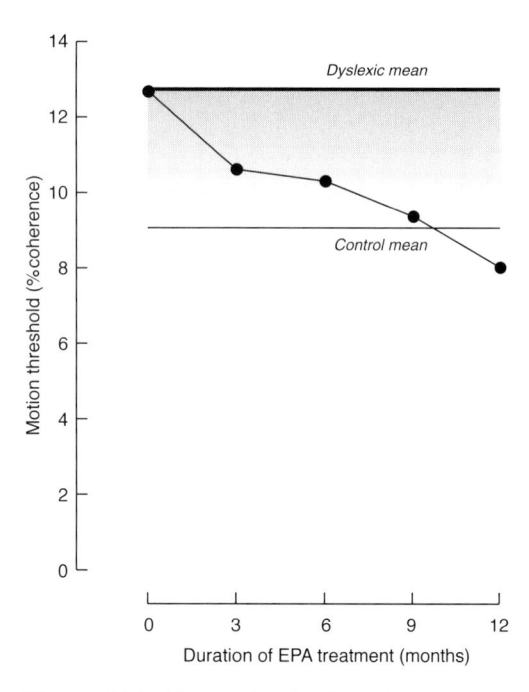

Figure 17.5. Changes in visual motion sensitivity in a single schizophrenic/dyslexic patient over a period of 12 months of treatment with EPA. Means for dyslexic and control subjects taken from earlier trials are shown for comparison.

unlikely that the remission was a consequence of extra attention and regular follow-up, as these had also been experienced during the two previous years with other research studies. Most noteworthy is that the improvement cannot be attributed at all to antipsychotic medication.

Following EPA treatment, clear improvements were also evident with respect to reading, spelling and other symptoms associated with the subject's dyslexia. A corresponding reduction was observed in clinical ratings of EFA deficiency signs, which were initially high. The results of this case study thus strongly support the idea that EFA deficiency is a common factor in the predisposition to dyslexia and schizophrenia (Horrobin et al., 1995). They further suggest that treatment with ω-3 fatty acids may be beneficial in reducing dyslexic symptoms, and double-blind trials are underway to address this issue.

Another interesting feature is the improvement in visual motion sensitivity, an index of magnocellular visual function. Although some contribution from learning effects cannot be ruled out, data from other (untreated) subjects have indicated little change in performance on repeated testing. It is known that ω-3 fatty acids are essential to visual function (Neuringer et al., 1988). Moreover, Stordy (1995) found visual deficits in dyslexic adults (specifically, an impairment of dark adaptation) that subsequently normalized following treatment with DHA. It is therefore plausible that treatment with ω-3 fatty acids could lead to improvements in other aspects of visual function, and the magnocellular deficits found in dyslexia and the schizophrenia spectrum are obviously of particular interest. The results of this single case study do suggest benefits from EPA treatment, but the double-blind trials of EFA supplementation in dyslexia should provide more definitive evidence.

The apparent shift in handedness accompanying EPA treatment in this case was an unexpected finding, but the particular improvement in left-hand performance would be consistent with improved right-hemisphere function. Although many of the symptoms of schizophrenia have been linked with left-hemisphere dysfunction, others have suggested that the primary problem may be a failure of attentional filtering by the right hemisphere (Venables, 1984; Cromwell, 1987;

Cutting, 1990). It is therefore interesting that the right hemisphere has been found to have a relatively higher rate of deacylation and reacylation of complex lipids and appears more active than the left in releasing AA under conditions of stress (Pediconi and Rodriguez de Turco, 1984; Ginobili de Martinez et al., 1985). The rationale for treatment with EPA was that this inhibits a PLA_2 enzyme that removes complex fatty acids, such as AA and DHA, from neuronal membranes (Finnen and Lovell, 1991). These observations suggest that there could perhaps be some asymmetry to its action in favour of the right hemisphere, although further investigation is clearly warranted.

CONCLUSIONS

Over two decades ago Horrobin (1977) put forward a membrane phospholipid hypothesis of schizophrenia, and supporting evidence has been accumulating since then, as discussed in other chapters of this book. One of the virtues of this hypothesis is that it makes specific predictions that are eminently testable. In particular, it predicts that a sustained remission of schizophrenic symptoms should follow treatment with EPA. The results described in this chapter are clearly entirely consistent with this prediction and offer further compelling evidence in support of the hypothesis.

So far as the history of the pharmacotherapy of schizophrenia is concerned, the first major development was the discovery of the efficacy of the archetypal typical antipsychotic chlorpromazine in the treatment of psychosis, particularly in reducing positive symptoms, although the drawbacks of such typical neuroleptics in terms of their adverse effects are very well known. A second major step forward took place with the report of good results in chronic schizophrenia from treatment with the archetypal atypical antipsychotic, clozapine (Gross and Langner, 1966; Kane et al., 1988). As pointed out earlier in this chapter, this beneficial action of clozapine may be a function of its action on membrane phospholipid composition (Glen et al., 1996; Horrobin, 1997). It is our belief that a third major step forward may now be taking place, with the finding of significant benefits from treatment with EPA on both positive and negative symptoms, without any adverse effects. Double-blind trials of EPA, in addition to routine medication in schizophrenia, have yielded promising results (Mellor et al., 1996; Peet et al., 1996; 1997). The remarkable and comprehensive benefits found in the case study reported here indicate a need for additional trials of EPA treatment in unmedicated patients with schizophrenia.

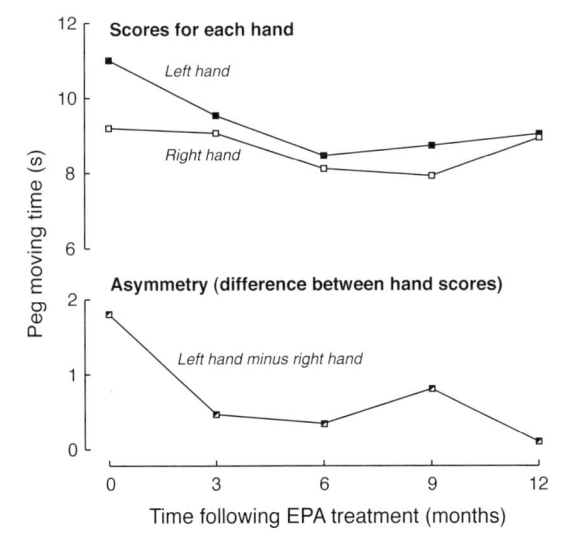

Figure 17.6. Laterality changes in a single schizophrenic/dyslexic patient over a period of 12 months of treatment with EPA. The upper panel shows the performances on a pegboard task for right and left hands, with the faster times being achieved by the right hand and thus indicating a preference for that hand. The asymmetry, indicated by the difference between right hand and left hand scores, is shown in the lower panel; a reduction of this asymmetry was noted over the period of EPA treatment.

REFERENCES

American Psychiatric Association. Diagnostic and statistical manual of mental disorders. 4th edn (DSM-IV). Washington, DC: American Psychiatric Association, 1994.

Andreasen NC. Scale for the assessment of negative symptoms (SANS). Iowa City, Iowa: University of Iowa, 1984a.

Andreasen NC. Scale for the assessment of positive symptoms (SAPS). Iowa City, Iowa: University of Iowa, 1984b.

Annett M. Left, right, hand and brain: the right shift theory. Hillsdale, New Jersey: Erlbaum, 1985.

Cornelissen PL, Richardson AJ, Mason AJS, Stein JF. Contrast sensitivity measured at photopic luminance levels and coherent motion detection in dyslexics and controls. Vision Res 1995; 35: 1483–1494.

Cromwell RL. An argument concerning schizophrenia: the left hemisphere drains the swamp. In: Glass A, ed. Individual differences in hemispheric specialisation. New York: Plenum Press, 1987: 349–356.

Crow TJ, Done DJ, Sacker A. Childhood precursors of psychosis as clues to its evolutionary origins. Eur Arch Psychiatry Clin Neurosci 1995; 245: 61–69.

Cutting J. The right cerebral hemisphere and psychiatric disorders. Oxford: Oxford University Press, 1990.

Erlenmeyer-Kimling L, Marcuse Y, Cornblatt B, Friedman D, Rainer JD, Rutschmann J. The New York high risk project. In: Watt NF, Anthony LC, Rolf JE, eds. Children at risk of schizophrenia: a longitudinal perspective. New York: Cambridge University Press, 1984: 169–189.

Finnen MJ, Lovell CR. Purification and characterisation of phospholipase A₂ from human epidermis. Biochem Soc Trans 1991; 19: 915.

Fish B. Infant predictors of the longitudinal course of schizophrenic development. Schizophr Bull 1987; 13: 395–409.

Ginobili de Martinez MS, Rodriguez de Turco EB, Barrantes FJ. Endogenous asymmetry of rat brain lipids and dominance of the right cerebral hemisphere in free fatty acid response to electroconvulsive shock. Brain Res 1985; 339: 315–321.

Glen AIM, Glen EMT, Horrobin DF et al. A red cell membrane abnormality in a subgroup of schizophrenic patients: evidence for two diseases. Schizophr Res 1994; 12: 53–61.

Glen AIM, Cooper SJ, Rybakowski J, Vaddadi K, Brayshaw N, Horrobin DF. Membrane fatty acids, niacin flushing and clinical parameters. Prostagland Leukotr Essent Fatty Acids 1996; 55: 9–15.

Gross H, Langner E. Das Wirkungsprofil eines chemisch Neuartigen Breitbandneuroleptikums der Dibenzodiazepingruppe. Wien Med Wochenschr 1966; 116: 814–816.

Horrobin DF. Schizophrenia as a prostaglandin deficiency disease. Lancet 1977; i: 936–937.

Horrobin DF. Schizophrenia as a membrane lipid disorder which is expressed throughout the body. Prostagland Leukotr Essent Fatty Acids 1996; 55: 3–7.

Horrobin DF. Clozapine: elevation of membrane unsaturated lipid levels as a new mechanism of action. Biol Psychiatry 1997; 42: 161S.

Horrobin DF. The membrane phospholipid hypothesis as a biochemical basis for the neurodevelopmental concept of schizophrenia. Schizophr Res 1998; 30: 193–208.

Horrobin DF, Ally AI, Karmali RA, Karmazyn M, Manku MS, Morgan RO. Prostaglandins and schizophrenia: further discussion of the evidence. Psychol Med 1978; 8: 43–48.

Horrobin DF, Glen AIM, Vaddadi K. The membrane hypothesis of schizophrenia. Schizophr Res 1994; 13: 195–207.

Horrobin DF, Glen AIM, Hudson CJ. Possible relevance of phospholipid abnormalities and genetic interactions in psychiatric disorders: the relationship between dyslexia and schizophrenia. Med Hypotheses 1995; 45: 605–613.

Hudson CJ, Lin A, Horrobin DF. Phospholipases: in search of a genetic basis of schizophrenia. Prostagland Leukotr Essent Fatty Acids 1996; 55: 115–118.

Kane J, Honigfeld G, Singer J, Meltzer H. Clozapine for the treatment-resistant schizophrenic. A double-blind comparison with chlorpromazine. Arch Gen Psychiatry 1988; 45: 789–796.

Marcus J. Cerebral functioning in offspring of schizophrenics: a possible genetic factor. Int J Ment Health 1974; 3: 57–73.

Mellor JE, Laugharne JDE, Peet M. Omega-3 fatty acid supplementation in schizophrenia patients. Hum Psychopharmacol 1996; 11: 39–46.

Neuringer M, Anderson GJ, Connor WE. The essentiality of n-3 fatty acids for the development and function of the retina and brain. Annu Rev Nutr 1988; 8: 517–541.

Pediconi MF, Rodriguez de Turco EB. Free fatty acid content and release kinetics as manifestations of cerebral lateralization in mouse brain. J Neurochem 1984; 43: 1–7.

Peet M, Laugharne JDE, Mellor J, Ramchand CN. Essential fatty acid deficiency in erythrocyte membranes from chronic schizophrenic patients, and the clinical effects of dietary supplementation. Prostagland Leukotr Essent Fatty Acids 1996; 55: 71–75.

Peet M, Laugharne JDE, Mellor J. Double-blind trial of fatty acid supplementation in the treatment of schizophrenia. International Congress on Schizophrenia Research, Colorado Springs, Colorado, USA, April, 1997.

Pettegrew JW, Keshavan MS, Panchalingam K et al. Alterations in brain high-energy phosphate and membrane phospholipid metabolism in first-episode drug-naïve schizophrenics. A pilot study of the dorsal prefrontal cortex by *in vivo* phosphorus-31 nuclear magnetic resonance spectroscopy. Arch Gen Psychiatry 1991; 48: 563–568.

Puri BK, Richardson AJ. Sustained remission of positive and negative symptoms of schizophrenia following treatment with eicosapentaenoic acid. Arch Gen Psychiatry 1998; 55: 188–189.

Richardson AJ. Dyslexia, handedness and syndromes of psychosis-proneness. Int J Psychophysiol 1994; 18: 251–263.

Richardson AJ. Dyslexia and schizotypy. In: Claridge GS, ed. Schizotypy: implications for illness and health. Oxford: Oxford University Press, 1997: 171–201.

Richardson AJ, Gruzelier JH, Puri BK. Reduced visual motion sensitivity in unmedicated schizophrenic patients. Schizophr Res 1996; 18: 217–218.

Richardson AJ, Cox IJ, Sargentoni J, Puri BK. Abnormal cerebral phospholipid metabolism in dyslexia indicated by phosphorus-31 magnetic resonance spectroscopy. NMR Biomed 1997; 10: 309–314.

Richardson AJ, Easton T, Gruzelier JH, Puri BK. Laterality changes accompanying symptom remission in schizophrenia after treatment with eicosapentaenoic acid. Schizophr Res 1999a, in press.

Richardson AJ, Easton T, Corrie AC, Clisby C, Stordy BJ. Is developmental dyslexia a fatty acid deficiency syndrome? Proc Nutr Soc 1999b, in press.

Rieder RO, Nichols PL. The offspring of schizophrenics. 3. Hyperactivity and neurological soft signs. Arch Gen Psychiatry 1979; 36: 665–674.

Stevens LJ, Zentall SZ, Deck JL, Abate ML, Lipp SR, Burgess JR. Essential fatty acid metabolism in boys with attention-deficit hyperactivity disorder. Am J Clin Nutr 1995; 62: 761–768.

Stordy BJ. Benefit of docosahexaenoic acid supplements to dark adaptation in dyslexics. Lancet 1995; 346: 385.

Venables PH. Cerebral mechanisms, autonomic responsiveness, and attention in schizophrenia. In: Spaulding WD, Cole JK, eds. Nebraska symposium on motivation. Lincoln: University of Nebraska Press, 1984: 47–92.

Wiederholt JL, Bryant BR. The Gray Oral Reading Tests, 3rd edn (GORT). Austin, Texas: Pro-Ed, 1992.

New Strategies for the Treatment of Schizophrenia: ω-3 Polyunsaturated Fatty Acids

Malcolm Peet

STRATEGIES FOR THE DEVELOPMENT OF NEW ANTIPSYCHOTIC DRUGS

The first antipsychotic drug to be discovered was chlorpromazine. This was developed from compounds with antihistaminic and sedative properties. It was originally used as part of a pre-anaesthetic cocktail and was found to induce a state of mind which was dubbed 'lobotomie pharmacologique' (Shepherd et al., 1968). This term was used because the condition of the patients after being given large doses of chlorpromazine resembled that seen in patients treated by frontal lobotomy, which was, at that time, a popular treatment for schizophrenia. Chlorpromazine was then tried in schizophrenia and was found to reduce the intensity of psychotic symptoms and behavioural disturbances.

Numerous controlled trials have since confirmed the therapeutic efficacy of chlorpromazine in schizophrenia, and many drugs with a similar pharmacology have been developed. It was recognized that these drugs share the common pharmacological property of blocking dopamine D_2 receptors. Indeed, a significant correlation was demonstrated between the clinical dosage of antipsychotic drugs and their potency in displacing labelled spiperone from striatal dopamine D_2 receptors (Seeman et al., 1976). This concept is probably flawed because clinical dosage is as much a reflection of adverse effect threshold as it is of efficacy. Nevertheless, as a result of this pharmacology the dopamine hypothesis of schizophrenia was born.

In its simplest form, the dopamine hypothesis states that schizophrenia is the result of dopaminergic hyperactivity. Early studies measuring dopamine receptors in the brains of schizophrenic patients appeared to support this hypothesis by showing increased D_2 receptor density in post-mortem brain tissue taken from schizophrenic patients (Owen et al., 1978). However, it is now recognized that this increased receptor density was due to previous antipsychotic drug treatment. Modern studies using receptor labels *in vivo*, carried out on unmedicated schizophrenic patients, have failed to show any consistent abnormality of dopamine D_2 receptors (Farde, 1997).

More recently, with the recognition that D_2 blockade was associated as much with adverse effects as with benefits, agents acting on other receptors have been sought. Such work was greatly stimulated by the clinical efficacy of clozapine which has very low affinity for the dopamine D_2 receptor. Other agents have been developed which are much less potent D_2 receptor blockers, but which are thought to act at other receptor sites such as the sites for 5-hydroxytryptamine (5-HT). These drugs, such as olanzapine and quetiapine, are commonly referred to as 'atypical' antipsychotic drugs (Reynolds, 1997). The precise meaning of this term is unclear, some taking it to mean that the drugs act through effects on other than D_2 receptors, others that these drugs cause fewer and less marked extrapyramidal effects, whilst still others take the cynical view that any new drug introduced in the present climate is dubbed atypical by the manufacturers.

All of this research has in common a focus on receptor modulation as the basis for treating schizophrenia. Until recently, little attention has been paid to cell membrane pathology in this context. It is well recognized that the composition of phospholipid in cell membranes alters many membrane functions, including those related to neurotransmitter receptors and second messengers. For example, there is experimental evidence that the n-6:n-3 balance modulates dopaminergic function in cat caudate slices (Davidson et al., 1988), and that dietary deficiency of α-linolenic acid, the ω-3 precursor, alters dopamine metabolism (Zimmer et al., 1998) as well as serotonin 5-HT$_2$ and dopamine D_2 receptor function (Delion et al., 1996) in rat frontal cortex. Receptor modulation by polyunsaturated fatty acids (PUFAs) has, for these and other reasons, clear relevance to potential new treatments for schizophrenia.

THE MEMBRANE HYPOTHESIS OF SCHIZOPHRENIA AS THE BASIS FOR DEVELOPING NEW TREATMENT STRATEGIES

The membrane hypothesis of schizophrenia is detailed elsewhere in this book. Essentially, it is proposed that abnormalities of cell membrane phospholipid metabolism are of aetiological importance in schizophrenia. Three abnormalities related to that hypothesis hold potential for new treatment strategies.

Low membrane PUFA levels

Several studies have reported reduced levels of PUFAs in phospholipid extracted from cell membranes of red blood cells (RBCs) and platelets from schizophrenic patients. Particularly low levels of docosahexaenoic acid (DHA) and arachidonic acid (AA) have been consistently found, and most authors also report reductions of linoleic acid and eicosapentaenoic acid (EPA) (Glen et al., 1994; Peet et al., 1995). These studies were mostly conducted in patients treated with antipsychotic medication, though no correlation was found between PUFA depletion and antipsychotic drug dosage. Nevertheless, there is one study suggesting that thrombocyte membrane PUFA depletion in phenothiazine-treated patients may be dose related, so that a drug effect cannot be ruled out (Fischer et al., 1992). Despite this reservation, treatment of schizophrenia by PUFA supplementation has a good theoretical base, particularly when considered in conjunction with evidence of receptor modulation by membrane PUFA composition.

Raised levels of phospholipase A_2

Another finding relating to phospholipid metabolism is the elevation of levels of phospholipase A_2 (PLA_2), an enzyme responsible for releasing PUFAs from phospholipids. The enzyme exists in several forms, and elevation of calcium-independent PLA_2 has been demonstrated in serum from schizophrenic patients (Gattaz et al., 1990; Ross et al., 1997). Strategies aimed at inhibiting PLA_2 can therefore be considered in the treatment of schizophrenia. Many, but not all, currently used antipsychotic drugs have an inhibitory effect on rat brain PLA_2 (Trzeciak et al., 1995). It is also of interest that PUFAs have been shown to inhibit PLA_2 activity differentially. Thus, Finnen and Lovell (1991), using human epidermal cells *in vitro* found that EPA inhibits PLA_2, whereas DHA does not. Strategies aimed at inhibiting calcium-independent PLA_2 may be worth investigation in the treatment of schizophrenia.

Increased oxidative stress

A third biochemical finding relates to an increase in oxidative stress in schizophrenic patients. If this finding is of aetiological importance, then strategies aimed at reinforcing antioxidant defence mechanisms may also be of therapeutic benefit. The free radical scavenger, vitamin E, has been shown to decrease oxidative stress in normal healthy adults (Cadenas et al., 1996) and in those under oxidative stress, such as diabetics (Jain et al., 1996). Vitamin E has been used with success in the treatment of tardive dyskinesia (Adler et al., 1998) but as yet there are no definitive data on its usefulness in the treatment of core schizophrenic symptoms.

DIETARY PUFAs AND SCHIZOPHRENIA

Whilst the membrane hypothesis of schizophrenia suggests at least three novel approaches to the treatment of schizophrenia, our group has focused on the use of PUFAs. There are two studies suggesting that the content of PUFAs, and in particular ω-3 PUFA, in the diet affects the outcome and severity of schizophrenia.

The World Health Organization (1979) studied the outcome of schizophrenia and found that long-term outcome was better in so-called underdeveloped countries than in western developed countries. This finding has been difficult to explain, particularly as modern treatments which should improve outcome are less available in underdeveloped countries. Christensen and Christensen (1988) investigated national diet in relation to the WHO figures for schizophrenia outcome. Dietary fat intake was expressed as the ratio between fat derived from land animals and birds (mostly saturated) to fat obtained from fish and plant sources (mostly unsaturated). They found a highly significant correlation between dietary fat ratios and schizophrenia outcome. It was noted that 97% of the variance in schizophrenia outcome could be explained by the combined variation in the percentages of fat from land animals and birds and from vegetables, fish and seafood, respectively, such that relatively less saturated fat and more PUFAs in the diet were associated with better outcome. This is by far the strongest explanation so far produced for the international variation in schizophrenia outcome.

Our group has investigated the severity of schizophrenic symptoms in relation to dietary intake of PUFA. The diet of 20 schizophrenic patients was investigated using the 7-day weighed intake method, and the patients' dietary intake of PUFAs was assessed using the FOODBASE programme. This gave us the opportunity to assess the importance of specific PUFAs in the diet. It was found that a greater dietary intake of ω-3

PUFAs, and particularly EPA, in the normal diet was associated with less severe schizophrenic symptoms, and particularly with less positive symptoms, as well as less tardive dyskinesia (Mellor et al., 1996).

Thus, both international outcome studies and between-patient studies have provided evidence that dietary PUFAs, and particularly ω-3 PUFAs, are related to schizophrenic pathology. The obvious next step is to investigate the possible therapeutic benefits of PUFA supplementation.

CLINICAL TRIALS OF PUFA SUPPLEMENTATION IN THE TREATMENT OF SCHIZOPHRENIA

A small number of previous studies have attempted to treat schizophrenia by PUFA supplementation. Vaddadi et al. (1986) treated 21 inpatients resistant to neuroleptics with either depot neuroleptic medication plus dihomo-γ-linolenic acid (DGLA), placebo depot medication plus DGLA, or a double placebo. There were no significant treatment effects on behaviour or schizophrenic symptomatology. In a subsequent study, Vaddadi et al. (1989) gave evening primrose oil to patients with movement disorders who were predominantly schizophrenic and who had long-term exposure to neuroleptic medication. There was a significant treatment effect on schizophrenic symptoms but no clinically important effect on tardive dyskinesia (TD). Wolkin et al. (1986) found that evening primrose oil did not benefit either schizophrenic symptoms or TD, but the study included only a small number of patients.

One previous open study has used ω-3 supplementation in the form of linseed oil (50% α-linolenic acid) which was given to five patients, with apparent benefit (Rudin, 1981).

We have conducted a series of studies using preparations with a high EPA content in the treatment of schizophrenia. In the first of these studies (Mellor et al., 1996) 20 schizophrenic patients who were still symptomatic despite their current antipsychotic drug treatment, were treated with 10 g daily of MaxEPA fish oil (Seven Seas Health Care Limited, Hull) each day for 6 weeks. Each capsule contained 171 mg of EPA and 114 mg of DHA. This treatment led to significant improvement of scores on rating scales for both schizophrenic symptomatology and TD. The total score on the Positive and Negative Syndrome Scale (PANSS) (Kay et al., 1987) fell from 78.9 ± 17.7 to 65.6 ± 9.0 ($p < 0.005$). The severity of TD as measured by the Abnormal Involuntary Movement Scale (AIMS) (Kane et al., 1992) fell from 20.2 ± 7.1 to 12.3 ± 5.3 ($p < 0.001$). RBC membrane levels of PUFAs were measured in patients from this study, and subsequent multiple regression analysis showed that changes in RBC membrane total ω-3 PUFAs were strongly associated with changes in total PANSS scores.

In a second open study, carried out in India, Shah et al. (1998) treated 10 schizophrenic patients for 3 months with EPA-enriched oil (Kirunal™, Laxdale Ltd, Stirling, Scotland). Again, all patients were symptomatic despite antipsychotic drug treatment which was continued throughout the study. Once more there was substantial improvement in the total PANSS scores, which fell from 75.3 ± 11.7 to 46.5 ± 12.3 ($p < 0.01$).

We were interested in defining more precisely the particular effects of different ω-3 PUFAs. We therefore carried out a double-blind trial comparing an EPA-enriched oil (Kirunal™, Laxdale Ltd, Stirling, Scotland), a DHA-enriched oil, and a corn oil placebo, for 3 months, given to a group of schizophrenic patients who were symptomatic despite their antipsychotic medication (which remained unchanged throughout the study). The patients were rated at the beginning and the end of treatment using the PANSS. A total of 45 patients completed the study. The greatest improvement in total PANSS, positive symptoms and general psychopathology was seen in the EPA group, there being no difference between the three treatment groups in the improvement in negative symptoms. The effect on positive symptoms reached statistical significance ($F = 3.34$; $p < 0.05$). The greatest difference was between the effect of EPA ($23.8 \pm 3.9\%$ improvement) and DHA ($3.3 \pm 6.8\%$ improvement), which was statistically significant ($t = 2.58$; $p < 0.05$).

These two open studies and the small double-blind trial, taken together with the epidemiological evidence, provide strong support for a therapeutic effect of EPA in the treatment of schizophrenia. Further large-scale controlled trials are now in progress, using EPA both as an addition to antipsychotic medication and also as the sole agent. Support for the use of EPA as a sole agent has come from a recent case report of a patient who showed a marked and sustained response to this treatment over a 1-year period (Puri and Richardson, 1998).

POSSIBLE MODEL OF ACTION OF EPA

The clear differential effect between EPA and DHA in the double-blind trial was unexpected. There is very little EPA in neuronal membranes, whereas there is a very large quantity of DHA. Furthermore, there is evidence that incorporation of DHA into cell membranes, at least in fibroblasts, has a substantially greater effect than EPA on membrane biophysical characteristics and function (Brown and Subbaiah, 1994). It is therefore possible that the EPA was having its effect through some mechanism other than direct incorporation into the cell membrane. One possibility is that EPA was acting through inhibition of PLA_2. There is evidence that, in some systems, EPA, but not DHA, is capable of inhibiting this enzyme (Finnen and Lovell, 1991).

CONCLUSION

The membrane hypothesis of schizophrenia has given rise to potential new treatment strategies for schizophrenia. We have explored one of these, using ω-3 PUFA supplementation, with encouraging preliminary results. Further clinical studies based on the hypothesis may give rise to novel treatment approaches which have moved away from current receptor-based treatments.

REFERENCES

Adler LA, Edson R, Lavori P et al. Long-term treatment effects of vitamin E for tardive dyskinesia. Biol Psychiatry 1998; 43: 868–872.

Brown ER, Subbaiah PV. Differential effects of eicosapentaenoic acid and docosahexaenoic acid on human skin fibroblasts. Lipids 1994; 29: 825–829.

Cadenas S, Rojas C, Mandez J, Herrero A, Barja G. Vitamin E decreases urine lipid peroxidation products in young healthy human volunteers under normal conditions. Pharmacol Toxicol 1996; 79: 247–253.

Christensen O, Christensen E. Fat consumption and schizophrenia. Acta Psychiatr Scand 1988; 78: 587–591.

Davidson BC, Kurstjens NP, Patton J, Cantrill RC. Essential fatty acids modulate apomorphine activity at dopamine receptors in rat caudate slices. Eur J Pharmacol 1988; 149: 317–322.

Delion S, Chalon S, Guilloteau D, Besnard JC, Durand G. Alpha-linolenic acid dietary deficiency alters age-related changes of dopaminergic and serotoninergic neurotransmission in the rat frontal cortex. J Neurochem 1996; 66: 1582–1591.

Farde L. Brain imaging of schizophrenia – the dopamine hypothesis. Schizophr Res 1997; 28: 157–162.

Finnen MJ, Lovell CR. Purification and characterisation of phosphokinase A_2 from human epidermis. Biochem Soc Trans 1991; 19: 91.

Fischer S, Kissling W, Kuss H-J. Schizophrenic patients treated with high-dose phenothiazine or thioxanthine become deficient in polyunsaturated fatty acids in their thrombocytes. Biochem Pharmacol 1992; 44: 317–323.

Gattaz WF, Hübner CK, Nevalainen TJ, Thuren T, Kinnunen PKJ. Increased serum phospholipase A_2 activity in schizophrenia: a replication study. Biol Psychiatry 1990; 28: 495–501.

Glen AIM, Glen EMT, Horrobin DF et al. A red cell membrane abnormality in a subgroup of schizophrenic patients: evidence for two diseases. Schizophr Res 1994; 12: 53–61.

Jain SK, McVie R, Jaramillo JJ et al. The effect of modest vitamin E supplementation on lipid peroxidation products and other cardiovascular risk factors in diabetic patients. Lipids 1996; 31 (Suppl): 587–590.

Kane JM, Jeste DV, Barnes TE et al. Tardive dyskinesia: a task force report of the American Psychiatric Association. Washington DC: APA, 1992, 265–268.

Kay SR, Fiszbein A, Opier LA. The positive and negative syndrome scale (PANNS) for schizophrenia. Schizophr Bull 1987; 13: 261–276.

Mellor JE, Laugharne JDE, Peet M. Omega-3 fatty acid supplementation in schizophrenia patients. Hum Psychopharmacol 1996; 11: 39–46.

Owen F, Cross AJ, Crow TJ, Longden A, Poulter M, Riley GT. Increased dopamine receptor sensitivity in schizophrenia. Lancet 1978; ii: 223–226.

Peet M, Laugharne JDE, Rangarajan N, Horrobin DF, Reynolds G. Depleted red cell membrane essential fatty acids in drug treated schizophrenic patients. J Psychiatr Res 1995; 29: 227–232.

Puri BK, Richardson AJ. Sustained remission of positive and negative symptoms of schizophrenia following treatment with eicosapentaenoic acid. Arch Gen Psychiatry 1998; 55: 188–189.

Reynolds GP. What is an atypical antipsychotic? J Psychopharmacol 1997; 11: 195–199.

Ross BM, Hudson C, Erlich J, Warsh JJ, Kish SJ. Increased phospholipid breakdown in schizophrenia: evidence for the involvement of a calcium-independent phospholipase A_2. Arch Gen Psychiatry 1997; 54: 487–494.

Rudin DO. The major psychoses and neuroses as omega-3 essential fatty acid deficiency syndrome: substrate pellagra. Biol Psychiatry 1981; 16: 837–850.

Seeman P, Lee T, Chau-Wong M, Wong K. Antipsychotic drug doses and neuroleptic/dopamine receptors. Nature 1976; 261: 717–719.

Shah S, Vankar GK, Telang SD, Ramchand CN, Peet M. Eicosapentaenoic acid (EPA) as an adjunct in the treatment of schizophrenia. Schizophr Res 1998; 29: 158.

Shepherd M, Lader M, Rodright R. Clinical psychopharmacology. London: English Universities Press, 1968: 87.

Trzeciak HI, Kalacinski W, Malecki A, Kokot D. Effect of neuroleptics on phospholipase A_2 activity in the brain of rats. Eur Arch Psychiatry Clin Neurosci 1995; 245: 179–182.

Vaddadi KS, Gilleard CJ, Mindham RHS, Butler RA. A controlled trial of prostaglandin E_1 precursor in chronic neuroleptic-resistant schizophrenic patients. Psychopharmacology 1986; 88: 362–367.

Vaddadi KS, Courtney P, Gilleard CJ, Manku MS, Horrobin DF. A double-blind trial of essential fatty acid supplementation in patients with tardive dyskinesia. Psychiatry Res 1989; 27: 313–323.

Wolkin A, Jordan B, Peselow E, Rubenstein M, Petrosen J. Essential fatty acid supplementation in tardive dyskinesia. Am J Psychiatry 1986; 143: 912–914.

World Health Organisation. Schizophrenia: an international follow-up study. New York: John Wiley and Sons, 1979.

Zimmer L, Hembert S, Durang G et al. Chronic n-3 polyunsaturated fatty acid diet-deficiency acts on dopamine metabolism in rat frontal cortex: a microdialysis study. Neurosci Lett 1998: 240: 177–181.

Part VII

DEPRESSION

Long-chain Polyunsaturated Fatty Acids in Depression and Related Conditions

Joseph R. Hibbeln

INTRODUCTION

The proposition that the intake of n-3 long-chain polyunsaturated fatty acids (LCPUFAs), and specifically eicosapentaenoic acid (EPA) and docosahexaenoic acid (DHA), may decrease the prevalence and severity of depressive illness offers a heuristic explanation for epidemiological aspects of major depression and many other biological findings. These inexpensive nutrients are potential biological treatments which are not only virtually free of any adverse effects, but which may also be associated with significant health benefits in a variety of areas: e.g., in reducing the risks of cardiovascular disease, cancer and osteoporosis.

Whilst the way in which n-3 LCPUFAs influences the neurobiology of depressive illness remains a matter of conjecture, five possible mechanisms can be identified which may either work alone or in combination, and which do not exclude other physiological and pharmacological pathways of interaction of n-3 LCPUFAs and central nervous system function. These putative mechanisms are: (1) alterations in the biophysical structure of membranes, and subsequent alterations in membrane-bound signal transduction, affecting multiple transmitter systems; (2) specific modulation of brain 5-hydroxytryptamine (5-HT; serotonin) levels which predict suicide-related and impulsive behaviours; (3) eicosanoid imbalances mediating neuroendocrine functions, including the hypothalamic–pituitary–adrenal (HPA) axis; (4) immune–neuroendocrine interactions; and (5) structural and functional neurological effects resulting from nutritional deprivation in early life.

It has been observed that cholesterol-lowering therapies may increase the risk of violent death from accidents or suicide. There are suggestions that the intake and alterations in tissue levels of n-3 LCPUFAs may have a crucial role in this aspect of behaviour; an understanding of how this could come about involves a comparison of the roles played by LCPUFAs and cholesterol in determining the biophysical properties of membranes.

LCPUFAs, NEUROTRANSMITTER FUNCTION AND DEPRESSION

Neuronal membrane LCPUFAs may be involved in influencing biogenic amine function, and specifically noradrenergic and serotonergic neurotransmission, at several levels: neurotransmitter synthesis, breakdown, synaptic release, presynaptic reuptake, and receptor binding. Evidence that n-3 LCPUFAs have a specific role in neurotransmission comes from a study by Toffano et al. (1976) in which it was found that dopamine, norepinephrine and epinephrine concentrations were increased following administration of phosphatidylserine when this had been obtained from brain cortex, and was therefore rich in 22:6n-3 (Salem et al., 1986; Salem, 1989), but not when it had been prepared from soybean and thus had low 22:6n-3 content. Patients with unipolar depression were found by Sengupta et al. (1981) to have reduced levels of total serum phosphatidylserine.

The n-3:n-6 balance may be important in modulating catecholamine function, particularly as the functions of n-3 LCPUFAs may not be duplicated by those of n-6 LCPUFAs (Salem and Niebylski, 1995). In this context it is interesting to note that tryptophan hydroxylase, which is involved in the rate-limiting step of catecholamine synthesis and has important effects on membrane order (Mandell, 1984), is activated in adrenal medullary cells by 20:4n-6. In rats, a diet low in n-3 and relatively rich in n-6 EFAs leads to reduced brain mitochondrial monoamine oxidase activity (Crane and Greenwood, 1987). Dietary deficiency in n-3 intake has been shown to lead to replacement of n-3 by n-6 LCPUFAs in frontal cortex and striatal brain regions of rats (Salem et al., 1986; Salem, 1989). Diets that have a high relative content of n-6 EFAs (e.g., sunflower oil) have been found to have marked and widespread effects on adrenergic systems (Rulka and Hamm, 1988; Semafuco et al., 1989; Nicolas et al., 1991). Membrane fluidity changes induced by 18-2:n-6 lead to changes in 5-HT binding *in vitro* (Heron et al., 1980). These and other studies indicate that neurotransmitter function that is directly linked to depressive symptoms can be modulated by neuronal membrane changes that are, in their turn, affected by the balance of n-3:n-6 LCPUFAs.

LCPUFAs AND 5-HT MODULATION

Cholesterol-lowering therapies and risk of violent death

In the early 1990s, a number of reports began to appear which implicated dietary essential fatty acids (EFAs), and specifically LCPUFAs, in a variety of behavioural and cognitive disturbances.

Muldoon et al. (1990) noted an increased mortality from suicide and homicide in individuals who, in order to decrease the risk of coronary artery disease (CAD), had been receiving treatment aimed at lowering their serum cholesterol levels. The reduced death rate from CAD was reported to be fully cancelled out by the increased mortality arising from self-inflicted injury or other forms of violence or accident.

This finding of an apparent relationship between cholesterol lowering and increased aggressiveness linked to depression, was in accord with the results of other studies in humans (Endelberg, 1992; Morgan et al., 1993) and in monkeys (Kaplan et al., 1991). Other investigators (Fowkes et al., 1992; Jacobs et al., 1992; Brown et al., 1994), however, failed to establish such a relationship, whilst still others (Pekkanen et al., 1989; Weidner et al., 1992; Irribaren et al., 1995) came to the opposite conclusion.

The resolution of these apparently contradictory findings came when it was noted that changes in hostility/depression were not, in fact, directly related to variations in serum cholesterol levels but to changes in the intake of n-3 LCPUFAs. In those studies in which the subjects' diets had been rich in fish, and hence in n-3 LCPUFAs (Connor and Connor, 1977), there were reductions in hostility, depression and suicide. This was clearly demonstrated by Weidner et al. (1992) in a 5-year prospective study. The relationship determined by Irribaren et al. (1995) between low rates of cholesterol intake and low rates of suicide may have been due to the fact that they studied an Hawaiian population in which there was a high consumption of fish. Whilst Pekkanen et al. (1989) found an association between serum cholesterol and reduced violence-related mortality in a population in a coastal region of Finland, where fish was a common dietary constituent, they failed to show the same relationship in the population of an inland region where fish was less frequently consumed.

The finding by Fowkes et al. (1992) of a relationship between measures of hostility and serum triglyceride levels, becomes understandable when it is known that n-3 LCPUFAs lead to reductions in serum triglycerides, according to an analysis carried out by Harris (1996) of the results from 72 placebo-controlled studies.

That cholesterol levels are only indirectly related to mood and hostility is well demonstrated by the argument that since reduced cholesterol appears to be linked to both increased hostility/depression (Muldoon et al., 1990) and lowered risk of CAD (Booth-Kewley and Friedman, 1987), it should follow that individuals with low risk of CAD would have a tendency to aggression or depression, whereas the opposite appears actually to be the case (Seigman and Smith, 1994). Hibbeln and Salem (1995) proposed that this apparent contradiction could be resolved if such behavioural and mood changes were related not to cholesterol, but to levels of DHA, an n-3 LCPUFA which is found in high concentrations in neuronal membranes where it appears to be critically important in neuronal functioning (Salem et al., 1986). The rationale behind this will be presented later in this chapter.

Direct support for the importance of n-3 LCPUFA levels in depression, is provided by the finding of significant linear correlations between the ratio of arachidonic acid (AA; an n-6 LCPUFA) and EPA (an n-3 LCPUFA), and two ratings of depressed mood (Adams et al., 1996). Similar findings have been reported by Edwards et al. (1996), Maes et al. (1996) and Edwards et al. (1998). In 6–10-year-old boys with attention deficit/hyperactivity disorder (ADHD), plasma 22:6n-3 levels were predictive of the degree of behavioural disturbance (Stevens et al., 1995). Virkkunen et al. (1987) showed that a plasma deficiency of n-3 LCPUFAs was characteristic of violent, impulsive offenders, and more recently Stevens et al. (1995) also reported that low n-3 LCPUFAs were predictive of impulsive behaviour. Hamazaki et al. (1996), in a double-blind, placebo-controlled trial, were able to prevent increases in induced aggression by supplementing the subjects' diet with 22:6n-3. The severity of depressed mood was found by Adams et al. (1996), Maes et al. (1996) and Peet et al. (1998) to be linked to low concentrations of n-3 LCPUFAs.

It seems reasonable, on the basis of such information, to assume that n-3 LCPUFAs are likely to be implicated in the expression of a range of behavioural and cognitive disturbances (including hostility, impulsiveness, aggression, suicidal ideation and acts, hyperactivity, attention deficits, and alcoholism) that are known to be associated with mood disorders. The question remains, however, as to the nature of the mechanism underlying this connection. Hibbeln et al. (1997) proposed that the answer to this almost certainly lies in the relationship between LCPUFAs and certain neurotransmitters, specifically 5-HT.

5-Hydroxyindoleacetic acid and behaviour

Concentrations of 5-hydroxyindoleacetic acid (5-HIAA) in cerebrospinal fluid (CSF) provide an index of 5-HT turnover in the frontal cortex (Stanley et al., 1985). The variety of behavioural disturbances noted above as being associated with mood disorder have all been linked to low CSF 5-HIAA levels and thus to low serotonergic activity in the brain.

Linnoila et al. (1983), for example, reported that individuals showing aggressive behaviour characterized by impulsivity – a combination which may be critically implicated in unprovoked aggression and suicide – are differentiated from those whose aggressivity is of a nonimpulsive nature, by having low CSF levels of 5-HIAA. This received support from a study by Roy et al. (1987, 1988) who reported that hostility in healthy males was predicted by low CSF 5-HIAA concentrations; the same group, in a later study (Roy et al., 1991), found increased risk of attempted and successful suicide in individuals with low CSF 5-HIAA. Other studies came to the same conclusion: low CSF 5-HIAA levels have been shown to be associated with impulsive and unprovoked violent behaviour in patients with affective disorders (Coccaro et al., 1989), impulsive behaviour in alcoholics (Virkkunen et al., 1994a; Fils-Aime et al., 1996), aggressive behaviour in patients with diagnoses of personality disorder (Brown et al., 1979), suicidal depression (Gibbons and Davis, 1986), and impaired impulse control (Mann, 1995). Animal studies are in accord with these findings: Higley et al. (1996) noted that low CSF 5-HIAA levels were predictive of aggressive behaviour and impaired social functioning amongst nonhuman primates.

The association between depression and markedly reduced serotonergic activity is certainly well established (for a review, see Meltzer and Lowey, 1987), and this has, indeed, been the stimulus for the development of the selective serotonin reuptake inhibiting (SSRI) and a number of other antidepressant drugs.

Relationship between LCPUFAs and serotonergic activity

Dietary intake of LCPUFAs

Evidence for the putative causal relationship between low dietary intake of LCPUFAs and correspondingly reduced serotonergic activity comes from a number of sources. Nizzo et al. (1978), for example, showed that CSF 5-HIAA levels were increased following an intravenous infusion of phospholipids rich in DHA. DeLion et al. (1994), using rats as experimental subjects, found an increase in 5-HT$_2$ receptor density, typical of reduced serotonergic transmission (Roy et al., 1991), as a result of n-3 LCPUFA deficiency induced during the animals' gestation and early development; binding affinity remained unchanged. Exactly the same changes had been reported some years earlier in a study of the frontal cortices of suicide victims (Stanley et al., 1983).

Muldoon et al. (1990) and Endelberg (1992) suggested that lowered serotonergic activity in patients with high risk of suicide was related to a reduction in dietary intake of cholesterol and hence of serum cholesterol levels, support for such a relationship being provided by subsequent work on Rhesus monkeys (Kaplan et al., 1994) in which reduced serum cholesterol levels, brought about by a cholesterol-low diet, were related to an increase in violent behaviour and low CSF levels of 5-HIAA. However, similar effects to those reported by Kaplan et al. (1994), i.e., low CSF 5-HIAA levels associated with aggression, had been reported earlier by the same group of workers (Kaplan et al., 1991), also in monkeys but using diets differing in fat composition and not only in cholesterol. Noting this, Hibbeln et al. (1997) examined plasma concentrations of both total cholesterol and EFAs in human subjects to determine which might predict CSF 5-HIAA concentrations.

Plasma LCPUFA levels

The study reported by Hibbeln et al. (1997) involved 45 healthy volunteers who were not given any special diet to change EFA or cholesterol intake. CSF levels of 5-HIAA, and also of the dopamine metabolite, homovanillic acid (HVA), were obtained and correlated with plasma total cholesterol, total fatty acids, various LCPUFAs (18:2n-6, 20:4n-6, 22:5n-6, 18:3n-3, 20:5n-3, and 22:6n-3), and total LCPUFAs (the sum of the 20 and 22 carbon fatty acids). There were statistically significant correlations between total LCPUFAs and the CSF levels of both 5-HIAA ($r = +0.41$; $p < 0.005$) and HVA ($r = +0.47$; $p < 0.001$); no relationships were noted between indices of serotonergic function and plasma cholesterol levels. This latter finding was in accord with conclusions reached in a variety of investigations conducted by other workers (e.g., Modai et al., 1995; Ansseau, 1996; Zale et al., 1996).

This work has subsequently been followed up by Hibbeln et al. (1998a) in a study involving a comparison between healthy volunteers, late-onset alcoholics, and early-onset alcoholics. There was no statistically significant correlation in any group between total plasma cholesterol level and CSF 5-HIAA or HVA concentrations. Plasma DHA level, however, predicted CSF 5-HIAA and concentrations in all three subject groups. The correlations with 5-HIAA were: for healthy volunteeers, $r = +0.32$ ($p < 0.05$); for late-onset alcoholics, $r = +0.08$ (nonsignificant); and for early-onset alcoholics, $r = -0.33$; ($p < 0.05$). With HVA, the correlations were: for healthy volunteeers, $r = +0.31$; for late-onset alcoholics, $r = +0.32$; and for early-onset alcoholics, $r = -0.31$; all correlation coefficients were statistically significant at $p < 0.05$. When the correlation coefficients were compared, it was found that, for both 5-HIAA and HVA, the values differed significantly between healthy volunteers and early-onset alcoholics, but not between the healthy volunteers and late-onset alcoholics. The importance of this distinction lies in the fact that early onset of alcoholism has been reported to be distinguished from alcoholism of late onset, by being associated with a variety of social difficulties, problems related to aggression and impulse control, and suicide attempts (Buydens-Branchey et al., 1989; Irwin et al., 1990; Virkkunen et al., 1994a,b; Sigvardsson et al., 1996). CSF 5-HIAA and HVA levels were best predicted by plasma concentrations of the n-3 LCPUFA, DHA.

The finding of a negative correlation between CSF concentrations of transmitter metabolites and plasma levels of LCPUFAs, particularly DHA, in early-onset alcoholics, suggests that dietary supplementary of n-3 LCPUFAs to this kind of patient would exacerbate the problems of violence and impulse control associated with alcohol intake; alternatively, these results may indicate that impulsive individuals have a defect in brain uptake or concentration of DHA, and may need a greater than normal dietary supply. It was therefore important to see whether or not this finding could be replicated. Hibbeln et al. (1998b) thus undertook a further study in which a comparison was made between violent and nonviolent subjects, the two groups each containing both healthy subjects and patients with a history of alcoholism and ongoing problems in this regard. The groups did not differ in terms of age, alcohol consumption or alcohol-related liver damage, all factors which could have acted as confounding variables in the earlier study (Hibbeln et al., 1998a). It was reported that the negative correlation between CSF 5-HIAA and plasma DHA was replicated in the violent subjects, a correlation coefficient of $r = -0.46$ ($p < 0.05$) being obtained and being of the same general magnitude as that obtained in the earlier study in early-onset alcoholics. There was no corresponding correlation between CSF 5-HIAA and plasma DHA in the nonviolent group. CSF HVA levels were not correlated with any LCPUFA measure in either violent or nonviolent subjects.

The work of Hibbeln et al. (1998a,b) indicates that the negative correlation between plasma DHA and CSF 5-HIAA is related to the tendency of the subjects to violent, impulsive behaviour and not to alcohol intake *per se*.

LCPUFAs AND CHOLESTEROL: ROLES IN DETERMINING BRAIN FUNCTION AND BEHAVIOUR

One salient observation in neurobiological studies of depression is that no one single transmitter or neuroendocrine function is likely to be exclusively responsible for the pathophysiology of the illness. A common link may be that alterations in the LCPUFA composition of the neuronal membrane, and subsequent disturbances in the biophysical environment, result in the kind of disturbances in the activity of multiple membrane-bound receptors, metabolic enzymes, and signal transduction systems, which have been described in depressed subjects.

In view of the observations, noted earlier in this chapter, that treatments aimed at lowering serum cholesterol levels appear to be associated with a variety of behavioural disturbances linked to serotonergic mechanisms, the question arises as to the relative importance of the roles played by cholesterol and LCPUFAs in determining this chain of events. Muldoon et al. (1990) and Endelberg (1992) argued that lowering dietary or plasma cholesterol could reduce the brain concentrations of 5-HT by altering membrane characteristics such as fluidity, receptor conformation and binding kinetics, and/or the activity of membrane-bound enzymes. When this hypothesis is examined closely, however, it seems less plausible than the alternative view that LCPUFAs are primarily responsible for the membrane effects underlying the behavioural effects brought about by changes in dietary and tissue cholesterol levels. The arguments for this view can be briefly summarized.

Dietary determinants of plasma cholesterol

Under normal human dietary conditions, altering cholesterol intake has only a marginal effect on plasma cholesterol concentrations. Changes in the intake of saturated, monounsaturated and polyunsaturated fatty acids, on the other hand, have a much greater effect on plasma cholesterol concentrations, according to large epidemiological studies in human populations (Keys et al., 1965).

Relationships between plasma and brain cholesterol levels

The concentrations of cholesterol in the brain are largely unrelated to those in the plasma. A few early studies in the 1950s and 1960s suggested that cholesterol might be able to cross the blood–brain barrier (e.g., Dobbing, 1963), but later, well-controlled studies demonstrated that these results were probably artifactual (Pardridge and Mietus, 1980). Cholesterol could not be detected crossing into the brain, despite controlling for preparation artifacts and equilibration with endogenous serum preparations (Pardridge and Mietus, 1980). Edmond et al. (1991) found that the consumption of artificial milk which contained either extremely high, low, or normal concentrations of cholesterol, led to profound alterations in plasma and lung cholesterol concentrations, but brain concentrations of cholesterol and sterols remained unaltered. It has also been shown that, during development, when the accumulation of cholesterol in the brain is occurring most rapidly, the full cholesterol requirement can be synthesized *in situ* (Jones et al., 1975a,b; Edmond et al., 1991). Thus, alterations in dietary intake of cholesterol or in plasma cholesterol concentrations are not likely to influence biophysical properties of neuronal membranes as predicted by Muldoon et al. (1990) and Endelberg (1992).

While the brain is capable of satisfying all its cholesterol requirements endogenously, it is entirely dependent upon exogenous dietary or maternal sources for polyunsaturated EFAs (Salem, 1989), and selectively concentrates DHA into synaptic neuronal membranes (Connor et al., 1990). Dietary deficiencies in n-3 EFAs during development result in deficiencies of DHA in brain tissues (Salem et al., 1986; Salem, 1989).

LCPUFA modulation of cholesterol effects on membranes

Although cholesterol is important in determining membrane order parameters (Mitchell and Litman, 1998), polyunsaturate composition is a powerful modulator of cholesterol-induced changes in membrane order. Cholesterol-induced condensation, measured by increasing order in hydrocarbon chains, is reduced in the presence of polyunsaturates, with greater unsaturation of surrounding acyl chains. Membranes containing the highly unsaturated fatty acid DHA, showed the lowest degree of cholesterol-induced condensation (J.A. Barry and K. Gawrisch, personal communication). Heron et al. (1980) demonstrated *in vitro* that linoleic acid, a polyunsaturated EFA with two double bonds, reduced membrane viscosity and decreased the number of high-affinity sites on 5-HT receptors.

The receptor rhodopsin and the 5-HT receptor are both members of the superfamily of G protein-coupled receptors, sharing both structural and functional similarities. Mitchel et al. (1992) demonstrated that the membrane phospholipid acyl chain composition was the primary determinant of the relationship between bulk membrane packing properties and the formation of metarhodopsin II (meta II), the active form of the receptor; cholesterol was found to have a secondary, modulating effect. In addition, highly unsaturated phospholipids, such as those containing di-docosahexaenoate, promoted the formation of meta II and markedly diminished cholesterol-induced inhibition of meta II formation. Highly unsaturated fatty acids, especially DHA, contribute unique biophysical properties to neuronal membranes, such as lateral domain formation (Litman et al., 1991; Litman and Mitchell, 1996); their effects cannot be reproduced by cholesterol, or by monounsaturated or diunsaturated fatty acids (Niebylski and Salem, 1994; Salem and Niebylski, 1995).

Species differences in cholesterol effects on brain 5-HT

Animal studies have produced conflicting results regarding the effects of dietary changes in cholesterol intake on brain 5-HT concentrations. When cholesterol intake was lowered as an isolated dietary variable, Rhesus monkeys exhibited an increase in violent behaviour, accompanied by a significant reduction in levels of CSF 5-HIAA and serum cholesterol (Kaplan et al., 1994). In gerbils, however, no relationships were found between in brain concentrations of tryptophan, 5-HT, or 5-HIAA, and levels of circulating cholesterol (Fernstrom et al., 1996). As noted earlier in this chapter, rats maintained on a diet deficient in n-3 LCPUFAs, which led to reduced brain concentrations of DHA, showed a 44% increase in 5-HT$_2$ receptor number in the frontal cortex (DeLion et al., 1994), a finding strikingly similar to the 44% increase in the 5-HT$_2$ receptor number in the frontal cortices of suicide victims (Stanley et al., 1983).

Relationships between cholesterol and LCPUFAs

Hibbeln and Salem (1995) suggested that plasma total cholesterol might be a surrogate marker for changes in LCPUFA intake or metabolism, which could have a primary role in influencing central 5-HT turnover rate. Consistent with this interpretation are the subsequent findings by Hibbeln et al. (1997) that CSF 5-HIAA appears to be robustly related to total LCPUFAs in plasma, despite corrections for age and measures of alcohol intake, and that total LCPUFAs also predicted CSF concentrations of HVA. It is, however, necessary to bear in mind that a causal relationship has not yet been demonstrated linking central serotonergic function and dietary or plasma lipids, including total cholesterol or highly unsaturated EFAs. Although plasma total cholesterol concentrations did not predict CSF 5-HIAA concentrations in the study of Hibbeln et al. (1997), such a relationship might be found in other, more impulsive, populations, such as subjects with a history of serious suicide attempts. Prospective studies are required in order to determine the relationship between the consumption of highly unsaturated EFAs, cholesterol metabolism, and violent and suicidal behaviour or central 5-HT turnover rate.

LCPUFAs AND THE IMMUNE–NEUROENDOCRINE SYSTEM IN DEPRESSION

Smith (1991) put forward the hypothesis that a low dietary intake of n-3 LCPUFAs might enhance interleukin 1b (IL-1b) secretion which would, in its turn, promote the release of corticotrophin releasing factor (CRF) and thus lead to hyperactivation of the HPA axis. The results of recent studies, reviewed below, lend substantial support to this view.

Increased release of interleukin 1b

It is suggested that, in humans, an increased ratio of the n-6 LCPUFA AA to the n-3 compounds DHA and EPA, leads to increased release of IL-1b. The tissue concentrations of both n-6 and n-3 LCPUFAs, the precursors of leukotrienes, prostaglandins and other eicosanoids which regulate immune function, are dependent upon dietary sources. Ingesting moderate amounts of fish-derived n-3 LCPUFAs markedly reduced IL-1b production, and within 6 months of EPA and DHA supplementation there was a marked reduction in unstimulated levels of IL-1b, prostaglandin E$_2$, and leukotriene B4, in patients with multiple sclerosis and normal controls (Gallai et al., 1995). In normal subjects, stimulated IL-1b production was significantly reduced by 40% ($p < 0.005$) by adding EPA and DHA to National Cholesterol Education Panel step-2 diets (Meydani et al., 1993), and IL-1b production was suppressed by 43% ($p < 0.05$) by daily supplementation with fish oil concentrate (Endres et al., 1989). In patients with rheumatoid arthritis (Kremer et al., 1990; Epersen et al., 1992), IL-1b production was reduced by 54%, and clinical improvements were noted in joint tenderness, following supplementation with EPA and DHA.

IL-1b and increased CRF secretion

Peripheral IL-1b is a potent stimulus for the secretion of CRF in the hypothalamus, thereby linking the neuroendocrine and immune systems by activation of the HPA axis (Berkenbosch et al., 1987; Sapolsky et al., 1987). Peripheral injection of IL-1b stimulates expression of mRNA for CRF and c-fos in CRF-containing neurones in the parvocellular cells of the paraventricular nucleus in the hypothalamus (Harbuz et al., 1992; Ericsson et al., 1994). IL-1b activation of the HPA axis may also occur *via* other mechanisms yet to be elucidated.

IL-1b stimulation of CRF release appears to be dependent upon eicosanoid release (Rivier and Vale, 1991) and may thus be modulated by an elevated ratio of n-6 to n-3 precursors in tissues. It has been reported (Maes et al., 1993) that, in patients with unipolar depression, IL-1b is elevated compared to controls ($p < 0.05$), and in both depressed patients and normal controls there was a positive correlation ($r = +0.50$; $p < 0.001$) between elevated levels of IL-1b and hyperactivity of the HPA axis as indicated by the dexamethasone suppression test (Shintani et al., 1993). These *ex vivo* measures of IL-1b release may model intermittent activation of monocytes. In addition, acute stimulation with IL-1b causes a 2–3-fold increase in 5-HT and norepinephrine release, and increases catabolism as demonstrated by a 1.2–1.5-fold elevation in 5-HIAA levels (Shinani et al., 1993). Depletion of central 5-HT and norepinephrine are central to current theories of the aetiology of depression (Meltzer and Lowey, 1987).

CRF, HPA activation and depressive symptoms

On the basis of many human and animal studies (for a review, see Kling et al., 1989), hypersecretion of CRF is believed to be directly related to clinical depression and to be responsible for the hyperactivity of the HPA axis in depression. CRF-like immunoreactive components were elevated nearly 2-fold in the CSF of depressed patients compared to neurological controls and schizophrenics in a study by Baki et al. (1987), confirming earlier findings (Nemeroff et al., 1984). Kling et al. (1989) have argued that an important aspect of the underlying pathophysiology of depression is an overdriven, generalized stress response, which leads to mutually reinforcing hyperactivity of the CRF and locus coeruleus norepinephrine systems: we suggest that the abnormally high set-point for CRF secretion and locus coeruleus activity could both be driven by excessive IL-1b secretion.

Although no data are available from studies on humans, in animals IL-1b administration elicits behaviour related to depression, including anorexia (Hallerstein et al., 1989; Uehara et al., 1989), sleep changes (Krueger et al., 1984; Payne et al., 1993), and decreased exploratory behaviour (Payne et al., 1993). CRF antagonists block induction of these behaviours by IL-1b (Uehara et al., 1989; Dunn et al., 1991; Payne et al., 1993). IL-1b-induced anorexia was found by Hallerstein et al. (1989) to be reversed by a diet rich in the n-3 LCPUFAs, DHA and EPA, derived from fish oil, compared with a matched corn oil diet that was rich in n-6 fatty acids.

Modulation of immune–neuroendocrine interactions by dietary n-3 LCPUFAs

Patients with depression may have low levels of n-3 LCPUFAs in their tissues. Adams, Sinclair and others (personal communication) have recently observed that unmedicated unipolar depressives have significantly decreased amounts of n-3 LCPUFAs in eythrocytes compared to controls. An increased ratio of the n-6 LCPUFA AA to the n-3 EPA in erythrocytes was highly correlated ($r = +0.73$; $p < 0.01$) with the severity of depressive symptoms. Although no treatment studies have been conducted with purified DHA or EPA, some results suggest that n-3 LCPUFAs may have an antidepressant effect. Of great interest in this regard are the results of a multicentre study (Cenacchi et al., 1993) in which 494 elderly patients were treated with about 90 mg/day of DHA contained in bovine cortex phosphatidylserine, which markedly improved scores of apathy and social withdrawal compared to treatment with corn oil (which typically contains less than 1% of n-3, but around 52% of n-6, LCPUFAs). An antidepressant effect was also noted for bovine phosphatidylserine in a placebo-controlled crossover study of 10 elderly women (Maggioni et al., 1990). Since n-3 LCPUFAs, such as DHA, are essential components of synaptic membranes (Salem et al., 1986; Salem, 1989; Salem and Ward, 1993) and, along with EPA, may modulate immune–neuroendocrine interactions, dietary n-3 LCPUFAs may decrease vulnerability to depression.

LCPUFAs AND DEPRESSION-RELATED CONDITIONS

Coronary artery disease

If, as appears to be the case, there is a causal relationship between depression and low dietary intake of n-3 LCPUFAs, and if such a dietary deficiency is also a contributory factor in coronary artery disease (CAD) (Connor, 1991), then it would follow that there should be a positive correlation between depression and CAD. This is, in fact, the case according to Booth-Kewley and Friedman (1987), on the basis of a meta-analysis of 83 studies which demonstrated that CAD correlated more strongly with depression than any other personality variable investigated. Fielding (1991), in a subsequent overview of findings in this area concluded that both the occurrence and the survival outcome of CAD were predicted by premorbid depression. There is clear evidence that major depression occurring near the time of myocardial infarction is a predictor of additional adverse cardiac events and cardiac mortality in the following 24 h, and after 6, 12 and 18 months (Sinclair, 1980; Hasegawa, 1985; Sinclair et al., 1987; Siguel and Lerman, 1994)

It is possible that CAD and depression or hostility are related because of a common nutritional cause, i.e., a low consumption of n-3 fatty acids.

Alcoholism

There is a well-known relationship between affective disorder and alcoholism (Weissman, 1983; Schuckit, 1986; Merikangas and Gelertner, 1990; Winokur, 1990). Alcoholics in whom there is an early onset of dependence, are particularly likely to demonstrate aggressive behaviour and to have a high risk of suicide (Mann, 1995). This may reflect an underlying commonality of mechanism between alcoholism, hostility and depression. Alcohol consumption is, in fact, a confounding factor in studies which compare suicide attempters and controls.

Pawlowsky and Salem (1995, 1996, 1997) reported that, in adult cats and Rhesus monkeys maintained on diets resembling those typical of alcoholics, alcohol consumption led to depletion of brain levels of DHA; this would be a particularly important observation if it were confirmed in humans, given that more than half of the adults committing violent crimes have consumed alcohol chronically (Miczek et al., 1996). Alcohol also contributes to an increase in symptoms of anxiety and, in extreme cases, to psychotic behaviour in schizophrenic patients.

It has been found that increased lipid peroxidation is associated with alcohol consumption (Rosenblum et al., 1989; Bjorneboe and Bjorneboe, 1993), and there is evidence (Salem and Ward, 1993) that this may result in a relative depletion of the n-3 LCPUFAs from neuronal membranes, thereby possibly facilitating the onset of depressive symptoms. Abstinence from alcohol allows the n-3 LCPUFAs to become reestablished in the neuronal membranes, and it may be that dietary supplementation with n-3 LCPUFAs could speed the process of recovery from alcoholism.

Multiple sclerosis

Schubert and Foliart (1993), on the basis of a meta-analysis of published studies, concluded that depression is highly associated with multiple sclerosis (MS), and that the extent of the relationship is greater than can be ascribed merely to the physical disabilities to which MS gives rise; moreover, the MS lesions are not localized in anatomical regions known to be involved in the production of depressive symptoms (Minden and Schiffer, 1990). It is now known that MS is characterized by a variety of changes in LCPUFAs in the central nervous system. Thus, 20:4n-6 and 22:6n-3 levels are lower in MS subjects than in healthy controls in the white matter (Gerstl et al., 1965; Kishimoto et al., 1967; Wilson and Tocher, 1991) and plasma (Cunnane et al., 1989; Holman et al., 1989), and 22;6n-3 is apparently completely absent from MS adipose stores (Nightingale et al., 1990).

The geographical distribution of affective disorders (Robins and Regier, 1991) is very similar to that of MS (Bernsohn and Stephanides, 1967), and it has been suggested that regional differences in 22:6n-3 consumption at critical times during neural development could explain the distribution pattern (Bernsohn and Stephanides, 1967). Whilst dietary supplementation with n-3 and n-6 mixtures leads to only a slight decrease in relapses of MS, there is a more marked improvement in quality of life (Bates, 1990), possibly reflecting improvements in associated depressive symptoms.

Postpartum depression

Postpartum depression (Gitlin and Pasnau, 1989; Robins and Regier, 1991) has been linked to plasma 22:6n-3 depletion (Holman et al., 1991) as a result of the diversion of this essential nutrient to the developing foetal nervous system, and there is evidence that the extent of this depletion increases with subsequent pregnancies (Al et al., 1994). If low n-3 levels are related to the risk of developing depression, this may be one of the reasons for the occurrence of depressive illness in the prenatal and postpartum periods. If this is so, then providing pregnant and lactating mothers with n-3 LCPUFA supplementation might help to prevent the emergence of both mild and more severe expressions of this condition. There is, indeed, some evidence to support this view, in that a cross-national study shows that there is a significant negative correlation ($r = -0.69$; $p < 0.001$) between the nearly 100-fold variance in point prevalence of postpartum depression and the nearly 200-fold variance in apparent fish consumption (Figure 19.1).

It should be noted, in interpreting the correlation illustrated in Figure 19.1, that cross-national comparisons of the point prevalence of postpartum depression are not as reliable as comparisons of structured interview diagnostic data on the prevalence of major depression. Although no diagnostic instrument is without its faults, the items for the Edinburgh Postpartum Depression scale rely on descriptions of biological changes such as sleep, weight, and appetite changes, and the scale has been validated across 17 countries against RDC and DSM-III or DSM-III-R diagnostic criteria; because of its reliability and wide international use, only studies using this scale, with validation for the culture and language of the population studied, were considered for this analysis. Insufficient data were available for analysis of the effects of social and family support, and of social class, both of which factors clearly influence the prevalence of postpartum depression (O'Hara, 1995).

Insulin resistance

Patients with major depression have been reported to show insulin resistance (Mueller et al., 1969; Koslow et al., 1982; Winokur et al., 1988), as has also been observed during alcohol withdrawal from chronic alcoholic patients (Andersen et al., 1983; Adner and Nygren, 1990). Insulin resistance in these cases is likely to be related to membrane insensitivity which has been found in several studies to be linked to raised levels of n-6 LCPUFAs (Storlien et al., 1991; Borkman et al., 1993).

Insulin binding in retinoblastoma cells is enhanced by 22:6n-3 which causes an increase in receptor number (Yorek et al., 1989).

Hypercalcaemia

Hypercalcaemia and a corresponding increase in intracellular calcium have been reported to be depressogenic (Dubovsky and Franks, 1983). Intracellular calcium may be decreased by administration of 22:6n-3, according to the results of an *in vitro* study of cultured myocytes (Hallaq et al., 1992), as a result of an inhibitory effect of the n-3 LCPUFA on L-type calcium channels. If a similar effect were to occur *in vivo*, then depletion of 22:6n-3 would be associated with increased passage of calcium through the L-type channels, resulting in an increase in intracellular calcium, and the consequent occurrence of depressive symptoms. It is interesting that verapamil, a calcium channel blocker, can have beneficial effects in treating affective disorder, possibly as a result of offsetting the consequences of DHA depletion.

STRESS-INDUCED DEPLETION OF LCPUFAs

Whilst in some depressed individuals the balance of n-6:n-3 LCPUFAs may be determined by genetic factors, and in others by the composition of the diet, it is possible that environmental influences unrelated to diet could also lead to polyunsaturate depletion. Hibbeln and Salem (1995) have suggested that reduction of neuronal LCPUFAs may occur as a result of repeated periods of emotional stress, and there is a body of information generally supportive of this idea. Thus, Gulyaeva et al. (1989) reported that a chronic (3-week) emotional/pain stress regimen in rats led to an increase in lipid peroxidation in the animals' brain tissue, with resultant neuronal phospholipid depletion and the appearance of depressive-like behaviour. Avdulov et al. (1990) noted the appearance of changes in synaptosomal membranes brought about by repeated immobilization stress. Various forms of stress have been reported to cause increases in brain levels of thiobar-

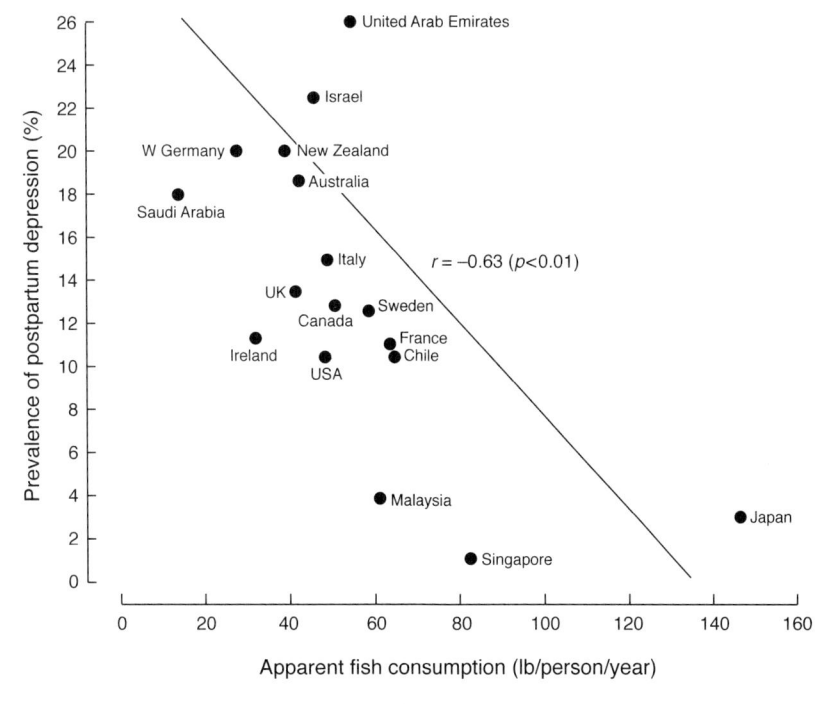

Figure 19.1. Relationship between point prevalence of postpartum depression in 19 countries and the apparent consumption of fish in the same countries. Information regarding the prevalence of postpartum depression was derived from a wide range of studies (Cox et al., 1993; Kok et al., 1994; Jadresic et al., 1995; MacLennan et al., 1996; Abou-Saleh et al., 1997; Bernazzini et al., 1997; Carpiniello et al., 1997; Fossey et al., 1997; Ghubash et al., 1997; Kit et al., 1997; Tamak et al., 1997; Wickberg et al., 1997; Yoshida et al., 1997; Bergant et al., 1998; Lee et al., 1998; Stuart et al., 1998). The values for apparent fish consumption are based on economic data relating to the disappearance of fish from economies (World Health Organisation, 1996), and are not direct dietary consumption data.

bituric acid reactive substances (TBARS) (Sosnovskii et al., 1992), changes indicative of depletion of protective antioxidants (Desole et al., 1990), and a reduction in superoxide dismutase (Sosnovskii et al., 1993). It is also possible that reactivity to stress may be further enhanced as a result of a stress-induced depletion of n-3 LCPUFAs, according to a study in Rhesus monkeys reported by Reisbeck et al. (1990).

DIETARY IMPLICATIONS
The evolutionary perspective

Whilst there are many possible reasons for the progressive rise, over the last 100 years, in the risk of developing major depression (Klerman and Weisman, 1989; Cross-National Collaborative Group, 1992; Weisman et al., 1996), exemplified by a nearly 100-fold increase in the lifetime prevalence of depression in North America, an intriguing suggestion is that such findings may be linked to a progressive increase over the same period in the consumption of saturated fatty acids and n-6 EFAs, coupled with a decreased consumption of n-3 EFAs. On the basis of the foregoing discussion, the dietary n-6:n-3 LCPUFA ratio is a crucial determinant of mood/hostility state and of vulnerability to depression.

Based on estimates of palaeolithic nutrition, and upon the diet typical of modern hunter-gatherer populations (Eaton et al., 1998), it has been suggested that the early evolution of humans took place under conditions which provided a diet that was lower in saturated fats, and higher in polyunsaturated fats, than the modern diet. The proportion of n-6 polyunsaturates in the diet has increased markedly in the last century due to reliance of agriculture upon a few plant species as sources for EFAs for the domestic food chain (Simopoulos, 1991). Wild and free-range animals have significantly more n-3 fatty acids in their tissues than do currently produced commercial livestock (Crawford et al., 1969). In models of palaeolithic diets reflecting arid high altitude and other environments, ratios of dietary n-6 to n-3 fatty acids range from 0.4 to 2.8, without assuming any intake of fish or seafood; these values may be compared with dietary n-6:n-3 ratios of between 10:1 and 25:1 estimated for modern diets (Eaton and Konner, 1985; Hunter, 1989; Simopoulos, 1991; Raper et al., 1992).

It has been proposed (Broadhurst et al., 1998) that the evolution of a large cranial capacity could have been facilitated by the ready availability of fish from inland lakes formed by the Rift Valley. This food source, rich in EPA, DHA and AA, would have influenced the composition of the entire food chain in the lake ecology. The composition of fatty acids in brain tissues does not vary much between species, but the size of the brain does. During early postnatal development in humans, the brain requires preformed DHA and AA to maintain the compositional patterns of fatty acids. Since adequate amounts of DHA and AA cannot be synthesized from linoleic and linolenic precursors (Salem et al., 1996), it may well have been the ready availability of DHA and AA from the environment that facilitated the differentiation of hominid species with large cranial capacity.

Fish consumption and depression

If n-3 LCPUFAs are, as Hibbeln and Salem (1996) have proposed, protective against depression, and if n-3 LCPUFA levels can be raised appreciably by a diet rich in fish, then one would expect to find the incidence of major depression to be lower in those countries in which fish form a major element of the normal diet than in other countries where fish consumption is relatively low. This prediction is borne out by the results of a number of studies. Low rates of depression and of depressive symptoms have, for example, been reported in Japan (Makiya, 1978; Sarai, 1979; Hasegawa, 1985) where fish consumption, and thus n-3 LCPUFA intake, are high (Hairi et al., 1987), compared with significantly higher rates in the USA (Zung, 1967; Blazer and Williams, 1980; O'Hara et al., 1985; Krause and Liang, 1992) where fish consumption and n-3 LCPUFA intake are correspondingly low (Jonnalagada et al., 1995).

Hibbeln (1998) has noted that the annual prevalence of major depression shows a nearly 60-fold variation across countries, and that this pattern is related to that of annual fish consumption across the same countries: a strong protective effect of fish consumption on the prevalence of major depression was described ($r = -0.84$; $p < 0.005$), which is very similar to the protective role of fish consumption in cardiovascular disease (Hibbeln, 1998).

Whilst it is prudent to regard these interpretations with caution, as many social and cultural factors may influence the occurrence and expression of depressive illness, the data nevertheless consistently suggest a strong protective relationship between fish consumption and major depression.

Cholesterol lowering and n-3 LCPUFAs

In an attempt to lower serum cholesterol levels, individuals are often advised to reduce their total intake of fat and to consume vegetable oils instead. However, many such oils have relatively high levels of n-6 LCPUFAs compared with their n-3 LCPUFA content; for example, the n-6:n-3 ratios in soybean oil and corn oil are 14:1 and 54:1, respectively (United States Department of Agriculture, 1979). Such dietary adjustments may therefore result in deficiencies in n-3 LCPUFA intake (Meydani et al., 1993; Siguel and Lerman, 1994). That this may have consequences for mood and behaviour was indicated by Kaplan et al. (1991) who found that monkeys given a low-fat diet with an n-6:n-3 LCPUFA ratio of around 33:1 showed greater aggression than others given a high-fat diet in which the n-6:n-3 ratio was 6:1.

Drugs designed to lower cholesterol levels may result in changes in tissue LCPUFAs (e.g., Agheli and Jacotot, 1991; Grøn et al., 1992; Delva et al., 1996; Hibbeln and Salem, 1996), with consequent increases in expressed anger and hostility (Strandberg et al., 1994), for the reasons outlined earlier in this chapter.

SUMMARY AND CONCLUSIONS

Whilst there is clearly much work still to be done in this area, the basic framework is already quite clear of what may be a powerful model linking diet, LCPUFAs, serotonergic neurotransmission, and mood disorders. Reductions in dietary intake of n-3 LCPUFAs (and particularly of DHA), associated with changes in the n-6:n-3 plasma ratio of LCPUFAs, may have profound effects upon serotonergic transmission at more than one level (including synthesis, release, reuptake, receptor affinity) and upon neuronal membrane order. These serotonergic effects, in their turn, are reflected in a range of behavioural and cognitive disturbances characteristic of mood disorder.

Whilst it is too early to give a definitive response to the question of whether dietary supplementation of n-3 PUFAs might, under the right circumstances, and in appropriately selected groups of patients, produce cognitive/behavioural corrections which will act to offset mood disturbance, such an outcome is strongly predicted by the available evidence. In other chapters in this book, evidence generally in line with this prediction is presented from a variety of studies, and this strongly argues for further, more extensive investigations to be set up in the future.

REFERENCES

Abou-Saleh MT, Ghubash R. The prevalence of early postpartum psychiatric morbidity in Dubai: a transcultural perspective. Acta Psychiatr Scand 1997; 95: 428–432.

Adams PB, Lawson S, Sanigorski A, Sinclair AJ. Arachidonic acid to eicosapentaenoic acid ratio in blood correlates positively with clinical symptoms of depression. Lipids 1996; 31 (Suppl): S167–S176.

Adner N, Nygren A. Insulin sensitivity in alcoholics in a withdrawal state. J Intern Med 1990; 228: 59–64.

Agheli N, Jacotot B. Effect of simvastatin and fenofibrate on the fatty acid composition of hypercholesterolaemic patients. Br J Pharmacol 1991; 4: 423–428.

Al M, Houwelingen AC, Honstra G. Docosahexaenoic acid, 22:6(n3), cervonic acid (CA), and hypertension in pregnancy: consequences for mother and child. Paper presented at the American Heart Association scientific conference on omega-3 fatty acids in nutrition, vascular biology and medicine, Houston, TX, 1994.

Andersen NB, Hagen C, Faber OK, Lindholm J, Boisen P, Worning H. Glucose tolerance and B cell function in chronic alcoholism: its relation to hepatic histology and exocrine pancreatic function. Metabolism 1983; 32: 1029–1032.

Avdulov NA, Eremenko AV, Valdman KM et al. Changes in synaprosomal membranes from cerebral cortex due to psychogenic stress in rats. Ann Ist Super Sanita 1990; 26: 31–36.

Baki CM, Bissette G, Arato M, O'Connor L, Nemeroff CM. CSF corticotrophin-releasing factor-like immunoreactivity in depression and schizophrenia. Am J Psychiatry 1987; 144: 73–77.

Bates D. Dietary lipids and multiple sclerosis. Ups J Med Sci 1990; S48: 173–187.

Bergant AM, Nguyen T, Heim K, Ulmer H and Dapunt O. Deutschsprachige Fassung und Validierung der 'Edinburgh postnatal' 'depression scale.' Dtsch Med Wochenschr 1998; 123: 35–40.

Berkenbosch F, van Oers J, del Ray A, Tilders F, Besedovsky H. Corticotrophin-releasing factor-producing neurons in the rat activated by interleukin-1. Science 1987; 238: 524–526.

Bernazzani O, Saucier JF, David H, Borgeat F. Psychosocial predictors of depressive symptomatology level in postpartum women. J Affective Disord 1997; 46: 39–49.

Bernsohn J, Stephanides LM. Aetiology of multiple sclerosis. Nature 1967; 215: 821–823.

Bjorneboe A, Bjorneboe GE. Antioxidant status and alcohol-related diseases. Alcohol Alcohol 1993; 28: 111–116.

Blazer D, Williams CD. Epidemiology of dysphoria and depression in an elderly population. Am J Psychiatry 1980; 137: 439–444.

Booth-Kewley S, Friedman HS. Psychological predictors of heart disease: a quantitative review. Psychol Bull 1987; 101: 343–362.

Borkman M, Storlien LH, Pan DA, Jenkins AB, Chisholm DJ, Cambell LV. The relationship between insulin sensitivity and the fatty acid composition of skeletal muscle phospholipids. N Engl J Med 1993; 328: 238–244.

Broadhurst CL, Cunnane SC, Crawford MA. Rift Valley lake fish and shellfish provided brain-specific nutrition for early *Homo*. Br J Nutr 1998; 79: 3–21.

Brown GL, Goodwin FK, Ballenger JC et al. Aggression in humans correlates with cerebral spinal fluid metabolites. Psychiatry Res 1979; 1: 131–139.

Brown LS, Salive ME, Harris TB et al. Serum cholesterol concentrations and severe depressive symptoms in elderly people. Br Med J 1994; 308: 1328–1332.

Buydens-Branchey L, Branchey MH, Noumair D. Age of alcoholism onset. Arch Gen Psychiatry 1989; 46: 225–230.

Carpiniello B, Pariante CM, Serri F, Costa G, Carta MG. Validation of the Edinburgh postnatal depression scale in Italy. J Psychosom Obstet Gynecol 1997; 18: 280–285.

Cenacchi T, Bertoldin T, Faarina C et al. Cognitive decline in the elderly. A double-blind, placebo-controlled multicenter study on efficacy of phosphatidylserine administration. Aging Clin Exp Res 1993; 5: 123–133.

Coccaro EF, Siever LJ, Klar HM et al. Serotonergic studies in patients with affective and personality disorders. Arch Gen Psychiatry 1989; 46: 587–599.

Connor WE. Evaluation of publicly available scientific evidence regarding certain nutrient disease relationships. 7. Omega-3 fatty acids and heart disease. Bethesda, MD: Life Sciences Research Office, 1991.

Connor WE, Connor SL. Dietary treatment of hyperlipidemia. In: Rifkind BM, Levy RI, eds. Hyperlipidemia: diagnosis and therapy. New York: Grune and Stratton, 1977: 281–326.

Connor WE, Neuringer M, Lin DS. Dietary effects upon brain fatty acid composition: the reversibility of n-3 fatty acid deficiency and turnover of docosahexaenoic acid in the brain, erythrocytes and plasma of Rhesus monkeys. J Lipid Res 1990; 31: 237–248.

Cox JL, Murray D, Chapman G. A controlled study of the onset, duration and prevalence of postnatal depression. Br J Psychiatry 1993; 163: 27–31.

Crane SB, Greenwood CE. Dietary fat source influences neuronal mitochondrial monoamine oxidase activity and macronutrient selection in rats. Pharmacol Biochem Behav 1987; 27: 1–6.

Crawford MA, Gale MM, Woodford MH. Linoleic and linolenic acid elongation products in muscle tissue of *Syncerus caffer* and other ruminant species. Biochem J 1969; 115: 25–27.

Cross National Collaborative Group. The changing rate of major depression: cross national comparisons. JAMA 1992; 268: 3098–3105.

Cunnane SC, Ho SY, Bore-Duffy P, Ells KR, Horrobin DF. Essential fatty acid and lipid profiles in plasma and erythrocytes in patients with multiple sclerosis. Am J Clin Nutr 1989; 50: 801–806.

DeLion S, Chalon S, Herault J, Guilloteau D, Besnard J, Durand G. Chronic dietary α-linolenic acid deficiency alters dopaminergic and serotonergic neurotransmission in rats. J Nutr 1994; 124: 2466–2476.

Delva NJ, Mathews DR, Cowen PJ. Brain serotonin (5-HT) neuroendocrine function in patients taking cholesterol lowering drugs. Biol Psychiatry 1996; 39: 100–106.

Desole MS, Meile M, Esposito G, Enrico P, De Natale G, Miele E. Analysis of immobilization stress-induced changes of ascorbic acid, noradrenaline and dopamine metabolism in discrete brain areas of the rat. Pharmacol Res 1990; 22 (Suppl 3): 43–44.

Dobbing J. The entry of cholesterol into rat brain during development. J Neurochem 1963; 10: 739–742.

Dubovsky SL, Franks RD. Intracellular calcium ions in affective disorders: a review and hypothesis. Biol Psychiatry 1983; 18: 781–797.

Dunn AJ, Antoon M, Chapman Y. Reduction of exploratory behavior by intraperitoneal injection of interleukin-1 involves brain corticotrophin-releasing factor. Brain Res Bull 1991; 26: 539–542.

Eaton SB, Konner M. Paleolithic nutrition: a consideration of its nature and current implications. N Engl J Med 1985; 312: 283–289.

Eaton SB, Sinlair AJ, Cordain L, Mann NJ. Dietary intake of long-chain polyunsaturated fatty acids during the paleolithic. World Rev Nutr Diet 1998; 83: 12–23.

Edmond J, Korsak RA, Morro JW, Torok-Both G, Catlin DH. Dietary cholesterol and the origin of cholesterol in the brain of developing rats. J Nutr 1991; 121: 1323–1330.

Edwards RhW, Peet M, Shay J, Horrobin DF. Omega-3 polyunsaturated fatty acid levels in the diet and in red blood cell membranes of depressed patients. J Affective Disord 1998; 48: 149–155.

Endelberg H. Low cholesterol and suicide. Lancet 1992; 339: 727–729.

Endres S, Ghorbani R, Kelly VE et al. The effect of dietary supplementation with n-3 polyunsaturated fatty acids on the synthesis of interleukin 1 and tumor necrosis factor by mononuclear cells. N Engl J Med 1989; 320: 265–271.

Eperson GT, Grunnet N, Lervang HH et al. Decreased interleukin-1β in plasma from rheumatoid arthritis patients after dietary supplementation with n-3 polyunsaturated fatty acids. Clin Rheumatol 1992; 11: 393–395.

Ericsson A, Krisztina KJ, Kovacs J, Sawchenko PE. A functional anatomical analysis of central pathways subserving the effects of interleukin-1-b on stress-related neuroendocrine neurons. J Neurosci 1994; 14: 897–913.

Fernstrom MH, Verrico CD, Ebaugh AI, Fernstrom JD. Diet-related changes in serum cholesterol concentrations do not alter tryptophan hydroxylase rate or serotonin concentrations in gerbil brain. Life Sci 1996; 58: 1433–1444:

Fielding R. Depression and acute myocardial infarction: a review and reinterpretation. Soc Sci Med 1991; 32: 1017–1028.

Fils-Aime M, Eckardt MJ, George DT et al. Early-onset alcoholics have lower cerebrospinal fluid 5-HIAA than late-onset alcoholics. Arch Gen Psychiatry 1996; 53: 216–221.

Fossey E, Papiernik E, Bydlowski M. Post-partum blues: a clinical syndrome and predictor of post-natal depression? J Psychosom Obstet Gynecol 1997; 18: 17–21.

Fowkes FGR, Leng GC, Donnan PT et al. Serum cholesterol, triglycerides, and aggression in the general population. Lancet 1992; 340: 995–998.

Gallai VG, Sarchielli P, Trequatrini A et al. Cytokine secretion and eicosanoid production in the peripheral mononuclear cells of MS patients undergoing dietary supplementation with n-3 polyunsaturated fatty acids. J Neuroimmunol 1995; 56: 143–153.

Gerstl B, Tavastjerna MG, Hayman RB, Eng LF, Smith JK. Alterations in myelin fatty acids and plasmalogens in multiple sclerosis. Ann NY Acad Sci 1965; 122: 405–407.

Ghubash R, Abou-Saleh MT, Daradkeh K. The validity of the Arabic Edinburgh postnatal depression scale. Soc Psychiatry Psychiatr Epidemiol 1997; 32: 474–476.

Gibbons RD, Davis JM. Consistent evidence for a biological subtype of depression characterized by low CSF 5-HIAA levels. Acta Psychiatr Scand 1986; 74: 8–12.

Gitlin M, Pasnau RO. Psychiatric syndromes linked to reproductive function in women: a review of current knowledge. Am J Psychiatry 1989; 146: 1413–1422.

Grøn M, Christensen E, Hagve T et al. Effects of clofibrate feeding on desaturation and oxidation in isolated rat liver cells. Biochim Biophys Acta 1992; 1123: 170–176.

Gulyaeva NV, Levshina IP, Obidin AB. Indices of free-radical oxidation of lipids and antiradical protection of the brain: neurochemical correlates of the development of the general adaptation syndrome. Neurosci Behav Physiol 1989; 19: 367–382.

Hairi T, Terano T, Saito H et al. Clinical and epidemiological studies of eicosapentaenoic acid in Japan. In: Lands WEM, ed. Proceedings of the AOCS short course on polyunsaturated fatty acids and eicosanoids. Biloxi MS: American Oil Chemists Society, 1987: 46–54.

Hallaq H, Smith TW, Leaf A. Modulation of dihydropyridine-sensitive calcium channels in heart cells by fish oil fatty acids. Proc Natl Acad Sci USA 1992; 89: 1760–1764.

Hallerstein MK, Meydani SN, Meyani M, Wu K, Dinarello CA. Interleukin-1-induced anorexia in the rat: influence of prostaglandins. J Clin Invest 1989; 84: 228–235.

Hamazak T, Sawazaki S, Itomura M et al. The effect of docosahexaenoic acid on aggression in young adults: a double-blind study. J Clin Invest 1996; 97: 1129–1133.

Harbuz MS, Stephanou A, Sarlis N, Lightman SL. The effects of recombinant human interleukin (IL)-1a, IL-1b or IL-6 on hypothalamo–pituitary–adrenal axis activation. J Endocrinol 1992; 133: 349–355.

Harris WS. n-3 Fatty acids and lipoproteins: comparison of results from human and animal studies. Lipids 1996; 31: 243–252.

Hasegawa K. The epidemiological study of depression in later life. J Affective Disord 1985; Suppl 1: S3–S6.

Heron D, Shinitzki M, Hershkowitz M, Samuel D. Lipid fluidity markedly modulates the binding of serotonin to mouse brain membranes. Proc Natl Acad Sci USA 1980; 77: 7463–7467.

Hibbeln JR. Fish consumption and major depression. Lancet 1998; 351: 1213.

Hibbeln JR, Salem N. Dietary polyunsaturated fatty acids and depression: when cholesterol does not satisfy. Am J Clin Nutr 1995; 62: 1–9.

Hibbeln JR, Salem N. Cholesterol lowering drugs alter polyunsaturated fatty acid levels. Biol Psychiatry 1996; 40: 686–687.

Hibbeln JR, Umhau JC, George DT, Salem N. Do plasma polyunsaturates predict hostility and depression? World Rev Nutr Diet 1997; 82: 175–186.

Hibbeln JR, Linnoila M, Umhau JC, Rawlings R, George DT, Salem N. Essential fatty acids predict metabolites of serotonin and dopamine in cerebrospinal fluid among healthy control subjects and early- and late-onset alcoholics. Biol Psychiatry 1998a; 44: 235–242.

Hibbeln JR, Umhau JC, Linnoila M et al. A replication study of violent and nonviolent subjects: cerebrospinal fluid metabolites of serotonin and dopamine are predicted by plasma essential fatty acids. Biol Psychiatry 1998b; 44: 243–249.

Higley JD, Mehlman PT, Poland RE et al. CSF testosterone and 5-HIAA correlate with different types of aggressive behaviors. Biol Psychiatry 1996; 40: 1067–1082.

Holman RT, Johnson SB, Kokman E. Deficiencies in polyunsaturated fatty acids and replacement by nonessential fatty acids in plasma lipids in multiple sclerosis. Proc Natl Acad Sci USA 1989; 86: 4720–4724.

Holman RT, Johnson SB, Ogburn PL. Deficiency of essential fatty acids and membrane fluidity during pregnancy and lactation. Proc Natl Acad Sci USA 1991; 88: 4835–4839.

Hunter JE. Omega-3 fatty acids from vegetable oils. In: Galli C, Simopoulos AP, eds. Dietary ω-3 and ω-6 fatty acids: biological effect and nutritional essentiality. New York: Plenum Press, 1989: 43–55.

Irribaren C, Reed DM, Wergowske G et al. Serum cholesterol and mortality due to suicide and trauma in the Honolulu heart program. Arch Intern Med 1995; 155: 695–700.

Irwin M, Schuckit M, Smith T. Clinical importance of the age of onset of alcoholism in type I and type 2 primary alcoholics. Arch Gen Psychiatry 1990; 47: 320–324.

Jacobs D, Blackburn H, Higgens M et al. Report on the conference on low blood cholesterol: mortality associations. Circulation 1992; 86: 1046–1060.

Jadresic E, Araya R, Jara C. Validation of the Edinburgh postnatal depression scale (EPDS) in Chilean postpartum women. J Psychosom Obstet Gynecol 1995; 16:1 87–191.

Jones JP, Nicholas HJ, Ramsay RB. Biosynthesis of cholesterol by brain tissues: distribution in subcellular fractions as a function of time after injection of [2-C-14] acetate and [U-C-14] glucose into 15-day-old rats. J Neurochem 1975a; 24: 117–121.

Jones JP, Nicholas HJ, Ramsay RB. Rate of sterol formation by rat brain glia and neurons in vitro and in vivo. J Neurochem 1975b; 24: 122–126.

Jonnalagada SS, Egan SK, Heimbach JT et al. Fatty acid consumption pattern of Americans: 1987–1988 USDA nationwide food consumption survey. Nutr Res 1995; 15: 1767–1781.

Kaplan JR, Manuck SB, Shively CA. The effects of fat and cholesterol on social behavior in monkeys. Psychosom Med 1991; 53: 634–642.

Kaplan JR, Shively CA, Fontenot MB et al. Demonstration of an association among dietary cholesterol, central serotonergic activity, and social behavior in monkeys. Psychosom Med 1994; 56: 479–484.

Keys A, Anderson J, Grande F. Serum cholesterol changes in response to diet. IV. Particular saturated fatty acids in the diet. Metabolism 1965; 14: 776–786.

Kishimoto Y, Radin NS, Tourtellotte WW, Parker JA, Itabashi HH. Gangliosides and glycephospholipids in multiple sclerosis white matter. Arch Neurol 1967; 16: 44–56.

Kit LK, Janet G, Jegasothy R. Incidence of postnatal depression in Malaysian women. J Obstet Gynaecol Res 1997; 23: 85–89.

Klerman GL, Weismann MM. Increasing rates of depression. JAMA 1989; 261: 2229–2235.

Kling MA, Perini GI, Demitrack MA et al. Stress-responsive neurohormonal systems and the symptom complex of affective illness. Psychopharm Bull 1989; 25: 312–318.

Kok, LP, Chan PS, Ratnam SS. Postnatal depression in Singapore women. Singapore Med J 1994; 35: 33–35.

Koslow SH, Stokes PE, Mendels J, Ramsey A, Casper R. Insulin tolerance test: human growth hormone response and insulin resistance in primary unipolar depressed, bipolar depressed and control subjects. Psychol Med 1982; 12: 45–55.

Krause N, Liang J. Cross cultural variations in depressive symptoms in later life. Int Psychogeriatr 1992; 4 (Suppl 2): 185–202.

Kremer JM, Lawrence DA, Jubitz W et al. Dietary fish oil and olive oil supplementation in patients with rheumatoid arthritis. Arthritis Rheum 1990; 33: 810–820.

Krueger JM, Walter J, Dinarello CA, Wolff SM, Chedid L. Sleep promoting effects of endogenous pyrogen (interleukin-1). Am Jm Physiol 1984; 246: R994–R999.

Lee DT, Yip SK, Chiu HF et al. Detecting postnatal depression in Chinese women. Validation of the Chinese version of the Edinburgh Postnatal Depression Scale. Br J Psychiatry 1998; 172: 433–437.

Linnoila M, Virkkunen M, Scheinn M et al. Low cerebrospinal fluid levels of 5-hydroxyindoleacetic acid concentrations differentiates impulsive from nonimpulsive violent behavior. Life Sci 1983; 33: 2609–2614.

Litman BJ, Mitchell DC. A role for phospholipid polyunsaturation in modulating membrane protein function. Lipids 1996; 31 (Suppl): S193–S197.

Litman BJ, Lewis EN, Levin IW. Packing characteristics of highly unsaturated bilayer lipids: Raman spectroscopic studies of multilamellar phosphatidylcholine dispersions. Biochemistry 1991; 30: 313–319.

MacLennan A, Wilson D, Taylor A. The self-reported prevalence of postnatal depression. Aust NZ J Obstet Gynaecol 1996; 36: 313.

Maes M, Bosmans E, Meltzer HY, Scharpe S, Suy E. Interleukin 1-b: a putative mediator of HPA axis hyperactivity in major depression? Am J Psychiatry 1993; 150: 1189–1193.

Maes M, Smith R, Christophe A, Cosyns P, Desnyder R, Meltzer H. Fatty acid composition in major depression: decreased ω3 fractions in cholesteryl esters and increased C20:4ω6/C20:5ω3 ratio in cholesteryl esters and phospholipids. J Affective Disord 1996; 38: 35–46.

Maggioni M, Picotti GB, Bondiolotti GP, Panerai A, Cenacchi T, Nobile P. Effects of phosphatidylserine therapy in geriatric patients with depressive disorders. Acta Psychiatr Scand 1990; 81: 265–270.

Makiya H. Epidemiological investigation of psychiatric disorders of old age in Sashiki-village, Okinawa. Keio J Med 1978; 55: 503.

Mandell AJ. Non-equilibrium behavior of some brain enzyme and receptor systems. Ann Rev Pharmacol Toxicol 1984; 24: 237–274.

Mann JJ. Violence and aggression. In: Bloom FE, Kupfer DJ, eds. Psychopharmacology: the fourth generation of progress. New York: Raven Press, 1995: 1919–1928.

Meltzer HY, Lowey MT. The serotonin hypothesis of depression. In: Meltzer HY, ed. Psychopharmacology: the third generation of progress. New York: Raven Press, 1987: 233–248.

Merikangas K, Gelertner G. Comorbidity for alcoholism and depression. Psychiatr Clin North Am 1990; 13: 613–632.

Meydani SN, Lichtenstein AH, Cornwell S et al. Immunologic effects of National Cholesterol Education Panel step-2 diets with and without fish derived n-3 fatty acid enrichment. J Clin Invest 1993; 92: 105–113.

Miczek KA, Weerts EM, DeBold JF. Alcohol, aggression and violence: biobehavioral determinants. In: Martin SE, ed. Alcohol and interpersonal violence: fostering multidisciplinary perspectives. NIAAA Research Monograph. Rockville, MD: National Institutes of Health, 1996: 83–119.

Minden SL, Schiffer RB. Affective disorders in multiple sclerosis. Arch Neurol 1990; 47: 98–104.

Mitchell DC, Litman B. Effect of cholesterol on membrane order and dynamics in highly polyunsaturated phospholipid bilayers. Biophys J 1998; 75: 896–908.

Mitchell DC, Straume M, Litman BJ. Role of sn-2-polyunsaturated phospholipids and control of membrane receptor conformational equilibrium: effects of cholesterol and acyl chain unsaturation on the metarhodopsin I–metarhodopsin II equilibrium. Biochemistry 1992; 31: 662–670.

Modai I, Valevski A, Kikinzon L et al. Lack of association between cholesterol blood levels and platelet serotonin uptake. Eur Psychiatry 1995; 10: 352–354.

Morgan RE, Palinkas LA, Barrett-Connor EL et al. Plasma cholesterol and depressive symptoms in older men. Lancet 1993; 341: 75–79

Mueller PS, Henninger GR, McDonald RK. Insulin tolerance test in depression. Arch Gen Psychiatry 1969; 21: 587–594.

Muldoon MF, Manuck SB, Matthews KA. Lowering cholesterol concentrations and mortality: a quantitative review of primary prevention trials. Br Med J 1990; 301: 309–314.

Nemeroff CB, Widerlov E, Bissette G et al. Elevated concentrations of CRF corticotrophin-releasing factor-like immunoreactivity in depressed patients. Science 1984; 226: 1342–1344.

Nicolas C, Lacasa D, Giudicelli Y et al. Dietary (n-6) polyunsaturated fatty acids affect β-adrenergic receptor binding and adenylate cyclase activity in pig adipocyte membrane. J Nutr 1991; 121: 1179–1186.

Niebylski CD, Salem N. A calorimetric investigation of a series of mixed-chain polyunsaturated phosphatidylcholines: effect of sn-2 chain length and degree of unsaturation. Biophys J 1994; 67: 2387–2393.

Nightingale S, Woo E, Smith AD et al. Red blood cell and adipose tissue fatty acids in mild inactive multiple sclerosis. Acta Neurol Scand 1980; 82: 43–50.

Nizzo MC, Tegos S, Gallamini A et al. Brain cortex phopspholipids liposomes effects on CSF HVA, 5-HIAA and on prolactin and somatotopin secretion in man. J Neural Transm 1978; 43: 93–102.

O'Hara MW. Postpartum depression. Causes and consequences. New York: Springer-Verlag, 1995.

O'Hara MW, Kohout FK, Wallace RB. Depression among the rural elderly: a study of prevalence and correlates. J Nerv Ment Disord 1985; 173: 582–589.

Pardridge WM, Mietus LJ. Palmitate and cholesterol transport through the blood–brain barrier. J Neurochem 1980; 34: 463–466.

Pawlowsky RJ, Salem N. Prolonged ethanol exposure causes a decrease in docosahexaenoic acid and an increase in docosapentaenoic acid in the feline brain and retina. Am J Clin Nutr 1995; 61: 1284–1289.

Pawlowsky RJ, Salem N. Chronic alcohol exposure in Rhesus monkeys alters electroretinograms and decreases levels of neural docosahexaenoic acid. Paper presented at the Research Society on Alcoholism, Washington DC, 22–27 June, 1996.

Pawlowsky RJ, Flynn BM, Salem N. The effects of low dietary levels of polyunsaturates on alcohol-induced liver disease in Rhesus monkeys. Hepatology 1997; 26: 1386–1392.

Payne LC, Ferenc O, Krueger JM. Hypothalamic releasing hormones mediating the effects of interleukin-1 on sleep. J Cell Biochem 1993; 53: 309–313.

Peet M, Murphy B, Edwards R, Shay J, Horrobin D. Depletion of docosahexaenoic acid in ethrythrocyte membranes of depressed patients. Biol Psychiatry 1998; 43: 315–319.

Pekkanen J, Nissinen A, Punsar S et al. Serum cholesterol and the risk of accidental or violent death in a 25 year follow-up: the Finnish cohorts of the seven countries study. Arch Intern Med 1989; 149: 1589–1591.

Raper NR, Cronin FJ, Exter J. Omega-3 fatty acid content of the US food supply. J Am Coll Nutr 1992; 11: 304–308.

Reisbeck S, Neuringer M, Hasmain R, Connor W. Polydipsia in Rhesus monkeys deficient in omega-3 fatty acids. Physiol Behav 1990; 47: 315–323.

Rivier C, Vale W. Stimulatory effect of interleukin-1 on ACTH secretion in the rat: is it modulated by prostaglandins? Endocrinology 1991; 129: 384–388.

Robins LN, Regier DA, eds. Psychiatric disorders in America: the epidemiologic catchment area study. New York: The Free Press, 1991.

Rosenblum ER, Gavaaler JS, van Thiel DH. Lipid peroxidation: a mechanism for alcohol-induced testicular injury. Free Radic Biol Med 1989; 7: 569–577.

Roy A, Virkkunen M, Linnoila M. Reduced serotonin turnover in a subgroup of alcoholics? Prog Neuropsychopharmacol Biol Psychiatry 1987; 43: 315–319.

Roy A, Adinoff B, Linnoila M. Acting out hostility in normal volunteers: negative correlation with levels of 5-HIAA in cerebral spinal fluid. Psychiatry Res 1988; 24: 187–194.

Roy A, Virkkunen M, Linnoila M. Serotonin in suicide, violence, and alcoholism. In: Coccaro E, Murphy P, eds. Serotonin in major psychiatric disorders. Washington: American Psychiatric Association, 1991: 187–208.

Rulka CA, Hamm MW. Dietary fat and the β-adrenergic mediated chronotropic response in the rat. J Nutr 1988; 118: 1304–1310.

Salem N Jr. Omega-3 fatty acids: molecular and biochemical aspects. In: Spiller G, Scala J, eds. New protective roles of selected nutrients in human nutrition. New York: Alan R. Liss, 1989: 109–228.

Salem N Jr, Niebylski CD. The nervous system has an absolute molecular species requirement for proper function. Mol Membr Biol 1995; 12: 131–134.

Salem N, Ward G. The effects of ethanol on polyunsaturated fatty acid composition. In: Alling C, Diamond I, Leslie SW, Sun GY, Wood WG, eds. Alcohol, cell membranes, and signal induction in brain. New York: Plenum Press, 1993: 33–46.

Salem N, Kim HY, Yergey JA. Docosahexaenoic acid: membrane function and metabolism. In: Simopoulos A, Kifer RR, Martin R, eds. Health effects of polyunsaturated fatty acids in seafoods. Vol. 15. New York: Academic Press, 1986: 263–317.

Salem N, Wegher B, Mena P, Uauy R. Arachidonic and docosahexaenoic acids are biosynthesized from their 18-carbon precursors in human infants. Proc Natl Acad Sci USA 1996; 93: 49–54.

Sapolsky R, Rivier C, Yamamoto G, Plotsky P, Vale W. Interleukin-1 stimulates the secretion of hypothalamic corticotrophin releasing factor. Science 1987; 238: 522–524.

Sarai K. The epidemiology of the depressive state. Seichinshinkeishi 1979; 81: 777–853.

Schubert DSO, Foliart RH. Increased depression in multiple sclerosis patients, a meta-analysis. Psychosomatics 1993; 34: 124–130.

Schuckit MA. Genetic and clinical implications of alcoholism and affective disorders. Am J Psychiatry 1986; 143: 140–147.

Seigman AW, Smith TW, eds. Anger, hostility and the heart. Hilldale: Lawrence Erlbaum, 1994.

Semafuco WEB, Rutledge CO, Dixon WR. Modulation of adrenergic neurotransmission in the rat tail artery by dietary lipids. J Cardiovasc Pharmacol 1989; 13: 138–145.

Sengupta N, Datta SC, Sengupta D. Platelet and erythrocyte membrane lipid and phospholipid patterns in different types of mental patients. Biochem Med 1981; 25: 267–275.

Shintani F, Kanba S, Nakaki T et al. Interleukin 1-b augments release of norepinephrine, dopamine and serotonin in the rat anterior hypothalamus. J Neurosci 1993; 13: 3574–3581.

Siguel EN, Lerman RH. Altered fatty acid metabolism in patients with angiographically documented coronary heart disease. Metabolism 1994; 43: 982–933.

Sigvardsson S, Bohmann M, Cloninger CR. Replication of the Stockholm adoption study of alcoholism. Confirmatory cross-fostering analysis. Arch Gen Psychiatry 1996; 53: 681–687.

Simopoulos AP. Omega-3 fatty acids in health and disease, growth and development. Am J Clin Nutr 1991; 54: 438–463.

Sinclair AJ, O'Dea K. Dunstan G, Ireland PD, Niall M. Effects on plasma lipids and fatty acid composition of very low fat diets enriched with fish or kangaroo meat. Lipids 1987; 22: 53–59.

Sinclair HM. Dietary facts and coronary heart disease. Lancet 1980; i: 414–415.

Smith RS. The macrophage theory of depression. Med Hypotheses 1991; 35: 298–306.

Sosnovskii AS, Tsvetlova MA, Uzunova PI et al. Lipid peroxidation in rats with emotional stress: correlation with open field behaviour. Byull Eksp Biol Med 1992; 113: 19–21.

Sosnovskii AS, Balashova TS, Pirogova GV, Kubatiev AA, Pertsov SS. Activity of antioxidant enzymes in the limbic reticular structures of rat brain after short-term immobilization. Byull Eksp Biol Med 1993; 115: 683–685.

Stanley M, Mann J, Durand G. Increased serotonin-2 binding in frontal cortex of suicide victims. Lancet 1983; i: 214–216.

Stanley M, Traskman-Bendz L, Dorovini-Zis K. Correlations between aminergic metabolites simultaneously obtained from human CSF and brain. Life Sci 1985; 37: 1279–1286.

Stevens LJ, Zentall SS, Deck JL, Abate ML, Lipp SR, Burgess JR. Essential fatty acid metabolism in boys with attention-deficit hyperactivity disorder. Am J Clin Nutr 1995; 62: 761–768.

Storlien L, Jenkins AB, Chisholm DJ, Pascoe WS, Khouri S, Kraegen EW. Influence of dietary fat composition on development of insulin resistance in rats. Relationship to muscle triglyceride and ω-3 fatty acids in muscle phospholipids. Diabetes 1991; 40: 280–289.

Strandberg TE, Raikkonen K, Partinen M et al. Associations of cholesterol lowering by statins with anger and hostility in hypercholesterolemic men. Biol Psychiatry 1994; 35: 575–577.

Stuart S, Couser G, Schilder K, O'Hara MW, Gorman L. Postpartum anxiety and depression: onset and comorbidity in a community sample. J Nerv Ment Dis 1998; 186: 420–424.

Tamaki R, Murata M, Okano T. Risk factors for postpartum depression in Japan. Psychiatry Clin Neurosci 1997; 1: 93–98.

Toffano G, Leon A, Benvegnu D, Boarato E, Azzone GF. Effect of brain cortex phospholipids on the catecholamine content of mouse brain. Pharmacol Res Commun 1976; 8: 581–590.

Uehara A, Sekiya C, Takasugi Y, Namiki M, Arimura A. Anorexia induced by interleukin-1: involvement of corticotrophin-releasing factor. Am J Physiol 1989; 26: R613–R617.

United States Department of Agriculture. Composition of foods: fats and oils. Agriculture handbook No. 8-4. Washington, US: US Department of Agriculture, 1979.

Virkkunen ME, Horrobin DF, Jenkins DK et al. Plasma phospholipids, essential fatty acids and prostaglandins in alcoholic, habitually violent and impulsive offenders. Biol Psychiatry 1987; 22: 1087–1096.

Virkkunen M, Rawlings R, Tokola R et al. CSF biochemistries, glucose metabolism, and diurnal activity rhythms in alcoholic violent offenders, fire setters, and healthy volunteers. Arch Gen Psychiatry 1994a; 51: 20–27.

Virkkunen M, Kallio E, Rawlings R et al. Personality profiles and state aggressiveness in Finish alcoholic, violent offenders, fire setters and healthy volunteers. Arch Gen Psychiatry 1994b; 51: 28–33.

Weidner G, Connor SL, Hollis JF. Improvements in hostility and depression in relation to dietary change and cholesterol lowering. Ann Intern Med 1992; 117: 820–823.

Weisman MM, Bland RC, Canino GJ et al. Crossnational epidemiology of major depression and bipolar disorder. JAMA 1996; 276: 293–299.

Weissman MW. The treatment of depressive symptoms secondary to alcoholism, opiate addiction and schizophrenia: evidence for the efficacy of tricyclics. In: Clayton PJ, Barret JE, eds. Treatment of depression: old controversies and new approaches. New York: Raven Press, 1983: 207–216.

Wickberg B, Hwang CP. Screening for post-natal depression in a population based Swedish sample. Acta Psychiatr Scand 1997; 95: 62–66.

Wilson R, Tocher DR. Lipid and fatty acid composition is altered in plaque tissue from multiple sclerosis brain compared with normal white brain matter. Lipids 1991; 26: 9–12.

Winokur G. The concept of secondary depression and its relationship to comorbidity. Psychiatr Clin North Am 1990; 13: 567–583.

Winokur A, Maislin G, Phillips JL, Amsterdam JD. Insulin resistance after oral glucose tolerance testing in patients with major depression. Am J Psychiatry 1988; 145: 325–330.

World Health Organisation. Fish and Fishery products. World apparent consumption based on food balance sheets (1961–1993) FAO Fisheries Circular No. 821 rev 3. Rome, Italy: Food and Agriculture Organization, 1996.

Yorek M, Leeney E, Dunlap J, Ginsberg B. Effect of fatty acid composition on insulin and IGF-1 binding in retinoblastoma cells. Invest Ophthalmol Vis Sci 1989; 30: 2087–2092.

Yoshida K, Marks MN, Kibe N, Kumar R, Nakano H, Tashiro N. Postnatal depression in Japanese women who have given birth in England. J Affective Disord 1997; 43: 69–77.

Zale CF, New AS, Trestman RL et al. Serum cholesterol and impulsive aggressive behavior in personality disorder patients. Paper presented at the American Psychiatric Association Annual Meeting, New York, 4–9 May, 1996.

Zung WWK. Depression in the normal aged. Psychosomatics 1967; 8: 287–292.

Essential Fatty Acid Intake in Relation to Depression

20

Rhian W. Edwards and Malcolm Peet

INTRODUCTION

The causal basis of major depression still remains elusive, despite the tremendous amount of research in this area. Biochemical, genetic and psychosocial factors have all been put forward as being involved in the pathogenesis of depression. However, each proposal is associated with limitations, including patient heterogeneity, problems in classifying major depression, and differences in laboratory assay techniques used to assess biological markers of depression. This has resulted in conflicting data and there is no unequivocal evidence-based theory of the aetiology of major depression.

Nevertheless, because of the effectiveness of antidepressants, which modulate primarily the serotonergic and adrenergic neurotransmitter systems of the brain, the most widely accepted concept of the cause of depression is biochemical, proposing that the neurotransmitter systems of the brain are dysfunctional. In particular, the biochemical evidence suggests that depletion of serotonin and noradrenaline may lead to depression (Heninger et al., 1996). Though the reasons for these depletions remain elusive, there is increasing evidence suggesting that they may be due to dysfunctions of pre- and postsynaptic receptors, G-proteins or secondary messenger systems. As supported by Noponen et al. (1993) and Bourin and Baker (1996), neurotransmitter function and regulation depends upon membrane receptors, which are, in turn, linked to G-protein and secondary messenger systems. The question still remains as to what causes the initial dysfunctions of the pre- and postsynaptic receptors, G-proteins or secondary messenger systems.

In this chapter it is proposed that abnormalities in the lipid composition of neurones may be responsible for the dysfunctions of neurotransmitter systems associated with major depression, and that the membrane lipid hypothesis of depression can bring together and support the other theories of the causes of depression. It is suggested how the biological theories could be linked to environmental and psychosocial theories of the cause of depression.

THE RELEVANCE OF LIPIDS TO PSYCHIATRY

There are three main reasons for considering the possibility that lipid abnormalities may be important in the pathogenesis of depression. First, membrane lipids participate directly in the structure and hence the function of cells (Bourre et al. 1989; Reisbick et al., 1990; Salem and Niebylski; 1995; Litman and Mitchell; 1996; Horrobin, 1997). Second, lipid derivatives not only regulate the activity of many enzymes and secondary messengers in neurones, but form many of the secondary messengers and play an important role in gene expression and hence protein synthesis (Zidovetski and Lester, 1992; Tanaka and Nishizuka, 1994; Horrobin, 1997). Third, neurones forming the brain, the spinal cord, and the peripheral nerves contain the highest concentration of lipids after adipose tissue (Bourre et al., 1989). However, unlike adipose tissue, the major components of neuronal membrane, especially in the brain, are structural phospholipids (Innis, 1993) which therefore play a major role in the function of the neurone.

NEURONAL MEMBRANE COMPOSITION AND ITS FUNCTIONAL IMPORTANCE

Brain phospholipids are especially rich in docosahexaenoic acid (DHA), an ω-3 essential fatty acid (EFA) and arachidonic acid (AA), an ω-6 EFA. Both ω-3 and ω-6 polyunsaturated fatty acids (PUFAs) are regarded as EFAs because their parent fatty acids, namely α-linolenic acid (ALA) and linoleic acid (LA), respectively, can be derived only from the diet (Garrow and James, 1993; Salem and Niebylski, 1995) and cannot be synthesized within the body.

Although AA is evenly distributed throughout mammalian tissue, DHA is highly concentrated only in the brain, retina and sperm, i.e., in cells that are highly metabolically active and whose functions involve the transfer of chemical information (Salem, 1989; Reisbick et al., 1990; Salem and Niebylski, 1995). DHA is thus regarded as a crucial structural component of the nervous system (Reisbick et al., 1990; Christensen and Hoy, 1997). The main effect of DHA is to increase fluidity (Bourre et al., 1989; Su et al., 1996). As a whole, however, ω-3 EFAs are reported to allow optimal function of the neurone membrane, by affecting membrane fusion (Sterner et al., 1985), increasing the fluidity of the membrane (Conroy et al., 1986), or by influencing protein interactions with either each other or the cell membrane (Hu et al., 1988; Stubbs, 1992). The composition, and hence fluidity, of the membrane therefore seems to be crucial in normal cellular functions.

Further evidence to support the importance of DHA for normal cell membrane function stems from the effects of cell membrane deficiencies of DHA. Deficiency of ω-3 DHA, especially, leads to behavioural changes in monkeys, such as polydipsia, aggression and isolation (Reisbick et al., 1994). Differences in performance on learning tasks in rats have also been found (Wainwright, 1992). Preterm infants receiving DHA supplementation or breast milk (which is high in ω-3 EFAs, especially DHA), have scored better on intelligence and development scales than infants fed on formula feeds, which are deficient in these PUFAs (Wainwright, 1992).

In addition, the crucial role of DHA in normal neuronal function is shown by the debilitating effects of Zellweger syndrome and other disorders of peroxisomal biogenesis. Zellweger syndrome, which has its onset in foetal life and which is more prevalent in early life, is characterized by feeble foetal activity; after birth (breech presentation is very common) there is marked generalized hypotonia (poor or absent Moro reflex); respiratory problems, failure to thrive, vomiting, mental retardation, variable seizures and visual impairment also occur (Magalini and Magalini, 1997). In these disorders, a profound deficiency of DHA exists and supplementation with DHA has been found to result in a significant improvement in the symptoms (Martinez, 1996).

Although these studies have some limitations, they consistently show that ω-3 EFAs, especially the longer chain ω-3 EFAs such as eicosapentaenoic acid (EPA) and DHA, are essential to normal membrane function. Given the effects that the ω-3 EFAs, especially DHA, have on neuronal cell function, it is not implausible to consider that disorders of the lipid membrane may play a role in the aetiology and pathogenesis of depression.

LIPID HYPOTHESIS OF MAJOR DEPRESSION

The lipid hypothesis of major depression postulates that reduced membrane fluidity, due to a depletion of DHA, results in membrane dysfunction (Smith, 1991; Hibbeln and Salem, 1995). The composition and hence fluidity of the membrane seems to be crucial in normal cellular functions, e.g., in receptor function, ion channel function, production of secondary messengers, enzyme activity, signal transmission, gene expression and secretion of neurotransmitters (Menon and Dhopeshwarkar, 1982; Clamp et al., 1997).

Relationship to 'orthodox' hypotheses of major depression

The mechanisms by which reduced membrane fluidity, or depletions in DHA, can potentially affect the biological processes that are implicated in major depression are described below.

Neurotransmitter receptors

The cell membrane lipid composition has been shown to regulate both neurotransmitter and hormone receptors (Loh and Law, 1980). Synaptic receptors of neural membranes are intrinsic proteins and are embedded in the lipid cell membrane (Stockert et al., 1992). Membranes that are rich in DHA are more fluid or destabilized (Stubbs, 1992). This fluidity allows the membrane to contract and expand with a minimal input of energy (Holte et al., 1996) thus enabling efficient membrane protein or receptor function (Stubbs, 1992). Increased fluidity of the membrane affects receptor function (Pelitz et al., 1991) by allowing protein or receptor conformational changes to occur more efficiently (Stubbs, 1992). Therefore, a change in the neuronal membrane fluidity will concomitantly affect the responsiveness of the receptor, which will impact upon cellular activity and function (Clandinin et al., 1992).

Diets chronically deficient in ALA, the precursor of DHA, were found to affect the dopaminergic and serotoninergic neurotransmission systems in the frontal cortex of male rats (Delion et al., 1996). Davidson et al. (1988) found that a deficiency of post-δ6-desaturation ω-3 and ω-6 EFAs attenuated the sensitivity of the function of presynaptic dopamine autoreceptors.

It is a widely accepted hypothesis that deficient cerebral monaminergic neurotransmitters play a pivotal role in depression (Westenburg, 1997). Bovine hypothalamic phospholipids (rich in DHA) were found to activate aminergic pathways *in vivo* and *in vitro* (Bruni et al. 1976; Leon and Toffano, 1976). Indeed, alterations in pre- and postsynaptic receptor function, neurotransmitter turnover rate, and alterations in cell firing, as a result of phospholipid administration, have accompanied changes in monoaminergic neurones after a prolonged antidepressant treatment (Drago et al., 1985). Preparations of bovine hypothalamic phospholipids potentiated the inhibitory effect of all antidepressant drugs in a despair test administered to male rats (Drago et al., 1985). The phospholipids also significantly reduced the latency between the administration of antidepressants and their effects (Casacchia et al., 1982; Drago et al., 1985). In a double-blind study (Casacchia et al., 1982), 26 depressed patients treated with 75 mg/day of clomipramine were supplemented with either 200 mg/day of phospholipids or 500 ml/day of isotonic saline solution for 21 days. Although the end-scores of the Hamilton Rating Scale (HAM-D) were not significantly different between the patients treated with phospholipids and those receiving only saline, the onset of action of the antidepressant seemed to be more rapid in the group supplemented with phospholipids, as by the seventh day of therapy the HRS scores were significantly lower in this treatment group than in saline-treated patients.

G-proteins

G-proteins play critical roles in the regulation of neuronal function (Manji, 1992; Lesch and Manji, 1992). Abnormalities in G-protein function, leading to dysfunctional transduction mechanisms, have been proposed in the pathophysiology of depression (Manji, 1992; Bourin and Baker, 1996). A number of studies have shown G-protein activity to be attenuated in major depression and that antidepressants stimulate G-protein activity (Ozawa and Rasenick, 1989; Chen and Rasenick, 1995). However, in a later study Young et al. (1996) could not replicate this finding. In bipolar depression, lithium was found to attenuate G-protein function (Avissar and Schreiber, 1992).

The activity of G-proteins has been found to be affected by the level of membrane fluidity or the levels of DHA in membrane phospholipids (Litman and Mitchell, 1996). Further, Litman and Mitchell (1996) discovered that more DHA in retinal tissue resulted in greater levels of production of the G-protein-activated photointermediate of rhodopsin, metarhodopsin II. Conversely, adding cholesterol, and thus reducing the fluidity of the membrane, resulted in a reduction of the amount of metarhodopsin II formed (Litman and Mitchell, 1996). Therefore, the evidence seems to suggest that reduced membrane fluidity may be associated with depression *via* its affects on G-protein function, and that G-protein dysfunction may be implicated in the pathogenesis of depression.

Secondary messengers and protein kinases

Secondary messengers and protein kinases are of major importance in signal transduction from outside the cell membrane receptors to the interior of the cell where they affect protein functions and gene expression (Clandinin et al., 1992; Slater et al., 1996). Their normal function is dependent on the composition of the neuronal synaptic membrane (Clandinin et al., 1992).

In particular, protein kinase C (PKC) activity may be implicated in the pathogenesis of depression. Recent evidence from animal studies suggests that protein kinases may be involved in neuroadaptive mechanisms occurring in the brain after repeated administration of antidepressants (Li and Hrdina, 1997). However, there is no consensus regarding how antidepressants affect PKC activity. Some evidence suggests that antidepressants (fluoxetine and desipramine) reduce PKC activity of rat brain synaptosomes (Mann et al., 1995), while other data suggest that PKC activity after antidepressants is not different from that of controls (Li and Hrdina, 1997).

Despite this lack of consensus concerning the effect of antidepressants upon the activity of PKC, the composition of the cell membrane plays an obligatory role in PKC activation (Zidovetski and Lester, 1992; Slater et al., 1996). Many kinases also interact with the cell membrane as part of the signal transduction process (Slater et al., 1996). In addition, the activities of protein kinases have been found to be affected by G-proteins through the products of the secondary messenger effector enzymes (Avissar and Schreiber, 1992), all of which are affected by the fluidity of the phospholipid bilayer (Litman and Mitchell, 1996). Hence, not only is the interaction with the membrane lipid-dependent, but it is also dependent upon the membrane lipid composition (Slater et al., 1996).

Further evidence of the importance of the fatty acid composition of cell membranes stems from studies of phosphatidylserine (PS), which is believed to be a prominent mediator of the interactions of protein kinases with the cell membrane (Slater et al., 1996), and contains high levels of DHA (Litman and Mitchell, 1996).

Red cell membrane EFAs and diet in depressive patients

The evidence presented above seems to indicate that neuronal membrane composition, especially in terms of its DHA content, affects a number of processes that are implicated in the cause of major depression. Although the evidence is circumstantial and indirect, the body of evidence seems to point to a disorder of synaptic membranes associated with reduced fluidity dysfunction due to a depletion of DHA. This biological evidence is supported by epidemiological data and a small number of clinical studies.

There is epidemiological evidence that diet may be a contributory factor to depression (Smith, 1991). There has been a substantial increase in the lifetime risk for major depression during this century (Cross-National Collaborative Group, 1992). The swiftness of this dramatic increase in the prevalence of depression suggests that an environmental factor is involved. Smith (1991) and Hibbeln and Salem (1995) hypothesized that the sharp rise in depression is due to increased consumption of ω-6 EFAs at the expense of ω-3 EFAs. This shift in diet is supported by Taylor et al. (1979), Rice (1984), Eaton and Konner (1985) and Leaf and Weber (1987). Indeed, compared to America and North Western Europe, where the ω-6:ω-3 EFA ratio is high, countries that have a high ω-3 intake, such as Japan, China and Taiwan have been found to have substantially lower rates of depression (Smith, 1991; Hibbeln and Salem, 1995; Hibbeln, 1998). This seems to suggest that a diet low in ω-3 EFAs is a risk factor for depression.

The epidemiological observations are also supported by recent clinical studies, which have also reported that major depression is associated with a deficiency of ω-3 fatty acids, in particular DHA. Despite lacking a control group and using a relatively crude method to assess dietary intake, Adams et al. (1996) reported that the AA:EPA ratio in plasma and red blood cell (RBC) membrane phospholipids, correlated positively with the severity of depression. Maes et al. (1996) reported a significant decrease of total ω-3 EFAs, and also reduced ALA and EPA in serum cholesterol esters, in major depressed patients compared to those with minor depression or healthy controls; they also found a significant increase of the ratio of AA to EPA in both cholesterol esters and phospholipids in the major depressives. Peet et al. (1998) also reported a significant depletion of total ω-3 EFAs, particularly DHA in the RBC membranes of drug-free depressives. However, this study did not fully control for possible confounding factors, such as stress, smoking habits, and dietary intake. More recently, in a Japanese study consisting of 47 elderly patients (Seko et al., 1997), significant negative correlations between RBC membrane ω-3 EFA levels and depression were found; in addition, the AA:EPA ratio of the serum and RBC membranes also showed a positive correlation with the severity of depression.

Supplementation with ω-3 EFAs has been found to affect human emotional state. In a 4-month double-blind, placebo-controlled trial, Stoll et al. (1997) found that, after supplementation with 9 g/day of ω-3 EFAs, bipolar depressives had a significantly longer period of remission compared to a placebo group. In another 3-month double-blind placebo-controlled trial, supplementation with 1.5 g/day of DHA stabilized aggression levels and prevented enhancement of aggression at times of mental stress (Hamazaki et al., 1996). These studies provide further support for the hypothesis that ω-3 EFAs modulate human emotional state.

While two earlier studies reported elevated levels of ω-3 EFAs in serum phospholipids of depressed people (Ellis and Sanders, 1977; Fehiley et al., 1981), the comparison groups were other psychiatric patients who are known to have very depleted levels of some EFAs (Peet et al., 1995).

In a recent carefully controlled study, Edwards et al. (1998) assessed not only RBC membrane fatty acid levels and correlated these with the severity of depression, but also past and current fatty acid intake and eating habits. 'Past', in this context, refers to the dietary habits or dietary intake consumed at a time when the depressives identified themselves as not feeling depressed, i.e., to their dietary intake or dietary habits prior to the onset of depression. The same point in time was then applied to the nondepressed subjects and used to identify their 'past' diet. 'Current' refers to the dietary intake and dietary habits of the subjects at the time of the study. Past diet history was assessed using a specifically designed and piloted food frequency questionnaire, and current diet was assessed using the 7-day weighed intake method which was validated with a 24-h diet recall.

The 10 depressed subjects, who were receiving antidepressant therapy, were matched with 14 healthy nondepressed controls. The two groups did not differ significantly in mean age, or in the distribution of sexes and membership of different social classes; in addition there were no differences between the groups in the distribution of a number of factors that have been proposed as modulators of ω-3 EFA levels, including body mass index, life events, smoking habits, alcohol intake and the number of children.

ω-3 EFAs, in particular DHA, were found to be significantly lower in the RBC membranes of depressives compared to controls (Table 20.1). Although not significantly different, the past and current dietary ω-3 EFA intake was lower in the depressives than in the controls, with no significant differences in energy intake (see Table 20.1). The RBC membrane fatty acid levels and the current dietary fatty acid levels were then correlated with the Beck Depression Inventory scores (Beck et al., 1981), which is a measure of the severity of depression. As shown in Table 20.2, significant negative correlations between both RBC membrane ω-3 EFA levels and current dietary intake of ω-3 EFA, and the Beck Depression Inventory scores were found only for the ω-3 EFA series. None of the ω-6 EFA series showed a significant correlation with the Beck Depression Inventory score. These correlations support the relationship between dietary intake and RBC membrane ω-3 EFA levels and depression.

As shown in Table 20.3, significant correlations were found between current ALA intake and the RBC membrane levels of EPA and DHA (Edwards et al., 1998), adding further evidence that dietary intake affects the fatty acid composition of the cell membranes.

Table 20.1. ω-3 PUFA levels in depressed patients and control subjects, in red cell membranes (expressed as mg/100 mg total phospholipid, and in the current diet (measured using the 7-day weighed intake method and expressed as mg/100 g absolute total energy intake [ATE] per day)[a]; means ± SEM.

PUFAs	Patients	Controls
RBC membranes		
18:3n-3	0.09 ± 0.03	0.12 ± 0.02
20:5n-3	0.52 ± 0.07*	0.73 ± 0.05
22:5n-3	1.52 ± 0.28*	2.03 ± 0.09
22:6n-3	3.25 ± 0.60*	4.72 ± 0.29
Total n-3	5.39 ± 0.93*	7.60 ± 0.38
Current diet[b]		
18:3n-3	1034.9 ± 100.4	1363.4 ± 100.7
20:5n-3	82.3 ± 23.2	140.3 ± 35.7
22:5n-3	55.7 ± 15.3	77.1 ± 11.8
22:6n-3	141.4 ± 38.5	210.7 ± 52.2
Total n-3	1331 ± 143.3	1807.7 ± 212.2

[a] Absolute total energy (ATE) intake: patients, 9153.73 ± 769.44 kJ; controls, 8478.21 ± 584.75 kJ (difference nonsignificant).
[b] Past dietary intake is not shown, as there were no significant differences between past and current intake on any PUFA. *In comparison with the corresponding value for control subjects, $p < 0.05$ (Student's t test); other differences are statistically nonsignificant.

Table 20.2. Correlations (Pearson's product-moment correlation coefficient) between Beck Depression Inventory scores in depressed patients, and PUFA levels in red cell membranes (mg/100 mg total phospholipid) and in the current diet (measured using the 7-day weighed intake method, and mg/100 g ATE/day)[a].

PUFAs	r
RBC membranes	
18:3n-3	−0.81**
20:5n-3	−0.33
22:5n-3	−0.64 [§]
22:6n-3	−0.80**
Total n-3	−0.75*
Current diet[b]	
18:3n-3	−0.83***
20:5n-3	−0.38
22:5n-3	−0.16
22:6n-3	−0.27
Total n-3	−0.75**

[a] Correlation between Beck Depression Inventory score and ATE, $r = +0.02$ (nonsignificant). $p <$: *0.05; **0.01; ***0.005.
[§] $0.1 > p > 0.05$ (borderline significance).

The eating habits of depressed patients

The eating habits of the depressed subjects differed from those of the nondepressed subjects. As expected, all the depressed subjects reported that their eating habits and diet had changed since the onset of their depression. Thus, the current diet and eating habits of the depressives were not the same as their past intake and habits.

Although medicated with antidepressants, the depressive cases felt unenthusiastic, unmotivated, apathetic and tired. These symptoms of depression were reflected in the current eating habits of the depressives in that they tended to eat more convenience and snack foods. When snacking was categorized as either up to three snacks per week or more than four snacks per week, the depressed patients were found to eat significantly more snacks than were eaten by the nondepressed control subjects ($p < 0.05$; Fisher's exact probability test).

Another interesting factor in relation to the consumption of snacks was that there was no significant difference between the past and current consumption of snacks within the depressive subjects, despite the significant difference between the depressives and nondepressives in the current consumption of snacks,

Table 20.3. Statistically significant correlations (Pearson's product-moment correlation coefficient) between dietary intake[a] of PUFAs and RBC membrane[b] PUFAs in depressed patients and control subjects.

Dietary PUFA	RBC PUFA	r
Depressed patients		
18:3n-3	18:3n-3	+0.70*
	20:5n-3	+0.71*
	22:5n-3	+0.76***
	22:6n-3	+0.81**
	Total n-3	+0.82**
Total n-3	AA:DHA	−0.84***
	Total n-6:total n-3	−0.69*
18:3n-6	18:3n-3	+0.68*
	AA:DHA	−0.68*
22:5n-6	AA:DHA	−0.69*
AA:EPA	22:5n-6	+0.81**
	AA:EPA	+0.75*
AA:DHA	22:5n-6	+0.70*
Total n-6:total n-3	AA:EPA	+0.78*
	AA:DHA	+0.70*
Control subjects		
22:5n-3	18:3n-3	+0.68**
22:6n-3	22:5n-3	+0.56*
20:3n-6	22:5n-3	+0.55*
	22:4n-6	+0.55*
	AA:EPA	+0.54*

[a] Measured using the 7-day weighed intake method, and expressed as mg/100 g ATE/day; [b] expressed as mg/100 mg total phospholipid. $p <$: *0.05; **0.01; ***0.005.

Table 20.4. Estimated current absolute nutrient intake, cholesterol intake, ATE, and total n6:total n3 ratio, in depressed patients ($n = 10$) and nondepressed control subjects ($n = 14$); means ± SEM.

Intake parameter	Depressed patients	Control subjects
Fat (% ATE[a])	30.75 ± 1.86	34.14 ± 1.84
Carbohydrate (% ATE)	50.94 ± 2.42	48.10 ± 2.10
Protein (% ATE)	14.41 ± 2.98	14.81 ± 0.70
Cholesterol (mg/g)	201.20 ± 26.59	241.60 ± 27.80
ATE (kJ)	9153.90 ± 769.44	8478.60 ± 594.75
Total n6:total n3	9.98 ± 2.25	6.34 ± 0.77

indicating that prior to their onset of depression, the depressed subjects generally ate more snacks than the nondepressed subjects.

The depressed subjects also reported eating more cold or uncooked foods after the onset of their depression: such foods require little or no preparation. Examples of such foods were confectionery, crisps, cereals, sandwiches, milk, cheese, yoghurts and ice cream. As the current dietary assessment was conducted in the summer, fruit and vegetables were also popular with the depressed patients. Snack foods (other than fruit and vegetables) are high in cholesterol, saturated, *trans-* and ω-6 fatty acids and are also a rich source of carbohydrates.

Nevertheless, despite this greater consumption of snack foods, and in contrast to what was expected, the results of the current 7-day weighed intake revealed that the depressives' current dietary intake appeared relatively healthy. As can be seen from Table 20.4, the depressed subjects consumed more energy, and carbohydrates, and less fat, protein and cholesterol, than the controls, though the differences were not statistically significant. The dietary ω-6:ω-3 total EFA ratio was also higher in the depressive group, though again the difference failed to attain statistical significance.

DIETARY DEFICIENCY AS AN EXPLANATORY PRINCIPLE IN DEPRESSION

We have reviewed the essential role that DHA plays in maintaining cell membrane fluidity and hence optimum cell function. Lower levels of cell membrane DHA seem to modulate the activity of the many factors implicated in the aetiology and pathogenesis of depression. Compared to healthy controls, depressives have been found to have significantly reduced levels of DHA, and ω-3 EFAs in general, in their red cell membranes. Further, there are significant correlations between both dietary ω-3 intake and RBC membrane ω-3 levels, and severity of depression. Despite these findings, it remains unclear how this deficiency of DHA occurs in depressives and, indeed, whether it is a cause or an effect of depression. A recent report of therapeutic benefit from ω-3 supplementation in unstable manic-depressive patients (Stoll et al., 1997) gives support to the hypothesis that ω-3 depletion may be a cause rather than an effect of depression. However, metabolic abnormalities of lipid metabolism affecting the incorporation of breakdown EFAs cannot be excluded.

DIETARY DEFICIENCY OF ω-3 EFAs AND CHRONIC PHYSICAL DISEASES

Further evidence to support the role of a high ω-6: ω-3 dietary ratio, hence DHA depletion, as a causative factor in depression relates to the relationship between depression and physical illnesses such as diabetes, coronary heart disease and hypertension. This has recently been reviewed by Peet and Edwards (1997).

Non-insulin-dependent diabetes mellitus

An association between depression and non-insulin-dependent diabetes mellitus (NIDDM) is recognized. It has been observed repeatedly that depressive patients show relative insulin resistance (Eaton et al., 1996; Storlien et al., 1996). Nine out of ten controlled studies have shown an association between depression and NIDDM (Jonas et al. 1997; Appel et al., 1993; Gavard et al., 1993).

From prospective data, the odds ratio for developing NIDDM was found to be 2.23 in people with a previous history of major depression (Eaton et al., 1996). In a 5-year follow-up study, Lustman et al. (1988) reported that, in patients with NIDDM, depression preceded the development of diabetes, while in IDDM diabetes precedes the depression.

Certain types of antidepressants, particularly the selective serotonin reuptake inhibitors (SSRIs), have been found to improve fasting blood sugar levels in laboratory and clinical studies (Goodnick et al., 1997). Another form of treatment in severe depression is electro-convulsive therapy (ECT). Except for a small earlier study (Schalch, 1967), ECT has also been found either to treat or to ameliorate NIDDM (Fakhri et al., 1980; Thomas et al., 1983; Finestone and Weiner, 1984; Nutt et al., 1988; Williams et al., 1992).

Insulin resistance, or the relative failure of insulin action and associated hyperinsulaemia, observed in depressed subjects, may be due to receptor insensitivity. This could suggest that NIDDM, like depression, is associated with cell membrane dysfunctions as a result of a deficiency of DHA in cell membranes. Indeed, supplementation with DHA has been found to ameliorate type-2 diabetes (Sullivan et al., 1990; Ikemoto et al., 1996; Storlien et al., 1996; Shimura et al., 1997). Further, decreased skeletal muscle concentration of DHA and docosapentaenoic acid are highly correlated ($r = +0.97$) with higher insulin receptor insensitivity (Storlien et al., 1991).

Thus, the membrane lipid abnormalities found in depression (Adams et al., 1996; Maes et al., 1996, Peet et al., 1998; Edwards et al., 1998) seem to mirror those which cause insulin resistance, i.e., high ω-6:ω-3 EFA ratio in the cell membranes with, in particular, low levels of DHA.

Coronary heart disease and hypertension

Low intake of ω-3 EFAs is also a risk factor for coronary heart disease (CHD) (McLennan, 1993; McLennan et al., 1985, 1988; Raheja et al., 1997). Depression has been found to be the strongest psychological predictor of CHD (Booth-Kewley and Friedman, 1987; Pratt et al., 1996). Dietary deficiency of ω-3 EFAs may be an aetiological factor in both depression and CHD.

Several clinical studies have demonstrated a beneficial relationship between ω-3 PUFAs and CHD (Kang and Leaf, 1996). Diets rich in fish and fish oil have been shown to be effective in both primary and secondary prevention of CHD (Burr et al., 1989; de Logneril et al., 1994). One study with a 20-year follow-up showed a 50% reduction in mortality from CHD in men who consumed at least 30 g of fish per day (Kromhout et al., 1985). Another showed that advice to eat fatty fish led to a 29% reduction in mortality in the two years following myocardial infarction (Burr et al., 1989). In the experimental group, who were receiving ω-3 EFAs, de Logneril et al. (1994) found a 70% reduction in cardiovascular deaths. Further, a low prevalence of cardiovascular disease has been observed in Greenland Eskimos who consume a diet high in ω-3 EFAs (Bang and Dyerberg, 1972, 1979; Dyerberg et al., 1975; Dyerberg and Bang, 1979).

Hypertension is an important risk factor for CHD (Bradlow, 1986). Given the well-established relationship between depression and CHD, it does not seem implausible that a relationship between depression and hypertension may exist. Indeed, Jonas et al. (1997) discovered a relationship between anxiety and depression and subsequent hypertension. In this prospective study, normotensive subjects ($n = 2992$) were rated for depression and anxiety and screened 9 years later for hypertension. After other risk factors, such as smoking and alcohol use had been taken into account, both anxiety and depression (with relative risks of 1.82 and 1.80, respectively) remained as independent predictors of hypertension.

As in depression, NIDDM, and CHD, the same dietary risk factors seem to play a role in the development of hypertension. The ω-3 EFAs have been reported to have an ameliorative effect upon hypertension. A number of studies have found that supplementation with ω-3 EFAs reduces blood pressure (Appel et al., 1993). A meta-analysis conducted by Appel et al. (1993) of 17 controlled trials (13 with a trial duration of less than 3 months) showed that supplementation with ω-3

EFAs (average dose >3 g/day) led to significant reductions in blood pressure in untreated hypertension. Of the six studies of untreated hypertension ($n = 291$), two found significant reductions in systolic blood pressure (mean reduction −5.5 mmHg) and four recorded significant reductions in diastolic blood pressure (mean reduction −3.5 mmHg) (Singer et al., 1986; Knapp and Fitzgerald, 1989; Meland et al., 1989; Bonaa et al., 1990; Levinson et al., 1990; Radack et al., 1991).

CONCLUSIONS

The lipid hypothesis of depression is a unifying concept for understanding the aetiology and the pathogenesis of depression, as well as other chronic diseases faced by westernized societies, namely, NIDDM, CHD and hypertension. The lipid hypothesis is based on one central observation that ω-3 EFAs, and particularly DHA, play a crucial role in cellular function. Depletions of cell membrane ω-3 EFAs lead to cellular dysfunctions. It has been put forward in this chapter that these cellular dysfunctions give rise to depression, NIDDM, CHD and hypertension. Also, evidence has been put forward that depression is not only related to these diseases but actually precedes them. Nevertheless, although preliminary studies do support the hypothesis, many unanswered questions remain. The hypothesis has substantial implications for the treatment of depression and the possible prevention of subsequent associated physical illnesses.

REFERENCES

Adams PB, Lawson S, Sanigorski A, Sinclair AJ. Arachidonic acid to eicosapentanoic acid ratio in blood correlates positively with clinical symptoms of depression. Lipids 1996; 31 (Suppl): S157–S161.

Appel LJ, Miller ER, Seidler AJ, Whelton PK. Does supplementation of diet with fish oil reduce blood pressure? A meta-analysis of controlled clinical trials. Arch Intern Med 1993; 153: 429–438.

Avissar R, Schreiber G. The involvement of guanine nucleotide binding G-proteins in the pathogenesis and treatment of affective disorders. Biol Psychiatry 1992; 31: 435–459.

Bang HO, Dyerberg J. Plasma lipids and lipoproteins in Greenlandic west coast Eskimos. Acta Med Scand 1972; 192: 85–94.

Bang HO, Dyerberg J. Lipid metabolism, atherogenesis, and haemostasis in Eskimos: the role of the prostaglandin-3 family. Haemostasis 1979; 8: 227–233.

Beck AT, Ward CH, Mendelson M, Mock J, Erbaugh J. An inventory for measuring depression. Arch Gen Psychiatry 1981; 4: 147–150.

Bonaa KH, Bjerve KS, Straume B, Gram IT, Thelle C. Effect of eicosapentaenoic and docosahexaenoic acids on blood pressure in hypertension. N Engl J Med 1990; 322: 795–801.

Booth-Kewley S, Friedman HS. Psychological predictors of heart disease: a quantitative review. Psychol Bull 1987; 101: 343–362.

Bourin M, Baker GB. The future of antidepressants. Biomed Pharmacother 1996; 50: 7–12.

Bourre J-M, Dumont O, Piciotti M, Pascal G, Durand G. Composition of nerve biomembranes and nutritional fatty acids. Nutrition 1989; 5: 266–270.

Bradlow BA. Thrombosis and omega-3 fatty acids: epidemiological and clinical aspects. In: Simopoulos AP, Kifer RR, Martin RE, eds. Health effects of polyunsaturated fatty acids in seafoods. Orlando: Harcourt Brace Jovanovich, 1986: 111–133.

Bruni A, Toffano G, Lenon A, Boarato E. Pharmacological effects of phosphatidylserine liposomes. Nature 1976; 260: 331–333.

Burr ML, Gilbert JF, Holliday RM et al. Effects of changes in fat, fish and fibre intakes on death and myocardial reinfarction: diet and reinfarction trial (DART). Lancet 1989; ii: 757–761.

Casacchia M, Meco G, Pirro R et al. Phospholipid liposomes in depression: a double blind study *versus* placbo. Int Pharmacopsychiatry 1982; 17: 274–279.

Chen J, Rasenick MM. Chronic treatment of C6 glioma cells with antidepressant drugs increases functional coupling between a G-protein (G-s) and adenylyl cyclase. J Neurochem 1995; 64: 727–732.

Christensen MM, Hoy C-E. Early dietary intervention with structured triacylglycerols containing docosahexaenoic acid. Effect on brain, liver and adipose tissue lipids. Lipids 1997; 32: 185–191.

Clamp AG, Ladha S, Clark DC, Grimble RF, Lund EK. The influence of dietary lipids on the composition and membrane fluidity of rat hepatocyte plasma membrane. Lipids 1997; 32: 179–184.

Clandinin MT, Suh M, Hargreaves K. Impact of dietary fatty acid balance on membrane structure and function of neural tissues. In: Bazán NG, Murphy MG, Toffano G, eds. Neurobiology of EFAs: advances in experimental medicine and biology. Vol 318. New York: Plenum Press 1992: 197–210.

Conroy DM, Stubbs CD, Belin J, Pryor CL, Smith AD. The effects of dietary (n-3) fatty acid supplementation on lipid dynamics and composition in rat lymphocytes and liver microsomes. Biochim Biophys Acta 1986; 861: 457–462.

Cross-National Collaborative Group. The changing rate of major depression: cross national comparisons. JAMA 1992; 268: 3098–3105.

Davidson BC, Cantrill RC, Kurstjens NP, Patton J. Polyenoic fatty acid deprivation of juvenile cats modulates ^{3}H-dopamine release from presynaptic receptors in caudate slices. In Vivo 1988; 2: 295–298.

de Logneril M, Renaud S, Mamelle N et al. Mediteranean alpha-linolenic acid-rich diet in secondary prevention of conronary heart disease. Lancet 1994; 143: 1454–1459.

Delion S, Chalon S, Guilloteau D, Besnard JC, Durand G. Alpha-linolenic acid dietary deficiency alters age-related changes of dopaminergic and serotoninergic neurotransmission in the rat frontal cortex. J Neurochem 1996; 66: 1582–1591.

Drago F, Continella G, Mason GA, Hernandez DE, Scapagnini U. Phospholipid liposomes potentiate the inhibitory effect of antidepressant drugs on immobility of rats in a despair test (constrained swim). Eur J Pharmacol 1985; 115: 179–184.

Dyerberg J, Bang HO. Haemostatic function and platelet polyunsaturated fatty acids in Eskimos. Lancet 1979; ii: 433–435.

Dyerberg J, Bang HO, Hjorne N. Fatty acid composition of the plasma lipids in Greenland Eskimos. Am J Clin Nutr 1975; 28: 958–966.

Eaton SB, Konner M. Paleolithic nutrition: a consideration of its nature and current implications. N Engl J Med 1985; 312: 283–289.

Eaton WW, Armenian H, Gallo J. Depression and risk for onset of type II diabetes. Diabetes Care 1996; 19: 1097–1102.

Edwards RhW, Peet M, Shay J, Horrobin D. Omega-3 polyunsaturated fatty acid levels in the diet and in red blood cell membranes of depressed patients. J Affective Disord 1998; 48: 149–155.

Ellis FR, Sanders TAB. Long-chain polyunsaturated fatty acids in endogenous depression. J Neurol Neurosurg Psychiatry 1977; 40: 168–169.

Fakhri O, Fadhli AA, El Rawi RM. Effect of electroconvulsive therapy on diabetes mellitus. Lancet 1980; ii: 775–777.

Fehily AMA, Bowey OAM, Ellis FR, Meade BW, Dickerson JWT. Plasma and erythrocyte membrane long chain polyunsaturated fatty acids in endogenous depression. Neurochem Internat 1981; 3: 37–42.

Finestone DH, Weiner RD. Effects of ECT on diabetes mellitus. Acta Psychiatr Scand 1984; 70: 321–326.

Garrow JS, James WPT. Human nutrition and dietetics. 9th edn, Churchill Livingstone, Edinburgh, 1993.

Gavard J, Lustman PJ, Clouse R. Prevalence of depression in adults with diabetes. Diabetes Care 1993; 16: 1167–1178.

Goodnick PJ, Kumar A, Henry JH, Buki VM, Goldberg RB. Sertraline in coexisting major depression and diabetes mellitus. Psychopharmacol Bull 1997; 33; 2: 261–264.

Hamazaki T, Sawazaki S, Itomura M et al. The effect of docosahexaenoic acid on aggression in young adults: a double-blind study. J Clin Invest 1996; 97: 1129–1133.

Heninger GR, Delgado PL, Charney DS. The revised monoamine theory of depression: a modulator role for monoamines, based on new findings from monoamine depletion experiments in humans. Pharmacopsychiatry 1996; 29: 2–11.

Hibbeln JR. Fish consumption and major depression. Lancet 1998; 351: 1213.

Hibbeln JR, Salem N. Dietary polyunsaturated fatty acidss and depression: when cholesterol does not satisfy. Am J Clin Nutr 1995; 62: 1–9.

Holte LL, Separovic F, Gawrisch K. Nuclear magnetic resonance investigation of hydrocarbon chain packing in bilayers of polyunsaturated phospholipids. Lipids 1996; 31 (Suppl): S199–S203.

Horrobin DF. Fatty acids, phospholipids and schizophrenia. In: Yehuda S, Mostofsky DI, eds. Handbook of EFA biology: biochemistry, physiology and behavioural neurobiology. Hummana Press Inc: Totawa, NJ, 1997: 245–256.

Hu J-S, James G, Olson EN. Protein fatty acylation: a novel mechanism for association of proteins with membranes and its role in transmembrane regulatory pathways. BioFactors 1988; 1: 219–226.

Ikemoto S, Takahashi M, Tsunoda N, Maruyama K, Itakura H, Ezaki O. High-fat diet-induced hypoglycemia and obesity in mice: differential effects of dietary oils. Metabolism 1996; 45: 1539–1546.

Innis SM. Insights into possible mechanisms of essential fatty acid uptake into developing brain from studies of diet, circulating lipids, liver and bran n6 and n3 fatty acids. In: Dobbing J, Benson JD, eds. Lipids, learning and the brain: fats in infant formulas. Report of the 103rd Ross Conference on Paediatric Research. Ross Laboratories: Ohio, 1993: 4–26.

Jonas BS, Franks P, Ingram DD. Are symptoms of anxiety and depression risk factors for hypertension? Longitudinal evidence from the National Health and Nutrition Examination/Epidemiologic follow-up study. Arch Fam Med 1997; 5: 44–48.

Kang JX, Leaf A. The cardiac antiarrhythmic effects of polyunsaturated fatty acid. Lipids 1996; 31: S41–S44.

Knapp HR, Fitzgerald GA. The antihypertensive effects of fish oil: a controlled study of polyunsaturated fatty acid supplements in essential hypertension. N Engl J Med 1989; 320: 1037–1043.

Kromhout D, Bosschieter EB, Coulander C de L. The inverse relation between fish consumtion and 20-year mortality from coronary heart disease. N Engl J Med 1985; 312: 1205–1209.

Leaf A, Weber PC. A new era for science in nutrition. Am J Clin Nutr 1987; 45: 1048–1053.

Leon A, Toffano G. Possible role of BC-PL in enhancing ^{32}P incorporation into mice brain phospholipids. Structural requirements for phospholipids in biological membranes. Adv Exp Med Biol 1976; 72: 307–313.

Lesch KP, Manji HK. Signal-transducing G-proteins and antidepressant drugs: evidence for modulation of alpha subunit gene expression in rat brain. Biol Psychiatry 1992; 32: 549–579.

Levinson PD, Iosiphidis AH, Saritelli AL, Herbert PN, Steiner M. Effects of n-3 fatty acids in essential hypertension. Am J Hypertens 1990; 3: 754–760.

Li Q, Hrdina PD. GAP-43 phosphorylation by PKC in rat cerebrocortical synaptosomes: effect of antidepressants. Res Commun Mol Pathol Pharmacol 1997; 96: 3–13.

Litman BJ, Mitchell DC. A role for phospholipid polyunsaturation in modulating membrane protein function. Lipids 1996; 31 (Suppl): S193–S197.

Loh HH, Law PY. The role of membrane lipids in receptor mechanisms. Annu Rev Pharmacol Toxicol 1980; 20; 201–234.

Lustman PJ, Griffith LS, Clouse RE. Depression in adults with diabetes: results and psychiatric patients. Psychosom Med 1988; 54: 602–611.

Maes M, Smith R, Christophe A, Cosyns P, Desnyder R, Mettzer H. Fatty acid composition in major depression: decreased ω3 fractions in cholesteryl esters and increased C20:4ω6/C20:5ω3 ratio in cholesteryl esters and phospholipids. J Affective Disord 1996; 38: 35–46.

Magalini SI, Magalini SC. Dictionary of medical syndromes. 4th edn. Lippincott-Raven, Philadelphia, 1997.

Manji HK. G-proteins: implications for psychiatry. Am J Psychiatry 1992; 149: 746–760.

Mann CD, Vu TB, Hrdina PD. Protein kinase C in rat brain cortex and hippocampus: effect of repeated administration of fluoxetine and desipramine. Br J Pharmacol 1995; 115: 595–600.

Martinez M. Docosahexaenoic acid therapy in docosahexaenoic acid-deficient patient with disorders of peroximal biogenesis. Lipids 1996; 31 (Suppl): S145–S152.

McLennan PL. Relative effects of dietary saturated, monounsaturated and polyunsaturated fatty acids on cardiac arrhythmias in rats. Am J Clin Nutr 1993; 57: 207–212.

McLennan PL, Abeywardena MY, Charnock JS. Influence of dietary lipids on arrhythmias and infarction after coronary artery ligation in rats. Can J Physiol Pharmacol 1985; 63: 1411–1417.

McLennan PL, Abeywardena MY, Charnock JS. Dietary fish oil prevents ventricular fibrilation following coronary artery occlusion and reperfusion. Am Heart J 1988; 16: 709–717.

Meland E, Fugelli P, Laerum E, Ronneberg R, Sandivk L. Effect of fish oil on blood pressure and blood lipids in men with mild to moderate hypertension. Scand J Prim Health Care Suppl 1989; 7: 131–135.

Menon NK, Dhopeshwarkar GA. Essential fatty acid deficiency and brain development. Prog Lipid Res 1982; 21: 309–326.

Noponen M, Sanfilipo M, Samanich K et al. Elevated PLA$_2$ activity in schizophrenics and other psychiatric patients. Biol Psychiatry 1993; 34: 641–649.

Nutt DJ, Gleiter CH, Linnoila M. Repeated electroconvulsive shock normalizes blood glucose levels in genetically obese mice (C57BL/6J ob/ob) but not in genetically diabetic mice (C57BL/KsJ db/db). Brain Res 1988; 448: 377–380.

Ozawa H, Rasenick MM. Coupling of the stimulatory GTP-binding-protein G-s to rat synaptic membrane adenylate cyclase is enhanced subsequent to chronic antidepressant treatment. Mol Pharmacol 1989; 36: 803–808.

Peet M, Edwards RhW. Lipids, depression and physical diseases. Curr Opin Psychiatry 1997; 10: 477–480.

Peet M, Laugharne JDE, Rangarnjan N, Horrobin DF, Reynolds G. Depleted red cell membrane essential fatty acids in drug-treated schizophrenic patients. J Psychiatr Res 1995; 29: 227–232.

Peet M, Murphy B, Shay J, Horrobin D. Depletion of omega-3 fatty acid levels in red blood cell membranes of depressive patients. Biol Psychiatry 1998; 43: 315–319.

Pelitz JE, Sarasyam N, Chotani M, Saran A, Halaris A. Relationship between membrane fluidity and adrenoreceptor binding in depression. Psychiatry Res 1991; 38: 1–12.

Pratt LA, Ford DE, Crum RM, Armenian HK, Gallo JJ, Eaton WW. Depression, psychotropic medication, and risk of myocardial infarction. Circulation 1996; 94; 3123–3129.

Radack K, Deck C, Huster G. The effects of low doses of n-3 fatty acid supplementation on blood pressure in hypertensive subjects. Arch Intern Med 1991; 151: 1173–1180.

Raheja BS, Bhoraskar AS, Narang SV. Refined cereal high fat urban diet: a major risk factor for diabetes mellitus and coronary heart disease. Are seed oils heart-friendly? J Diabet Assoc India 1997; 37: 1–6.

Reisbick S, Neuringer M, Hasnain R, Connor WE. Polydipsia in rhesus monkeys deficient in omega-3 fatty acids. Physiol Behav 1990; 47: 315–323.

Reisbick S, Neuringer M, Hasnain R, Connor WE. Home cage behavior of rhesus monkeys with long-term deficiency of omega-3 fatty acids. Physiol Behav 1994; 55: 231–239.

Rice RD. The effects of low doses of MaxEPA for long periods. Br J Clin Pract 1984; 38 (Suppl): 85–88.

Salem N Jr. Omega-3 fatty acids: molecular and biochemical aspects. In: Spiller G, Scala J, eds. New protective roles of selected nutrients in human nutrition. New York: Alan R Liss, 1989: 109–228.

Salem N Jr, Niebylski CD. The nervous system has an absolute molecular species requirement for proper function. Mol Membr Biol 1995; 12: 131–134.

Schalch DS. The influence of physical stress and exercise on growth hormone and insulin secretion in man. J Lab Clin Med 1967; 69: 256–269.

Seko C, Ninno N, Nakamura K. Relationship between fatty acid composition in blood and depressive symptoms in the elderly. Jpn J Hyg 1997; 52: 330.

Shimura T, Miura T, Usami M et al. Docosahexaenoic acid (DHA) improved glucose and lipid metabolism in KK-A^y mice with genetic non-insulin-dependent diabetes mellitus (NIDDM). Biol Pharm Bull 1997; 20: 507–510.

Singer P, Berger I, Luck K, Taube C, Naumann E, Godicke W. Long-term effect of mackerel diet on blood pressure, serum lipids and thromboxane formation in patients with mild essential hypertension. Atherosclerosis 1986; 62: 259–265.

Slater SJ, Kelly M, Yeager MD, Larkin J. Polyunsaturation in cell membranes and lipid bilayers and its effects on membrane proteins. Lipids 1996; 31 (Suppl): S189–S192.

Smith RS. The macrophage theory of depression. Med Hypotheses 1991; 35: 298–306.

Sterner DC, Zaks WJ, Creutz CE. Stimulation of the Ca^{2+}-dependent polymerization of synexin by *cis*-unsaturated fatty acids. Biochem Biophys Res Commun 1985; 132: 505–512.

Stockert M, Zieher LM, Medina JH. Interactions of phospholipids and free fatty acids with antidepressant recognition bending sites in rat brain. In: Bazan NG, Murphy MG, Toffano G, eds. Advances in experimental medicine and biology. Vol 318. Neurobiology of essential fatty acids. New York: Plenum Press, 1992.

Stoll AL, Severus E, Marangell L, Freeman MP, Ruster S, Diamond E. Four month, prospective, double-blind, placebo-controlled study comparing the long-term efficacy of omega-3 fatty acids. Poster Presentation, American College of Neuropsychopharmacologist Annual Meeting, Hawaii. December, 1997.

Storlien LH, Jenkins AB, Chisholm DJ, Pascoe WS, Khouri S, Kreagen EW. Influence of dietary fat composition on development of insulin resistance in rats. Relationship to muscle triglyceride and ω-3 fatty acids in muscle phospholipids. Diabetes 1991; 40: 280–289.

Storlien LH, Pan DA, Kriketos AD et al. Skeletal muscle membrane lipids and insulin resistance. Lipids 1996; 31 (Suppl): S261–S265.

Stubbs CD. The structure and function of docosahexaenoic acid in membranes. In: Sinclair A, Gibson R, eds. Third International Congress on Essential Fatty Acids and Eicosanoids. Campaign: American Oil Chemists Society 1992: 116–121.

Su H-M, Keswick LA, Brenna JT. Increasing dietary linoleic acid in young rats increases and then decreased docosahexaenoic acid in retina but not in brain. Lipids 1996; 31: 1289–1298.

Sullivan DR, Yue DK, Capogreco C et al. The effects of dietary n-3 fatty acid in animal models of type 1 and type 2 diabetes. Diabetes Res Clin Pract 1990; 9: 225–230.

Tanaka C, Nishizuka Y. The protein kinase C family for neuronal signaling. Annu Rev Neurosci 1994; 17: 551–567.

Taylor TG, Gibney MJ, Morgan JB. Homeostatic function and polyunsaturated fatty acids. Lancet 1979; ii: 8156–8157.

Thomas A, Goldney R, Phillips P. Depression, electroconvulsive therapy and diabetes mellitus. Aust N Z J Psychiatry 1983; 17: 289–291.

Wainwright PE. Do essential fatty acids play a role in brain and behavioural development? Neurosci Biobehav Rev 1992; 16: 193–205.

Westenburg HGM. Studies on the biochemistry of depression. Presented at the 6th World Congress of Biological Psychiatry meeting, Nice, France. June, 1997.

Williams K, Smith J, Glue P, Nut D. The effects of electroconvulsive therapy on plasma insulin and glucose in depression. Br J Psychiatry 1992; 161: 94–98.

Young LT, Li PP, Kamble A, Siu KP, Warch JJ. Lack of effect of antidepressants on mononuclear leukocyte G-protein levels or function in depressed outpatients. J Affective Disord 1996; 39: 201–207.

Zidovetski R, Lester DS. The mechanism of activation of protein kinase C: a biophysical perspective. Biochim Biophys Acta 1992; 1134: 261–272.

Part VIII

DYSLEXIA AND DYSPRAXIA

Essential Fatty Acids in Dyslexia: Theory, Evidence and Clinical Trials

Alexandra J. Richardson, Terese Easton, Ann Marie McDaid, Jacqueline A. Hall, Paul Montgomery, Christine Clisby and Basant K. Puri

INTRODUCTION

There is substantial and mounting evidence that subtle abnormalities of membrane phospholipid metabolism may underlie a wide range of neurodevelopmental disorders. A membrane hypothesis of schizophrenia is now well established (Horrobin et al., 1994), and ample evidence for this is discussed in many other chapters of this book. A more recent suggestion is that abnormalities of phospholipid metabolism may also be a contributory factor in developmental dyslexia (Horrobin et al., 1995), probably involving deficiencies in one or more of certain long-chain, polyunsaturated fatty acids, such as eicosapentaenoic acid (EPA) docosahexaenoic acid (DHA) and arachidonic acid (AA).

In this chapter, a brief outline is given of the clinical features of dyslexia and its association with other disorders, followed by an overview of what is already known of its biological basis. It is shown that a disorder of membrane fatty acid metabolism is highly compatible with existing knowledge about the biological predisposition to dyslexia, and the current evidence for this proposal is discussed.

The suggestion that membrane phospholipid abnormalities may play a role in dyslexia and related developmental disorders clearly has important implications for new treatment possibilities. Large-scale double-blind trials of essential fatty acid (EFA) treatment in dyslexia are now underway, and these are described here. Results from these studies are not yet available, but some preliminary data from baseline assessments are presented, and these findings are consistent with the proposal that fatty acid deficiency is a factor in dyslexia.

THE DYSLEXIA SYNDROME

Clinical features of dyslexia

Developmental dyslexia is defined by difficulties in learning to read and write, despite adequate general ability, opportunity and motivation. It is constitutional, and affects at least 5% of the general population, although it is more common in males. Dyslexia occurs at similar rates across cultures, and problems persist into adulthood (Miles, 1986; Kinsbourne et al., 1991). The effects can be devastating in countries where literacy is essential to full participation in society.

As well as specific problems with reading and writing, dyslexia typically involves a particularly uneven profile of cognitive strengths and weaknesses. The precise pattern may vary between individuals, but characteristic features include specific deficits in working memory (particularly for verbal material) and particular problems with sequencing, orientation and direction (Miles, 1994). There are usually persistent problems in distinguishing left from right, in remembering telephone numbers or complex instructions, and in learning by rote sequences such as the months of the year and multiplication tables.

Poor phonological skills, i.e., difficulties in appreciating and manipulating the sound-structure of words, are another classic feature which some maintain to be the core problem in dyslexia (Snowling, 1987). However, phonological deficits may sometimes be a consequence rather than a cause of poor reading, as they are found in adults who are illiterate for socio-economic reasons (Morais, 1985). More fundamentally, they simply cannot account for the full range of findings in dyslexia: problems are manifest in skills quite independent of phonological processing, such as handwriting and copying, learning to tie shoelaces, hopping and skipping, clapping in rhythm, learning to ride a bicycle, and throwing and catching a ball (Augur, 1985; Miles, 1994). An interesting proposal which does address this broader picture is that dyslexia involves a more general difficulty in the automatization of skills, which is most evident for complex, highly demanding, multimodal tasks such as learning to read and write (Nicolson and Fawcett, 1990, 1994).

A similarly broad range of problems persists into adulthood. Kinsbourne et al. (1991) used a battery of neuropsychological tests and found that dyslexic adults showed a wide range of difficulties that were by no means confined to the language domain. Particularly striking were their problems with tasks where performance could not be expected to depend in any way on reading or educational experience, such as neuromotor performance and simple temporal order judgements in both visual and auditory domains.

There is considerable clinical heterogeneity within dyslexia, but little progress has been made in the identification of clear subtypes (Hooper and Willis, 1989; Seymour, 1994). Analogies with acquired dyslexia and the study of patterns of reading errors have led to a 'surface' *versus* 'phonological' distinction (Castles and Coltheart, 1993), while the most common delineation *via* clinical or neuropsychological testing has been in terms of 'visuo-spatial' *versus* 'auditory-linguistic' problems. However, in most cases visual and phonological problems co-occur (Lovegrove, 1991; Slaghuis et al., 1993); and it is possible that they may even have a common physiological basis, as discussed further below. It should also be emphasized that variation in the clinical picture by no means precludes some common underlying factor at the biological level.

A wide range of additional features are more loosely associated with dyslexia, although their relevance has been much debated. These include a variety of 'soft' neurological signs and minor physical anomalies (Critchley, 1970), an excess of left- or mixed-handedness (Eglington and Annett, 1994) and other indications of unusual cerebral lateralization as well as higher rates of atopic conditions such as asthma and eczema and other autoimmune disorders (Geschwind and Galaburda, 1987; Tonnessen et al., 1993). Although these factors may, on the surface, appear to have little or nothing to do with reading *per se*, they may nonetheless provide possible clues to the biological mechanisms underlying dyslexia. At the very least, an appraisal of the full range of features associated with dyslexia suggests that it involves much more than simply a disorder of reading, and should therefore be considered as part of a much broader neurodevelopmental syndrome.

Associations between dyslexia and other developmental disorders

Language disorders

Clinically, there is some overlap between dyslexia and other developmental disorders. Children with dysphasia (problems with spoken language) almost inevitably go on to experience dyslexic difficulties, and in such overt, but much rarer cases, dysphasia would be the primary diagnosis. However, more transient problems in learning spoken language are very common in dyslexic children, and subtle language impairments are often still evident in adulthood, although these may be apparent only on explicit testing (Denckla, 1993).

Attentional disorders

Attention-deficit/hyperactivity disorder (ADHD) also co-occurs with dyslexia. The clinical overlap is estimated at 30–50% in both directions (Conners, 1990; Dykman and Ackerman, 1991), and the association with dyslexia appears to be stronger for attentional disorder without overt hyperactivity than it is for a predominantly hyperkinetic form of ADHD (Dykman and Ackerman, 1991; Hynd et al., 1991). There is already evidence for EFA deficiency in ADHD (Colquhoun and Bunday, 1981; Mitchell et al., 1987; Stevens et al., 1995). It therefore seems likely that the investigation of fatty acid metabolism in dyslexia could help to elucidate further the similarities and differences between these two conditions.

Movement disorders

Developmental coordination disorder (dyspraxia) is another associated condition. As noted above, general clumsiness and visuomotor problems are classic in dyslexic children (Augur, 1985), and evidence from both experimental and random population studies strongly supports the clinical picture of motor problems as a fundamental weakness (Haslum, 1989; Nicolson and Fawcett, 1994). This relationship between dyslexia and poor motor coordination is also compatible with a phospholipid hypothesis, as movement disorders in the general population have been linked with deficiencies in highly unsaturated fatty acids such as AA and DHA (Nilsson et al., 1996). Moreover, there is already evidence that children with dyspraxia may benefit from EFA supplementation (Stordy, personal communication).

Schizophrenia spectrum of disorders

Although these are clearly disorders of a different nature, there appear to be many connections between dyslexia and the so-called schizophrenia spectrum of disorders, ranging from similarities in their clinical and experimental associations to common features at the level of biological predisposition (Richardson, 1994, 1997). Both conditions run in the same families (Marcus, 1974; Rieder and Nichols, 1979; Erlenmeyer-Kimling et al., 1984; Fish, 1987), which points to common or interactive genetic factors. There is now compelling evidence for disordered membrane phospholipid metabolism in schizophrenia, as discussed elsewhere in this book. It has therefore been suggested that the familial associations with dyslexia, as well as some of the other features common to dyslexia and schizophrenia, could plausibly be explained by separate but interactive predispositions to fatty acid deficiency in both of these conditions (Horrobin et al., 1995; Horrobin, 1996).

Clinical observations suggest that dyslexia is often accompanied by an unusual perceptual and cognitive style. When this was first investigated using personality measures, dyslexic adults were found to score very highly on a scale designed to assess a broad range of schizotypal personality traits in the general population (Richardson and Stein, 1993; Richardson, 1994). However, as with clinical schizophrenia, the personality traits involved in schizotypy or psychosis-proneness appear to involve three, if not four, overlapping syndromes or dimensions (Vollema and Van den Bosch, 1995; Claridge et al., 1996). Further investigation showed that dyslexia in adults was strongly associated with a primary positive dimension of schizotypy that involves unusual perceptual experiences and unconventional beliefs, resembling a much milder, nonpsychotic form of the hallucinations and delusions found in clinical schizophrenia (Richardson, 1994, 1997). Associations were also found with other positive traits, such as hypomanic tendencies and attentional problems, but dyslexia did not appear to relate either to the more negative, anhedonic features of schizotypy, or to an antisocial, impulsive dimension of psychosis-proneness.

This association of dyslexia with positive, but not negative, schizotypal traits is interesting in view of suggestions that dyslexia may involve a particular deficiency of n-3 (rather than n-6) fatty acids (Stordy, 1995). A particular improvement in the positive symptoms of schizophrenia has been reported following treatment with n-3 fatty acids (Peet et al., 1996, 1997), while other evidence suggests that the more negative, withdrawn and anhedonic features of schizophrenia may particularly relate to deficiency in AA, the most important of the n-6 fatty acids in the brain (Glen et al., 1996). It may also be relevant that n-3 deficiency has recently been implicated in clinical depression (Peet et al., 1998). Depression – often with cyclic tendencies – is frequently associated in clinical practice with both dyslexia and ADHD, but where the connection with dyslexia has been noted, depression has usually been regarded as secondary to the life-adjustment problems that often follow from this condition (Saunders and Barker, 1972).

FATTY ACIDS AND DYSLEXIA: AN EVALUATION OF THE EVIDENCE

As discussed above, the idea that fatty acids may play a role in dyslexia has initial plausibility given both the clinical features associated with this condition, and the fact that dyslexia is associated with other disorders in which phospholipid abnormalities have already been implicated. In this section, brief consideration is given to what is already known about the biological predisposition to dyslexia, allowing further evaluation of the lipid hypothesis. This is followed by a summary of the direct evidence for abnormal fatty acid metabolism in dyslexia which provided the rationale for clinical treatment trials.

Biological factors in dyslexia

Genetics

There is a substantial genetic contribution to dyslexia, with heritable variation estimated at around 50% (Pennington, 1995). However, no clear mode of transmission has been identified, and no single genetic model can accommodate all of the data, as might be expected given the complexity and variability of the phenotype. Molecular genetic studies suggest linkage to a region on the short arm of Chromosome 6 (Cardon et al., 1994, 1995; Grigorenko et al., 1997), and the proximity of this site to the HLA region has generated interest in view of the much-debated association between dyslexia and autoimmune disorders, although no candidate gene has yet been identified. This would obviously help to focus the search for biological mechanisms; but equally, hypotheses about potential mechanisms would assist in narrowing the search for candidate genes. Recently the lipid hypothesis has provided some interesting new genetic evidence with respect to schizophrenia (Hudson et al., 1996); and in view of the proposal that there may be interactive genetic effects in the predispositions to dyslexia and schizophrenia (Horrobin et al., 1995), those investigating the genetics of dyslexia might do well to consider the possibility of abnormal lipid metabolism in this disorder.

Sex differences

The sex ratio in dyslexia also awaits proper explanation. Although this may well have been over-estimated in some early reports, around three or four males are affected for every female (James, 1992). In some respects, this looks like an exaggeration of the normal slight advantage of females for language-related skills (Hyde and Linn, 1988). However, males are over-represented to varying degrees across a whole range of developmental disorders, encompassing developmental dysphasia, dyslexia and dyspraxia, ADHD, Tourette's syndrome, schizophrenia, Asperger's syndrome, and autism; moreover, all of these disorders show some degree of clinical overlap or aggregation within families. Little progress has been made in the obvious search for X-linked genes underlying these conditions; rather, it would seem that in females a higher genetic loading is required for the clinical expression of disorder. The fact that phospholipid abnormalities appear to be implicated in many of these conditions offers an interesting new possibility to explain the sex ratio, because males appear to be more vulnerable than females to the effects of EFA deficiency (Pudelkewicz et al., 1968; Huang et al., 1990).

Neuroanatomical features

Neuroanatomical studies have provided some support for the longstanding view that unusual cerebral lateralisation is part of the predisposition to dyslexia. The usual gross structural asymmetries are more often reduced or reversed in dyslexic subjects (Hynd and Semrud-Clikeman 1989), and dyslexic brains typically show an unusual symmetry (rather than the usual leftward asymmetry) of the planum temporale, an auditory association area implicated in language processing (Galaburda et al., 1985). This planum symmetry appears to distinguish dyslexic from ADHD children (Hynd et al., 1990) and has also been related to poor phonological skills (Larsen et al., 1990), but as this 'abnormal' symmetry is shared by up to a quarter of the general population (Galaburda et al., 1987) it is clearly not a feature which is specific to dyslexia.

More specific are the various microscopic abnormalities of neuronal organization that have been reported in studies of dyslexic brains post-mortem (Drake, 1968; Galaburda et al., 1985; Humphreys et al., 1990). These primarily include ectopias (collections of misplaced cells) and dysplasias (abnormalities of neuronal layering), which clearly arise during prenatal development and are typically accompanied by an unusually rich pattern of cortical connectivity (Rosen et al., 1993). Although these focal abnormalities are often particularly concentrated in left perisylvian regions, their distribution is actually widespread and bilateral, and it varies between individual cases. If these anomalies are of aetiological significance, then this individual variation in their distribution might certainly help to explain some of the clinical heterogeneity in dyslexia.

The reasons for their origin in dyslexic brains are unknown, but similar abnormalities are found in association with certain autoimmune conditions, such as systemic lupus erythematosus (SLE), suggesting a possible autoimmune basis, and dyslexia occurs at strikingly high rates (around 45%) in the children of mothers with SLE (Lahita, 1988). Similar ectopias are also found in certain strains of mouse which have congenital autoimmune dysfunction, further supporting the idea that these cortical anomalies may reflect abnormal autoimmune influences on the developing brain (Rosen et al., 1993). If so, this could well be relevant to the current hypothesis of abnormal lipid metabolism in dyslexia. Essential fatty acids are known to play a crucial role in regulating normal immune function, and Clausen and Møller (1967) first showed that the susceptibility of the rat brain to autoimmune attack can be increased by depleting its membranes of essential fatty acids *via* dietary deprivation.

Physiological features

A similar speculation about autoimmune influences *in utero* has arisen from physiological studies of dyslexia. This is *via* the so-called 'magnocellular hypothesis', that dyslexia involves a neurodevelopmental disorder which specifically affects a subset of large (magnocellular) neurones specialized for very rapid temporal processing in the nervous system. Psychophysical and physiological studies have provided compelling evidence of low-level visual deficits in dyslexia for tasks involving very rapid temporal coding, such as the perception of motion and flicker, implicating the subcortical magnocellular visual pathway (Stein and Walsh, 1997). Consistent with this, post-mortem studies have revealed neuroanatomical abnormalities specific to this visual subsystem (Livingstone et al., 1991). Moreover, these authors noted that, in histological studies, visual magnocellular neurones are selectively stained by certain antibodies, suggesting a possible specific vulnerabilty of these cells to autoimmune attack.

Such selective staining extends to other brain regions, including known auditory pathways, suggesting that the same vulnerability might also affect modalities other than vision. Deficits in auditory temporal coding have been found in dyslexia which may contribute to phonological problems (Tallal et al., 1993; McAnally and Stein, 1996; Witton et al., 1998); and although there is no such clear anatomical distinction in the auditory system as there is in the visual system between fast (magnocellular) and slow (parvocellular) subsystems, psychophysical measures of visual and auditory temporal processing do show strong intercorrelations (Witton et al., 1998).

The motor coordination problems often associated

with dyslexia are also consistent with a generalized deficit in neural timing (Wolff, 1993), and it has been suggested that this (as well as many other features of dyslexia) could be explained by mild cerebellar dysfunction (Nicolson et al., 1995; Fawcett et al., 1996). The cerebellum has long been recognized as a 'timing' device extraordinaire, with a critical role in the control and guidance of movement (Stein and Glickstein, 1992), and it receives massive input from the visual magnocellular system. However, only recently has the cerebellum also been implicated in sequential learning, attention and other aspects of cognitive function (see Braitenberg et al., 1997), which adds a great deal to the plausibility of a role for this structure in dyslexia.

In summary, current evidence suggests that a key feature of the biological predisposition to dyslexia may be a multimodal disorder of rapid temporal processing, possibly arising from abnormal autoimmune influences on the developing brain. It is easy to see that this is compatible with a lipid hypothesis, given the importance of fatty acids in brain development, in regulation of the immune system, and in cognitive (and especially visual) function. It is quite remarkable that, so far, almost no research into dyslexia has been conducted from a biochemical perspective, but the existing evidence suggests that the study of phospholipid metabolism could well be a fruitful line of investigation.

How might EFA deficiency contribute to dyslexia?

It is clear that the predisposition to dyslexia is shaped during prenatal development, and there can be no doubts about the importance of fatty acids during this period. Lipids are quantitatively the most important component of brain structure, and in the central nervous system two fatty acids are particularly important: AA and DHA, between them making up around 15% of the dry mass of the brain. The fatty acids of membrane phospholipids play a crucial role in membrane structure, the functioning of membrane-bound and membrane-associated proteins, and cell signalling responses (Nunez, 1993). Free fatty acids play a host of functional roles *via* their prostaglandin and leukotriene derivatives, and are known to influence both cardiovascular and immune function. EFA metabolism can therefore influence many aspects of brain development, including neuronal migration, axonal and dendritic growth, and the creation, remodelling and pruning of synaptic connections (Crawford, 1992).

It is at least possible that EFA deficiency during prenatal development could be a contributory factor in the cytoarchitectonic abnormalities reported in dyslexic brains post-mortem. Detailed studies of ectopias suggest that these may arise following an initial breach in the pial–glial membrane, through which migrating neurones then pass beyond their usual target locations (Rosen et al., 1993). This kind of event could plausibly reflect an abnormal fragility of membranes, and/or a particular susceptibility to autoimmune attack, either of which is a potential consequence of EFA deficiency. As animal models of these ectopias are available, these kinds of possibilities are certainly open to experimental study.

More generally, animal studies have already shown that both neural integrity and function can be permanently disrupted by deficits of n-6 and n-3 fatty acids during foetal and neonatal development (Yamamoto et al., 1987; Neuringer et al., 1988; Bourre et al., 1989). Short-term nutritional deficiencies may have permanent effects if they occur during certain 'critical periods' of neurodevelopment (Lucas, 1994), and although these kinds of relationship are obviously very difficult to investigate in humans, particular time-windows of vulnerability have been identified in animal studies (e.g., Budowski et al., 1987). Both n-6 and n-3 fatty acids are essential, but the n-3 fatty acids such as DHA are thought to play a special role in highly active sites, such as the synapses and photoreceptors, and have particularly been linked to visual and cognitive deficits. By contrast, deficiencies of AA have been associated more with general growth indices, such as low birth weight and reduced head circumference. The subtle visual and cognitive anomalies associated with dyslexia could plausibly reflect a relative deficiency of n-3 fatty acids in particular, and there is already some evidence for this, as discussed below.

Adequate supplies of EFAs are also required throughout development and adult life in order to maintain normal function. The truly essential fatty acids are linoleic acid (18:2n-6) and α-linolenic acid (18:3n-3), because these cannot be synthesized within the body. *Via* processes of elongation and desaturation these EFAs can be converted into the longer-chain fatty acids, such as AA and DHA, that are most important in neuronal membranes. However, various environmental or constitutional factors can act to interfere with these conversion processes, resulting in a relative deficiency of the longer-chain polyunsaturated fatty acids (LCPUFAs) despite adequate availability of their EFA precursors. Consistent with this, there is evidence that infants may benefit from the LCPUFAs that are present in breast-milk but absent from many formula feeds. Thus Makrides et al. (1995) showed that the advantage to visual development that has often been reported for breast-fed over formula-fed infants was eliminated when DHA was added to formula milk. There is already ample evidence for the importance of this fatty acid in vision, as it is a major component of retinal cells (Bazan et al., 1986), and more recently it has been implicated in other aspects of neurotransmitter metabolism and receptor function (Delion et al., 1994; Nishikawa et al., 1994).

Provision of the precursor EFAs alone should usually be sufficient to meet requirements for DHA and other LCPUFAs if normal conversion mechanisms are effective. The effects of early nutrition on development are a major focus of current research (see Dobbing, 1997), but as yet there is no clear consensus on the requirement for LCPUFAs in infant formula, and the methodological problems are considerable. Individual differences are particularly difficult to identify, but in one recent study the benefits from direct supplementation with LCPUFAs appeared to be confined to a subgroup of infants who initially showed poor attention control (Willatts et al., 1996). In older children there is already evidence that n-3 fatty acid deficiency relates to attentional, behavioural and learning problems (Stevens et al., 1995, 1996), and it is not unreasonable to propose that constitutional factors (e.g., a particular problem in converting EFAs to LCPUFAs) might increase the requirement for dietary LCPUFAs in conditions such as ADHD and dyslexia.

Direct evidence for EFA deficiency in dyslexia

There is already some direct evidence of fatty acid deficiency in dyslexia. Baker (1985) reported a case study of a dyslexic child, which involved biochemical investigations, and his insightful observations are worth reporting in detail. Clinical signs had provided strong indications of fatty acid deficiency, as the child had 'very dry, patchy, dull skin ... his hair was easily tousled ... and had a straw-like texture rather than a normal silky feel. He had dandruff. The skin on the backs of his arms was raised in tiny closed bumps like chicken skin. His fingernails were soft and frayed at the ends .... All of these findings point to an imbalance of fatty acids' (p. 583). This was confirmed by blood biochemical analyses, and following nutritional therapy, it was reported that 'improvement in [his] school work coincided with the return of normal lustre and texture to his skin and hair. If he had been a cocker spaniel his family would have accepted the connection between his "glossier coat" and better disposition more readily. The timing was convincing .... With a twinkle in his eye, he told his grandmother that dandruff had been the cause of his dyslexia' (p. 583).

Fatty acid deficiency as a contributory factor in dyslexia was explicitly proposed by Stordy (1995), who found an impairment of dark adaptation in dyslexic adults which then normalized rapidly following DHA supplementation. There are other reports of reduced dark adaptation in dyslexia (Carroll et al., 1994; MacDonell et al., 1997), and although it is not yet clear whether this relates to the other visual deficits associated with dyslexia, this certainly warrants investigation. As noted above, DHA in particular is crucial for normal visual (and cognitive) development (Neuringer et al., 1994; Makrides et al., 1995); and it is an attractive speculation that EFA deficiency may perhaps particularly affect the fast 'magnocellular' systems implicated in dyslexia.

Further direct evidence of phospholipid abnormalities in dyslexia came from a study using cerebral ^{31}P-magnetic resonance spectroscopy (^{31}P-MRS) to investigate membrane lipid turnover (Richardson et al., 1997). The results suggested problems with phospholipid synthesis in dyslexia, as was proposed by Horrobin et al. (1995), and this is consistent with fatty acid deficiency, although further elucidation will be sought from blood biochemical studies now underway. In addition, ^{31}P-MRS is being conducted on a subset of volunteers from the adult clinical trials described below, to find out whether EFA treatment will affect these measures of brain lipid metabolism.

The rationale for clinical trials

The most important implication of Stordy's (1995) study is that it has raised new treatment possibilities. The visual deficit she found in dyslexic subjects was no longer evident following just 1 month of DHA supplementation, suggesting an abnormality of phospholipid metabolism which is relatively mild. The important issue, of course, is whether EFA treatment can affect other, arguably more central, aspects of dyslexia. There was anecdotal evidence of broader benefits in Stordy's adult subjects, and the case study by Baker (1985) very much supports this idea. However, formal double-blind trials involving a wide range of assessments are clearly required in order to substantiate these reports, and this was the rationale for setting up the clinical trials reported here.

CLINICAL TRIALS OF FATTY ACID TREATMENT IN DYSLEXIA

Clinical treatment trials are now underway, involving both children and adults, to assess the therapeutic potential of EFA supplementation in dyslexia. The supplement used in these trials is Efalex™ (supplied by Efamol Ltd, UK), and this actually provides LCPUFAs directly, rather than the precursor EFAs (see above), but the term EFA will nonetheless be used here for simplicity. The basic design and measures used in these trials are described below, and some preliminary data from baseline assessments are presented.

Study design and measures

Two large-scale randomized, double-blind placebo-controlled trials are in progress. One involves up to 80 dyslexic adults aged 18–55 years and 80 matched controls. The second involves up to 120 dyslexic children aged 8–12 years, recruited from referrals to a specialist dyslexia research clinic. The basic design of each of these studies is similar, involving an initial double-blind, fixed-dose, parallel groups study for 6 months with random allocation of subjects to the treatments (Efalex™ or placebo: dosage is eight capsules per day, to be taken in a divided dose morning and evening with food; the placebo treatment is olive oil). This stage is followed by a second 6-month period involving a one-way crossover of treatment (placebo to Efalex™). Participants are thus followed for 12 months from baseline, and follow-up visits are scheduled at 3-month intervals. Assessments carried out at baseline and each follow-up point include:

Interview/checklist measures

Interviews and checklists are used both for screening (medical history, general health, and minimal details of nutritional habits and substance use) and to assess traits and symptoms associated with dyslexia (including handedness, personality, and a range of symptoms encompassing visual, auditory, linguistic and motor function). Ratings include a scale designed to assess clinical signs of fatty acid deficiency, described in detail below.

Psychometric measures of cognitive function

These include standardized assessments of reading, spelling, general ability (both verbal and non-verbal), working memory for sequential material (auditory-verbal and visuo-spatial), and phonological skills.

Experimental measures of visual and auditory function

Visual function (sensitivity to coherent motion, visual search) and auditory function (discrimination of changes in the frequency and duration of tones) are assessed.

Biochemical measures

Blood samples are being collected, where possible, for analysis of the fatty acid composition of red cell membranes and plasma, and some adult subjects are also being assessed using ^{31}P-MRS.

Subject samples to date

For the preliminary analyses reported here, baseline assessments were available on 95 adult subjects (61 dyslexic, 34 control) of whom 73 went on to take part in the full treatment trial (the remaining 22 met the entry criteria but did not take part in the treatment study for other reasons). Most of the dyslexic subjects had previously been identified as such by educational psychologists, but in all cases their specific difficulties with written language were confirmed using standardized tests of reading, spelling and general ability (see Table 21.1). Controls were required to have no history of difficulties with either reading or spelling, but again their written language skills and general ability were assessed to confirm this. Subjects were also assessed using a simple dyslexia screening checklist for adults (Vinegrad, 1994). This scale has 20 items, each scored 'yes' or 'no', and validation studies have shown that scores of 9 or more are indicative of dyslexia, although diagnosis always requires confirmation *via* psychometric assessments.

As Table 21.1 shows, the two groups were well matched for sex and age and did not differ on verbal or nonverbal tests of general ability, but the performance of the dyslexic group was very significantly inferior for both single word reading and spelling and for passage reading ($p < 0.0001$, in all cases). The dyslexic subjects also showed characteristic deficits on tests of both digit span, assessing working memory for auditorily presented material ($p < 0.0001$) and digit–symbol substitution, involving the matching and copying of numbers to abstract symbols ($p < 0.0001$). As expected, scores on the dyslexia screening checklist showed hardly any overlap between the two groups ($p < 0.0001$).

From the children's study, data were available for 66 dyslexic subjects (48 male, 18 female) aged 8–12 years, all of whom subsequently entered the treatment trial. Children were judged to meet dyslexic criteria if their word reading on the British Ability Scales (BAS) (Elliott, 1983) was more than two standard deviations below the level expected for their general ability as assessed by the BAS similarities or matrices subtests. The psychological assessment battery also included the BAS subtests of spelling and recall of digits.

Table 21.1. Psychological test scores in 61 dyslexic adults (29.8 ± 9.9 years of age; mean ± SD) and 34 adult control subjects (32.1 ± 9.8 years of age). Results are given as means ± SD.

Test	Control	Dyslexic
General ability [a]		
Similarities	13.3 ± 2.2	13.1 ± 2.5
Vocabulary	13.4 ± 2.7	12.4 ± 2.5
Block design	13.4 ± 2.9	13.1 ± 3.2
Picture arrangement	11.8 ± 2.4	11.9 ± 2.7
Reading and spelling [b]		
Word reading	116.7 ± 5.3	95.2 ± 14.4†††
Spelling	114.7 ± 7.3	85.0 ± 16.2†††
Passage reading	125.2 ± 5.5	86.0 ± 17.7†††
Other measures [c]		
Digit span	12.4 ± 2.0	8.5 ± 2.4†††
Digit symbol	11.9 ± 2.9	9.6 ± 2.7†††
Dyslexia screening	2.8 ± 2.1	13.4 ± 3.5†††

[a] All tests in this category were taken from the Wechsler Adult Intelligence Scales (WAIS-R), UK edition (Psychological Corporation, 1994); [b] the tests for word reading and spelling were taken from the Wide Range Achievement Test – Revised (Jastak and Wilkinson, 1984), and the test for passage reading was taken from the Gray Oral Reading Tests, third edition (GORT3) (Wiederholt and Bryant, 1992); [c] the tests for digit span and digit–symbol substitution were taken from the WAIS-R (Psychological Corporation, 1994), and dyslexia screening was based on the Revised Adult Dyslexia Check List (Vinegrad, 1994). Statistical analysis for group comparisons employed the t test, except for the dyslexia screening scores for which a Mann-Whitney test (two-tail) was used; †††in comparison with the corresponding value for control subjects, $p < 0.0001$.

Ratings of EFA deficiency signs

Baseline assessments in both the adults' and children's trials include interview/checklist ratings of clinical signs of possible EFA deficiency (Stevens et al., 1995). Specifically, these ratings comprise seven indicators which have been linked with EFA deficiency (namely thirst, frequent urination, dry skin, dry hair, brittle nails, dandruff and follicular keratosis), although it is acknowledged that each of these symptoms can have other causes. The applicability of each item is rated on a four-point scale (0 = not at all; 1 = just a little; 2 = quite a lot; 3 = very much). Stevens et al. (1995) found that ADHD boys had higher scores than controls on these putative EFA deficiency signs, both in total, and especially on the items concerning thirst, frequent urination and dry skin. This was consistent with the biochemical evidence they also reported for fatty acid deficiency in ADHD, involving reductions of AA, DHA and total n-3 fatty acids in plasma.

Most important for our purposes was that significant associations were found in their study between high EFA deficiency scores, as measured by this scale, and the blood biochemical measures. Thus high scores on these clinical signs were related to low concentrations of AA and DHA in plasma, and subjects with high EFA deficiency scores also showed a lower concentration of total n-3 fatty acids. Thus, despite its simplicity, and the acknowledged lack of specificity of the symptoms it includes, this scale nonetheless appears to provide a reasonably reliable index of deficiency in those fatty acids that have been implicated in dyslexia. As results from our own blood biochemical analyses are not yet available, these EFA deficiency ratings at baseline have been examined in relation to other study measures in both adults and children.

Preliminary results from baseline assessments

EFA deficiency signs and dyslexic status

Our primary question was whether EFA deficiency signs would be higher in dyslexic than in nondyslexic subjects. This could be addressed only with the adult data, as all the subjects in the children's treatment trial are dyslexic. Initial comparisons were made using the Mann-Whitney test (two-tail) as the distributions of both item and total scores were inevitably abnormal. As illustrated in Figure 21.1, total EFA deficiency signs

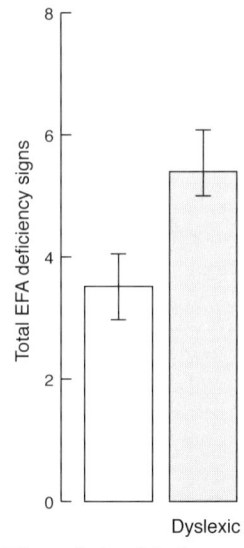

Figure 21.1. The relationship between total fatty acid deficiency signs and dyslexic status; means ± SEM for 34 control adults and 61 dyslexic adults.

(i.e., the sum of scores across all seven items) were significantly higher in the dyslexic group ($p < 0.05$) than in the controls.

Scores for each individual item were then compared in the same way (Mann-Whitney test, two-tail). Significant group differences were found for ratings of excessive thirst ($p < 0.05$), frequent urination ($p < 0.01$), dry hair ($p < 0.05$) and brittle nails ($p < 0.05$), with higher scores for the dyslexic group in all cases. Individual item scores were then further examined according to the method used by Stevens et al. (1995), namely a comparison using Fisher's exact test of the proportion of individuals in each group with scores of either 2 or 3 (the two highest degrees of severity). As Table 21.2 shows, on this less sensitive but arguably stricter analysis, ratings of dry hair and brittle nails did not differ between groups, but endorsements of excessive thirst and frequent urination were still significantly higher in the dyslexic group ($p < 0.05$ and $p < 0.005$, respectively).

In addition, scores on the adult dyslexia screening checklist were examined in relation to total EFA deficiency scores using rank-order correlations (Spearman's ρ). These scores were not available for two control and seven dyslexic subjects, and hence these analyses involved 86 rather than 95 subjects. As illustrated in Figure 21.2, dyslexia screening checklist scores were strongly associated with total EFA deficiency signs both for the whole sample ($\rho = 0.38$; $p < 0.0005$) and within the dyslexic group ($\rho = 0.37$; $p < 0.001$). A weaker, statistically nonsignificant, correlation was seen for control subjects ($\rho = 0.20$), although variance on both measures was also much reduced.

Table 21.2. Prevalence of a variety of signs of moderate or severe fatty acid deficiency (i.e., percentages of subjects showing a score of 2 or 3) amongst dyslexic ($n = 61$) and control ($n = 34$) adults.

Sign	Control	Dyslexic
Excessive thirst	8.8	27.9*
Frequent urination	2.9	26.2***
Dry skin	35.3	27.9
Dry hair	11.8	18.0
Brittle nails	14.7	19.7
Dandruff	5.9	14.8
Follicular keratosis	8.8	16.4

In comparison with the corresponding value for control subjects, $p <$: *0.05; ***0.005 (Fisher's exact probability test).

EFA deficiency signs and psychometric measures

For the children's study, control data is not yet available, but EFA deficiency ratings were examined in relation to standardized measures of reading, spelling and general ability (see Table 21.3). The sample was divided on median scores into high EFA deficiency (total scores 0–2) and low EFA deficiency (total scores ≥ 3). High EFA deficiency was associated with more severe reading deficits, measured both in terms of the reading lag in months and as age-standardized scores ($p < 0.05$), but no other differences were found between the two groups. In the adult sample no significant relationships were found between psychometric test scores and EFA deficiency signs. Thus there was no evidence to suggest that EFA deficiency is characteristic of only a particular subgroup of dyslexic individuals as defined by psychometric measures.

EFA deficiency signs and other measures of dyslexic symptomatology

Both adults and children were assessed using interview checklist ratings of a range of symptoms typically associated with dyslexia in clinical experience (Table 21.4).

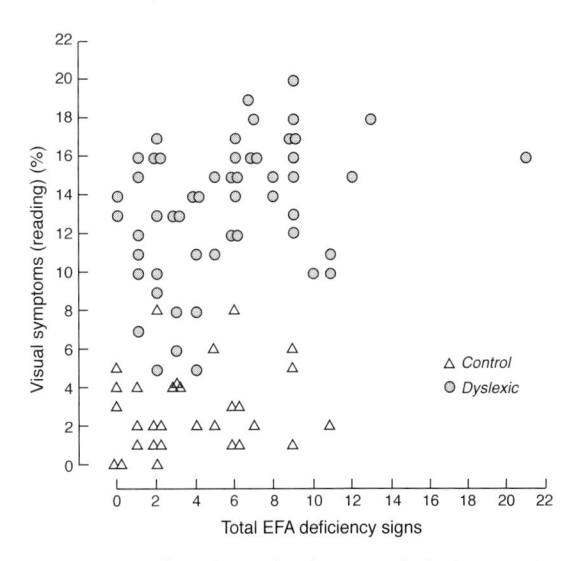

Figure 21.2. The relationship between dyslexia screening checklist scores and fatty acid deficiency signs in 54 dyslexic adults and 32 control adults. Dyslexia scores were obtained using the Revised Adult Dyslexia Checklist (Vinegrad, 1994). Correlations between dyslexia screening scores and total EFA deficiency signs were calculated using Spearman's rank correlation coefficient: for all subjects, $\rho = 0.38$, $p < 0.0005$; or dyslexic subjects, $\rho = 0.37$, $p < 0.001$; and for controls, $\rho = 0.20$, nonsignificant.

Categories include visual symptoms experienced during reading, auditory-perceptual language confusions, spoken language difficulties and problems with motor coordination.

As a validation of these symptom measures, scores from dyslexic and control adults at baseline were first compared. There were highly significant differences across all symptom categories as illustrated in Figure 21.3, with higher scores for the dyslexic group in all cases (all comparisons $p < 0.0001$, Mann-Whitney, two-tail). With confirmation that scores on these global symptom measures are indeed associated with dyslexia, symptom scores were then explored in relation to total EFA deficiency signs in both adults and children. Rank-order correlations are shown in Table 21.5.

In children, high EFA deficiency signs were significantly correlated only with visual symptoms when reading ($\rho = 0.34$, $p < 0.05$), although it should be noted that many of these ratings were provided mainly by parents; the only exception to this was for visual symptoms during reading, which are so subjective that the child's own opinion was always sought and given precedence.

Table 21.3. Psychological test scores, based upon the British Ability Scales, in 33 children (117.5 ± 16.5 months of age; mean ± SD) with low EFA deficiency, and 33 children (120.8 ± 17.4 months of age) with high EFA deficiency. Results are given as means ± SD.

Test	EFA deficiency group Low	EFA deficiency group High
Reading		
Reading age (months)	94.8 ± 14.2	90.4 ± 10.9[a]
Reading lag (months)	22.7 ± 13.0	30.4 ± 14.4*
Reading T-score[b]	39.8 ± 5.0	37.0 ± 4.9*
Spelling		
Spelling age (months)	95.7 ± 14.3	93.3 ± 11.8[a]
Spelling T-score[b]	40.3 ± 5.1	38.8 ± 6.3
Other measures		
Similarities[b] (verbal reasoning)	61.4 ± 6.2	59.4 ± 7.6
Matrices[b] (nonverbal reasoning)	54.2 ± 6.6	51.8 ± 8.9[a]
IQ[c]	109.1 ± 30.1	105.5 ± 32.0[a]
Recall of digits	40.6 ± 6.8	38.8 ± 9.2[a]

[a] Statistical analysis employed a Mann-Whitney test (two-tail) owing to a non-normal distribution of scores, whilst for other group comparisons a t test was employed; [b] age standardized score, with a mean of 50 and standard deviation of 10; [c] pro-rated from the similarities and matrices scores. *In comparison with the corresponding value for low EFA deficiency subjects, $p < 0.05$.

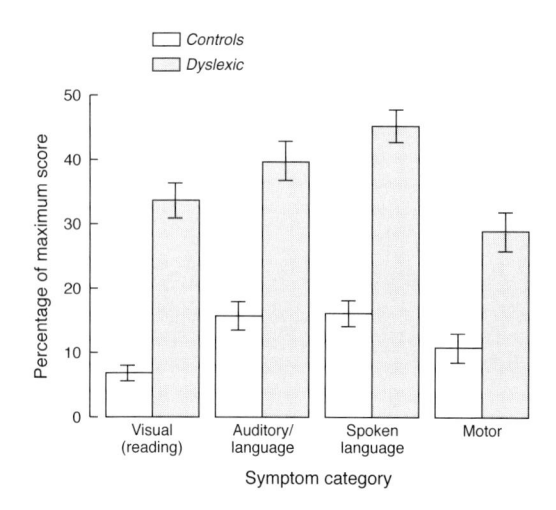

Figure 21.3. Dyslexia-related symptoms in 34 control adults and 58 dyslexic adults. The items used to derive the symptom scales are shown in Table 21.4; total scores for each symptom category are shown as a percentage of the maximum possible score. Means ± SEM; all group differences were statistically significant at $p < 0.0001$ (Mann-Whitney, two tail).

In adults, EFA deficiency signs were associated with the full range of measures of dyslexic symptomatology (see Figures 21.4–21.7), including not only visual problems but also auditory – linguistic, spoken language and motor coordination difficulties ($p < 0.005$ in all cases). When dyslexic and control groups were considered separately, these relationships were significant within the dyslexic group ($p < 0.05$ in all cases), and a particularly strong association was seen between EFA deficiency signs and motor problems ($p < 0.005$). No significant associations were found within the control group, although here the variance on both measures was also much reduced.

EFA deficiency signs and schizotypal traits

In adults, a range of schizotypal personality traits was assessed using the Oxford-Liverpool Inventory of Feelings and Experiences (Mason et al., 1995). This includes scales assessing four global dimensions of schizotypy (unusual experiences, cognitive disorganization, introvertive anhedonia and impulsive nonconformity) as well as the STA schizotypy scale – an earlier broad measure of positive schizotypal traits (Claridge and Broks, 1984). Scores on these measures were available for 52 dyslexic and 27 control subjects.

EFA deficiency signs were significantly correlated with two of the positive dimensions, namely unusual experiences, indexing anomalous perceptions and

Table 21.4. The dyslexia symptom interview checklist. Respondents rate the applicability of each item to themselves as 0 (not at all), 1 (just a little), 2 (quite a lot), or 3 (very much).

Visual symptoms experienced during reading
(When you try to read, how much are you bothered by the following?)

1. Headaches or eye strain.
2. Losing your place on the page.
3. Particular problems with small, crowded print.
4. 'Double vision,' i.e., letters and words splitting into two.
5. Print becoming blurred or out of focus (even with glasses).
6. Letters or words moving around on the page or board.
7. Letters or words moving 'in and out' of the page or board.
8. A distorted (stretched or twisted) appearance to the print.
9. 'Glare' or discomfort from reading in bright light.
10. The appearance of a 'fringe,' 'halo,' or 'aura' around words.
11. Problems or discomfort from reading a computer screen[a].
12. On TV or cinema, difficulty reading subtitles to a film[a].

Auditory–perceptual problems with language.
(When listening to language, how much are you bothered by the following?).

1. Difficulty following and understanding very rapid speech.
2. Problems decoding speech against background noise (e.g., music, traffic, machinery or other environmental sounds).
3. Difficulty following speech when you can't see the speaker's face or expressions (e.g., on the telephone).
4. Particular problems in concentrating when more than one person is talking (e.g., in a crowded room or party).
5. Difficulty hearing clearly in a large (but quiet) lecture or school hall.
6. Trouble understanding if the speaker has a strong accent.

Difficulties with spoken language
(When using language, how much are you bothered by the following?)

1. Word-finding difficulties (e.g., in rapid naming, or recall).
2. Using too few words when explaining something (i.e., not giving enough detail or elaboration).
3. A tendency to give long, complicated or 'roundabout' explanations (i.e., too much detail, not enough structure).
4. Talking very fast, with a tendency to 'ramble on'.
5. Talking very slowly and carefully, but often missing the chance to 'join in' or say what you want as a result.
6. Stuttering, or getting tongue-tied.
7. Pronunciation problems, especially with multi-syllabic words.

Motor coordination problems
(Please rate any problems you may have in the following areas.)

1. General clumsiness (e.g., tripping, knocking things over).
2. Difficulty with balance (e.g., riding a bicycle, climbing, reaching or leaning).
3. Problems in catching or hitting a ball at speed (e.g., tennis, badminton, squash, rounders, batting and fielding in cricket).
4. Problems with fine motor coordination (e.g., threading a needle, sewing, sorting beads, making models, skilled carpentry, etc.).
5. Difficulty automatizing a *new* set of movements (e.g., learning to drive, driving a different car, learning a new keyboard routine, sporting or dance sequence, etc.).

This is a preliminary instrument; the items were designed for administration by interview, thus allowing for further discussion or explanation if needed. Items and categories will be reviewed when data from larger samples of subjects have been collected and analyzed in detail. [a] These items were included for the adult subjects only.

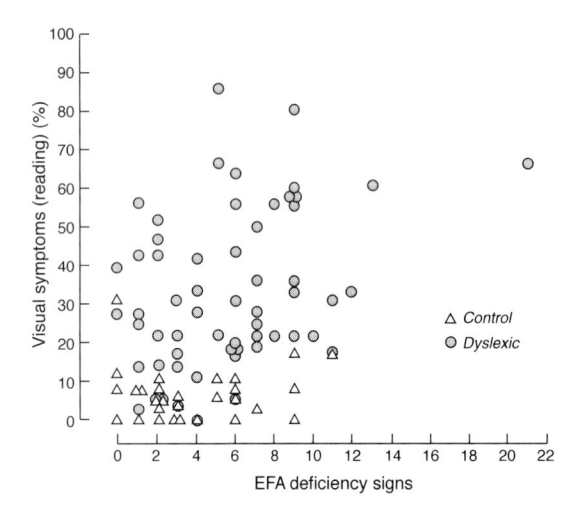

Figure 21.4. The relationship between visual symptoms (reading) and fatty acid deficiency signs in 34 control adults and 58 dyslexic adults. The items used to derive the visual symptom score are shown in Table 21.4. The correlation between visual symptoms (reading) scores and total EFA acid deficiency signs is given in Table 21.5.

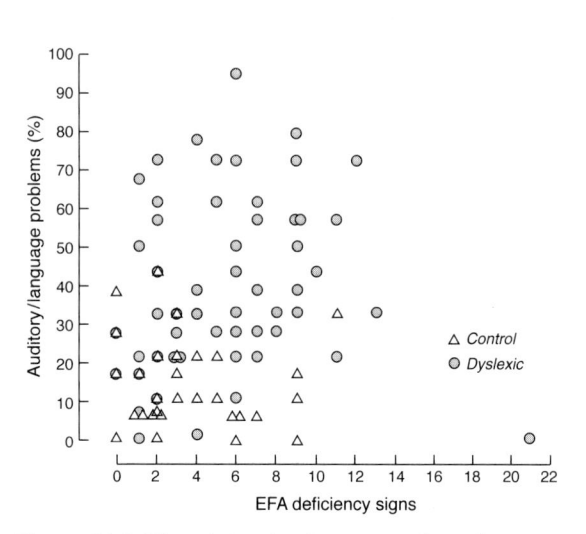

Figure 21.5. The relationship between auditory/language problems and fatty acid deficiency signs in 34 control adults and 58 dyslexic adults. The items used to derive the auditory/language problems score are shown in Table 21.4. The correlation between auditory/language problems and total EFA acid deficiency signs is given in Table 21.5.

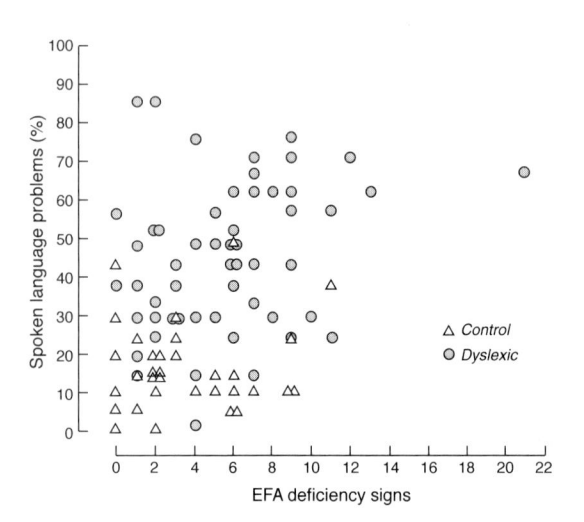

Figure 21.6. The relationship between spoken language problems and fatty acid deficiency signs in 34 control adults and 58 dyslexic adults. The items used to derive the spoken language problems score are shown in Table 21.4. The correlation between spoken language problems and total EFA acid deficiency signs is given in Table 21.5.

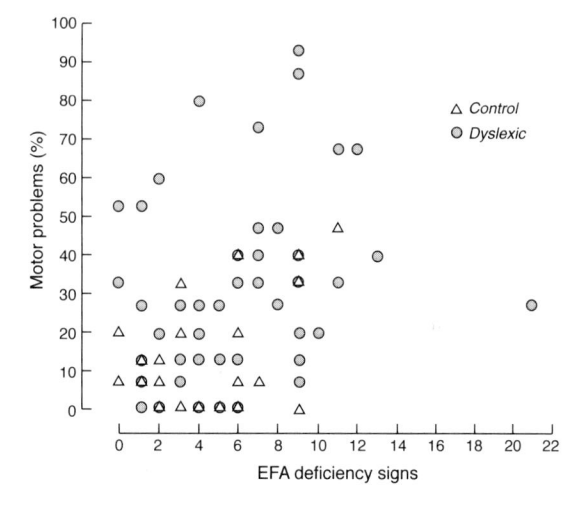

21.7. The relationship between motor problems and fatty acid deficiency signs in 34 control adults and 58 dyslexic adults. The items used to derive the motor problems score are shown in Table 21.4. The correlation between motor problems and total EFA acid deficiency signs is given in Table 21.5.

Table 21.5. Correlations (Spearman's rank order correlation coefficient) between total EFA deficiency signs and dyslexic symptom ratings in children ($n = 50$) and adults ($n = 92$); the adults were subdivided into those with dyslexia ($n = 58$) and others (controls) without dyslexia ($n = 34$).

Symptoms	Children All	Adults Dyslexic	Adults Control	Adults All
Visual symptoms (reading)	+0.34*	+0.32*	+0.15	+0.37†
Auditory/language problems	+0.19	+0.39*	0.00	+0.31**
Spoken language problems	+0.02	+0.30*	+0.01	+0.33**
Motor problems	−0.04	+0.35**	+0.10	+0.41†

$p <$: *0.05; **0.01; †0.001 (two-tail significance levels).

cognitions ($\rho = 0.29$; $p < 0.01$), and cognitive disorganization, assessing attentional problems and social anxiety ($\rho = 0.24$; $p < 0.05$). A similar relationship was therefore seen with the STA schizotypy scale which assesses a combination of these traits ($\rho = 0.29$, $p < 0.05$), but no associations were found between EFA deficiency signs and the third positive dimension of impulsive nonconformity, nor between EFA deficiency and the negative dimension of introvertive anhedonia.

Associations with EFA deficiency were therefore found for exactly the same positive schizotypal traits previously shown to be associated with dyslexia (Richardson, 1994). The same relationship between dyslexia and positive schizotypy was apparent in this sample: higher scores for the dyslexic group were found only for unusual experiences, cognitive disorganization and the STA scale ($p < 0.0005$ in all cases, Mann-Whitney or t test, two-tail).

To determine whether the relationships between these schizotypal traits and EFA deficiency were simply incidental to the strong dyslexia-schizotypy association, separate analyses were carried out for control and dyslexic groups. No relationships were found in controls, but within the dyslexic group EFA deficiency signs were very strongly associated with positive schizotypal traits (unusual experiences, $\rho = 0.40, p < 0.005$; cognitive disorganization, $\rho = 0.29, p < 0.05$; STA scale $\rho = 0.43, p < 0.005$). This finding is interesting in view of the proposal by Horrobin et al. (1995) of separate, but potentially interactive, deficiencies in EFA metabolism in dyslexia and schizophrenia. EFA deficiency signs do not appear to relate to schizotypal traits in nondyslexic subjects, yet within a group of dyslexic subjects (who may perhaps have an additional predisposing vulnerability), the same indices of fatty acid deficiency are highly correlated with positive schizotypal traits.

SUMMARY AND CONCLUSIONS

Evidence has been considered here for the proposal that an abnormality of phospholipid metabolism, involving deficiencies in certain LCPUFAs, may be a contributory factor in developmental dyslexia (Horrobin et al., 1995; Stordy, 1995). It has been shown that this would be perfectly compatible with what is already known about the biological basis of dyslexia. Moreover, there are similarities between dyslexia and the schizophrenia spectrum which suggest shared features at the level of biological predisposition. As discussed elsewhere in this book, there is now substantial evidence of phospholipid abnormalities in schizophrenia (Horrobin et al., 1994; Horrobin 1996, 1998), and it is therefore plausible that a similar (but probably independent) abnormality may be operating in dyslexia. In other, related conditions, such as ADHD, there is already some evidence for EFA deficiency, particularly of n-3 fatty acids (Stevens et al., 1995, 1996).

The direct evidence for phospholipid abnormalities in dyslexia remains relatively limited to date, but this includes an early and compelling case report of a dyslexic child in whom biochemical investigation did reveal EFA deficiency; and moreover, treatment to correct this was followed by marked improvements in schoolwork (Baker, 1985). Clear improvements in visual function have been shown in dyslexic adults following supplementation with n-3 fatty acids (Stordy, 1995), with anecdotal reports of wider benefits. In addition, brain imaging with ^{31}P-MRS has revealed abnormalities in membrane lipid turnover in dyslexic adults that are consistent with fatty acid deficiency (Richardson et al., 1997).

An EFA hypothesis of dyslexia clearly has implications for new treatment possibilities. Double-blind clinical trials of fatty acid treatment in dyslexia are underway, and some preliminary results from baseline assessments have been presented here. Clinical signs of EFA deficiency were examined in relation to dyslexia and associated traits in both children and adults. Consistent with the hypothesis, dyslexic adults showed significantly more EFA deficiency signs than matched controls; and in children, for whom control data is not yet available, EFA deficiency was associated with more severe reading deficits. Otherwise, the available data showed no significant associations between EFA deficiency signs and any particular psychometric profile. These signs were, however, associated with a wide range of dyslexic symptomatology as assessed by interview checklist measures, including visual symptoms when reading, auditory and spoken language confusions, and motor coordination difficulties.

In dyslexic adults, but not in controls, EFA deficiency signs were also associated with positive schizotypal traits, primarily those involving unusual perceptual experiences and associated odd beliefs. These traits have already been shown to relate to dyslexia (Richardson 1994, 1997), as they did in this sample, and the current findings could help to elucidate this. If EFA deficiency (perhaps particularly for n-3 fatty acids) is a risk factor for these unusual experiences, it may be that dyslexic individuals have a particular independent vulnerability to such deficiency. This would be consistent with the interactive genetic model proposed by Horrobin et al. (1995) to explain the familial aggregation of dyslexia, schizophrenia and related disorders.

In conclusion, it is already known that n-3 fatty acids such as DHA are particularly important in neuronal membranes, and that adequate levels are essential for normal visual and cognitive development as well as the maintenance of these functions (Crawford, 1992; Neuringer et al., 1994; Makrides et al., 1995). It is thus not at all unreasonable to propose that a mild abnormality of fatty acid metabolism could contribute to subtle developmental conditions such as dyslexia. The clinical treatment trials described here should provide further evidence with which to evaluate this proposal.

ACKNOWLEDGEMENTS

This research is supported by a project grant from the Sue Fowler Dyslexia Research Trust. Thanks are also due to Professor John Stein at the University Laboratory of Physiology, Oxford for providing additional staff and resources, and to Efamol Ltd for supplying the treatments used in the clinical trials. In collection of the data reported here, the particular contributions of Joel Talcott, Liz Westwood, Janet Walter and Gillian Hebb to the children's study, and those of Anna Corrie, Claire Higgins and Catherine Calvin to the adult study, are gratefully acknowledged. Special thanks are also offered to Jonathan Winter and Peter Hansen of the University Laboratory of Physiology, Oxford, for their technical support and advice.

REFERENCES

Augur J. Guidelines for teachers, parents and learners. In: Snowling M, ed. Children's written language difficulties. Windsor: NFER-Nelson, 1985; 147–169.

Baker SM. A biochemical approach to the problem of dyslexia. J Learn Disabil 1985; 18: 581–584.

Bazán NG, Reddy TS, Bazan HEP, Birkle DL. Metabolism of arachidonic and docosahexaenoic acids in the retina. Prog Lipid Res 1986; 25: 595–606.

Bourre J-M, Marianne F, Youyou A et al. The effects of dietary α-linolenic acid on the composition of nerve membranes, enzymatic activity, amplitude of electrophysiological parameters, resistance to poisons and performance of learning tasks in rats. J Nutr 1989; 119: 1880–1891.

Braitenberg V, Heck D, Sultan F. The detection and generation of sequences as a key to cerebellar function: experiments and theory. Behav Brain Sci 1997; 20: 229–277.

Budowski P, Leighfield MJ, Crawford MA. Nutritional encephalomalacia in the chick: an exposure of the vulnerable period for cerebellar development and the possible need for both ω-6 and ω-3 fatty acids. Br J Nutr 1987; 58: 511–520.

Cardon LR, Smith SD, Fulker DW, Kimberling WJ, Pennington BF, DeFries JC. Quantitative trait locus for reading disability on chromosome 6. Science 1994; 266: 276–279.

Cardon LR, Smith SD, Fulker DW, Kimberling WJ, Pennington BF, DeFries JC. Quantitative trait locus for reading disability: a correction. Science 1995; 268: 5217.

Carroll TA, Mullaney P, Eustace P. Dark adaptation in disabled readers screened for scotopic sensitivity syndrome. Percept Mot Skill 1994; 78: 131–141.

Castles A, Coltheart M. Varieties of developmental dyslexia. Cognition 1993, 47: 149–180.

Claridge GS, Broks P. Schizotypy and hemisphere function. I. Theoretical considerations and the measurement of schizotypy. Person Individ Diff 1984; 5: 633–648.

Claridge G, McCreery C, Mason PO et al. The factor structure of 'schizotypal traits': a large replication study. Br J Clin Psychol 1996; 35: 103–115.

Clausen J, Møller D. Allergic encephalomyelitis induced by brain antigen after deficiency in polyunsaturated fatty acids during myelination. Is multiple sclerosis a nutritive disorder? Acta Neurol Scand 1967; 43: 375–388.

Colquhoun I, Bunday S. A lack of essential fatty acids as a possible cause of hyperactivity in children. Med Hypotheses 1981; 7: 673–679.

Conners CK. Dyslexia and the neurophysiology of attention. In: Pavlidis GTh, ed. Perspectives on dyslexia, Vol 1. Chichester: John Wiley & Sons, 1990: 163–195.

Crawford MA. Essential fatty acids and neurodevelopmental disorder. In: Bazan NG, Toffano G, Horrobin DF et al., eds. Neurobiology of essential fatty acids. New York: Plenum Press, 1992: 307–314.

Critchley M. The dyslexic child. London: Heinemann, 1970.

Delion S, Chalon S, Herault J, Guilloteau D, Besnard J-C, Durand G. Chronic dietary α-linolenic acid deficiency alters dopaminergic and serotonergic neurotransmission in rats. J Nutr 1994; 124: 2466–2476.

Denckla MB. A neurologist's overview of developmental dyslexia. Ann N Y Acad Sci 1993; 682: 23–26.

Dobbing J, ed. Developing brain and behaviour: the role of lipids in infant formula. London: Academic Press, 1997.

Drake W. Clinical and pathological findings in a child with developmental learning disability. J Learn Disabil 1968; 1: 486–502.

Dykman RA, Ackerman PT. Attention deficit disorder and specific reading disability: separate but often overlapping disorders. J Learn Disabil 1991; 24: 96–103.

Eglington E, Annett M. Handedness and dyslexia: a meta-analysis. Percept Mot Skill 1994; 79: 1611–1616.

Elliott CD. British ability scales. Revised edn. Windsor: NFER–Nelson, 1983.

Erlenmeyer-Kimling L, Marcuse Y, Cornblatt B, Friedman D, Rainer JD, Rutschmann J. The New York high risk project. In: Watt NF, Anthony EJ, Wynne LC, Rolf JE, eds. Children at risk for schizophrenia: a longitudinal perspective. New York: Cambridge University Press 1984; 169–189.

Fawcett AJ, Nicolson RI, Dean P. Impaired performance of children with dyslexia on a range of cerebellar tasks. Ann Dyslexia 1996; 46: 259–283.

Fish B. Infant predictors of the longitudinal course of schizophrenic development. Schizophr Bull 1987; 13: 395–409.

Galaburda AM, Sherman GF, Rosen GD, Aboitiz F, Geschwind, N. Developmental dyslexia: four consecutive patients with cortical anomalies. Ann Neurol 1985; 18: 222–233.

Galaburda AM, Corsiglia J, Rosen GD, Sherman GF. Planum temporale asymmetry: reappraisal since Geschwind and Levitsky. Neuropsychologia 1987; 25: 853–868.

Geschwind N, Galaburda AM. Cerebral lateralization: biological mechanisms, associations and pathology. Cambridge, MA: MIT Press, 1987.

Glen AIM, Glen EMT, MacDonell LEF, Skinner FK, Sutherland J, Ward PE. Learning difficulties in familial schizophrenia. Schizophr Res 1996; 18: 171.

Grigorenko EL, Wood FB, Meyer MS et al. Susceptibility loci for distinct components of developmental dyslexia on chromosomes 6 and 15. Am J Hum Genet 1997; 60: 27–39.

Haslum MN. Predictors of dyslexia? Irish J Psychol 1989; 10: 622–630.

Hooper S, Willis WG. Learning disability subtyping: neuropsychological foundations, conceptual models and issues in clinical differentiation. New York: Springer, 1989.

Horrobin DF. A possible relationship between dyslexia and schizophrenia, two disorders in which membrane phospholipid metabolism is disturbed. Schizophr Res 1996; 18: 156.

Horrobin DF. The membrane phospholipid hypothesis as a biochemical basis for the neurodevelopmental concept of schizophrenia. Schizophr Res 1998; 30: 193–208.

Horrobin DF, Glen AIM, Vaddadi K. The membrane hypothesis of schizophrenia. Schizophr Res 1994; 13: 195–207.

Horrobin DF, Glen AIM, Hudson CJ. Possible relevance of phospholipid abnormalities and genetic interactions in psychiatric disorders: the relationship between dyslexia and schizophrenia. Med Hypotheses 1995; 45: 605–613.

Huang Y-S, Horrobin DF, Watanabe Y, Bartlett ME, Simmons VA. Effects of dietary lineleic acid on growth and liver phospholipid fatty acid composition in intact and gonadectomized rats. Biochem Arch 1990; 6: 47–54.

Hudson CJ, Kennedy JL, Gotowiec A et al. Genetic variant near cytosolic phospholipase A_2 associated with schizophrenia. Schizophr Res 1996; 21: 111–116.

Humphreys P, Kaufman WE, Galaburda AM. Developmental dyslexia in women: neuropathological findings in three patients. Ann Neurol 1990; 28: 727–738.

Hyde JS, Linn MC. Gender differences in verbal ability: a meta-analysis. Psychol Bull 1988; 104: 53–69.

Hynd GW, Semrud-Clikeman M. Dyslexia and brain morphology. Psychol Bull 1989; 106: 447–482.

Hynd GW, Semrud-Clikeman M, Lorys AR, Novey ES, Eliopoulos D. Brain morphology in developmental dyslexia and attention deficit disorder/hyperactivity. Arch Neurol 1990; 47: 919–926.

Hynd GW, Lorys AR, Semrud-Clikeman M, Nieves N, Huettner MIS, Lahey BB. Attention-deficit disorder without hyperactivity: a distinct behavioural and neurocognitive syndrome. J Child Neurol 1991; 6 (Suppl): 35–41.

James WH. The sex ratios of dyslexic children and their sibs. Devel Med Child Neurol 1992; 34: 530–533.

Jastak S, Wilkinson G. The wide range achievement test – revised. Wilmington: Jastak Associates Inc., 1984.

Kinsbourne M, Rufo DT, Gamzu E, Palmer RL, Berliner AK. Neuropsychological deficits in adults with dyslexia. Devel Med Child Neurol 1991; 33: 763–775.

Lahita RG. Systemic lupus erythematosus: learning disability of the male offspring of female patients and relationship to laterality. Psychoneuroendocrinology 1988; 13: 385–396.

Larsen JP, Høien T, Lundberg I, Ødegaard H. MRI evaluation of the size and symmetry of the planum temporale in adolescents with developmental dyslexia. Brain Lang 1990; 39: 289–301.

Livingstone MS, Rosen GD, Drislane FW, Galaburda AM. Physiological and anatomical evidence for a magnocellular defect in developmental dyslexia. Proc Natl Acad Sci USA 1991; 88: 7943–7947.

Lovegrove W. Spatial frequency processing in dyslexic and normal readers. In: Stein JF, ed. Vision and visual dyslexia. London: Macmillan, 1991: 148–154.

Lucas A. Role of nutritional programming in determining adult morbidity. Arch Dis Child 1994; 71: 288–290.

MacDonell L, Skinner FK, MacDonald MA et al. Neuropsychological, visual and essential fatty acid assessments of adults with dyslexic-type problems. Fourth World Congress on Dyslexia, Macedonia: 23–26 September, 1997.

Makrides M, Newmann M, Simmer K, Pater J, Gibson R. Are long-chain polyunsaturated fatty acids essential nutrients in infancy? Lancet 1995; 345: 1463–1468.

Marcus J. Cerebral functioning in offspring of schizophrenics: a possible genetic factor. Int J Ment Health 1974; 3: 57–73.

Mason O, Claridge G, Jackson M. New scales for the assessment of schizotypy. Person Individ Diff 1995; 18: 7–13.

McAnally K, Stein J. Auditory temporal coding in dyslexia. Proc R Soc Lond [Biol] 1996; 263: 961–965.

Miles TR. On the persistence of dyslexic difficulties into adulthood. In: Pavlidis GTh, Fisher DF, eds. Dyslexia: its neuropsychology and treatment. London: Wiley, 1986: 149–163.

Miles TR. Dyslexia: the pattern of difficulties. Oxford: Blackwell, 1994.

Mitchell EA, Aman MG, Turbott SH, Manku M. Clinical characteristics and serum essential fatty acid levels in hyperactive children. Clin Paediatr 1987; 26: 406–411.

Morais J. Literacy and awareness of the units of speech: implications for research on the units of perception. Linguistics 1985; 23: 707–721.

Neuringer M, Anderson GJ, Connor WE. The essentiality of n-3 fatty acids for the development and function of the retina and brain. Annu Rev Nutr 1988; 8: 517–541.

Neuringer M, Reisbeck S, Janowsky J. The role of n-3 fatty acids in visual and cognitive development: current evidence and methods of assessment. J Pediatr 1994; 125: S39–S47.

Nicolson RI, Fawcett AJ. Automaticity: a new framework for dyslexia research? Cognition 1990; 30: 159–182.

Nicolson RI, Fawcett AJ. Comparisons of deficits in cognitive and motor skills among children with dyslexia. Ann Dyslexia 1994; 44: 147–164.

Nicolson RI, Fawcett AJ, Dean P. Time estimation deficits in developmental dyslexia: evidence for cerebellar involvement. Proc Roy Soc 1995; 259: 43–47.

Nilsson A, Horrobin DF, Rosengren A, Waller L, Adlerberth A, Wilhelmson L. Essential fatty acids and abnormal involuntary movements in the general male population: a study of men born in 1933. Prostagland Leukotr Essent Fatty Acids 1996; 55: 83–87.

Nishikawa M, Kimura S, Akaitke N. Facilitatory effect of docosahexaenoic acid on N-methyl-D-aspartate response in pyramidal neurones of rat cerebral cortex. J Physiol 1994; 475: 83–93.

Nunez EA, ed. Fatty acids and cell signalling. Prostagland Leukotr Essent Fatty Acids 1993; 48: 1–122.

Peet M, Laugharne JDE, Mellor J, Ramchand CN. Essential fatty acid deficiency in erythrocyte membranes from chronic schizophrenic patients, and the clinical effects of dietary supplementation. Prostagland Leukotr Essent Fatty Acids 1996; 55: 71–75.

Peet M, Laugharne JDE, Mellor J. Double-blind trial of n-3 fatty acid supplementation in the treatment of schizophrenia. International Congress on Schizophrenia Research, Colorado Springs, April, 1997.

Peet M, Murphy B, Shay J, Horrobin D. Depletion of omega-3 fatty acid levels in red blood cell membranes of depressive patients. Biol Psychiatry 1998; 43: 315–319.

Pennington BF. Genetics of learning disabilities. J Child Neurol 1995; 10 (Suppl 1): S69–S77.

Psychological Corporation. The Wechsler Adult Intelligence Scales (WAIS-R), UK edition. San Antonio, Texas: Harcourt-Brace, 1994.

Pudelkewicz C, Seufert J, Holman RT. Requirements of the female rat for linoleic and linolenic acids. J Nutr 1968; 64: 138–147.

Richardson AJ. Dyslexia, handedness and syndromes of psychosis proneness. Int J Psychophysiol 1994; 18: 251–263.

Richardson AJ. Dyslexia and schizotypy. In: Claridge GS, ed. Schizotypy: relations with illness and health. Oxford: Oxford University Press, 1997: 171–201.

Richardson AJ, Stein JF. Personality characteristics of adult dyslexics. In: Wright SF, Groner R, eds. Facets of dyslexia and its remediation. North Holland: Elsevier Science Publishers, 1993: 411–423.

Richardson AJ, Cox IJ, Sargentoni J, Puri BK. Abnormal cerebral phospholipid metabolism in dyslexia indicated by phosphorus-31 magnetic resonance spectroscopy. NMR Biomed 1997; 10: 309–314.

Rieder RO, Nichols PL. The offspring of schizophrenics. 3. Hyperactivity and neurological soft signs. Arch Gen Psychiatry 1979; 36: 665–674.

Rosen GD, Sherman GF, Galaburda AM. Dyslexia and brain pathology: experimental animal models. In: Galaburda AM, ed. Dyslexia and development: neurobiological aspects of extraordinary brains. Cambridge, MA: Harvard University Press, 1993: 89–111.

Saunders WA, Barker MG. Dyslexia as a cause of psychiatric disorder in adults. Br Med J 1972; 4, 759–761.

Seymour P. Variability in dyslexia. In: Hulme C, Snowling M, eds. Reading development and dyslexia. London: Whurr, 1994: 65–85.

Slaghuis WL, Lovegrove WJ, Davidson JA. Visual and language processing deficits are concurrent in dyslexia. Cortex 1993; 29: 601–615.

Snowling M. Dyslexia. A cognitive developmental perspective. New York: Blackwell, 1987.

Stein JF, Glickstein M. Role of the cerebellum in visual guidance of movement. Physiol Rev 1992; 72: 972–1017.

Stein J, Walsh V. To see but not to read; the magnocellular theory of dyslexia. Trends Neurosci 1997; 20: 147–152.

Stevens LJ, Zentall SZ, Deck JL, Abate ML, Lipp SR, Burgess JR. Essential fatty acid metabolism in boys with attention-deficit hyperactivity disorder. Am J Clin Nutr 1995; 62: 761–768.

Stevens LJ, Zentall SS, Abate ML, Kuczek T, Burgess JR. Omega-3 fatty acids in boys with behaviour, learning, and health problems. Physiol Behav 1996; 59: 915–920.

Stordy BJ. Benefit of docosahexaenoic acid supplements to dark adaptation in dyslexics. Lancet 1995; 346: 385.

Tallal P, Miller S, Fitch RH. Neurobiological basis of speech: a case for the preeminence of temporal processing. Ann N Y Acad Sci 1993; 682: 27–47.

Tonnessen FE, Lokken A, Hoien T, Lundberg I. Dyslexia, left-handedness, and immune disorders. Arch Neurol 1993; 50: 411–416.

Vinegrad M. A revised adult dyslexia check list. Educare 1994; 48: 21–23.

Vollema MG, Van den Bosch RJ. The multidimensionality of schizotypy. Schizophr Bull 1995; 21: 19–31.

Wiederholt JL, Bryant BR. The Gray Oral Reading Tests, 3rd end. (GORT-3). Austin, TX: Pro-Ed, 1992.

Willats P, Forsyth JS, DiMondugno MK, Varma S, Colvin M. The effects of long chain polyunsaturated fatty acids on infant habituation at three months and problem solving at nine months. PUFA in infant nutrition: consensus and controversies. Proceedings of American Oil Chemists Society, Barcelona. Champaign, IL: American Oil Chemists Society, 1996: 42A.

Witton C, Talcott JB, Hansen PC et al. Sensitivity to dynamic auditory and visual stimuli predicts nonword reading ability in both dyslexic and normal readers. Curr Biol 1998; 8: 791–797.

Wolff PH. Impaired temporal resolution in developmental dyslexia. Ann N Y Acad Sci 1993; 682: 87–103.

Yamamoto N, Saitoh M, Moriuchi A, Nomura M, Okuyama H. Effect of dietary α-linolenate/linoleate balance on brain lipid composition and learning ability in rats. J Lipid Res 1987; 28: 144–151s.

22

Brain Phospholipid Metabolism in Dyslexia Assessed by Magnetic Resonance Spectroscopy

Basant K. Puri and Alexandra J. Richardson

INTRODUCTION

Magnetic resonance spectroscopy (MRS) is a powerful technique that can be used to monitor metabolic processes in the living human brain in a noninvasive way. In particular, 31-phosphorus MRS (^{31}P MRS) can be used to study brain phospholipid metabolism. The first study of developmental dyslexia using this technique was carried out by Richardson et al. (1997), to investigate the hypothesis that abnormalities of phospholipid metabolism may be a factor in this condition. In this chapter the use of ^{31}P MRS is first briefly described. There follow details of its application to the study of brain phospholipid metabolism in dyslexia. The implications of these findings are then discussed, with reference to findings from cerebral ^{31}P MRS studies of schizophrenia. Finally, future directions for the use of ^{31}P MRS in the study of dyslexia are outlined.

PHOSPHORUS-31 MRS

The ^{31}P isotope possesses the property of paramagnetism when in a static magnetic field, thus making it suitable for use in MRS studies. At the magnetic field strength that is used in clinical investigations (typically 1.5 T), seven principal metabolites are detectable in the living human brain using ^{31}P MRS. These are: phosphomonoester (PME), inorganic phosphorus (Pi), phosphodiester (PDE), phosphocreatine (PCr), and γ-, α- and β-nucleotide triphosphate (γ-, α- and β-NTP). These are illustrated in Figure 22.1.

The PME and PDE peaks from ^{31}P MRS spectra are the ones which specifically provide information relevant to the study of membrane phospholipid metabolism. The PME peak includes precursors to the synthesis of membrane phospholipids (Pettegrew et al., 1995). The main components of this peak are phosphorylethanolamine, phosphorylcholine, and phosphorylserine, which are precursors of myelin and membrane phospholipids such as phosphatidylethanolamine PE, phosphatidylcholine (PC; lecithin), and phosphatidylserine (PS) (Gyulai et al., 1984). By contrast, the PDE peak can provide an index of membrane phospholipid breakdown (Pettegrew et al., 1995). Although 90% of the PDE peak in the brain is believed to come from the phospholipid bilayer of myelin sheaths, the remainder derives from membrane degradation products such as

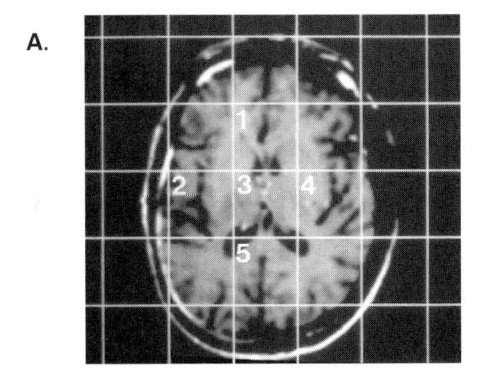

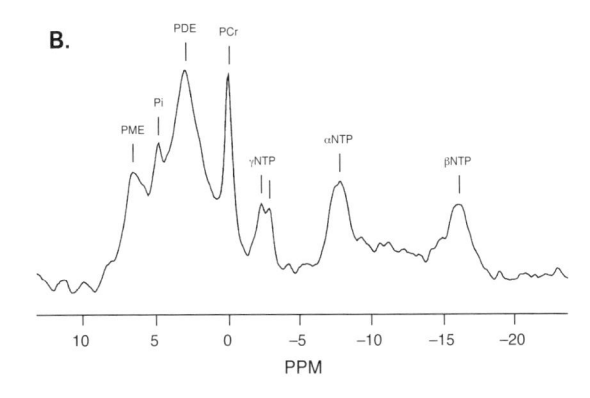

Figure 22.1. Representative MR results from a 33-year-old male. **A.** A T$_1$-weighted transverse image (SE 600/22) at the level of the basal ganglia, showing the voxels selected at this level. **B.** A representative ^{31}P MR spectrum from voxel No. 3 of **A**. After Richardson et al. (1997).

glycerophosphorylcholine and glycerophosphorylethanolamine. Information about energy metabolism is provided by the NTP resonances of ^{31}P spectra, of which the predominant contribution is from ATP, and also by the PCr and Pi resonances. In addition, intracellular pH can be determined from the relative positions of the Pi and PCr peaks (Petroff et al., 1985).

^{31}P MRS IN THE STUDY OF DYSLEXIA

Background and rationale

The membrane phospholipid hypothesis of schizophrenia is well established (see Horrobin, 1977; Horrobin et al., 1994) and is described in detail in other chapters of this book. It is now becoming clear that abnormalities of phospholipid metabolism may also play a role in a much wider range of neurodevelopmental disorders, and a recent suggestion is that this includes developmental dyslexia (Horrobin et al., 1995).

Richardson (1994, 1997) drew attention to the many similarities between developmental dyslexia and schizophrenia, which suggest that there may be common elements in the biological predisposition to these disorders. In both groups, right-handedness occurs less firmly and consistently than in the general population, and studies using structural magnetic resonance imaging have shown abnormal asymmetry of the cerebral planum temporale in both conditions (Larsen et al., 1990; Petty et al., 1995). Dyslexia is associated with a particular pattern of visual deficits for tasks such as fine spatial localization, motion, and flicker perception, pointing to a dysfunction of the fast magnocellular stream of visual processing for which there is now good evidence (see Stein and Walsh, 1997). Similar visual abnormalities have been reported in schizophrenia (Green et al., 1994a,b), and also in nonpsychotic subjects who show schizotypal personality traits (Richardson and Stein, 1993; Richardson and Gruzelier, 1994).

Dyslexic subjects themselves score very highly on scales designed to assess positive schizotypal personality traits in the general population (Richardson, 1994, 1997), primarily owing to their high endorsement of items relating to unusual perceptual experiences and associated unconventional beliefs. These traits have some validity in predicting psychotic breakdown (Chapman et al., 1994), and are common in the nonpsychotic first-degree relatives of patients with schizophrenia (Claridge et al., 1983), although they are by no means incompatible with normal healthy functioning. Other traits associated with an increased risk of schizophrenia include anhedonia and poor social or interpersonal rapport (Kendler et al., 1985), but it is notable that dyslexia does not appear to be associated with these characteristics (Richardson, 1994).

Probably the most compelling evidence for a link between dyslexia and schizophrenia is the consistent finding that, compared with the children of nonpsychotic parents, the children of schizophrenic parents are at higher risk of dyslexia (Marcus, 1974; Rieder and Nichols, 1979; Erlenmeyer-Kimling et al., 1984; Fish, 1987), and it is notable that similar attentional abnormalities and visuomotor problems during early development are associated with both disorders. A substantial genetic contribution is already well established for dyslexia (DeFries et al., 1987), as for schizophrenia (Gottesman, 1991), but these findings suggest a genetic component to dyslexia that is carried by those with schizophrenia. Horrobin and colleagues (1995) have proposed that a membrane phospholipid abnormality also occurs in dyslexia, and have put forward a model whereby genetic interactions in this domain could help to explain the aggregation of dyslexia, schizophrenia and other disorders within families.

Although there has been a remarkable lack of research into dyslexia from a biochemical perspective, the idea of a phospholipid abnormality is backed by some direct evidence. In an insightful case study of a dyslexic child, Baker (1985) cited essential fatty acid deficiency as an apparent key factor. More recently, Stordy (1995) found defective dark adaptation in adult dyslexic subjects, which then normalized following a high intake of docosahexaenoic acid (DHA). Further details of this work, and of the potential relevance of fatty acids in dyslexia and associated conditions, are given in Chapters 21 and 23 of this book (Richardson et al., 1999; Stordy, 1999).

^{31}P MRS has been used in several studies of schizophrenia (e.g., Pettegrew et al., 1991, 1995; Williamson et al., 1991, 1995; and see also Chapter 5 in this book, Williamson and Drost, 1999). This technique has provided strong evidence for an increased rate of breakdown of brain phospholipids in both medicated and unmedicated patients with this disorder (reduced PME and/or increased PDE). This is consistent with evidence for an increased rate of loss in schizophrenia of DHA and arachidonic acid (AA) from membranes, which has been attributed to enhanced phospholipase A$_2$ activity (Gattaz et al., 1990; Horrobin, 1996). By contrast, Horrobin et al. (1995) proposed that the predisposition to dyslexia might involve the opposite problem of reduced synthesis and/or incorporation of phospholipids into cell membranes. On this hypothesis, the prediction would be for ^{31}P MRS studies of dyslexia to yield the opposite pattern of results to that found in schizophrenia, namely increased PME and/or reduced PDE.

A study to investigate this was therefore carried out by Richardson et al. (1997).

Subjects and methods

The subjects were 22 adults (12 male, 10 female). Twelve had previously been identified by educational psychologists as dyslexic, and for this study their specific problems with literacy were confirmed by standardized reading and spelling measures compared with general ability. These subjects also showed the significant deficits in working memory and phonological skills that are characteristic of dyslexia (see Table 22.1). The remaining ten subjects were controls, selected as having no current or previous reading difficulties. These two groups were matched with respect to sex and age. There were seven male and five female dyslexic subjects, and five male and five female controls: $\chi^2 = 0.15$ (ns). The dyslexic subjects were aged 34.1 ± 9.5 years (mean ± SD), and the controls 28.3 ± 7.2 years: $t\,(df, 20) = 1.58$ (ns). Standard MR exclusion criteria were applied, such as ferromagnetic implants, claustrophobia or pregnancy. Other exclusion criteria were neurological or other significant medical disorder, psychoactive substance abuse, and regular use of essential fatty acid supplements.

This study was carried out at Hammersmith Hospital, London, where cerebral MRS data were obtained using a Picker prototype spectroscopy system (Picker International, Cleveland, Ohio, USA) based on a whole-body magnet (Oxford Magnet Technology, Oxford, UK) operating at 1.5 T. A set of localized ^{31}P MRS spectra were simultaneously obtained from an $8 \times 8 \times 8$ grid covering the entire head using a four-dimensional chemical shift imaging (4D-CSI) technique (Coutts et al., 1989), with a nominal spatial resolution of 4 cm × 4 cm × 4 cm and a repetition time of 5 s. The data set was filtered using a cosine filter in each spatial dimension and an exponential filter of 10.6 Hz in the spectral dimension, prior to four-dimensional Fourier transformation. Voxel positions were precisely matched across subjects, using high-resolution proton MR images obtained during the same scanning sessions. Ten voxels from comparable cerebral regions were selected for each subject and the spectrum from each voxel was individually and manually phased. Spectral resolutions and signal:noise ratios were visually assessed, and between seven and ten spectra from each subject were thus identified for further analysis. Phosphorus peaks were identified in each spectrum; relative peak areas were then calculated by fitting the signals to inverse polynomial functions. Figure 22.2 shows a representative fitted ^{31}P MRS spectrum.

Relative levels of each metabolite were calculated as a percentage of the total phosphorus signal (the sum of all peak areas). Metabolite ratios, as conventionally used in ^{31}P MRS studies, were also calculated

Table 22.1. The results of psychological assessment of the two groups of subjects involved in the ^{31}P MRS study of dyslexia; means ± SD.

	Study group		
Performance area and test	Dyslexia (n = 12)	Control (n = 10)	F^a
General ability[b]			
Similarities	14.4 ± 1.8	14.3 ± 1.7	0.03
Vocabulary	12.8 ± 2.3	13.2 ± 2.3	0.20
Block design	14.8 ± 3.6	12.6 ± 2.6	2.64
Picture arrangement	12.9 ± 3.6	12.3 ± 2.8	0.34
Reading and spelling[c]			
Reading	95.3 ± 13.8	117.1 ± 4.0	23.05†††
Spelling	85.3 ± 19.3	115.1 ± 5.7	22.13†††
Other test areas			
Non-word reading[d]	87.2 ± 13.1	109.6 ± 2.6	25.19†††
Digit span[b]	8.2 ± 2.2	13.1 ± 2.1	25.13†††

[a] One-way analysis of variance; [b] WAIS-R subtests (The Wechsler Adult Intelligence Scales (WAIS-R), UK edition, 1994); [c] scores on the Wide Range Achievement Test (Jastak and Wilkinson, 1984); [d] composite measures of errors and time taken to read 46 nonsense words (standard scores).
†††$p < 0.0001$ (other F values are statistically nonsignificant).

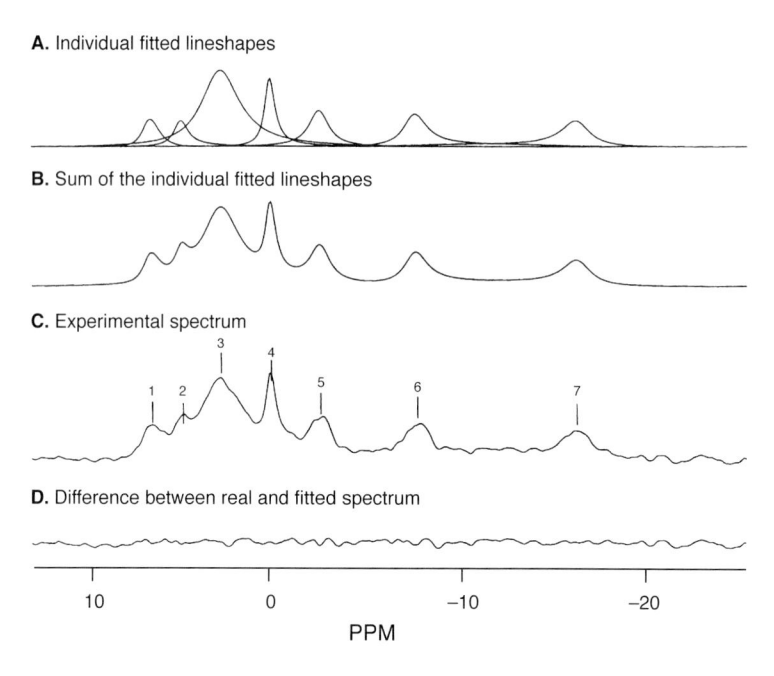

Figure 22.2. A representative curve fit of an MR spectrum from a 27-year-old control subject (male). The peaks were fitted to inverse polynomial lineshape functions using NMR1® (New Methods Research Inc., E. Syracuse, USA). **A.** The individual lineshapes. **B.** The fitted lineshapes are summed. **C.** The experimental plot. **D.** Difference between the experimental and fitted spectra. After Richardson et al. (1997).

(namely PME/βNTP, Pi/βNTP, PDE/βNTP, PME/PDE and PCr/Pi), and intracellular pH was calculated from the difference in the chemical shifts of Pi and PCr. For each subject, the spectral information from all the selected voxels was averaged to produce a single set of cerebral parameters. After confirmation that all variables yielded a normal distribution of values, group comparisons were carried out using a one-way ANOVA.

Results

The results of the study are shown in Table 22.2. Compared with the controls, the dyslexic group showed a significant elevation in both the PME/βNTP ratio ($p < 0.001$), as illustrated in Figure 22.3, and in the PME/PDE ratio ($p < 0.02$). Consistent with these results, the relative level of PME as a proportion of the total phosphorus signal was significantly higher in the dyslexic subjects ($p < 0.006$) than in the controls. The relative levels for all other metabolites did not differ significantly between the two groups; neither did any other metabolite ratios, nor did pH (see Table 22.2). No significant sex differences were found.

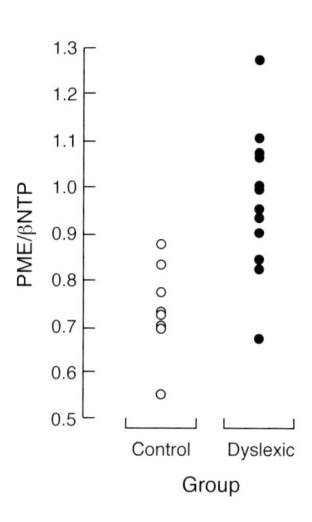

Figure 22.3. Scatterplot showing individual values for the PME/βNTP ratio in the two subject groups (dyslexic and control). After Richardson et al. (1997).

Table 22.2. Levels of phosphorus metabolites (expressed as a percentage of the total ^{31}P signal), metabolite ratios, and pH, in the two groups of subjects involved in the ^{31}P MRS study of dyslexia; means ± SD.

	Study group		
Parameter	Dyslexia ($n = 12$)	Control ($n = 10$)	F^a
Phosphorus metabolites			
PME	9.96 ± 1.51	8.39 ± 0.59	9.47**
Pi	6.46 ± 0.67	6.26 ± 0.77	0.43
PDE	36.76 ± 1.89	37.45 ± 1.66	0.82
PCr	10.09 ± 0.82	10.27 ± 1.11	0.19
γNTP	9.17 ± 1.27	9.00 ± 0.96	0.13
αNTP	16.12 ± 1.30	16.10 ± 1.56	0.00
βNTP	10.94 ± 1.37	11.89 ± 1.04	3.21
Metabolite ratios			
PME/βNTP	0.97 ± 0.16	0.74 ± 0.09	17.52††
Pi/βNTP	0.63 ± 0.14	0.55 ± 0.08	3.18
PDE/βNTP	3.56 ± 0.56	3.28 ± 0.29	2.00
PME/PDE	0.28 ± 0.05	0.23 ± 0.02	6.94*
PCr/Pi	1.63 ± 0.20	1.72 ± 0.34	0.54
pH	7.03 ± 0.03	7.03 ± 0.02	0.06

[a] One-way analysis of variance. $p <$: *0.05; **0.01; ††0.0005 (other F values are statistically nonsignificant).

Discussion

The first study of dyslexia using ^{31}P MRS revealed a significant elevation of phosphomonoesters in adult dyslexic subjects relative to matched controls. As noted earlier, the PME peak is multicomponent but includes major contributions from PC, PE, and L-phosphorylserine, which are important precursors of membrane phospholipids. This elevation of PMEs in dyslexia is therefore consistent with difficulties in the biosynthesis of phospholipids and/or their incorporation into membranes (where they become essentially invisible to MRS) and is in line with the prediction of the membrane hypothesis put forward by Horrobin et al. (1995).

Separation of the PME peak into its different components cannot be achieved with the methodology used here, and other metabolites, including sugar phosphates, can contribute to this region of the spectrum, so a definitive interpretation of these findings is not possible at this stage. However, the fact that there is already some other evidence for a phospholipid abnormality in dyslexia (Horrobin et al., 1995; Stordy, 1995) makes this appear to be the most probable explanation. Numerous different enzyme systems are involved in the biosynthesis of phospholipids and their incorporation into membranes (Dawson, 1985), so it is equally premature to attempt to attribute these findings to a specific phospholipid abnormality. However, possible enzymatic explanations for increased PME would include an increase in the activity of phosphodiesterase, phospholipase-C or kinase, or a decrease in phosphatase activity.

An elevation of cerebral PMEs is typically found during early brain development (Pettegrew et al., 1987, 1995). This is thought to reflect a major contribution from PE and may be associated with cell growth. In adults, raised levels of PMEs are not often found, although they are found in association with certain types of tumour (Negendank, 1992; Ruiz-Cabello and Cohen, 1992), and have also been reported in Alzheimer's disease (Pettegrew et al., 1987). None of these observations readily explains our finding of raised PMEs in adults with developmental dyslexia.

A raised cerebral PME peak has also been reported in patients with bipolar mood disorder while in the manic phase (Kato et al., 1991). While this finding might have resulted from accumulation of inositol 1-phosphate in the brain following pharmacotherapy with lithium, it may also at least partly be related to the findings reported in this chapter, in view of the report by Richardson (1994) of an association between dyslexia and hypomanic traits. This is in keeping with the general association found between dyslexia and positive, but not negative, schizotypal traits.

Finally, it should be noted that the metabolism of membrane phospholipids is heavily influenced by their essential fatty acid composition. Hence the findings reported in this chapter are consistent with essential fatty acid deficiency in dyslexia. As mentioned above, the importance of the long-chain polyunsaturated fatty acids, such as DHA, for visual and cognitive development is increasingly being recognized, and therefore it is conceivable that they may play some role in dyslexia and other neurodevelopmental disorders.

IMPLICATIONS AND FUTURE MRS STUDIES

The MRS study by Richardson et al. (1997) provides direct evidence in favour of some kind of abnormality of membrane lipid metabolism in dyslexia, and further investigation is clearly warranted to confirm and elucidate these findings. In particular, it would be helpful to use ^{31}P MRS in conjunction with other biochemical measures of phospholipid metabolism, as there are inevitably some uncertainties over the precise significance of the PME and PDE peaks in ^{31}P spectra as indices of membrane turnover (Ruiz-Cabello and Cohen, 1992). The findings of Stordy (1995) are consistent with a deficiency in dyslexia of certain ω-3 fatty acids. This would suggest that direct measures of the fatty acid composition of red cell membranes and plasma might provide useful additional information, an avenue which is currently being explored. Although it is possible that these kinds of MRS measures could ultimately prove to be of value in the identification of dyslexia and/or in evaluating treatment possibilities, there remains much additional work to be done before this can properly be evaluated. Assuming that these findings are replicable at a group level, both the reliability of MRS measures for individual subjects and their discriminative power would still require further investigation.

Given the clinical heterogeneity of dyslexia, it also makes sense to investigate associations between these MRS parameters and psychological test scores in a larger sample, to determine whether abnormalities may be confined to a particular subgroup. Moreover, the case for membrane abnormalities as a contributory factor in dyslexia would obviously be strengthened if these biochemical measures could be shown to relate to specific aspects of perceptual and cognitive function that are already known to be important in the acquisition of reading skills. This issue is under investigation in an extended sample of dyslexic and control adults, together with an examination of regional variation in these MRS measures.

As emphasized by Horrobin et al. (1995), the improvement in visual function in dyslexia reported by Stordy (1995) following essential fatty acid treatment indicates that at least some of the abnormalities associated with dyslexia may be quite easily reversible. Richardson and colleagues have therefore embarked on several double-blind placebo-controlled trials of essential fatty acid supplementation in dyslexia in order to assess whether this treatment leads to clinical improvement in other respects. As part of these studies in adults, ^{31}P MRS assessments are taking place at baseline and follow-up, to find out whether these measures will be sensitive to treatment effects. From an individual case study involving the successful treatment of schizophrenia with ω-3 fatty acids (Puri and Richardson, 1998; and see Chapter 21) the authors already have strong indications that clinical improvement is indeed mirrored by changes in ^{31}P MRS parameters; however, at the time of writing, the dyslexia treatment trials are still taking place and therefore results are not yet available.

REFERENCES

Baker SM. A biochemical approach to the problem of dyslexia. J Learn Disabil 1985; 18: 581–584.

Chapman LJ, Chapman JP, Kwapil TR, Eckblad M, Zinser MC. Putatively psychosis-prone subjects 10 years later. J Abnorm Psychol 1994; 103: 171–183.

Claridge GS, Robinson DL, Birchall PMA. Characteristics of schizophrenics' and neurotics' relatives. Per Individ Dif 1983; 4: 651–664.

Coutts GA, Cox IJ, Gadian DG, Sargentoni J, Bryant DJ, Collins AG. Phosphorus-31 magnetic resonance spectroscopy of the normal human brain: approaches using four-dimensional chemical shift imaging and phase mapping techniques. NMR Biomed 1989; 1: 190–197.

Dawson RMC. Enzymatic pathways of phospholipid metabolism in the nervous system. In: Eichberg J, ed. Phospholipids in nervous tissues. New York: John Wiley, 1985: 45–78.

DeFries JC, Fulker DW, La Buda MC. Evidence for a genetic aetiology in reading disability of twins. Nature 1987; 329: 537–539.

Erlenmeyer-Kimling L, Marcuse Y, Cornblatt B, Friedman D, Rainer JD, Rutschmann J. The New York high risk project. In: Watt NF, Anthony LC, Rolf JE, eds. Children at risk of schizophrenia: a longitudinal perspective. New York: Cambridge University Press, 1984: 169–189.

Fish B. Infant predictors of the longitudinal course of schizophrenic development. Schizophr Bull 1987; 13: 395–409.

Gattaz WF, Hübner CK, Nevalainen TJ, Thuren T, Kinnunen PKJ. Increased serum phospholipase-A$_2$ activity in schizophrenia: a replication study. Biol Psychiatry 1990; 28: 495–501.

Gottesman II. Schizophrenia genesis: the origins of madness. New York: WH Freeman and Co., 1991.

Green MF, Neuchterlein KH, Mintz J. Backward masking in schizophrenia and mania. I. Specifying a mechanism. Arch Gen Psychiatry 1994a; 51: 939–944.

Green MF, Neuchterlein KH, Mintz J. Backward masking in schizophrenia and mania. II. Specifying the visual channels. Arch Gen Psychiatry 1994b; 51: 945–951.

Gyulai L, Bolinger L, Leigh JS, Barlow C, Chance B. Phosphorylethanolamine: the major constituent of the phosphomonoester peak observed by ^{31}P NMR on developing dog brain. FEBS Lett 1984; 178: 137–142.

Horrobin DF. Schizophrenia as a prostaglandin deficiency disease. Lancet 1977; i: 936–937.

Horrobin DF. Schizophrenia as a membrane lipid disorder which is expressed throughout the body. Prostagland Leukot Essent Fatty Acids 1996; 55: 3–7.

Horrobin DF, Glen AIM, Vaddadi K. The membrane hypothesis of schizophrenia. Schizophr Res 1994; 13: 195–207.

Horrobin DF, Glen AIM, Hudson CJ. Possible relevance of phospholipid abnormalities and genetic interactions in psychiatric disorders: the relationship between dyslexia and schizophrenia. Med Hypotheses 1995; 45: 605–613.

Jastak S, Wilkinson G. The wide range achievement test – revised. Wilmington: Jastak Associates, 1984.

Kato T, Shioiri T, Takahashi S, Inubushi T. Measurement of brain phosphoinositide metabolism in bipolar patients using *in vivo* ^{31}P-MRS. J Affective Disord 1991; 22: 185–190.

Kendler KS, Gruenberg AM, Tsuang MT. Psychiatric illness in first-degree relatives of schizophrenic and surgical control patients. A family study using DSM-III criteria. Arch Gen Psychiatry 1985; 42: 770–779.

Larsen JP, Høien T, Lundberg I, Ødegaard H. MRI evaluation of the size and symmetry of the planum temporale in adolescents with developmental dyslexia. Brain Lang 1990; 39: 289–301.

Marcus J. Cerebral functioning in offspring of schizophrenics: a possible genetic factor. Int J Ment Health 1974; 3: 57–73.

Negendank W. Studies of human tumors by MRS: a review. NMR Biomed 1992; 5: 303–324.

Petroff OA, Prichard JW, Behar KL, Alger JR, den Hollander JA, Shulman RG. Cerebral intracellular pH by ^{31}P nuclear magnetic resonance spectroscopy. Neurology 1985; 35: 781–788.

Pettegrew JW, Kopp SJ, Minshew NJ et al. ^{31}P Nuclear magnetic resonance studies of phosphoglyceride metabolism in developing and degenerating brain: preliminary observations. J Neuropathol Exp Neurol 1987; 46: 419–430.

Pettegrew JW, Keshavan MS, Panchalingam K et al. Alterations in brain high-energy phosphate and membrane phospholipid metabolism in first-episode drug-naïve schizophrenics. A pilot study of the dorsal prefrontal cortex by *in vivo* phosphorus-31 nuclear magnetic resonance spectroscopy. Arch Gen Psychiatry 1991; 48: 563–568.

Pettegrew JW, Keshavan MS, Minshew NJ, McClure RJ. ^{31}P-MRS of metabolic alterations in schizophrenia and neurodevelopment. In: Nasrallah HA, Pettegrew JW, eds. NMR spectroscopy in psychiatric brain disorders. Washington, DC: American Psychiatric Press, 1995: 45–77.

Petty RG, Barta PE, Pearlson GD et al. Reversal of asymmetry of the planum temporale in schizophrenia. Am J Psychiatry 1995; 152: 715–721.

Puri BK, Richardson AJ. Sustained remission of positive and negative symptoms of schizophrenia following treatment with eicosapentaenoic acid. Arch Gen Psychiatry 1998; 55: 188–189.

Richardson AJ. Dyslexia, handedness and syndromes of psychosis-proneness. Int J Psychophysiol 1994; 18: 251–263.

Richardson AJ. Dyslexia and schizotypy. In: Claridge GS, ed. Schizotypy: implications for illness and health. Oxford: Oxford University Press, 1997: 171–201.

Richardson AJ, Gruzelier J. Visual processing, lateralization and syndromes of schizotypy. Int J Psychophysiol 1994; 18: 227–239.

Richardson AJ, Stein JF. Dyslexia, schizotypy and visual direction sense. Ann N Y Acad Sci 1993; 682: 400–401.

Richardson AJ, Cox IJ, Sargentoni J, Puri BK. Abnormal cerebral phospholipid metabolism in dyslexia indicated by phosphorus-31 magnetic resonance spectroscopy. NMR Biomed 1997; 10: 309–314.

Richardson AJ, Easton T, McDaid AM, Hall JA, Montgomery P, Clisby C, Puri BK. Essential fatty acids in dyslexia: theory, evidence and clinical trials. In: Glen I, Peet M, Horrobin DF, eds. Phospholipid spectrum disorder in psychiatry. Carnforth: Marius Press, 1999: 225–241.

Rieder RO, Nichols PL. The offspring of schizophrenics. 3. Hyperactivity and neurological soft signs. Arch Gen Psychiatry 1979; 36: 665–674.

Ruiz-Cabello J, Cohen JS. Phospholipid metabolites as indicators of cancer cell function. NMR Biomed 1992; 5: 226–233.

Stein JF, Walsh V. To see but not to read: the magnocellular theory of dyslexia. Trends Neurosci 1997; 20: 147–152.

Stordy BJ. Benefit of docosahexaenoic acid supplements to dark adaptation in dyslexics. Lancet 1995; 346: 385.

Stordy BJ. Essential fatty acids in the management of dyslexia and dyspraxia. In: Glen I, Peet M, Horrobin DF, eds. Phospholipid spectrum disorder in psychiatry. Carnforth: Marius Press, 1999: 251–260.

The Wechsler Adult Intelligence Scales (WAIS-R), UK edition. San Antonio, Texas: Harcourt-Brace, 1994.

Williamson PC, Drost DJ. ^{31}P-magnetic resonance spectroscopy in the assessment of brain phospholipid metabolism in schizophrenia. In: Glen I, Peet M, Horrobin DF, eds. Phospholipid spectrum disorder in psychiatry. Carnforth: Marius Press, 1999: 45–55.

Williamson PC, Drost D, Stanley J, Carr T, Morrison S, Merskey H. Localized phosphorus-31 magnetic resonance spectroscopy in chronic schizophrenic patients and normal controls. Arch Gen Psychiatry 1991; 48: 578.

Williamson PC, Drost DJ, Stanley JA, Carr TJ. ^{31}P-MRS in the study of schizophrenia. In: Nasrallah HA, Pettegrew JW, eds. NMR spectroscopy in psychiatric brain disorders. Washington, DC: American Psychiatric Press, 1995: 107–129.

Long-chain Fatty Acids in the Management of Dyslexia and Dyspraxia

B. Jacqueline Stordy

INTRODUCTION

A substantial body of research has established that many processes in the brain and visual system are related to certain long-chain polyunsaturated fatty acids (LCPUFAs). The brain, the most membrane-rich of all the body tissues, is composed largely (60%) of lipids, half of which are LCPUFAs. Docosahexaenoic acid (DHA) of the n-3 series, and arachidonic and adrenic acids (AA and ADrA) of the n-6 series, are the most prevalent of these LCPUFAs.

Dietary origins and metabolism of LCPUFAs

The essential fatty acids (EFAs), linoleic acid (LA) and α-linolenic acid (ALA), which are found in many foods (seeds, nuts, and the oils which they provide, being the richest dietary sources), give rise to most of the AA, ADrA and DHA in the tissues as the result of processes of elongation and desaturation. It is characteristic of modern dietary habits that we consume substantially increased quantities of hydrogenated and partially hydrogenated vegetable oils, which are used in the manufacture of processed foods such as margarine, as well as appearing in cooking fats, snacks and baked goods. The *trans* isomers of fatty acids, which are produced in the hydrogenation process, differ from the *cis* isomers in both structure and metabolism, and the results of studies carried out using rat and human fibroblasts have indicated that the *trans* fatty acids impair the desaturation and elongation of EFAs, and hence lower the production of LCPUFAs.

Whilst the complete desaturation and elongation pathways of EFA metabolism have not yet been fully elucidated, Infante and Huszagh (1997) have proposed that these processes may take place in three cell organelles, i.e., the microsomes, the mitochondria, and the peroxisomes. Figure 23.1 illustrates the conventional and putative pathways.

It was suggested until relatively recently that there was competition between n-6 and n-3 series EFAs for the same desaturase and elongase enzymes. That does indeed appear to be the case in some organelles, but the dual sets of enzymes for n-3 and n-6 series which are found in the proposed mitochondrial system, indicates that under some conditions only one of the EFA series may be affected.

The LCPUFAs, AA, eicosapentaenoic acid (EPA), and DHA, are available ready-formed only in foods of animal origin (Table 23.1). Because of the small amount of fish consumed in affluent, westernized societies, the usual diet in such societies is relatively deficient in LCPUFAs, particularly those of the n-3 series. Even if an adequate supply of EFAs is consumed in the diet, this is not, in itself, a guarantee that there will then be an adequate supply of LCPUFAs to the tissues. Certain medical conditions (e.g., diabetes, eczema and atopy), are characterized by defects of the conversion processes. Interference with EFA metabolism also results from the excess consumption of alcohol, hydrogenated or partially hydrogenated fats, and from zinc deficiency.

Developmental importance of LCPUFAs

An adequate supply of LCPUFAs in early life appears to be directly linked to the development of visual and intellectual capacities. LCPUFAs are present in human milk, though there can be substantial variability in the DHA content depending upon the diet of the mother (Sanders and Reddy, 1992) (Table 23.2), being very low if the mother adopts a vegan (strictly vegetarian) dietary style. Children aged 8 years, who had been born prematurely, were investigated by Lucas et al. (1992) who found that those premature infants to whom breast milk had been given had an 8-point IQ advantage over other premature infants who had received formula which did not contain LCPUFAs. This finding is in accord with the results of numerous other studies in which the development of visual acuity and/or behaviour has been

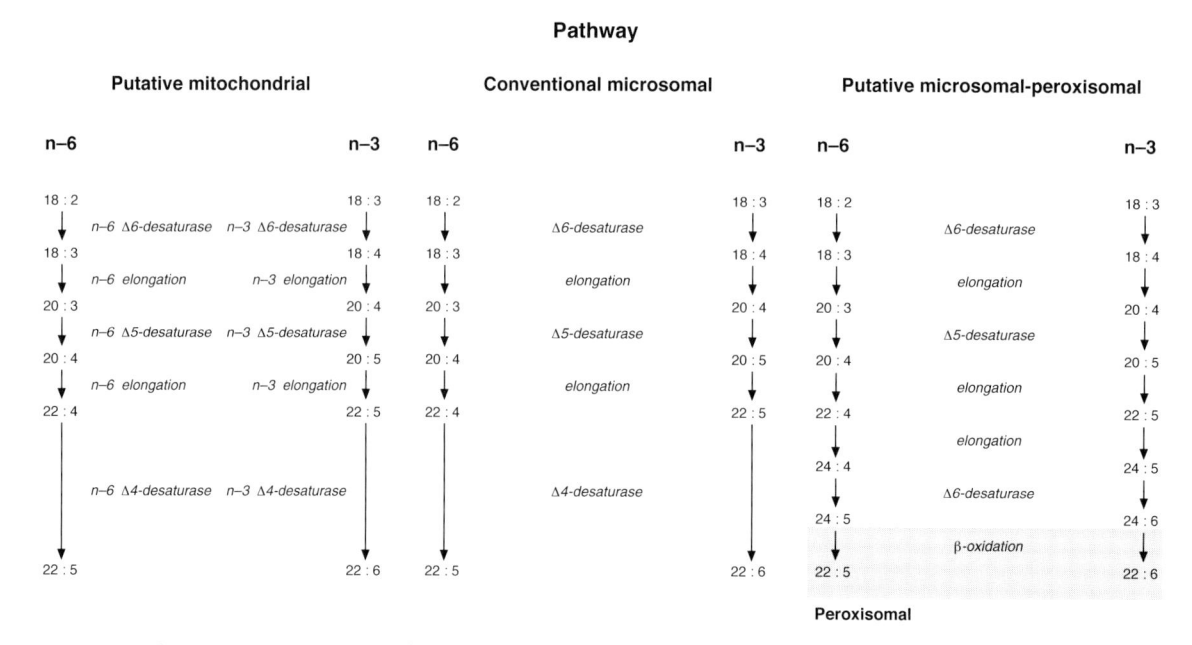

Figure 23.1. Conventional and putative pathways for desaturation and elongation of EFAs.

examined in term infants fed either breast milk or formula with and without LCPUFAs (Andraca and Uauy, 1995; Makrides et al., 1995; Heird et al., 1997; Horrwood and Fergusson, 1998). Investigations have also been extensively reported in which the dietary depletion of n-3 fatty acids or DHA has been found to affect learning and behaviour in animals. The interpretation of the results of such studies is complicated by difficulties in determining whether the learning and behavioural consequences of an LCPUFA-deficient diet are, at least in part, secondary consequences of the visual or of the central processing deficits (or both).

LCPUFAs and specific learning disorders

Several factors were responsible for my own research interest in the role played by LCPUFAs in the aetiology of learning disorders. In the first place, I wished to examine further the importance which LCPUFAs seemed to have for the development of visual and neural systems. Secondly, I was intrigued by an observation that the dyslexia which had occurred in many members of a large family in the course of three generations, appeared to be distinctly less severe, and also to have later onset, in those individuals in whom breast feeding had been continued for the longest times. Thirdly, it was becoming increasingly clear that three specific learning disorders – dyslexia, attention deficit/hyperactivity disorder (ADHD) and dyspraxia – were likely to have a common genetic origin and a common biological basis:

not only did they run in the same families, but they also frequently showed comorbidity in an individual.

The close relationships between these developmental disorders have tended to be obscured by differences in the way in which they have been treated or otherwise managed. Dyslexia has, for example, until relatively recently, been primarily the province of the educational psychologist; consequently, attempts to treat the condition, or at least to reduce its impact, have relied almost exclusively on educational techniques, including such procedures as structured multisensory learning. ADHD and attention deficit disorder (ADD), on the other hand, whilst usually initially identified in children by the educational psychologist, are likely to be treated, following referral to the paediatrician, using stimulant medication, behaviour therapy, or both. Dyspraxia may follow a similar referral route to the paediatrician, but subsequent intervention usually involves a combination of physiotherapy and occupational therapy.

It is largely as a result of the application of these very different types of intervention, and also because different categories of health care professional have been involved, that scant consideration has been given to those features which dyslexia, dyspraxia, ADHD, and other developmental learning deficits, may have in common. Certainly, there has been relatively little interest in any fundamental chemical differences which there might be in the tissues of these individuals which would distinguish them from other children not affected by the same

Table 23.1. Food sources of n-6 and n-3 fatty acids.

Fatty acid	Food source	% of total fatty acid
n-6		
Linoleic	Sunflower	20–75
	Corn	30–62
	Olive	11
γ-Linolenic	Borage	20
	Blackcurrant	17–20
	Evening primrose	10
Arachidonic	Beef	1
	Mackerel	4
	Turkey	5
n-3		
α-Linolenic	Green leaves	56
	Linseed	45–60
	Rapeseed	10–11
Eicosapentaenoic	Freshwater fish	5–13
	Mackerel	8
	Sardine	3
Docosahexaenoic	Freshwater fish	1–5
	Mackerel	8
	Sardine	9–13

Table 23.2. Fatty acid composition of human milk in vegans, vegetarians and omnivores.

Fatty acid	Diet group	% of total fatty acids
Linoleic	Vegans	23.8
	Vegetarians	19.5
	Omnivores	10.9
α-Linolenic	Vegans	1.36
	Vegetarians	1.25
	Omnivores	0.49
Arachidonic	Vegans	0.32
	Vegetarians	0.38
	Omnivores	0.38
Docosahexaenoic	Vegans	0.14
	Vegetarians	0.30
	Omnivores	0.37

developmental deficits, and which could possibly also indicate the interrelatedness of the conditions, despite their phenomenological differences.

Deficits in visual processing, particularly related to the magnocellular pathway, have been revealed as a result of extensive research in the neurophysiology of dyslexia. In addition, differences have been reported in the central processing of language (both written and auditory aspects) between dyslexic and nondyslexic individuals. Important questions are raised by such work, regarding what determines alternative pathways for processing, and whether this involves differences in anatomy, differences in cell chemistry, or possibly both.

That alterations in cell chemistry may be linked to ADHD is strongly suggested by the successful use of pharmaceutical intervention in that condition. Anatomical differences have been described in the brain of dyslexics, i.e., a decrease in left–right hemisphere asymmetry and an increase in ectopias (small groups of neurones that have migrated early in development to regions where they would not normally be found). The second of these features is particularly interesting in view of the fact that the fatty acid composition of the nerve cell membrane is one of the factors influencing neuronal migration.

These and other observations have led to the hypothesis that it may be a phospholipid membrane defect which provides the biological link between several developmental learning disorders. Strong evidence in favour of such a hypothesis has come from brain imaging studies (Richardson et al., 1997).

DYSLEXIA

The British Dyslexia Association (Crisfield, 1996) define and describe dyslexia in the following way:

Dyslexia is a complex neurological condition which is constitutional in origin. The symptoms may affect many areas of learning and function, and may be described as a specific difficulty in reading, spelling and written language. One or more of these areas may be affected.

Numeracy, notational skills (music), motor function and organizational skills may also be involved. However, it is particularly related to mastering written language, although oral language may be affected to some degree.

Dyslexia is a relatively common condition, and there is some evidence that it may be becoming more prevalent, though whether this simply reflects better diagnosis and recognition of the condition is unclear. Roush (1995) has noted a threefold increase in the prevalence of learning disabilities between 1976 and 1993 in the USA; dyslexia accounted for 80% of those with a learning disability. In the UK and the USA, according to the results of government sponsored studies, an estimated 10% of the population suffer from dyslexia to some extent, with 4% being severely affected. An accurate assessment of the true prevalence of dyslexia is made more difficult by confusion surrounding the precise definition of the condition, and by the denial by some that it actually exists.

Dyslexia poses great difficulties for the individual and can be a disabling condition which carries significant social and economic implications resulting from the loss of human potential.

Dyslexia has a number of characteristic features. These include: difficulties, often unexpected, in learning to read and write; problems with remembering sequences or tasks involving sequences, as, for example, multiplication tables and the alphabet; confusion between left and right; mirror reversals of letters and words; and poor short-term memory.

Poor phonological processing seems to be associated with the reading impairment in dyslexia, syllables often being broken down into phonemes, i.e., the smallest components of speech that are distinguishable acoustically. Dyslexic individuals appear to have deficits in accurate auditory perception and frequency analysis; this poses problems in learning to read unfamiliar words by breaking them down into phonemes before interpreting their meaning. That an impairment of visual processing is also involved is suggested by the difficulty which dyslexics show in reading short, familiar words of one syllable that are usually recognized visually as a totality without having to be broken down into phonemic components.

There is some overlap between certain features of dyslexia and those of ADHD and dyspraxia (developmental coordination disorder). Both ADHD and dyslexia are characterized by distractibility, poor attention and impulsive behaviour. A marked impairment in the development of motor coordination is the central feature of dyspraxia, an impairment which significantly interferes with academic achievement or activities of daily life (American Psychiatric Association, 1994). Impairments of ball skills and balance are shown by individuals with this disorder, as also are physical and ideational aspects of handwriting. Predictors for dyslexia have been examined by the British Birth Cohort Study on over 17 000 children. A total of 43 variables were identified showing statistically significant binary associations with dyslexia; of these, six survived the application of logistic regression techniques. Membership of the dyslexic group was predicted by the failing-to-catch-a-ball test (throwing a ball up, clapping a specified number of times and catching it) (Haslum, 1989), indicating that the motor coordination problems which comprise the core feature of dyspraxia are also a primary characteristic of dyslexia as well (Wolff et al., 1990).

The families with developmental disorders have also been shown to share certain conditions which appear to be linked to altered EFA metabolism; these include autoimmune disorders, allergies, autism and schizophrenia. Such a finding further reinforces the belief that there is a common biological basis to the developmental deficit syndromes (Horrobin et al., 1995). Disorders of fatty acid metabolism, clinical features of EFA deficiency, or improvements following dietary supplementation with specific fatty acids, have been reported in all of these conditions, indicating that this common biological basis is almost certainly related to fatty acid metabolism.

FATTY ACID SUPPLEMENTATION IN DYSLEXIA

The visual system in dyslexia

The role played by visual factors in dyslexia has been a matter of considerable debate. The magnocellular transient system is that component of the visual system which processes rapid stimuli. There is evidence from anatomical (Livingstone et al., 1991), psychophysical (Lovegrove et al., 1980), and functional magnetic resonance imaging (Eden et al., 1996) studies, that this system is impaired in dyslexia.

Fatty acids in the visual system

Input from all cone types and from rod cells is received by the magnocellular ganglion cells, which have large receptive fields (Lehmkuhle, 1993) and are also important for motion detection. Dark adaptation and vision in light of low intensity are mediated by the rod cells. In the outer segments of the rod cell are stacks of about 1000 discs of phospholipid membrane. These discs, which are continually renewed, and have a life of between 10 days and 1 month, have DHA as a major constituent of their membranes. The DHA accounts for up to 50% of all fatty acids, depending on the phospholipid class (Fleisler and Anderson, 1983). Similar enrichment with DHA is characteristic of synaptic membranes and neuronal growth cones, suggesting that this fatty acid plays an important role in neurotransmission (Breckenridge et al., 1972; Sastry, 1985) and dendrite arborisation.

The suggestion that there may be visual and central processing deficits in dyslexia makes it particularly pertinent to investigate fatty acid metabolism and requirements in this condition. I chose rod cell function in my own studies because the high requirement which these cells have for DHA provides a potentially sensitive biological indicator of deficiency.

Studies of dark adaptation in dyslexics

A Friedmann Visual Field Analyzer 2 was used to measure scotopic vision in 10 young adult dyslexics (six

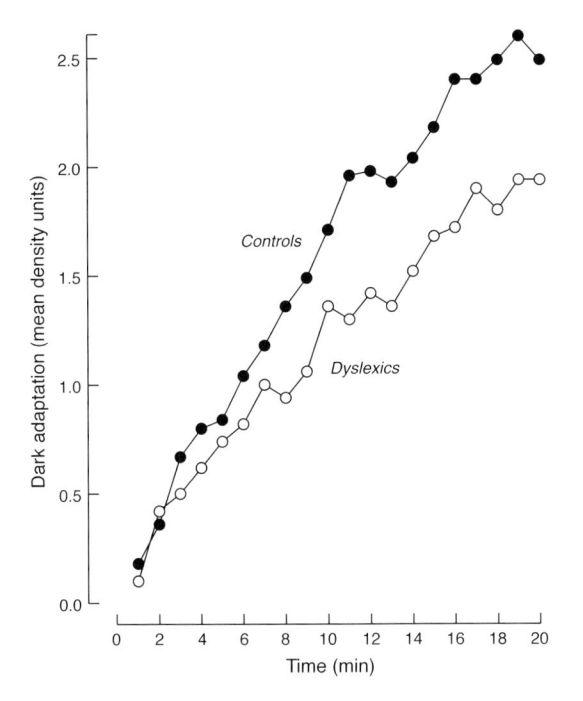

Figure 23.2. Dark adaptation in 10 young dyslexics and 10 nondyslexic controls.

men and four women), and 10 controls (six women and four men) (Stordy, 1995), the instrument being set for the dark adaptation function. It was found that there was poorer dark adaptation in members of the dyslexic group than amongst the control subjects (repeated measures ANOVA, $p < 0.05$) (Figure 23.2). The greatest effect was shown in the latter part of the adaptation curve, corresponding to adaptation in the rod cells.

A separate study (Stordy, 1995) examined dark adaptation in five young adult dyslexics and five controls, both before and after supplementation for 1 month with a high-DHA fish oil providing 480 mg of DHA daily. No change in dark adaptation was observed in the control group. In the dyslexic subjects, dark adaptation was found to be poor, but following dietary DHA supplementation scotopic vision in this group was consistently and significantly improved (paired t test on final rod threshold, $p < 0.04$) (Figure 23.3).

There are several biochemical states which may be associated with poor dark adaptation, including poor vitamin A status, zinc deficiency, and possibly deficiencies of vitamin C, riboflavin, nicotinic acid or thiamin (McClaren, 1963; Morrison et al., 1978). To examine whether there might be any dietary correlate of performance in the two studies briefly described above, the subjects were required to complete 7-day food records, in household measures; nutrient intakes were then estimated using food composition tables. No evidence was found of any inadequacy in the dietary

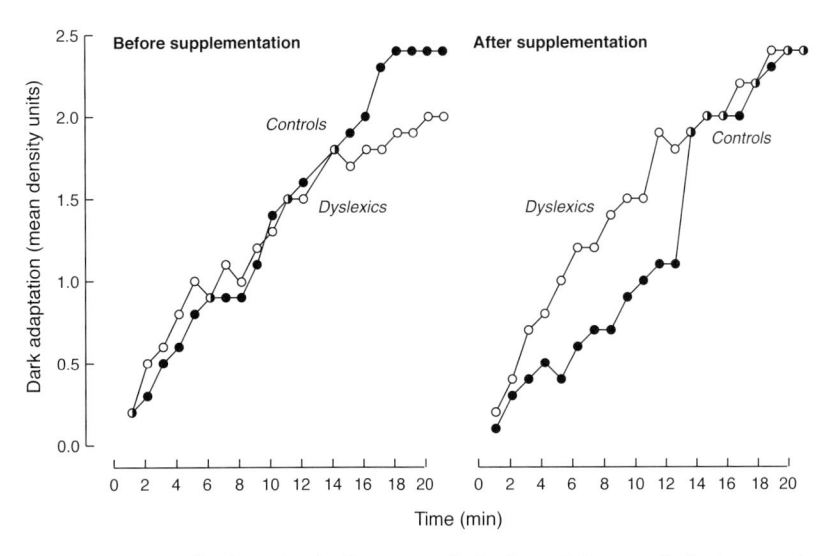

Figure 23.3. Dark adaptation in five young dyslexics and five nondyslexic controls, before and after supplementation with a high-DHA fish oil for 1 month.

supply of vitamin A or other nutrients, nor did the dyslexic and control groups show any differences in intake. Whilst 7-day food consumption records are not ideal for estimating vitamin A intakes, the dyslexic subjects were thought unlikely to complete longer food records satisfactorily.

It is of interest that, in the supplementation study, poor dark adaptation was initially exhibited by one of the control subjects, who was a vegetarian. Following supplementation in this subject, however, there was a substantial improvement in this function, suggesting that the low DHA content of his normal diet may have be a contributary factor in his condition.

The improvement that was observed in dark adaptation following 1 month of dietary supplementation with a DHA-rich fish oil is in accord with what is known about the physiology and turnover of rod cell phospholipid membranes.

The findings from these studies, though preliminary, were sufficiently clear-cut to justify setting up double-blind, placebo-controlled trials of fatty acid supplements in dyslexia. Baseline data from one of the studies that are currently in progress have already been reported elsewhere (Richardson et al., 1998).

FATTY ACID SUPPLEMENTATION IN DYSPRAXIA

Investigatory procedure

LCPUFA supplementation was used successfully by a member of a local group affiliated to the Dyspraxia Foundation, and, as a consequence, we were invited by the group to investigate whether improvements might be produced in the children of other members. An open study was therefore instituted in which the children were assessed before and after receiving dietary supplementation with a mixture of n-3 and n-6 fatty acids (Stordy, 1996, 1997). No placebo-treated control group was used.

In total, 17 families volunteered for the study, and written informed consent was sought from both the children and their parents. Baseline assessments were completed by all the children; two, however, did not attend for the final assessment and their baseline measurements have thus been excluded from the analysis. Of the 15 subjects for whom both baseline and final values were obtained, 11 were boys and four were girls; ages ranged between 5 and 12 years.

The ABC Movement Assessment Battery for Children (Henderson and Sugden, 1992) was used to assess the children's motor skills. One part of the test comprised a checklist that had to be completed by an adult who was familiar with the child (in this study it was completed by a parent). The check list was designed to evaluate complex interactions between the child and the physical environment; it can be used as a screening device in assessing children with problems or, as in this study, to evaluate the impact of some form of intervention (Henderson and Sugden, 1992). A second part of the test consisted of a series of objective measures of motor skills; these provided indices of manual dexterity, ball skills, and static and dynamic balance. The effects of intervention can also be studied by their effects on the movement tests. This test battery was developed to evaluate movement difficulties and the efficacy of treatment procedures instituted by physical education professionals and occupational therapists, under conditions where, for various reasons, it cannot be ensured that the child, parent or therapist are blind to the nature of the intervention.

Completion of the full test battery took place at the commencement of the study and again after 4 months of supplementation with a patented mixture of tuna oil, evening primrose oil, thyme oil and vitamin E (Efalex®, Efamol Ltd), which provided daily quantities of 480 mg DHA, 35 mg AA, 96 mg γ-linolenic acid, 80 mg vitamin E, and 24 mg of thyme oil. Thyme oil is extracted from the herb thyme by steam distillation; it is a volatile oil, rich in antioxidants, including thymol and carvacrol (Aeschbach et al., 1994).

Findings

Checklist scores above the 15th percentile were obtained for all children at baseline, indicating that all the subjects who were entered into this study presented initially with a marked degree of movement difficulty. The objective measures of movement performance

Table 23.3. ABC Movement assessment scores [a] in 15 dyspraxic children, before and after 4 months of dietary supplementation with n-3 and n-6 fatty acids; means ± SD.

Test	Time relative to supplementation	
	Before	After
Manual dexterity	9.93 ± 2.85	6.95 ± 3.76**
Ball skills	6.03 ± 2.94	3.90 ± 2.13*
Static dynamic balance	8.23 ± 4.47	5.88 ± 4.09*
Total impairment	24.20 ± 6.83	16.73 ± 8.16†††
Checklist [b]	87.14 ± 29.61	65.07 ± 28.63†

[a] High scores indicate poor performance; [b] records incomplete for one child, and so $n = 14$. In comparison with the corresponding score before supplementation, $p <$: *0.05; **0.01; †0.001; †††0.0001.

supported this evaluation: the total impairment score, defined as the sum of the scores for manual dexterity, ball skills and static and dynamic balance (high scores indicating poor performance) was in excess of the 1st percentile for all children except one. The remaining child, aged 12 years, was on the 8th percentile. Manual dexterity, ball skills, and static and dynamic balance were individually poor at baseline. Improvements were seen in all functional areas following supplementation. Statistically significant improvements were noted in overall total impairment scores and checklist scores ($p < 0.001$ in each case; sign test) following supplementation (see Table 23.3 and Figures 23.4 and 23.5), the variation in response between individuals being clearly illustrated in the figures.

The Conners' rating scales (Conners, 1990) for assessing ADHD were also used to assess any change that might be associated with supplementation with LCPUFAs, because many (though not all) dyspraxics score highly on ADHD rating scales. We were able to report a statistically significant improvement in the overall Conners' parent rating scale ($p < 0.05$) and a trend towards improvement on the Conners' teacher rating scale ($0.1 > p > 0.05$). A statistically significant reduction in anxiety was also seen on the Conners' parent subscales (Figure 23.6).

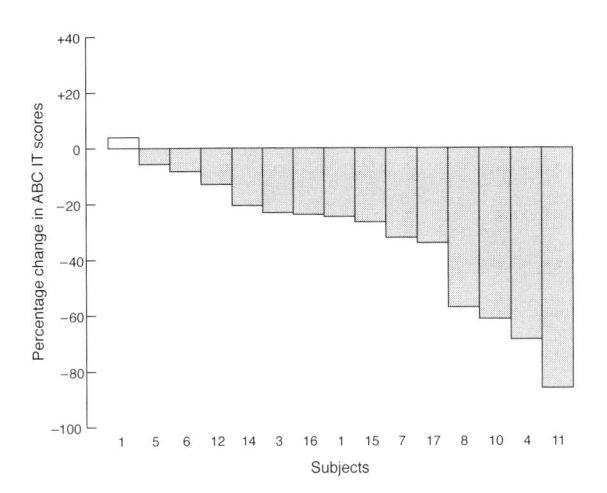

Figure 23.4. Distribution of ABC total impairment (TI) scores (summation of scores of objective tests for manual dexterity, ball skills and static and dynamic balance) in a group of 14 dyspraxic children. The score after supplementation with LCPUFAs is expressed as a percentage change from the score before treatment, for each child. Negative values indicate improvement.

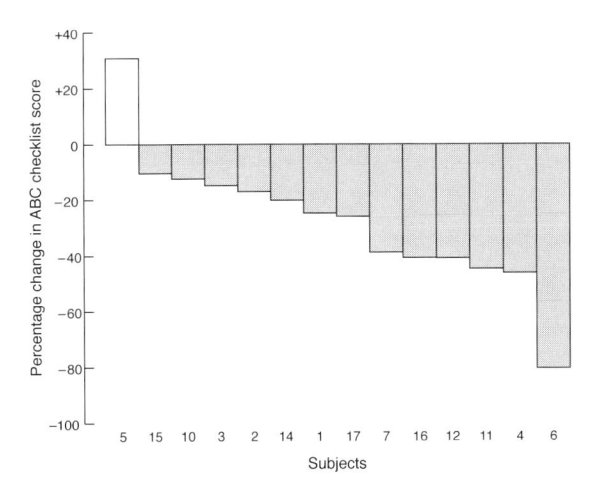

Figure 23.5. Distribution of ABC check list scores (an assessment of the child's day-to-day motor functioning, completed by the parent) in a group of 14 dyspraxic children. The score after supplementation with LCPUFAs is expressed as a percentage change from the score before treatment, for each child. Negative values indicate improvement.

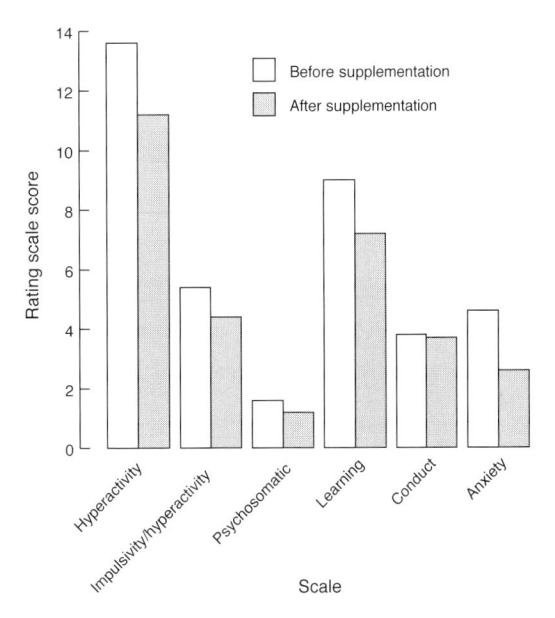

Figure 23.6. Conners parent rating scale scores (means) in 15 dyspraxic children, before and after n-3/n-6 fatty acid supplementation.

257

THE IMPORTANCE OF DIETARY PUFAs

Considerable interest has been expressed in the provision of adequate quantities of LCPUFAs for the foetus, the premature infant and the full-term infant. Uauy et al. (1996) suggested that the LCPUFA derivatives of elongation and desaturation of the EFAs may be essential nutrients for infants and for individuals with genetic defects in EFA metabolism, such as Zellweger syndrome, Batten's disease and retinitis pigmentosa. It is demonstrated by the studies described in this chapter that LCPUFAs are also likely to be essential nutrients for older children and also even for adults who possess specific learning disorders.

Stevens et al. (1995) showed that, in boys with ADHD, there are detectable clinical and biochemical signs of EFA deficiency, and they argued that that these children may show an impairment of the processes whereby the EFAs, LA and ALA, are converted to their long-chain derivatives, AA and DHA, respectively.

Children with good n-3 fatty acid status were also noted by Stevens et al. (1996) to show improved overall academic achievement and ability in mathematics. The same investigators also reported evidence that n-3 fatty acid status is related to behaviour in both monkeys (Reisbick et al., 1994) and man (Stevens et al., 1996). The improvements reported following supplements which provide AA and DHA are not surprising if individuals with dyslexia and dyspraxia have poorer conversion of LA to AA and of ALA to DHA.

The studies described above are, of course, preliminary. They are also small and their design faults do not permit allow firm conclusions to be made at the present time. Nevertheless, the findings are in line with what one might have predicted on the basis of current knowledge about the involvement of LCPUFAs in membrane function, and the possible relationships between membrane function and developmental disorders of learning. Further studies are in progress. These have been specifically designed to provide definitive assessments of the value, or otherwise, of LCPUFA supplements in dyslexia, ADHD and dyspraxia, and include double-blind, placebo-controlled trials.

Dietary management of dyslexia and dyspraxia

The importance of good nourishment, in every respect, for all women before and during pregnancy and when lactating, is now universally accepted. On the basis of the studies described above, it would appear prudent for pregnant women from families with a history of dyslexia, dyspraxia and ADHD to take particular care to ensure that their daily diet includes foods or food supplements which will provide adequate amounts of LCPUFAs.

Energy supply

Whilst all fatty acids are potentially subject to β-oxidation, this does not occur at the same rate for all of them. Under normal circumstances, LCPUFAs and EFAs may, in fact, be relatively spared so as to be available to serve their more important physiological roles. When the diet has low energy content, or when growth, reproduction, or high levels of physical activity make particularly high demands upon the body's energy reserves, fatty acids may need to be used as energy substrates. To ensure that EFAs or LCPUFAs are conserved for structural or metabolic purposes rather than used up as emergency energy substrates, it is important that an adequate energy supply is provided in the diet. It is not unusual for there to be some degree of deterioration in motor coordination during growth spurts; whilst the exact reasons for this are not known, it may be surmised, in the light of current research, that a deficiency of LCPUFAs is a contributory factor. If there is a high demand for LCPUFAs for nerve growth, coupled with a high demand for energy substrates, the supply of LCPUFAs may be diverted for such purposes. Parents may be advised that it is useful practice to check their children's height and body fat (using a measure such as body mass index), and to compare the results with suitable reference data so as to provide an assessment of energy status (Department of Health, 1991; Cole et al., 1995).

The parents of some children with developmental learning disorders report that their children are very choosy about their food. When this occurs, and is accompanied by evidence of poor growth and excessive thinness, it is appropriate, and indeed important, that advice on the desirability of energy-dense foods and snacks between meals should be given. Unfortunately, there is a modern tendency for such foods and snacks to be discouraged, and for concepts of healthy eating to be misunderstood by some parents; as a result, undesirable dietary restraint may be imposed. Instruction may also need to be given to schools to allow children to consume energy-rich snacks, such as buns, at breaktime, rather than just pieces of fruit.

Foods to include and foods to avoid

The studies discussed in this chapter appear to show that there is a special requirement for dietary supplementation of the LCPUFAs, particularly DHA, in individuals with dyslexia and dyspraxia. The foods required to provide these necessary nutrients are all of animal origin (see Table 23.1). While strict vegetarianism may be suitable for some individuals, it is not a suitable diet for those who come from families with a history of dyslexia, dyspraxia, or ADHD.

The small studies that have so far been completed suggest that substantial amounts of LCPUFAs are required to produce appreciable changes in those who suffer from developmental learning disorders. In order to obtain 480 mg of DHA, for example, it would be necessary for an individual to consume daily in excess of 500 g of fish; in many regions of the world this would represent both an unlikely and an expensive dietary scenario.

More *in vivo* conversion of EFAs to LCPUFAs might occur if hydrogenated and partially hydrogenated fats were to be avoided. To do this would involve carefully examining food labels to determine the ingredients in all purchased food, avoiding hard margarines and shortenings, and reducing the intake of such foodstuffs as ice-cream, chocolate, biscuits, pastry, and snack foods, all of which usually contain hydrogenated fats. In practice, however, avoiding hydrogenated and partially hydrogenated fats is very difficult, and there is, in fact, no evidence that even if total avoidance were achieved it would result in a sufficient enhancement of the availability of LCPUFAs to bring appreciable benefit to the dyslexic or dyspraxic individual. Moreover, children, and even those adults, who suffer from these conditions already have sufficient problems to cope with in their everyday life, without also having to undertake rigorous dietary monitoring.

Any kind of dietary restraint is difficult to achieve and maintain. It also imposes quite serious restrictions on social interaction. Unless the strict control of diet can be shown to be essential in managing a disorder, a simpler, and probably more effective, strategy would be to provide LCPUFAs, and particularly DHA, as dietary supplements, in the same way as folic acid supplementation is given in pregnancy, and in other cases where certain nutrients have been shown to be critical for well-being.

Ideally, such LCPUFA supplements should be based on fish oils with a high DHA content. Adequate antioxidant protection is also important. Because most fish liver oils provide relatively more EPA than DHA they are probably not ideal as supplements. Whilst these oils are relatively richer in vitamins A and D, this is not as advantageous as, superficially, it might appear to be: there is, for example, a possibility that the fat-soluble vitamins might be consumed in excess in view of the need to take LCPUFA supplementation as a long-term dietary strategy.

CONCLUSIONS

The specific learning disorders, dyslexia and dyspraxia, appear to be associated with an inborn error of metabolism affecting the conversion of EFAs to LCPUFAs. This leads to a deficiency of the LCPUFAs which are required for incorporation into membranes. This view is supported by the observation that amelioration of these conditions may be achieved by increasing the dietary supply of LCPUFAs.

The apparent increases, over the last few decades, in the prevalence of dyslexia and dyspraxia may have been brought about by dietary changes which have led to high levels of consumption of hydrogenated fat and low consumption of fish. These changes, together with a reduction in breast feeding, can exacerbate any LCPUFA deficiency which may already be present in genetically predisposed individuals.

ACKNOWLEDGEMENTS

The dyslexia studies were carried out with the active collaboration and technical skills of Katrina Searle, Liam Trow and Katy Wood; and the dyspraxia study with the assistance of Monica Wolff-Kleinman.

REFERENCES

Aeschbach R, Loliger J, Scott BC et al. Antioxidant actions of thymol, carvacrol, 6-gingerol, gingerone and hydroxytyrosol. Food Chem Toxicol 1994; 32: 31–36.

American Psychiatric Association. Diagnostic and statistical manual of mental disorders. 4th edn (DSM-IV). Washington, DC: American Psychiatric Association, 1994.

Andraca I, Uauy R. Breast feeding for optimal mental development. World Rev Nutr Diet 1995; 78: 1–27.

Breckenridge WC, Gombos G, Morgan IG. The lipid composition of adult rat brain synaptosomal plasma membranes. Biochim Biophys Acta 1972; 266: 695–707.

Cole TJ, Freeman JV, Preece MA. Body mass index reference curve for the United Kingdom, 1990. Arch Dis Child 1995; 73: 25–29.

Conners CK. Conners' rating scales manual. Toronto: Multi Health Systems, 1990.

Crisfield J. The dyslexia handbook 1996. Reading: British Dyslexia Association, 1996.

Department of Health. Report on health and social subjects 41. Dietary reference values for food and energy and nutrients for the United Kingdom. London: HMSO, 1991.

Eden GF, VanMeter JW, Rumsey JM, Maisog JM, Woods RP, Zeffiro TA. Abnormal processing of visual motion in dyslexia revealed by functional brain imaging. Nature 1996; 382: 66–69.

Fleisler SJ, Anderson RE. Chemistry and metabolism of lipids in the vertebrate retina. Prog Lipid Res 1983; 22: 79–131.

Haslum MN. Predictors of dyslexia? Irish J Psychol 1989; 10: 622–630.

Heird WC, Prager TC, Anderson RE. Docosahexaenoic acid and the development and function of the infant retina. Curr Opin Lipidol 1997; 8: 12–16.

Henderson SE, Sugden DA. Movement assessment battery for children. London: The Psychological Corporation, Harcourt Brace and Company, 1992.

Horrobin DF, Glen AIM, Hudson CJ. Possible relevance of phospholipid abnormalities and genetic interactions in psychiatric disorders: the relationship between dyslexia and schizophrenia. Med Hypotheses 1995; 45: 605–613.

Horrwood LJ, Fergusson DM. Breast feeding and later cognitive and academic outcomes. Pediatrics 1998; 101: 1–7.

Infante JP, Huszagh VA. On the molecular aetiology of decreased arachidonic (20:4n-6), docosapentaenoic (22:5n-6) and docosahexaenoic (22:6n-3) acids in Zellweger syndrome and other peroxisomal disorders. Mol Cell Biochem 1997; 168: 101–115.

Lehmkuhle S. Neurological basis of visual processes in reading. In: Willows DM, Kruk RS, Corcos E, eds. Visual processes in reading and reading disabilities. Hillsdale, New Jersey: Lawrence Erlbaum Associates 1993: 77–94.

Livingstone MS, Rosen GD, Drislane FW, Galaburda AM. Physiological and anatomical evidence for a magnocellular deficit in developmental dyslexia. Proc Natl Acad Sci USA 1991; 88: 7943–7947.

Lovegrove W, Bowling A, Badcock D, Blackwood M. Specific reading disability: differences in contrast sensitivity as a function of spatial frequency. Science 1980; 210: 439–440.

Lucas A, Morley R, Cole TJ, Lister G, Leeson-Payne C. Breast milk and subsequent intelligence quotient in children born preterm. Lancet 1992; 339: 261–264.

Makrides M, Neumann M, Simmer K, Pater J, Gibson R. Are long-chain polyunsaturated fatty acids essential nutrients in infancy? Lancet 1995; 345: 1463–1468.

McClaren DS. Malnutrition and the eye. New York: Academic Press, 1963.

Morrison SA, Russell RM, Carney EA, Oaks EV. Zinc deficiency, a cause of abnormal dark adaptation in cirrhotics. Am J Clin Nutr 1978; 31: 276–281.

Reisbick S, Neuringer M, Hasnain R, Conner WE. Home cage behaviour in rhesus monkeys with long-term deficiency of omega-3 fatty acids. Physiol Behav 1994; 55: 231–239.

Richardson AJ, Cox IJ, Sargentoni J, Puri BK. Abnormal cerebral phospholipid metabolism in dyslexia indicated by phosphorus-31 magnetic resonance spectroscopy. NMR Biomed 1997; 10: 309–314.

Richardson AJ, Easton T, Corrie AC, Clisby C, Stordy BJ. Is developmental dyslexia a fatty acid deficiency syndrome? Nutrition Society Summer Meeting, Guildford, UK 30 June–3 July, 1998.

Roush W. Arguing over why Johnny can't read. Science 1995; 267: 1896–1898.

Sanders TAB, Reddy S. The influence of a vegetarian diet on the fatty acid composition of breast milk and the essential fatty acid status of the infant. J Pediatrics 1992; 120: S71–S77.

Sastry PS. Lipids of the nervous tissue: composition and metabolism. Prog Lipid Res 1985; 24: 169–176.

Stevens LJ, Zentall SZ, Deck JL, Abate ML, Lipp SR, Burgess JR. Essential fatty acid metabolism in boys with attention-deficit hyperactivity disorder. Am J Clin Nutr 1995; 62: 761–768.

Stevens LJ, Zentall SS, Abate ML, Watkins BA, Kuczek T, Burgess JR. Omega-3 fatty acids in boys with behaviour, learning, and health problems. Physiol Behav 1996; 59: 915–920.

Stordy BJ. Benefit of docosahexaenoic acid supplements to dark adaptation in dyslexia. Lancet 1995; 346: 385.

Stordy BJ. Dark adaptation, motor skills, docosahexaenoic acid and dyslexia. Paper presented at the Fats of Life Symposium, Barcelona, 1996.

Stordy BJ. The fats of life. Paper presented at the 30th International Convention of the Australian Institute of Food Science and Technology, Perth, Western Australia, 4–8 May, 1997.

Uauy R, Peirano P, Hoffman D, Mena P, Birch D, Birch E. Role of essential fatty acids in the function of the developing nervous system. Lipids 1996; 31: S167–S176.

Wolff PH, Michel GF, Ovrut M, Drake C. Rate and timing precision of motor co-ordination in developmental dyslexia. Dev Psychol 1990; 26: 349–359.

Part IX

OTHER NEUROPSYCHIATRIC DISORDERS

Essential Fatty Acids in Children with Attention-Deficit/Hyperactivity Disorder

24

Laura J. Stevens and John R. Burgess

INTRODUCTION

Children who have problems paying attention, listening to instructions, completing tasks, fidgeting and squirming, or interrupting others, may have a condition known as attention-deficit/hyperactivity disorder (ADHD) (American Psychiatric Association, 1994). For children, ADHD is the most prevalent psychiatric problem, estimated to afflict from 5% to 10% of the school-age population (Szatmari, 1992). These behaviours may severely affect school performance, family relationships, and social interactions with peers. Roughly 20–25% of children with ADHD show one or more specific learning disabilities in mathematics, reading, and/or spelling (Barkley, 1990). Children with ADHD often have trouble performing academically and paying attention, and may show problems with disorganization, poor self-discipline, and low self-esteem.

Treatments for ADHD include behaviour therapy and medications (Hoza et al., 1995). Psychostimulant drugs and antidepressants are often used to calm children with ADHD at about a 75% effectiveness rate (Swanson et al., 1993). The advantages of using these medications include rapid response, ease of use, effectiveness, and relative safety. The disadvantages include possible adverse effects, such as decreased appetite and impaired growth, insomnia, increased irritability, and rebound hyperactivity when the drug wears off (Ahmann et al., 1991). Although the medications appear to treat the symptoms, and their efficacy is used as a basis for mechanistic studies, the aetiology of ADHD is still unknown. Thus, studies to elucidate the potential contributors to the behaviour problems in children with ADHD may lead to more effective treatment strategies in the future.

The exact causes of ADHD are unknown, but are theorized to involve both biological and environmental factors (Zametkin and Rapoport, 1987). Differences in brain function between children with ADHD and children without ADHD are a focus of research into the aetiology of this disorder (Castellanos, 1997). The underlying factors contributing to differences in brain function are under investigation and include genetic determinants (Goodman and Stevenson, 1989; Faraone et al., 1997), imbalances in neurotransmitter signalling pathways (Raskin et al., 1981; Pliska et al., 1996; Ballard et al., 1997) and receptor function (Cook et al., 1995), as well as hormonal (Hauser et al., 1993), environmental (Needleman et al., 1979), and developmental factors (Ucles et al., 1996). As behavioural patterns are complex, being influenced by genes as well as many facets of the environment, the causative factors for this disorder will differ markedly from one child to the next. Finding consistencies in other health characteristics among groups of children within the ADHD population should provide some clues as to why some children develop these behavioural characteristics and others do not.

Several environmental factors related to diet have been pursued as causative factors in the development of ADHD. These include food sensitivities (Carter et al., 1993), lead toxicity (Needleman et al., 1979), and deficiencies of iron (Sever et al., 1997), zinc (Toren et al., 1996), and magnesium (Kozielec and Starobrat-Hermelin 1997; Starobrat-Hermelin and Kozielec 1997). Our work has focused on the essential fatty acids (EFAs) and the status of the longer chain and highly polyunsaturated products that carry out many functions in the body.

Linoleic acid (18:2n-6) and α-linolenic acid (18:3n-3) are EFAs and must be consumed in the diet because humans and most other mammals lack the ability to synthesize these fatty acids (Holman, 1992). The EFAs are converted to a variety of longer, more highly polyunsaturated products (long-chain, polyunsaturated fatty acids, LCPUFAs) that function throughout the body. The n-6 fatty acids serve as a source of material for the formation of localized hormones, called eicosanoids, which are involved in a wide range of biologically significant processes in the body (Smith, 1992). The n-3 fatty acid series is specifically implicated in maintaining central nervous system function. Deficiency of n-6 fatty acids leads to impaired growth, dry and scaly skin, polydipsia and polyuria, among other symptoms (Burr and Burr 1930; Hansen et al., 1958). In addition to polydipsia, deficiency of n-3 fatty acids in rats and monkeys is associated with behavioural, sensory, and neurological dysfunction as well (Enslen et al., 1991; Yehuda and Carasso, 1993; Reisbick et al., 1994).

FATTY ACID STATUS IN BOYS WITH ADHD, AND RELATION TO BEHAVIOUR

A few studies have focused on EFA metabolism in children with ADHD. Children with hyperactivity have been reported to be more thirsty, and to be more likely to show symptoms of eczema, asthma, and other allergies, than children with normal activity levels (Mitchell et al., 1987). We have shown that 53 subjects with ADHD had a significantly lower composition of key fatty acids in the plasma polar lipids (20:4n-6, 20:5n-3 and 22:6n-3) and in red blood cell total lipids (20:4n-6 and 22:4n-6) than 43 control subjects (Stevens et al., 1995). This agrees with a previous report (Mitchell et al., 1987). However, a further finding was that a subgroup of 21 subjects with ADHD (40% of the sample), who exhibited a greater frequency of EFA deficiency symptoms (thirst, frequent urination, and dry hair), had significantly lower plasma composition of 20:4n-6, 22:6n-3, and total n-3 fatty acids than the remaining 32 subjects with ADHD (60% of the sample) with few EFA deficiency symptoms (Figure 24.1). This subgroup was designated L-ADHD, to indicate the low levels of LCPUFA in the blood. Moreover, the fatty acid composition of the plasma phospholipids for the subjects with few symptoms was not different from the control sample population. This is important, because previous studies that have tested the role of fatty acid supplementation in treating ADHD have not reported selection based on EFA status or frequency of symptoms (Aman et al., 1987; Arnold et al., 1989).

The relationship between the type of fatty acid (n-3 or n-6) and behaviour symptoms has not previously been studied in children with ADHD. We have found, by further analysis of all the subjects in the study, an inverse relationship between total n-3 fatty acid concentrations in the plasma and scores on behavioural assessment measures, i.e., Conners' Parent Rating Scale and teacher scores of academic abilities (Stevens et al., 1996). This was not the case for n-6 fatty acids. However, low blood concentration of both types of fatty acid was associated with a higher frequency of symptoms indicative of EFA deficiency. These results support a relationship between n-3 fatty acid status and behaviour in children, which parallels observations in

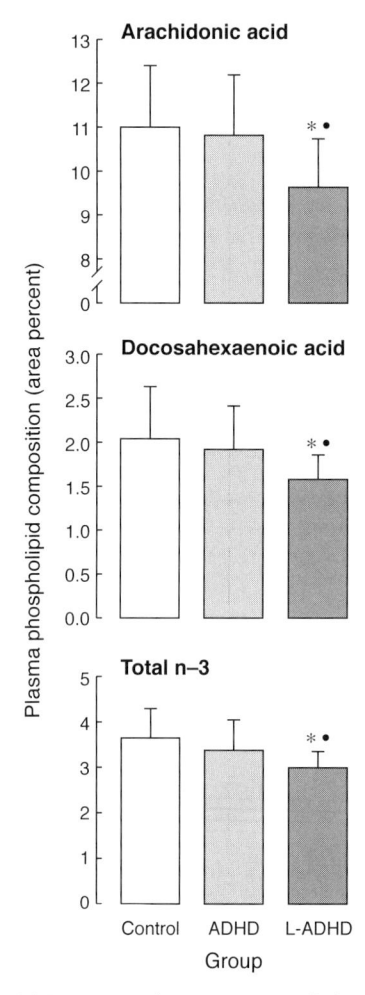

Figure 24.1. Fatty acid composition of plasma phospholipids from children with (ADHD) and without (control) attention-deficit/hyperactivity disorder. Children with ADHD were subdivided according to the reported frequency of symptoms indicative of EFA deficiency: L-ADHD report many symptoms of EFA deficiency; ADHD report few symptoms of EFA deficiency. *In comparison with the control value, $p < 0.05$; •in comparison with the value for ADHD, $p < 0.05$ (Newman-Keuls test following analysis of variance). Data from Stevens et al. (1995).

rats and monkeys (Yehuda and Carasso, 1993; Reisbick et al., 1994). Previous intervention studies have used a source of n-6 fatty acids (evening primrose oil) to treat behaviour problems and have reported variable and unsuccessful results (Aman et al., 1987; Arnold et al., 1989, 1994). However, since the n-3 fatty acids appear to be the important type for brain and visual function (Yehuda and Carasso, 1993; Reisbick et al., 1994), and n-6 fatty acid supplementation does not improve n-3 fatty acid status, evening primrose oil supplementation alone would not be expected to improve behaviour.

RELATIONSHIP BETWEEN LCPUFA STATUS AND BEHAVIOUR PROBLEMS

The cells of the nervous system are rich in LCPUFAs, playing a primary structural role, and influencing normal cerebral development (Bourre et al., 1989). Limited cellular pools of 20:4n-6, 22:6n-3 and total n-3 fatty acids could adversely affect brain function and influence behaviour in several ways (Murphy and Pearce, 1981; Neuringer et al., 1988). Depleted substrate, 20:4n-6, for eicosanoid biosynthesis could decrease production of the lipid mediators of nerve transmission in the central nervous system (Murphy and Pearce, 1981). Also, since 22:6n-3 is the predominant LCPUFA in the polar lipids of the cerebral cortex and retina (especially in cell membranes that are the most fluid and metabolically active), suboptimal levels of this fatty acid might negatively affect the function of the retina and cerebral cortex by decreasing membrane fluidity and impairing transport processes (Neuringer et al., 1988). Indeed, studies in animals have demonstrated that dietary intake of fatty acids can affect the amount of brain LCPUFAs. Feeding rats and primates diets deficient in 18:3n-3 for extended periods of time not only leads to depleted levels of 22:6n-3, but also results in compromised visual function and the development of abnormal behaviours (Yoshida et al., 1997, and references therein).

We hypothesize that the lower composition of arachidonic acid (AA), eicosapentanoic acid (EPA) and docosahexaenoic acid (DHA), observed in the blood of children with ADHD exhibiting symptoms of EFA deficiency, may reflect a subclinical deficit of these key fatty acids throughout the body. If this depleted status is manifested in central nervous system tissue, then the resulting ultrastructural changes that would occur may underlie the abnormal brain patterns that these children exhibit. Testing the validity of this hypothesis awaits further study.

CAUSATIVE FACTORS FOR LOWER LCPUFA IN SOME CHILDREN WITH ADHD

One would not expect that a single cause, or even a small number of factors, will be found to explain why ADHD appears to be so rampant in our society. As it is accepted that both genetic and environmental factors play a role in ADHD, so too could many factors, both intrinsic and extrinsic, influence an individual's fatty acid status. Applying this argument to the L-ADHD group of children, we have considered several factors that might contribute to the lower LCPUFA status observed in the subpopulation of children with ADHD. Although many other potential explanations are possible, we have considered: (1) intake-related factors, such as marginal consumption of EFAs and other nutrients; (2) disturbance in LCPUFA membrane incorporation; (3) inefficient conversion of EFAs to LCPUFAs; or (4) enhanced metabolism.

Primary nutrient deficiency

There are many studies that relate protein or total energy deficit to behavioural or cognitive problems. A deficiency of specific micronutrients has also been related to behavioural changes, i.e., iron, iodine, and vitamin A (Pollit et al., 1989; Garcia et al., 1990; McCullough et al., 1990; Schurch, 1995). These studies are generally reported on populations at risk in developing countries and may be confounded by other factors, such as parental socioeconomic status, education or intelligence. Environmental factors, such as general living conditions, repeated infections, and nutrient interactions may also confound results. Poor quality of the total diet in these groups is probably more of a problem than specific nutrient deficiencies. A diet low in calories and/or protein would probably be low in specific long-chain fatty acids as well.

Malnutrition in the prenatal or immediate postnatal period of the rat is sufficient to produce permanent alterations in the brain structure, resulting in enduring changes in behaviour (Levitsky and Strupp, 1995). Supplementation of human infants with LCPUFAs has shown beneficial results on cognitive function (Pollit et al., 1989; Grantham-McGregor, 1993). Studies have shown enduring effects on performance when comparing children who had formerly received mother's milk to those who had not (Lozoff et al., 1991). It has been suggested that malnutrition leaves the brain sufficiently intact to function under stable conditions, but enduring changes are evident under stressful conditions that may alter an individual's susceptibility to affective disorders (Strupp and Levitsky, 1995).

Although there is no lack of nutrients available in the Western world, a primary deficiency may occur due to lack of intake. With the emphasis on low fat diets for control of various chronic diseases, intake of foods containing long-chain fatty acids may be unnecessarily restricted. For children with ADHD, psychostimulant medications can suppress appetite, leading to decreased food intake and slower growth (Ahmann et al., 1991). Also, nutrient intake may be affected by poor food choices or food allergy/intolerance, resulting in a primary deficiency of these essential nutrients. For children with ADHD, deficiency of nutrients has been explored as a contributing factor in the development of behavioural problems. However, our initial analysis indicated that primary deficiency of EFAs appeared unlikely to explain the high frequency of EFA-deficiency symptoms and lower LCPUFAs for the L-ADHD subjects as a group. This conclusion was reached because dietary PUFA intake was greater in the ADHD group, and plasma linoleic acid composition did not differ between the groups (Stevens et al., 1995). However, evaluation of the fatty acid profiles and food intake results for individual subjects did reveal evidence of subclinical primary deficiency in a small subset of children within the L-ADHD group (Burgess et al., 1999). For these subjects, linoleic acid composition in both the plasma phospholipids and red blood cells was well below the mean for the control population, and 20:3n-9, a marker of primary EFA deficiency (Holman, 1992), was elevated in the plasma samples.

Other nutrients that have been explored as possible contributors to behaviour problems in children with ADHD include iron (Sever et al., 1997), magnesium (Kozielec and Starobrat-Hermelin, 1997), zinc (Toren et al., 1996), and vitamin B_6 (Bhagavan et al., 1975). Zinc has been postulated to be involved as a cofactor in the conversion of EFAs to LCPUFAs *via* desaturation reactions (Eder and Kirchgessner, 1996). Although the exact mechanism of its involvement with EFA metabolism remains controversial (Kramer et al., 1984; Eder and Kirchgessner, 1995, 1996), zinc status is under investigation in children with ADHD (Arnold et al., 1990; Sandyk, 1990; Toren et al., 1996). A positive correlation between serum zinc levels and free fatty acid levels was recently reported in a population of children with ADHD, but the relationship between the two types of nutrients was not clear (Bekaroglu et al., 1996). We have not observed a difference in zinc intake between control children and children with ADHD (Stevens et al., 1995). Nevertheless, the interaction between zinc status and EFA status needs to be considered in future studies of children with ADHD.

Magnesium status is also proposed to affect the conversion of EFAs to LCPUFAs *via* the Δ-6-desaturation step (Galland, 1985). Recent studies have explored the issue of magnesium status in children with ADHD and have reported that as many as 95% of the children with ADHD exhibited magnesium deficiency, as assessed by analysis of hair, red blood cells, or serum (Kozielec and Starobrat-Hermelin, 1997). In a follow-up study, magnesium status and behaviour improved with magnesium supplementation (Starobrat-Hermelin and Kozielec, 1997). We have not observed any difference in magnesium intake between children with or without ADHD, but have not assessed status (Stevens et al., 1995), partly, because of the variation in the clinical literature concerning magnesium status assessment (Shils, 1996).

Disturbance in LCPUFA membrane incorporation

A second possible cause for the lower LCPUFA composition of plasma phospholipids may be due to a disturbance in the mechanisms that direct incorporation of specific LCPUFAs into cellular phospholipids. Given the high composition of LCPUFAs in brain and retinal membranes, the mechanisms that direct this incorporation would have a strong influence on the overall fatty acid composition. A disruption could dramatically alter the phospholipid composition, leading to ultrastructural changes that affect function. A consideration of the role that fatty acid binding proteins (FABPs) play in this process is warranted. Recent studies have characterized a brain lipid-binding protein which has a high affinity for 22:6n-3 and a probable role in brain DHA utilization (Xu et al., 1996). This binding protein is a member of a family of fatty acid-binding proteins that is highly expressed during development of the central nervous system (Kurtz et al., 1994). Understanding the role that cellular binding proteins play in LCPUFA homeostasis in the nervous system might reveal whether disturbances in membrane incorporation into phospholipids contribute to lower levels of fatty acids in the L-ADHD.

Inefficient conversion of EFA to LCPUFA

A third possible cause for the low LCPUFA status of the L-ADHD group may be impaired conversion of the fatty acid precursors, linoleic acid and α-linolenic acid, to their longer and more highly unsaturated products. The conversion of linoleic acid and α-linolenic acid to LCPUFAs takes place in liver and a few other tissues by a series of desaturation, elongation, and β-oxidation reactions involving enzymes in the mitochondria and endoplasmic reticulum (Infante and Huszagh, 1997), as well as the peroxisomes (Sprecher, 1996). Possible sites of this inefficiency include the desaturase steps, the malonylCoA-dependent elongation steps, or the peroxisomal β-oxidation steps. Indirect evidence for such inefficiencies comes from studies with newborn infants, peroxisomal diseases, neural ceroid-lipofucsinosis, and retinitis pigmentosa (Uauy et al., 1996). A likely bottleneck in the conversion process is the Δ-6-desaturase catalyzed reaction, which is the initial step in the conversion process (Horrobin, 1993). In the analysis of blood fatty acid composition, the ratio of precursors to LCPUFA products is a commonly used index to assess the efficiency of this metabolic step, with higher values of the ratio indicating inefficient conversion. In our studies of children with ADHD exhibiting frequent symptoms of EFA deficiency we observed that the ratio of 18:2n-6 to all of its metabolites was greater in the L-ADHD children than in the control children or in children with ADHD reporting no EFA symptoms (Burgess et al., 1999). This result would indicate that, for many children in the L-ADHD group, inefficient conversion of precursors to LCPUFA products may be the primary reason for the lower 20:4n-6 and 22:6n-3 composition of the plasma phospholipids.

Enhanced metabolism

Another possible explanation for the lower composition of blood LCPUFAs in the L-ADHD is enhanced cellular metabolism of these fatty acids through oxidation mechanisms. Enhanced nonenzymatic oxidation due to impaired cellular defence systems has been shown to lead to depletion of many LCPUFAs in rat liver (Buttriss and Diplock, 1988). As many of the subjects in the L-ADHD group exhibited a pattern of lower LCPUFA composition, relative to controls, enhanced metabolism by oxidation may be a contributing factor to fatty acid status in these children. Oxidative stress can lead to over-utilization of endogenous cellular antioxidants and deplete status (Kehrer, 1993). Vitamin E is the main lipid-soluble antioxidant, and plasma levels reflect status throughout the body (Niki, 1996). We analyzed the α-tocopherol concentrations in blood plasma and red blood cells from children in our previous study (Stevens et al., 1995) and found no differences between the L-ADHD subjects and subjects with ADHD exhibiting normal fatty acid status with no symptoms of EFA deficiency (Burgess et al., 1999). Although these results were negative, evaluation of the role of enhanced metabolism in the L-ADHD population is still warranted for several reasons. First, assessment of antioxidant nutrient status may be insensitive to chronic oxidative metabolism of fatty acids that is marginally elevated; more sensitive markers of oxidative stress should be utilized to test this possibility in future studies. Second, enhanced enzymatic oxidation of LCPUFA would not influence antioxidant nutrient status, and if this situation occurred in some of the children it would not be detected. Measurements of eicosanoid production by white blood cells, or of the urinary excretion of metabolites, are useful indicators of this process and could be used in future studies to determine whether enhanced enzymatic metabolism is a contributing factor in the L-ADHD population.

CAUSATION OR ASSOCIATION: QUESTIONS TO ADDRESS FOR FUTURE RESEARCH

As indicated previously, the differences in LCPUFA composition between the L-ADHD and the control subjects was significant, but the values did not indicate clinical deficiency. Moreover, the relationship between the LCPUFA status and the behavioural problems that these children exhibit is not clear. We hypothesize that the lower composition of AA, EPA and DHA observed in the blood of these children with ADHD may reflect a subclinical deficiency of these key fatty acids throughout the body. Since n-3 fatty acids, and especially DHA, are enriched in the retina of the eye and certain regions of the brain, depletion of DHA from these regions may compromise sensory and brain function. A subclinical deficiency of DHA may be responsible for the abnormal behaviour of these children. Throughout the rest of the body, depletion of n-3 and n-6 LCPUFAs may be responsible for the outward symptoms of deficiency that these children report. However, establishing whether this association is causative is not a straightforward task. Supplementation with preformed LCPUFAs would seem to be the most efficient approach to testing the hypothesis, but, depending on the cause for the lower LCPUFA status, supplementation may not overcome the theoretical imbalance existing in the brains of these children. Nevertheless, as an initial step to test the biological significance of fatty acid status in the L-ADHD, we have begun a double-blind, placebo-controlled, intervention study using preformed LCPUFA supplementation, and testing the effects on the frequency of EFA deficiency symptoms as well as behaviour measures. The answer to the cause or association question awaits the results of this and other similar intervention studies.

REFERENCES

Ahmann PA, Waltonen SJ, Olson KA, Theye FW, Van Erem AJ, LePlant RJ. Placebo-controlled evaluation of Ritalin side effects. Pediatrics 1991; 91: 1101–1106.

Aman MG, Mitchell EA, Turbott SH. The effects of essential fatty acid supplementation by Efamol in hyperactive children. J Abnorm Child Psychol 1987; 15: 75–90.

American Psychiatric Association. Diagnostic and statistical manual of mental disorders. 4th edn (DSM-IV). Washington, DC: American Psychiatric Association, 1994.

Arnold LE, Kleykamp D, Votolato NA, Taylor WA, Kontras SB, Tobin K. Gamma-linolenic acid for attention-deficit hyperactivity disorder: placebo-controlled comparison to d-amphetamine. Biol Psychiatry 1989; 25: 222–228.

Arnold LE, Votolato NA, Kleykamp D, Baker GB, Bornstein RA. Does hair zinc predict amphetamine improvement of ADD/hyperactivity? Int J Neurosci 1990; 50: 103–107.

Arnold LE, Kleykamp D, Votolato N, Gibson RA, Horrocks L. Potential link between dietary intake of fatty acids and behavior: pilot exploration of serum lipids in attention-deficit hyperactivity disorder. J Child Adolesc Psychopharmacol 1994; 4: 171–182.

Ballard S, Bolan M, Burton M, Snyder S, Pasterczyk-Seabolt C, Martin D. The neurological basis of attention-deficit/hyperactivity disorder. Adolescence 1997; 32: 855–862.

Barkley RA. Attention-deficit hyperactivity disorder. A handbook for diagnosis and treatment. New York: Guilford Press, 1990.

Bekaroglu M, Aslan Y, Gedik Y et al. Relationship between serum free fatty acids and zinc, and attention-deficit hyperactivity disorder: a research note. J Child Psychol Psychiatry 1996; 37: 225–227.

Bhagavan H, Coleman M, Coursin DB. The effect of pyridoxine hydrochloride on blood serotonin and pyridoxal phosphate contents in hyperactive children. Pediatrics 1975; 55: 437–441.

Bourre J-M, Francois M, Youyou A et al. The effects of dietary α-linolenic acid on the composition of nerve membranes, enzymatic activity, amplitude of electrophysiological parameters, resistance to poisons and performance of learning tasks in rats. J Nutr 1989; 119: 1880–1892.

Burgess JR, Stevens LJ, Zhang W, Peck L. Long-chain polyunsaturated fatty acids in children with attention-deficit/hyperactivity disorder. Am J Clin Nutr 1999, in press.

Burr GO, Burr MM. On the nature and role of the fatty acids essential in nutrition. J Biol Chem 1930; 86: 587–621.

Buttriss JL, Diplock AT. The alpha-tocopherol and phospholipid fatty acid content of rat liver subcellular membranes in vitamin E and selenium deficiency. Biochim Biophys Acta 1988; 963: 61–69.

Carter CM, Urbanoqicz M, Hemsley R et al. Effects of a few food diet in attention deficit disorder. Arch Dis Child 1993; 69: 564–568.

Castellanos FX. Toward a pathophysiology of attention-deficit/hyperactivity disorder. Clin Pediatr 1997; 36: 381–393.

Cook EH, Stein MA, Krasowski MD et al. Association of attention-deficit disorder and the dopamine transporter gene. Am J Hum Genet 1995; 56: 993–998.

Eder K, Kirchgessner M. Activities of liver microsomal fatty acid desaturases in zinc-deficient rats force-fed diets with a coconut oil/safflower oil mixture of linseed oil. Biol Trace Element Res 1995; 48: 215–229.

Eder K, Kirchgessner M. Zinc deficiency and the desaturation of linoleic acid in rats force-fed fat-free diets. Biol Trace Element Res 1996; 54: 173–183.

Enslen M, Milon H, Malnoe A. Effect of low intake of n-3 fatty acids during the development of brain phospholipid, fatty acid composition and exploratory behavior in rats. Lipids 1991; 26: 203–208.

Faraone SV, Biederman J, Jetton JG, Tsuang MT. Attention deficit disorder and conduct disorder: longitudinal evidence of a familial subtype. Psychol Med 1997; 27: 291–300.

Galland L. Impaired essential fatty acid metabolism in latent tetany. Magnesium 1985; 4: 333–338.

Garcia SE, Kaiser LL, Dewey KG. Self-regulation of food intake among rural Mexican preschool children. Eur J Clin Nutr 1990; 44: 371–380.

Goodman R, Stevenson J. A twin study of hyperactivity – I. An examination of hyperactivity scores and categories derived from Rutter teacher and parent questionnaires. J Child Psychol Psychiatry 1989; 30: 571–589.

Grantham-McGregor SM. Assessments of the effects of nutrition on mental development and behavior in Jamaican studies. Am J Clin Nutr Suppl 1993; 57: 303S–309S.

Hansen AE, Haggard ME, Boelsche AN, Adam DJD, Wiese HF. Essential fatty acids in infant nutrition. III. Clinical manifestations of linoleic acid deficiency. J Nutr 1958; 66: 565–576.

Hauser P, Zametkin AJ, Mertinez P et al. Attention deficit-hyperactivity disorder in people with generalized resistance to thyroid hormone. N Engl J Med 1993; 328: 997–1001.

Holman RT. A long scaly tale – the study of essential fatty acid deficiency at the University of Minnesota. In: Sinclair A, Gibson R, eds. Essential fatty acids and eicosanoids: invited papers from the third international congress. Champagne, IL: AOCS Books, 1992: 3–17.

Horrobin DF. Fatty acid metabolism in health and disease: the role of Δ-6-desaturase. Am J Clin Nutr 1993; 57 (Suppl 5): 732S–737S.

Hoza B, Vallano G, Pelham WE. Attention-deficit hyperactivity disorder. In: Ammerman RT, Hersen M, eds. Handbook of child behavior therapy in the psychiatric setting. New York: Wiley, 1995: 181–198.

Infante JP, Huszagh VA. On the molecular aetiology of decreased arachidonic (20:4n-6), docosapentaenoic (22:5n-6) and docosahexaenoic (22:6n-3) acids in Zellweger syndrome and other peroxisomal disorders. Mol Cell Biochem 1997; 168: 101–115.

Kehrer J. Free radicals as mediators of tissue injury and disease. Crit Rev Toxicol 1993; 23: 21–48.

Kozielec T, Starobrat-Hermelin B. Assessment of magnesium levels in children with attention deficit hyperactivity disorder (ADHD). Magnesium Res 1997; 10: 143–148.

Kramer TR, Briske-Anderson M, Johnson SB, Holman RT. Influence of reduced food intake on polyunsaturated fatty acid metabolism in zinc-deficient rats. J Nutr 1984; 114: 1224–1230.

Kurtz A, Zimmer A, Schnutgen F, Bruning G, Spener F, Muller T. The expression pattern of a novel gene encoding brain-fatty acid binding protein correlates with neuronal and glial cell development. Development 1994; 120: 2637–2649.

Levitsky DA, Strupp BJ. Malnutrition and the brain: changing concepts, changing concerns. J Nutr 1995; 125: 2212S–2220S.

Lozoff B, Jimenez E, Wolf, A. Long-term developmental outcome of infants with iron deficiency. N Engl J Med 1991; 325: 687–694.

McCullough AL, Kirksey A, Wachs TD et al. Vitamin B-6 status of Egyptian mothers: relation to infant behavior and maternal-infant interactions. Am J Clin Nutr 1990; 51: 1067–1074.

Mitchell EA, Aman MG, Turbott SH, Manku M. Clinical characteristics and serum essential fatty acid levels in hyperactive children. Clin Pediatr 1987; 26: 406–411.

Murphy S, Pearce B. Eicosanoids in the CNS: sources and effects. Prostagland Leukotr Essent Fatty Acids 1981; 31: 163–170.

Needleman HL, Gunnoe C, Leviton A et al. Deficits in psychologic and classroom performance of children with elevated dentine lead levels. N Engl J Med 1979; 300: 689–695.

Neuringer M, Anderson GJ, Connor WE. The essentiality of n-3 fatty acids for the development and function of the retina and brain. Annu Rev Nutr 1988; 8: 517–541.

Niki E. α-Tocopherol. In: Cadenas E, Packer L, eds. Handbook of antioxidants. New York: Marcel Dekker Inc., 1996; 3–25.

Pliska SR, McCracken JT, Maas JW. Catecholamines in attention-deficit hyperactivity disorder: current perspectives. J Am Acad Child Adolesc Psychiatry 1996; 35: 264–272.

Pollit E, Hathirat P, Kotchabhakdi N, Missel L, Valyasvu A. Iron deficiency and educational achievement in Thailand. Am J Clin Nutr Suppl 1989; 50: 687–697.

Raskin LA, Shaywitz SE, Shaywitz BA, Anderson GM, Cohen DJ. Neurochemical correlates of attention deficit disorder. Pediatr Clin North Am 1981; 31: 387–396.

Reisbick S, Neuringer M, Hasnain R, Connor WE. Home cage behavior of rhesus monkeys with long-term deficiency of omega-3 fatty acids. Physiol Behav 1994; 55: 231–239.

Sandyk R. Zinc deficiency in attention-deficit hyperactivity disorder. Int J Neurosci 1990; 52: 239–241.

Schurch B. Malnutrition and behavioral development: the nutrition variable. J Nutr 1995; 125: 2255S–2262S.

Sever Y, Ashkenazi A, Tyano S, Weizman A. Iron treatment in children with attention-deficit hyperactivity disorder. Neuropsychobiology 1997; 35: 178–180.

Shils ME. Magnesium. In: Ziegler EE, Filer LJ, Jr, eds. Present knowledge in nutrition. Washington: ILSI Press, 1996; 256–264.

Smith WL. Prostanoid biosynthesis and mechanisms of action. Am J Physiol 1992; 263: F181–F191.

Sprecher H. New advances in fatty-acid biosynthesis. Nutrition 1996; 12 (Suppl 1): S5–S7.

Starobrat-Hermelin B, Kozielec T. The effects of magnesium physiological supplementation on hyperactivity in children with attention deficit hyperactivity disorder (ADHD). Positive response to magnesium oral loading test. Magnesium Res 1997; 10: 149–156.

Stevens LJ, Zentall SS, Deck JL, Abate ML, Lipp SR, Burgess JR. Essential fatty acid metabolism in boys with attention-deficit hyperactivity disorder. Am J Clin Nutr 1995; 62: 761–768.

Stevens LJ, Zentall SS, Abate ML, Kuczek T, Burgess JR. Omega-3 fatty acids in boys with behavior, learning, and health problems. Physiol Behav 1996; 59: 915–920.

Strupp BJ, Levitsky DA. Enduring cognitive effects of early malnutrition: a theoretical reappraisal. J Nutr 1995; 125: 2221S–2232S.

Swanson JM, McBurnett K, Wigal T et al. Effect of stimulant medication on children with attention deficit disorder: a 'review of reviews'. Except Child 1993; 60: 154–162.

Szatmari P. The epidemiology of attention-deficit hyperactivity disorder. Child Adolesc Psychiatr Clin N Am 1992; 1: 361–371.

Toren P, Eldar S, Sela B-A et al. Zinc deficiency in attention-deficit hyperactivity disorder. Biol Psychiatry 1996; 40: 1308–1310.

Uauy R, Peirano P, Hoffman D, Mena P, Birch D, Birch E. Role of essential fatty acids in the function of the developing nervous system. Lipids 1996; 31: S167–S176.

Ucles P, Lorente S, Rosa F. Neurophysiological methods for testing the psychoneural basis of attention deficit hyperactivity disorder. Childs Nerv Sys 1996; 12: 215–217.

Xu LZ, Sanchez R, Sali A, Heintz N. Ligand specificity of brain lipid-binding protein. J Biol Chem 1996; 271: 24711–24719.

Yehuda S, Carasso RL. Modulation of learning, pain thresholds, and thermoregulation in the rat by preparations of free purified alpha-linolenic acids: determination of the optimal n-3 to n-6 ratio. Proc Natl Acad Sci USA 1993; 90: 919–925.

Yoshida S, Yasuda A, Kawazato H et al. Synaptic vesicle ultrastructural changes in the rat hippocampus induced by a combination of α-linolenate deficiency and a learning task. J Neurochem 1997; 68: 1261–1268.

Zametkin AJ, Rapoport JL. Neurobiology of attention deficit disorder with hyperactivity: where have we come in 50 years? J Am Acad Child Adolesc Psychiatry 1987; 26: 676–686.

A Possible Role for Phospholipases in Autism and Asperger's Syndrome

25

David F. Horrobin

INTRODUCTION

Autism and the related, but milder, condition of Asperger's syndrome, are perhaps the least investigated of the major psychiatric disorders with regard to lipid metabolism. This article is therefore highly speculative and its aim is to stimulate thought and further research.

There is now strong evidence that autism has a substantial genetic component (Gillberg, 1993; Rapin, 1997). If this is so, there must be a biochemical factor which either causes or predisposes to autism. There are few clues as to what that biochemical factor may be, but some clinical observations are of interest (Gillberg, 1993; Rapin, 1997), and these may be summarized as follows: boys are affected much more frequently than girls; there is often a reduced need for sleep; hypotonia and clumsiness are common; epilepsy is common; there may be detailed abnormalities in the architecture of the brain, especially in the cerebellum, amygdala and hippocampus; the brain tends to be large (Piven et al., 1995; Davidovitch et al., 1996); thermoregulation may be abnormal, with a reduced ability to respond to heat or cold (Gerland, 1997); there may be an unusual resistance to pain (Prior and Werry, 1986; Gerland, 1997; Sher, 1997); and autistic behaviour frequently shows a substantial improvement when a child has a febrile illness (Sullivan, 1980; Cotterill, 1985).

OBSERVATIONS

I have had the opportunity to perform niacin flushing tests and to assay red cell phospholipid fatty acid compositions in two patients with mild Asperger's syndrome. In both patients the flushing response to the topical application of graded concentrations of methyl nicotinate to the forearm was seriously impaired (Ward et al., 1998; Ward and Glen, 1999). The flushing response depends on the release of arachidonic acid (AA) from cell membrane phospholipids and its subsequent conversion to prostaglandin D_2, an effective cutaneous vasodilator.

In schizophrenia, niacin flushing is impaired, and this is frequently associated with a reduced level of AA in red cell membranes (Glen et al., 1994, 1996; Ward et al., 1998). One possible explanation for this is chronic overactivity of one or more phospholipases, such as phospholipase A_2 or C (Horrobin, 1998). This would lead to depletion of the pool of AA released by niacin and hence to impairment of niacin flushing.

I therefore expected that in the two individuals with mild Asperger's syndrome there would be low normal or subnormal levels of AA in red cell membranes. I was surprised to find that, instead of being low, the red cell levels of AA and of docosahexaenoic acid (DHA), the n-3 fatty acid which is present in large amounts in red cell membranes, were both elevated. Thus, in schizophrenia this tends to be associated with low AA, while in Asperger's syndrome the two patients investigated to date both had unusually high red cell AA concentrations. These observations need to be tested in a much larger group of autistic and Asperger patients.

There has been one report of a study of red cell fatty acids in autism (Kane and Schauss, 1997). This also reported elevations of both AA and DHA as well as longer chain fatty acids, a phenomenon which was reasonably attributed to a possible peroxisomal disorder.

HYPOTHESIS

The high AA levels, coupled with a subnormal response to niacin, represent a puzzle. One possible explanation might be an abnormality opposite to that postulated in schizophrenia, namely a reduced, rather than an increased, activity of phospholipases, such as phospholipase A_2. In this case, one might expect membrane AA and DHA levels to be increased and there to be resistance to the effects of niacin which requires activation of phospholipase for its vasodilating effect.

If this were true, then there would be a reduced rate of release of AA, and probably of other fatty acids, leading to reduced levels of the free acids and of their derivatives, such as prostaglandins and other eicosanoids, anandamide and oleamide. This could account for a number of the features of autism summarized in above.

1. Since males have a much higher requirement than females for AA and essential fatty acids, a deficit of free essential fatty acids might be expected to have a greater impact on males than on females (Pudelkewicz et al., 1968).

2. Derivatives of fatty acids, such as anandamide and oleamide, may be natural sedating and sleep-inducing agents and so deficits might lead to a reduced need for sleep (Berdyshev et al., 1996; Thomas et al., 1997).

3. Extreme clumsiness (dyspraxia) seems to be associated with deficits of AA and DHA (Stordy, 1997).

4. Free fatty acids, particularly DHA, are important in controlling abnormal electrical discharges from neurones (Vreugdenhil et al., 1996). A deficit of free fatty acids could therefore lead to an increased risk of epilepsy.

5. Phospholipases and the cyclooxygenases which convert the fatty acids to eicosanoids are of critical importance in making and breaking normal synaptic junctions (Negre-Aminou et al., 1996; Smalheiser et al., 1996). Abnormalities in phospholipases could therefore lead to the observed detailed changes in brain cellular architecture.

6. Arachidonic acid seems to be a key regulator of brain size in normal infants (Koletzko, 1992). A high level of brain AA could therefore lead to a large brain.

7. The normal release of AA is critical to normal thermoregulatory mechanisms, both in the brain and in the periphery. A failure to release AA could therefore lead to problems with temperature control.

8. Release of AA is important in pain, and so a reduced ability to mobilize AA could lead to impaired pain sensation.

9. One of the things which happens in fever is activation of phospholipases. A fever might therefore lead to a move towards normal in a situation where phospholipases are subnormally activated at normal temperatures.

This concept is, of course, at this stage highly speculative. But it is amenable to testing and, if correct, could lead to novel approaches to treatment involving activation of phospholipases.

REFERENCES

Berdyshev EV, Boichot E, Lagente V. Anandamide – a new look on fatty acids ethanolamides. J Lipid Mediat Cell Signal 1996; 15: 49–67.

Cotterill RMJ. Fever in autistics. Nature 1985; 323: 426.

Davidovitch M, Patterson B, Gartside P. Head circumference measurements in children with autism. J Child Neurol 1996; 11: 389–393.

Gerland G. A real person: life on the outside. London: Souvenir Press, 1997.

Gillberg C. Autism and related behaviours. J Intellect Disabil Res 1993; 37: 343–372.

Glen AIM, Glen EMT, Horrobin DF et al. A red cell membrane abnormalilty in a subgroup of schizophrenic patients: evidence for two diseases. Schizophr Res 1994; 12: 53–61.

Glen AIM, Cooper SJ, Rybakowski J, Vaddadi K, Brayshaw N, Horrobin DF. Membrane fatty acids, niacin flushing and clinical parameters. Prostagland Leukotr Essent Fatty Acids 1996; 15: 9–15.

Horrobin DF. The membrane phospholipid hypothesis as a biochemical basis for the neurodevelopmental concept of schizophrenia. Schizophr Res 1998; 30: 193–208.

Kane PC, Schauss MA. Peroxisomal disturbances in children with epilepsy, hypoxia, and autism. Prostagland Leukotr Essent Fatty Acids 1997; 57: 265.

Koletzko B. Fats for brains. Eur J Clin Nutr 1992; 46 (Suppl 1): S51–S62.

Negre-Aminou P, Nemenoff RA, Wood MR, de la Houssaye BA, Pfenninger KH. Characterization of phospholipase A_2 activity enriched in the nerve growth cone. J Neurochem 1996; 67: 2599–2608.

Piven J, Arndt S, Bailey J, Havercamp S, Andreasen NC, Palmer P. An MRI study of brain size in autism. Am J Psychiatry 1995; 152: 1145–1149.

Prior M, Werry JS. Autism, schizophrenia and allied disorders. In: Quay HC, Werry JS, eds. Psychopathological disorders of childhood. New York: John Wiley, 1986: 156–210.

Pudelkewicz C, Seufert J, Holman RT. Requirements of the female rat for linoleic and linolenic acids. J Nutr 1968; 94: 138–146.

Rapin I. Autism. N Engl J Med 1997; 337: 97–104.

Sher L. Autistic disorder and the endogenous opioid sysgtem. Med Hypotheses 1997; 48: 413–414.

Smalheiser NR, Dissanayake S, Kapil A. Rapid regulation of neurite outgrowth and retraction by phospholipase A_2-derived arachidonic acid and its metabolites. Brain Res 1996; 721: 39–48.

Stordy BJ. Dyslexia, attention deficit disorder, dyspraxia: do fatty acid supplements help? Dyslexia Rev 1997; 9: 5–7.

Sullivan RC. Why do autistic children…? J Autism Dev Disorders 1980; 10: 231–241.

Thomas EA, Carson MJ, Neal MJ, Sutcliffe JG. Unique allosteric regulation of 5-hydroxytryptamine receptor-medicated signal transduction by oleamide. Proc Natl Acad Sci USA 1997; 94: 14115–14119.

Vreugdenhil M, Bruehl C, Voskuyl RA, Kang JX, Leaf A, Wadman WJ. Polyunsaturated fatty acids modulate sodium and calcium currents in CA1 neurons. Proc Natl Acad Sci USA 1996; 93: 12559–12563.

Ward PE, Glen I. Oral and topical niacin flush testing in schizophrenia. In: Glen I, Peet M, Horrobin DF, eds. Phospholipid spectrum disorder in psychiatry. Carnforth: Marius Press, 1999: 139–144.

Ward PE, Sutherland J, Glen EMT, Glen AIM. Niacin skin flush in schizophrenia: a preliminary report. Schizophr Res 1998; 29: 269–274.

Decreased Brain and Platelet Phospholipase A$_2$ Activity in Alzheimer's Disease

Wagner F. Gattaz, Nigel J. Cairns, Raymond Levy, Hans Förstl, Dieter F. Braus and Athanasios Maras

INTRODUCTION

Alterations in the processing of the amyloid precursor protein (APP) may give rise to the β-amyloid peptide (βA), the major component of the amyloid plaque in Alzheimer's disease (AD). Phospholipase A$_2$ (PLA$_2$) is the key enzyme in the metabolism of membrane phospholipids, cleaving the Sn2-fatty acid ester to produce lysophospholipids and free fatty acids. Emmerling et al. (1993) reported that the inhibition of PLA$_2$ decreased the carbachol-stimulated secretion of APP from cells transfected with the human M$_1$ muscarinic receptor, whereas the activation of PLA$_2$ increased APP secretion. Experimental evidence suggests that increased APP secretion by cells reduces the production of amyloidogenic peptides (Caporaso et al., 1992).

In view of these findings we investigated in two studies the activity of PLA$_2$ in brain tissue and in platelets from AD patients compared to nondemented controls. AD patients showed in both tissues a significant reduction of the enzyme activity. The data presented here on brain tissue have already been published elsewhere (Gattaz et al., 1995a).

EXPERIMENTAL PROCEDURES

The methods for tissue preparation and determination of PLA$_2$ activity have been described in detail elsewhere (Gattaz et al., 1995a,b, for brain and platelets, respectively). Data were analyzed by the nonparametric Mann-Whitney and Wilcoxon tests and the Spearman rank-order correlation coefficient (r_s).

Brain samples

Autopsied brain samples of parietal and frontal cortex (Brodmann areas 7 and 32, respectively) were obtained from the Medical Research Council Alzheimer's Disease Brain Bank, Institute of Psychiatry, London, UK. Samples from 23 cases of neuropathologically confirmed AD (seven male, 16 female; age 81.0 ± 7.5 years, mean ± SD) and 20 nondemented controls (10 male, 10 female; age 75.6 ± 9.8 years) were investigated. The degree of dementia was assessed in all but two AD patients within 12 months before death, using the Mini Mental State Examination (MMSE) (Folstein et al., 1975). None of the AD patients had received therapy for the disease. The causes of death were similar in AD patients and controls and were usually due to a terminal circulatory or respiratory failure. In AD patients, the age at disease onset was 72.9 ± 6.9 years, the duration of illness 9.5 ± 5.8 years, and the MMSE score 3.1 ± 4.9 (means ± SD in all cases).

Histological counts were obtained from 16 AD patients. Histological and counting methods for senile plaques (SPs) and neurofibrillary tangles (NFTs) have been described elsewhere (Förstl et al., 1992). The counts/mm^2 (means ± SD, with the range given in parentheses) were: SPs, parietal 5.0 ± 6.3 (0–22); SPs, frontal 4.1 ± 7.2 (0–27); NFTs, parietal 4.7 ± 4.6 (0.4–18); NFTs, frontal 5.9 ± 7.6 (0.1–24).

The demographic and biochemical data and the post-mortem interval are given in Table 26.1. There was a trend for AD patients to have a higher age at death than the patients in the control group, though this attained only borderline statistical significance ($0.10 > p > 0.05$). The difference in post-mortem interval, with shorter mean time from death to storage in the AD group, did not reach statistical significance ($p = 0.15$).

Platelets

We determined the platelet PLA$_2$ activity in 16 patients with a diagnosis of probable AD, as compared to 13 healthy controls and to 14 psychiatric patients with a major depression (Table 26.2). There were no significant differences between the three groups regarding age and sex distribution. In the AD patients the cognitive performance was assessed with the CAMCOG and the MMSE.

Table 26.1. Demographic and neurochemical data in Alzheimer's disease patients ($n = 23$) and nondemented controls ($n = 20$); means ± SD.

Parameter	Alzheimer's disease	Controls
Sex (M:F)	7:16	10:10
Age (years)	81.0 ± 7.5§	75.6 ± 9.8
Post-mortem time (h)	30.7 ± 14.5	38.1 ± 11.1
p-PLA$_2$[a]	27.4 ± 20.2***	43.4 ± 23.8
f-PLA$_2$[a]	26.9 ± 16.4§	37.9 ± 19.8

[a] Units of measurement of activity of PLA$_2$, pmol arachidonic acid/mg protein/45 min. In comparison with the corresponding value for control subjects, ***$p < 0.005$; §$0.10 > p > 0.05$ (borderline significance).

Table 26.2. Demographic and neurochemical data in Alzheimer's disease patients (n = 16), healthy controls (n = 13) and psychiatric (depressed) controls (n = 14); means ± SD.

Parameter	Alzheimer's disease	Healthy controls	Psychiatric controls
Sex (M:F)	4:8	9:4	6:8
Age (years)	70.2 ± 11.3	62.6 ± 9.7	62.3 ± 12.2
PLA$_2$[a]	14.3 ± 4.6*	19.4 ± 6.4	23.1 ± 6.0

[a] Units of measurement of activity of PLA$_2$, pmol arachidonic acid/mg protein/min. *In comparison with the corresponding value for Alzheimer's disease patients, $p < 0.05$.

PLA$_2$ ACTIVITY

Brain tissue

AD patients showed significantly lower parietal PLA$_2$ activity (p-PLA$_2$) than was seen in controls ($p < 0.005$). Frontal PLA$_2$ activity (f-PLA$_2$) was also reduced in AD patients, but the difference just failed to reach statistical significance ($p = 0.051$; Table 26.1). There was a significant correlation between p-PLA$_2$ and f-PLA$_2$ in AD patients ($r_s = +0.55; p < 0.005$), but not in controls ($r_s = +0.28$; ns).

In the AD group, both p-PLA$_2$ and f-PLA$_2$ correlated positively with age at death ($r_s = +0.37; p < 0.05$, and $r_s = +0.25$; ns). In controls, the correlations with age were negative and statistically nonsignificant. Because the AD patients tended to be older than controls, PLA$_2$ values were corrected for age by the regression coefficient in both patients and controls for further comparisons and partial correlations. Age-correction increased the significance of the difference for p-PLA$_2$ ($p < 0.001$) and the decrement of f-PLA$_2$ in AD patients became significant ($p < 0.05$).

Both p-PLA$_2$ and f-PLA$_2$ correlated positively with age at disease onset ($r_s = +0.60; p < 0.005$, and $r_s = +0.58; p < 0.005$, respectively). F-PLA$_2$ correlated negatively with counts of NFTs ($r_s = -0.56; n = 16; p < 0.01$) and SPs ($r_s = -0.47; n = 16; p < 0.05$). No significant correlations were found between p-PLA$_2$ and histological counts.

No correlations were found between both p-PLA$_2$ and f-PLA$_2$ and MMSE scores, duration of illness, or post-mortem interval. No significant differences were found between p-PLA$_2$ and f-PLA$_2$ within the AD group or within the control group (Table 26.1). Within both groups there were also no differences in the enzyme activity between males and females.

Platelets

Platelet PLA$_2$ activity was significantly reduced in AD patients as compared with healthy ($p < 0.03$) and psychiatric controls ($p < 0.002$) (Table 26.2). The reduction of the enzyme activity showed borderline correlation with an early onset of disease ($r_s = +0.43; 0.10 > p > 0.05$), and correlated significantly with the cognitive impairment as indexed by the score on the CAMCOG ($r_s = +0.55; p < 0.05$). AD patients with MMSE scores lower than 10 (median) showed significantly ($p < 0.05$) lower PLA$_2$ activity (11.8 ± 3.1) than patients with MMSE scores higher than 10 (16.2 ± 4.6).

DISCUSSION

Our finding of reduced PLA$_2$ activity in the brain suggests a decreased breakdown of membrane phospholipids by PLA$_2$ in AD patients. Moreover, our results indicate that the degree of the PLA$_2$ reduction was related to the severity of the pathological process, as in our AD sample the low enzyme activity was correlated with an earlier onset of the disease, higher NFT and SP numbers, and earlier age at death.

Our assumption of a decreased breakdown of membrane phospholipids in AD is supported by the results of an *in vivo* ^{31}P NMR spectroscopy investigation of the phosphomonoesters and phosphodiesters in AD patients (Brown et al., 1989). Phosphomonoesters are the precursors, and phosphodiesters are the breakdown products, of membrane phospholipids in the brain. AD patients showed increased phosphomonoesters and phosphomonoester/phosphodiester ratio in the temporoparietal region. Reduced PLA$_2$ activity, as demonstrated in our study, may contribute to this increment of phosphomonoesters in AD.

In the brain, docosahexanoate (22:6n-3) is one of the principal free fatty acids released by the deacylation of membrane phospholipids through PLA_2 (Bazan et al., 1986). Skinner et al. (1989) found a marked reduction in the proportion of docosahexanoate in the parietal cortex (but not in the frontal cortex) from AD patients, which is compatible with reduced PLA_2 as observed in the present study. Changes in the activity of other enzymes related to the membrane phospholipid turnover have already been described in AD brains, such as increased lipases and lysophospholipase activity (Farooqui et al., 1990) and decreased phospholipase D activity (Kanfer et al., 1986). The present finding of reduced PLA_2 activity provides new evidence for a disordered membrane phospholipid metabolism in AD.

A characteristic neuropathological finding in AD is the deposition of fibrillar aggregates of the β-amyloid protein, a 39–43 amino acid peptide produced by the cleavage of a large, membrane-bound APP (Dyrks et al., 1988). Emmerling et al. (1993) reported that the inhibition of PLA_2 decreased the carbachol-stimulated secretion of APP from cells transfected with the human M_1 muscarinic receptor, whereas the activation of PLA_2 increased APP secretion. Experimental evidence suggests that increased APP secretion by cells reduces the production of amyloidogenic peptides (Caporaso et al., 1992). It is therefore conceivable that, conversely, the reduction of APP secretion, as caused by decreased PLA_2 activity, may represent one possible route for amyloidogenesis in AD. This assumption is also supported by our finding of a correlation between the reduction of PLA_2 activity and the counts of SPs.

Because PLA_2 activity is under genetic control (Sharp et al., 1991), it is conceivable that the enzyme activity in the brain is related to the activity in blood cells. To test this assumption we investigated the enzyme activity in platelet membranes from AD patients compared to healthy and psychiatric controls. Platelets are interesting peripheral models in AD research, because they contain and secrete APP (Smith et al., 1990). Our finding of reduced PLA_2 activity in platelets is in line with the results in brain tissue. In both studies, decreased PLA_2 activity was related to a more severe form of AD (early onset, more cognitive impairment and higher numbers of plaques and tangles). Moreover, reduced platelet PLA_2 activity was specific for AD as compared to age-matched psychiatric controls. Further studies should clarify whether PLA_2 activity in platelets could be useful as a peripheral marker for a subgroup of AD.

SUMMARY

PLA_2 is a key enzyme in the metabolism of membrane phospholipids; it influences the processing and secretion of the APP, which gives rise to the βA, the major component of the amyloid plaque in AD. We investigated the PLA_2 activity in two samples: in post-mortem brains from 23 patients with AD and 20 nondemented elderly controls; and in platelets from 16 patients with probable AD, 13 healthy controls and 14 elderly patients with a major depression. In AD brains, PLA_2 activity was significantly decreased in the parietal, and to a lesser degree in the frontal, cortex. Lower PLA_2 activity correlated significantly with an earlier onset of the disease, higher counts of NFTs and SPs, and an earlier age at death. Also, PLA_2 activity in platelets was significantly reduced in AD patients as compared to healthy and to depressed controls. The reduction of the enzyme activity in platelets correlated with an early onset of disease and with cognitive impairment, thus indicating a relationship between abnormally low PLA_2 activity and a more severe form of the illness. The present results provide new evidence for disordered phospholipid metabolism in AD brains, and suggest that reduced PLA_2 activity may contribute to the production of amyloidogenic peptides in the disease. Moreover, it remains to be clarified in further studies whether PLA_2 activity in platelets may be useful as a peripheral marker for a subgroup of AD.

ACKNOWLEDGEMENTS

We are indebted to Professor W. Müller, Central Institute for Mental Health, Mannheim, to Professor E. Ferber, MaxPlanck-Institut für Immunbiologie-Freiburg, and to Professor A. Burns, Institute of Psychiatry, London, for the support given to this work. This work was supported by the Deutsche Forschungsgemeinschaft, SFB 258, Projects S4 and K2.

REFERENCES

Bazan HEP, Ridenour B, Birkle DL, Bazan NG. Unique metabolic features of docosahexanoate metabolism related to functional roles in brain and retina. In: Horrocks LA, Freysz L, Toffano G, eds. Phospholipid research and the nervous system. Biochemical and molecular pharmacology. Fidia Research Series, Vol. 4. Padova: Liviana Press, 1986: 67–78.

Brown GG, Levine SR, Gorell JM et al. *In vivo* ^{31}P NMR profiles of Alzheimer's disease and multiple subcortical infarct dementia. Neurology 1989; 39: 1423–1427.

Caporaso GL, Gandy SE, Buxbaum JD, Ramabhadran TV, Greengard P. Protein phosphorylation regulates secretion of Alzheimer βA4 amyloid precursor protein. Proc Natl Acad Sci USA 1992; 89: 3055–3059.

Dyrks T, Weidemann A, Multhaup G et al. Identification, transmembrane orientation and biogenesis of the amyloid A4 precursor of Alzheimer's disease. EMBO J 1988; 7: 949–957.

Emmerling MR, Moore CJ, Doyle PD, Carroll RT, Davis RE. Phospholipase A_2 activation influences the processing and secretion of the amyloid precursor protein. Biochem Biophys Res Commun 1993; 197: 292–297.

Farooqui AA, Liss L, Horrocks LA. Elevated activities of lipases and lysophospholipase in Alzheimer's disease. Dementia 1990; 1: 208–214.

Folstein M, Folstein S, McHugh P. Mini-Mental State. J Psychiatr Res 1975; 12: 189–198.

Förstl H, Burns A, Levy R, Cairns NJ, Luthert P, Lantos P. Neurologic signs in Alzheimer's disease: results of a prospective clinical and neuropathologic study. Arch Neurol 1992; 49: 1038–1042.

Gattaz WF, Maras A, Cairns NJ, Levy R, Förstl H. Decreased phospholipas A_2 activity in Alzheimer brains. Biol Psychiatry 1995a; 37: 13–17.

Gattaz WF, Schmitt A, Maras A. Increased platelet phospholipas A_2 activity in schizophrenia. Schizophr Res 1995b; 16: 1–6.

Kanfer JN, Hattori H, Orihel D. Reduced phospholipase D activity in brain tissue samples from Alzheimer's disease patients. Ann Neurol 1986; 20: 265–267.

Sharp JD, White DL, Chiou XG et al. Molecular cloning and expression of human Ca^{2+}-sensitive cytosolic PLA_2. J Biol Chem 1991; 266: 14850–14853.

Skinner ER, Watt C, Besson JAO, Best PV. Lipid composition of different regions of the brain in patients with Alzheimer's disease. Biochem Soc Trans 1989; 17: 213–214.

Smith RP, Higuschi DA, Broze GJ. Platelet coagulation factor Ixa-inhibitor, a form of Alzheimer amyloid precursor protein. Science 1990; 248: 1126–1128.

Phospholipids and Abnormal Involuntary Movements in the General Male Population

Agneta Nilsson, David F. Horrobin and Annika Rosengren

DYSKINETIC SYNDROMES IN SCHIZOPHRENIA

Tardive dyskinesia

Tardive dyskinesia (TD), the syndrome of involuntary, hyperkinetic abnormal movements that may occur during or after treatment with neuroleptic drugs, has generally been regarded as an unfortunate, and largely unexplained, adverse effect of such treatment. There is an enormous spread in the prevalence rates reported in neuroleptic-treated patients, with figures ranging between 5% and 70%, and even higher rates being reported in a few studies (Casey, 1987). These variations may be ascribed to differences in the methods used to assess dyskinesia and in the types of populations included in the studies.

The most consistently reported risk factor throughout all studies is advanced age (Smith and Baldessarini, 1980; Kane and Smith, 1982); alcoholism (Dixon et al., 1992) and diabetes mellitus (Mukherjee et al., 1985; Ganzini et al., 1991) have also been implicated. Previously reported higher prevalence rates among women (Kane and Smith, 1982; Richardson et al., 1984) have been questioned in more recent studies (Saltz et al., 1991; Morgenstern and Glazer, 1993). Of great interest are also the clear, and repeatedly demonstrated, associations with the negative syndrome of schizophrenia (Brown and White, 1991; Davis et al., 1992).

Vaddadi et al. (1989) (see also Vaddadi, 1992) have noted abnormalities in red cell membrane phospholipid essential fatty acids (EFAs) in neuroleptic-treated patients with schizophrenia and TD. These abnormalities consisted of progressively decreasing levels of the highly unsaturated fatty acids (HUFAs) concomitant with increasing severity of TD. Their findings are congruent with observations suggesting that TD may be linked to free radical formation in the brain (Lohr et al., 1988; Cadet and Kahler, 1994), since the molecules most susceptible to free radical damage are the HUFAs, particularly those with 3–6 double bonds. These fatty acids are not only damaged by free radicals, but in the process they generate further free radicals in a chain reaction which can be stopped only by chainbreaking antioxidants such as vitamin E. Many studies have demonstrated that vitamin E is an effective treatment for TD, at least in cases of moderate severity and duration (Lohr et al., 1988; Egan et al., 1992; Adler et al., 1993; Peet et al., 1993).

Spontaneous dyskinesia

Spontaneous dyskinesia (SD), which, by definition, occurs in individuals never exposed to neuroleptic drugs, is clinically indistinguishable from TD. SD has received far less research attention than TD, but a recent accumulation of studies suggests that SD is a fairly common phenomenon in schizophrenic patients without previous exposure to neuroleptics. This has been demonstrated in treatment settings where neuroleptics have not been part of the prevailing treatment policies (Owens-Cunningham et al., 1982), and in studies based partly on case notes from the preneuroleptic era (Fenton et al., 1994). Advanced age and cognitive impairment remain risk factors also for SD (Fenton et al., 1994).

Prevalence of dyskinesia

For a long time, TS and SD have been regarded as two separate entities, but in recent years the possibility has been recognized that dyskinesia might be attributable to the schizophrenic disease process rather than to its treatment, and a putative organic vulnerability associated with schizophrenia, as well as with this particular motor disorder, has been postulated (Waddington, 1989). There is, however, a remarkable lack of knowledge about the baseline levels of dyskinesia, i.e., the prevalence rates in the absence of risk factors, such as exposure to neuroleptics and schizophrenia. The basic idea behind our studies of abnormal involuntary movements (SD and TD) in the general population has therefore been to study dyskinetic phenomena without making any *a priori* assumptions about their cause. This approach might increase our understanding of the risk factors and pathological processes involved, and help to establish to what extent the different risk factors contribute to the prevalence rates.

DYSKINESIA AND FREE RADICALS

In our first study on dyskinesia in the general male population, we were able to show that cigarette smoking and exposure to neuroleptics were independently associated with dyskinesia (Nilsson et al., 1997). Since cigarette smoke is very rich in free radicals (Church and Pryor, 1985), and since neuroleptic drugs are known to enhance free radical formation, with consequent peroxidation of unsaturated lipids (Pall et al., 1987), we wanted to explore the possibility that neuronal depletion of HUFAs by free radicals might represent the common path whereby TD and SD had been produced in our sample. Such a possibility seems plausible in view of the work on TD and membrane phospholipids by Vaddadi (1992), mentioned earlier; it is further supported by the observations that the rates of formation of HUFAs within the body decline with age (Horrobin, 1992), and that the red cell membranes of schizophrenic patients with a predominantly negative syndrome are seriously depleted of HUFAs as compared with either normal controls or schizophrenic patients with a predominantly positive syndrome (Glen et al., 1994). A similar depletion of HUFAs is associated with alcoholism (Glen et al., 1990) as well as with diabetes mellitus (Jones et al., 1983; van Doormaal et al., 1988).

DYSKINESIA AND PHOSPHOLIPIDS: A GENERAL POPULATION STUDY

Structure of the study

The Department of Preventive Cardiology at Göteborg University has been conducting large investigations in successive cohorts of middle-aged men. These investigations have focused mainly on cardiovascular health and have involved the collection of large amounts of data (Welin et al., 1985; Rosengren et al., 1990). The cohort of men born in 1933 was investigated at age 59 years. This examination was extended to include analysis of fatty acid levels in plasma and videotaped sessions for the assessment of dyskinesia. The 602 participants comprised a random sample of all men born in 1933 and living in the city of Göteborg. Videotaped assessments and fatty acid levels were available in 487 (80.9%) of the original sample; drop-out was due to administrative reasons only, and no systematic bias was observed. Detailed descriptions of the cohort and the study protocol have been presented previously (Rosengren et al., 1990; Nilsson et al., 1996).

Findings

Prevalence of dyskinesia

The Abnormal Involuntary Movement Scale (AIMS) (Guy, 1976) was used for quantifying dyskinetic movements. The AIMS scores were 0 in 76.5% ($n = 372$), 1 in 8.4% ($n = 41$) and ≥ 2 in 15.1%. Since an AIMS score of 1 is considered inconclusive, men with this score were excluded from further analysis, which thus involved 74 dyskinetic men (i.e., AIMS score ≥ 2) and 372 nondyskinetic men (i.e., AIMS score = 0). Table 27.1 shows a univariate comparison of dyskinetic and nondyskinetic men.

The 15% prevalence rate of dyskinesia in 59-year-old men might seem high, but since no other general population survey of dyskinesia exists, it is not possible to say whether it is unexpectedly high. Comparisons can only be made with studies of healthy controls: McCreadie et al. (1996) found figures similar to ours in a somewhat older population in Madras, India.

Cigarette smoking and exposure to neuroleptics were independently associated with the present of dyskinesia in our sample. Since exposure to neuroleptics is a very rare event in the general population, cigarette smoking, with its higher prevalence, must be regarded as much more of a health hazard in terms of dyskinesia, at least in a sample such as ours. Our findings might also provide psychiatrists with a reason to modify the information that they give to their patients about the risk of dyskinesia as an adverse effect of treatment with neuroleptics.

Fatty acid levels

Table 27.2 presents the direction of the significant differences in plasma fatty acids between dyskinetic and nondyskinetic men. The striking, and most consistent, finding was that dyskinetic men had significantly lower arachidonic acid (AA) levels than found in nondyskinetic men in every fraction. Table 27.3 shows the distribution of the AA levels in the three different fractions of plasma. The AA levels were approximately 10% lower in a dyskinetic men, and Table 27.4 covers a logistic regression model with dyskinesia as dependent variable. In the first logistic model, containing seven variables, five factors separating dyskinetic from nondyskinetic

Table 27.1. Comparison of men with ($n = 74$) and without ($n = 372$) dyskinesia, on the basis of several psychiatric and biomedical variables.

Variable	Dyskinetic	Nondyskinetic
Psychiatric morbidity		
n (%)	13 (17.6)	30 (8.0)*
Parkinsonian symptom score [a]		
Mean ± SD	1.6 ± 2.0	1.0 ± 1.9*
Daily cigarette smoking score [b]		
Mean ± SD	0.72 ± 1.16	0.41 ± 0.93*
Diabetes mellitus		
n (%)	5 (6.8)	26 (7.0)
Exposure to neuroleptics		
n (%)	6 (8.1)	4 (1.1)**
Average alcohol consumption [c]		
Mean ± SD	5.1 ± 1.8	5.0 ± 2.2

[a] According to the scale proposed by Simpson and Angus (1970); [b] 0 = no cigarettes smoked per day, 1 = 1–10/day, 2 = 11–19/day, 3 = ≥ 20/day; [c] units/week (for definition, see Nilsson et al., 1986). In comparison with the corresponding value for dyskinetic men, $p <$: *0.05; **0.01; other values nonsignificant (Fisher's exact probability test and the Mann-Whitney U-test).

Table 27.2. Direction of significant differences in fatty acid levels between men with ($n = 74$) and without ($n = 372$) dyskinesia.

Fatty acid	Cholesterol	Triglycerides	Phospholipids
Palmitic	↑*	–	↑*
Oleic	↑*	–	↑
DGLA	–	↑**	–
AA	↓†††	↓***	↓†††

↑ = Significantly higher in dyskinetic than in nondyskinetic men; ↓ = significantly lower in dyskinetic than in nondyskinetic men; – = no significant difference; $p <$: *0.05; **0.01; ***0.001; †††0.0001.

Table 27.3. Plasma levels (mg/100 mg total lipid) of compounds incorporating arachidonic acid, in men with ($n = 74$) and without ($n = 372$) dyskinesia; means ± SD.

Group	Dyskinetic	Nondyskinetic
Cholesterolesters	4.3 ± 1.0	4.8 ± 1.1†††
Triglycerides	0.76 ± 0.25	0.86 ± 0.29***
Phospholipids	7.9 ± 1.7	8.8 ± 1.7†††

In comparison with the corresponding value for dyskinetic men, p: <***0.005; †††0.0001 (Mann-Whitney U-test).

Table 27.4. Logistic regression analysis of dyskinesia as a dependent variable.

	Seven variables		Three variables	
Variable	Odds ratio[b]	95% CI	Odds ratio	95% CI
1. Score for number of cigarettes per day	1.3	1.1–1.7*	1.4	1.1–1.7**
2. Exposure to neuroleptics (Yes or No)	6.2	1.1–36.2*	11.1	2.9–43.2††
3. Arachidonic acid phospholipids	0.26	0.15–0.46†††	0.25	0.15–0.44†††
4. Psychiatric morbidity (Yes or No)	1.05	0.4–2.8		
5. Parkinsonian symptoms (Simpson & Angus score)	1.1	0.99–1.3		
6. Diabetes mellitus (Yes or No)	1.1	0.3–3.2		
7. Average alcohol consumption (units/day)	1.0	0.9–1.2		

[a] The seven-variable model includes all psychiatric and biomedical variables of interest; the three-variable model includes only those variables attaining statistical significance. $p <$: *0.05; **0.01; ††0.0005; †††0.0001 (in the case of a continuous variable, p values are calculated on nondichotomized variables). [b] The odds ratio compares the 75th and 25th percentiles of the cumulative distribution.

men were included (i.e., psychiatric morbidity; parkinsonian symptom score; daily cigarette smoking score; exposure to neuroleptics; and AA levels in the phospholipid fraction in plasma), but we also chose to enter a further two factors which have been associated with dyskinesia in other studies (i.e., diabetes mellitus; alcohol intake). The three variables found to be significantly associated with dyskinesia in the seven variable model (i.e., daily cigarette smoking score; exposure to neuroleptics; and AA phospholipid level in plasma) were thus identified as the most interesting for further study and were therefore entered into the three-variable model, which demonstrated that they were all independent predictors of dyskinesia. Substituting AA levels in the phospholipid fraction for AA levels in cholesterolesters or AA levels in triglycerides did not alter the results; i.e., the score for number of cigarettes smoked per day, exposure to neuroleptics, and AA levels, all remained independently associated with dyskinesia. Table 27.5 presents the indicators of the EFA metabolism, where the rate-limiting steps are the conversion of the linoleic acid (LA) to γ-linolenic acid (GLA) and the conversion of dihomo-γ-linolenic acid (DGLA) to AA. The ratio is an indicator of the Δ-5-desaturase activity. Both ratios were significantly higher in dyskinetic than in nondyskinetic men, indicating impaired conversion of LA to AA in dyskinesia.

Implications

Exposure to neuroleptics is undeniably a strong risk factor for the development of dyskinesia, but its importance may hitherto have been exaggerated because of lack of knowledge of baseline rates of dyskinesia. We are now in the process of examining other cohorts of men, both younger and substantially older than in the present study, in the hope of further extending our knowledge of the epidemiology of dyskinesia.

We were also able to demonstrate a strong association between dyskinesia and low plasma levels of one of the important HUFAs in the brain, AA. These abnormalities were present also in dyskinetic individuals who had no psychiatric disorder and who had not been exposed to neuroleptics. Our results are consistent with the idea that depletion of one or more HUFAs may be an important factor in predisposing to the development of dyskinesias. This may prove to have important therapeutic implications. In randomized controlled trials of low doses of either of two other HUFAs, GLA and DGLA, Vaddadi et al. (1986) noted modest improvement in TD, but Wolkin et al. (1986) saw no such effect. Further trials with higher doses may be required, and it

Table 27.5. Indicators of EFA metabolism in dyskinesia in men with ($n = 74$) and without ($n = 372$) dyskinesia; means ± SD.

Indicator	Dyskinetic	Nondyskinetic
LA:AA	3.14 ± 0.8	2.84 ± 0.7[†]
DGLA:AA	0.36 ± 0.1	0.33 ± 0.1[**]

In comparison with the corresponding value for dyskinetic men, $p <$:**0.01; [†]0.001 (Mann-Whitney U-test).

may be particularly appropriate to consider combined trials with HUFAs and vitamin E, since it is possible that the HUFAs alone might partially restore brain HUFA levels while not reducing ongoing damage due to free radicals. Vitamin E alone might reduce ongoing damage while not being able to restore already lost HUFAs.

The finding of approximately 10% lower AA levels in dyskinesia lends further support to the hypothesis that TD and SD are produced through neuronal depletion of HUFAs. The lower levels could obviously be the result of free radical damage, which would be in agreement with the free radical hypothesis of dyskinesia as already mentioned, but our results also indicate that impaired conversion of LA to AA is involved in the development of dyskinesia.

REFERENCES

Adler LA, Peselow E, Rotrosen J et al. Vitamin E treatment of tardive dyskinesia. Am J Psychiatry 1993; 150: 1405–1407.

Brown KW, White T. The association between negative symptoms, movement disorders and frontal lobe psychological deficits in schizophrenic patients. Biol Psychiatry 1991; 30: 1182–1190.

Cadet JL, Kahler LA. Free radical mechanisms in schizophrenia and tardive dyskinesia. Neurosci Behav Rev 1994; 18: 457–467.

Casey DE. Tardive dyskinesia. In: Meltzer HY, ed. Psychopharmacology: the third generation of progress. New York: Raven Press, 1987: 1411–1419.

Church DF, Pryor WA. Free-radical chemistry of cigarette smoke and its toxicological implications. Environ Health Perspect 1985; 64: 111–126.

Davis EJB, Borde M, Sharma LN. Tardive dyskinesia and type II schizophrenia. Br J Psychiatry 1992; 160: 253–256.

Dixon L, Weiden PJ, Haas G, Sweeney J, Frances AJ. Increased tardive dyskinesia in alcohol-abusing schizophrenic patients. Compr Psychiatry 1992; 33: 121–122.

Egan MF, Hyde TM, Albers GW et al. Treatment of tardive dyskinesia with vitamin E. Am J Psychiatry 1992; 149: 773–777.

Fenton WS, Wyatt RJ, McGlashan TH. Risk factors for spontaneous dyskinesia in schizophrenia. Arch Gen Psychiatry 1994; 51: 643–650.

Ganzini L, Heintz RT, Hoffman WF, Casey DE. The prevalence of tardive dyskinesia in neuroleptic-treated diabetics. A controlled study. Arch Gen Psychiatry 1991; 48: 259–263.

Glen AIM, Glen EMT, MacDonnell LEF, Skinner FK. Essential fatty acids and alcoholism. In: Horrobin DF, ed. Omega-6-essential fatty acids: pathophysiology and roles in clinical medicine. New York: Wiley-Liss 1990: 321–332.

Glen AIM, Glen EMT, Horrobin DF et al. A red cell membrane abnormality in a subgroup of schizophrenic patients: evidence for two diseases. Schizophr Res 1994; 12: 53–61.

Guy W. ECDEU assessment manual for psychopharmacology. Washington, DC: US Department of Health, Education and Welfare; US Government Printing Office 1976: 534–537.

Horrobin DF. Nutritional and medical importance of gamma-linolenic acid. Prog Lipid Res 1992; 31: 163–194.

Jones DB, Carter RD, Haitas B, Mann JI. Low phospholipid arachidonic acid values in diabetic platelets. Br Med J [Clin Res] 1983; 286: 173–175.

Kane JM, Smith JM. Tardive dyskinesia: prevalence and risk factors. 1959–1979. Arch Gen Psychiatry 1982; 39: 473–481.

Lohr JB, Cadet JL, Lohr MA et al. Vitamin E in the treatment of tardive dyskinesia: the possible involvement of free radical mechanisms. Schizophr Bull 1988; 14: 291–296.

McCreadie RG, Thara R, Kamath S et al. Abnormal movements in never-medicated Indian patients with schizophrenia. Br J Psychiatry 1996; 168: 221–226.

Morgenstern H, Glazer WM. Identifying risk factors for tardive dyskinesia among long-term outpatients maintained with neuroleptic medications. Results of the Yale tardive dyskinesia study. Arch Gen Psychiatry 1993; 50: 723–733.

Mukherjee S, Wisniewski A, Bilder R, Sackheim H. Possible association between tardive dyskinesia and altered carbohydrate metabolism. Arch Gen Psychiatry 1985; 42: 205.

Nilsson A, Horrobin DF, Rosengren A, Waller L, Adlerberth A, Wilhelmsen L. Essential fatty acids and abnormal involuntary movements in the general male population: a study of men born in 1933. Prostagland Leukotr Essent Fatty Acids 1996; 55: 83–87.

Nilsson A, Waller L, Rosengren A, Adlerberth A, Wilhelmsen L. Cigarette smoking is associated with abnormal involuntary movements in the general male population – a study of men born in 1933. Biol Psychiatry 1997; 41: 717–723.

Owens-Cunningham DG, Johnstone EG, Frith DC. Spontaneous involuntary disorders of movements. Their prevalence, severity and distribution in chronic schiozphrenics with and without treatment with neuroleptics. Arch Gen Psychiatry 1982; 39: 452–461.

Pall HS, Williams, AC, Blake DR, Lunec J. Evidence of enhanced lipid peroxidation in cerebrospinal fluid of patients taking phenothiazines. Lancet 1987; ii: 596–599.

Peet M, Laugharne J, Rangarajan N, Reynolds GP. Tardive dyskinesia, lipid peroxidation, and sustained amelioration with vitamin E treatment. Int Clin Psychopharmacol 1993; 8: 151–153.

Richardson MA, Pass R, Craig TJ, Vickers E. Factors influencing the prevalence and severity of tardive dyskinesia. Psychopharmacol Bull 1984; 20: 33–38.

Rosengren A, Wilhelmsen L, Eriksson E, Risberg B, Wedel H. Lipoprotein (a) and coronary heart disease: a prospective case-control study in a general population sample of middle-aged men. Br Med J 1990; 301: 1248–1251.

Saltz BL, Woerner MG, Kane JM et al. Prospective study of tardive dyskinesia in the elderly. JAMA 1991; 266: 2402–2406.

Simpson GM, Angus JWS. Drug-induced extrapyramidal disorder – a rating scale for extrapyramidal side effects. Acta Psychiatr Scand Suppl 1970; 212: 20–27.

Smith JM, Baldessarini RJ. Changes in prevalence, severity, and recovery in tardive dyskinesia with age. Arch Gen Psychiatry 1980; 37: 1368–1373.

Vaddadi KS. Essential fatty acids and alpha-tocopherol supplementation in tardive dyskinesia. In: Packer L, Prilipko L, Christen Y, eds. Free radicals in the brain: aging, neurological and mental disorders. Berlin: Springer-Verlag, 1992: 74–90.

Vaddadi KS, Gilleard CJ, Mindham RHS, Butler RA. A controlled trial of prostaglandin E1 precursor in chronic neuroleptic-resistant schizophrenic patients. Psychopharmacology 1986; 88: 362–367.

Vaddadi KS, Courtney P, Gilleard CJ, Manku MM, Horrobin DF. A double-blind trial of essential fatty acid supplementation in patients with tardive dyskinesia. Psychiatry Res 1989; 27: 313–323.

Van Doormaal JJ, Idema IG, Muskiet FAJ, Martini IA, Dorenbos H. Effects of short-term high dose intake of evening primrose oil on plasma and cellular fatty acid compositions, α-tocopherol levels and erythropoiesis in normal and type I (insulin-dependent) diabetic men. Diabetologia 1988; 31: 576–584.

Waddington JL. Schizophrenia, affective psychoses, and other disorders treated with neuroleptic drugs: the enigma of tardive dyskinesia, its neurological determinants, and the conflicts of paradigms. In: Smythies JR, Bradley RJ, eds. International review of neurobiology, Vol. 31. San Diego: American Press, 1989: 297–353.

Welin L, Svärdsudd K, Ander-Peciva S et al. Prospective study on social influences on mortality: the study of men born in 1913 and 1923. Lancet 1985; i: 915–918.

Wolkin A, Jordan B, Peselow E, Rubenstein M, Petrosen J. Essential fatty acid supplementation in tardive dyskinesia. Am J Psychiatry 1986; 143: 912–914.

Essential Fatty Acids and Movement Disorders

28

Krishna S. Vaddadi

INTRODUCTION

There is a considerable overlap in the clinical presentation of some of the neurological and psychiatric disorders. For example, abnormal involuntary movements were reported among schizophrenic patients, before the era of neuroleptics (Farran-Ridge, 1926), while depression and psychoses are known to occur in both Huntington's disease and Parkinson's disease. It is, therefore, plausible that treatment of one aspect of clinical presentation of a disorder might give clues to the causation of another condition in the same population. Reductions in abnormal involuntary movements were noted during experimental treatment of schizophrenia with essential fatty acids (EFAs) (Vaddadi, 1984).

NEURONAL MEMBRANES AND ESSENTIAL FATTY ACIDS

Neuronal membranes are largely composed of phospholipids which are rich in EFAs, including dihomo-γ-linolenic acid (DGLA) and arachidonic acid (AA). These phospholipids provide the membranes with suitable fluidity and permeability properties (Porcellati, 1983; Farooqui and Horrocks, 1985).

The phospholipids are arranged in two layers and are penetrated by receptors, enzymes, and ion channels, which differentially protrude through the membrane or may be localized predominantly on the intracellular or extracellular membrane surface (Farooqui and Horrocks, 1991).

The neural membranes are highly interactive and dynamic and therefore the interaction of a ligand with its receptor may markedly affect neural membrane phospholipid metabolism (Farooqui and Horrocks, 1991). The biochemical actions of membrane associated proteins, such as receptors, ion channels and enzymes, can be modulated by the lipid composition of the membrane in which they are embedded (Horrobin and Manku, 1990).

EFAs must be taken in the diet, as the body cannot synthesize them. They constitute 20% of the solid matter in the brain (Horrobin, 1982). There are two types of EFAs, the n-6 series derived from linoleic acid (18:2n-6) and n-3 series derived from α-linolenic acid (18:3n-3). A variety of short-lived derivatives, such as eicosanoids, prostaglandins (PGs) and leukotrienes are formed from their metabolism. PGs modulate nerve conduction, neurotransmitter release and postsynaptic transmitter actions (Horrobin, 1982).

In relation to dopamine, which is involved in movement disorders (Parkinson's disease) and psychoses the interaction between dopamine and PGs is interesting. PGs of the E type and dopamine exert a physiological antagonism in the regulation of cyclic adenosine monophosphate (cAMP), PGE_1 increasing it and dopamine lowering it (Myers et al., 1978). Thus a deficit of PGE_1 will produce an apparent overactivity of the dopaminergic system whilst an excess of PGE_1 will result in reduced activity of the same system. PGEs are metabolic products of EFAs; therefore, the availability of EFAs (n-6 and n-3 series) can influence dopamine metabolism, in part by the formation of PGs and other metabolic products. The interaction between dopamine and eicosapentaenoic acid (EPA) has been demonstrated by Davidson et al. (1988) in animal studies in which both linoleic and α-linolenic acid (n-6 and n-3 series) fatty acids are essential for normal dopaminergic function of the cat caudate nucleus. Application of dopamine causes release of large amounts of AA (an n-6 series EFA) in Chinese hamster ovary cells transfected with both D_1 and D_2 receptors (Piomelli et al., 1991). AA and its metabolites have a major role to play in neuronal signal transduction (Shimuzu and Wolfe, 1990).

In presynaptic terminals, following depolarization there is intracellular calcium increase which triggers dopamine release and may, at the same time, enable the D_2 autoreceptors to release AA and its metabolites (Piomelli et al., 1991). These, in turn, are involved in the autoinhibitory actions of dopamine, by regulating K^+ and Ca^{2+} channel activities or protein phosphorylation.

It is therefore clear that EFAs, the components of neural membrane and their metabolites (e.g., PGs) may significantly influence dopamine receptor function in the striatum and elsewhere in the brain. This could then have a significant influence in abnormal involuntary movement disorder pathophysiology and its treatment.

ESSENTIAL FATTY ACIDS IN TARDIVE DYSKINESIA

Tardive dyskinesia (TD) is relatively common among psychiatric patients who have been exposed to neuroleptic medication (e.g., haloperidol, fluphenazine decanoate) for long periods, and may be defined as a syndrome of abnormal involuntary movements, usually of a choreoathetoid type and sometimes stereotyped, which principally affect the mouth and facial musculature, and sometimes the extremities and trunk (Jeste and Caliguiri, 1993).

Horrobin (1979) first suggested that a deficiency of PGE_1 may play an important role in the aetiology of schizophrenia. Attempts had been made to increase PGE_1 synthesis to alleviate symptoms of schizophrenia by giving a PGE_1 synthesis stimulator (penicillin), and or PGE_1 precursors, namely γ-linolenic acid (Vaddadi, 1979, 1984). Kaiya (1984) gave PGE_1 intravenously to alleviate symptoms of chronic schizophrenia. It was during these early open clinical studies that a reduction was observed in the intensity of abnormal involuntary movements in neuroleptic-treated schizophrenic patients (Vaddadi, 1984). Kaiya (1984) also reported a reduction in the extrapyramidal symptoms in schizophrenic patients who were infused with PGE_1. This led us to set up an animal model study of TD.

Animal studies

We studied the effect of evening primrose oil (linoleic acid 72%, and γ-linolenic acid 9%) on perioral movements induced by 2-(N, N-dipropyl)amino-5,6-dihydroxytetralin (tetralin) in guinea pigs. The treatment with EFAs abolished tongue protrusion completely; the reductions in grimacing, munching, and biting behaviour were small, but statistically significant. We concluded that EFAs, by increasing brain PG production, which in turn may reduce the dopaminergic function or alter GABA-ergic or serotonergic function, can reduce tetralin-induced perioral movements (Nohria and Vaddadi, 1982).

Costall et al. (1984) studied the antidyskinetic action of synthetic DGLA in the rodent model of dyskinesias, induced by tetralin and dopamine. DGLA is the precursor of PGE_1. They gave DGLA intraperitoneally or directly injected into the striatum (guinea pig model), and also orally. They were able to demonstrate that the DGLA was able to reduce dyskinesias or to abolish them completely. This effect was also seen in 10–14 days when the animals' diet was supplemented with DGLA. DGLA did not modify other behavioural paradigms of striatal dopamine dysfunction. Aspirin, a cyclooxygenase inhibitor, was able to block the action of DGLA. The authors suggested that DGLA, by becoming incorporated into lipid membranes and being converted to PGs, exerted an antidyskinetic effect.

Human studies

These successful animal experiments prompted us to study the therapeutic potential of orally administered fatty acids supplements in psychiatric patients exhibiting abnormal involuntary movements (Vaddadi et al., 1989). We used Efamol™ capsules containing linoleic acid 360 mg, γ-linolenic acid (45 mg), and vitamin E 10 IU as an antioxidant. This was a double-blind, placebo-controlled trial, with a crossover design, with each active and placebo phase lasting for 16 weeks. At the end of 16 weeks on each arm (active and placebo) there was an open phase of 4 weeks in which all patients were switched to receive 4-week active treatment with Efamol. In addition, they were also given Efavit™ tablets, containing ascorbic acid 125 mg, pyridoxine hydrochloride 25 mg, nicotinic acid 7.5 mg and zinc sulphate 4.4 mg. These micronutrients are known co-factors in the metabolism of EFAs to PGs.

We found that all patients had values of red blood cells (RBC) membrane cis-linoleic acid (n-6 series) below those of normal controls; patients who had severe dyskinesia as assessed by the AIMS score (Guy, 1976), had the lowest values of n-3 and n-6 series EFAs when compared either with psychiatric control patients without TD or with normal controls (Table 28.1). Since 81.3% of all these patients had schizophrenia, the results suggest a close association between schizophrenia, TD and EFA levels. Supplementation with EFA alone did not lessen the severity of dyskinesia, but the addition of micronutrients in the final open phase of the trial produced clinically significant improvement in movement disorder and in Weschler memory scale scores.

Inadequate dosage of EFAs, inadequate length of the trial, chronicity of the patient's illness, irreversibility of TD, and the lack of supplementation with α-linolenic acid and its metabolites, such as EPA, docosahexaenoic

Table 28.1. Levels of essential fatty acids in n-3 and n-6 series phospholipids of red blood cell membranes in mild, moderate and severe tardive dyskinesia compared with psychiatric controls and healthy controls; means ± SD. Data from Vaddadi et al. (1989).

Group	n	Age (years)	Essential fatty acid series n-3	Essential fatty acid series n-6
Tardive dyskinesia				
Mild	12	50.9	8.37 ± 4.48[a*]	14.50 ± 7.28[a**]
Moderate	11	52.4	7.37 ± 5.02[a*]	14.03 ± 8.19[a**]
Severe	14	50.3	4.41 ± 4.39[a**,b*,c*]	9.12 ± 7.14[a**,b**]
Psychiatric controls	17	43.1	7.72 ± 4.62[a*]	16.00 ± 7.28[a*]
Normal controls	20	52.3	11.17 ± 1.74	22.00 ± 2.42

Severity of was defined by the AIMS score: mild <10; moderate 10–12; severe >12. In comparison with the corresponding value for normal controls, $p <$: [a*]0.05; [a**]0.01. In comparison with the corresponding value for psychiatric controls, $p <$: [b*]0.05; [b**]0.01. In comparison with the corresponding value for mild TD, $p <$: [c*]0.05.

acid (DHA) (n-3 series EFAs), may well have contributed to nonsignificant therapeutic outcome in the blind phase of the trial. Peet et al. (1995) and Glen et al. (1994) reported depleted n-3 and n-6 series essential fatty acids in the RBC membranes of patients suffering from schizophrenia. There is evidence to suggest that RBC membrane fatty acid levels reflect those in the brain (Carlson et al., 1986; Connor et al., 1993).

Magnetic resonance spectroscopy studies have shown evidence of increased breakdown of membrane phospholipids in the prefrontal cortex of drug-naïve schizophrenics (Pettegrew et al., 1992). Increased activity of phospholipase A_2 enzymes, involved in splitting AA and DHA from neuronal membrane phospholipids has been shown in medication-free schizophrenics compared to healthy control subjects (Gattaz et al., 1987, 1990).

Peet et al. (1995) demonstrated, in a group of 23 drug-stable chronic schizophrenic patients, significant reductions in linoleic acid, AA, EPA (20:5n-3) and DHA compared to healthy controls in RBC membranes. These observations provide further evidence for abnormal membrane phospholipid metabolism in schizophrenia.

Mellor et al. (1995) treated a group of 20 chronic schizophrenic patients with 10 g/day of MAX-EPA™ (which contains n-3 series EFAs), for a period of 6 weeks. They were able to show a significant reduction in the patients' AIMS scores (Guy, 1976) and also noticed a significant reduction in their mental symptoms as assessed by positive and negative syndrome scale (PANSS) scores (Table 28.2).

However, studies of this nature, involving abnormal movements as symptoms, need to be conducted longer term; a period of at least 1–2 years is required to see the stability of perceived improvement, as it is well known that TD ratings tend to fluctuate.

There are no larger controlled, long-term trials of n-6 or n-3 fatty acids, with or without antioxidants, in TD patients. Preliminary findings are, however, encouraging.

A prevalence study of abnormal involuntary movements in the general male population from Sweden has been reported by Nilsson et al. (1996). This is an interesting large-scale study. A cohort of men born in 1933 was selected for the dyskinesia study. The men were assessed in 1963 and then followed up regularly. In 1992, a follow-up investigation was conducted on 602 men (68% of the original sample). Videotaped assessments were made of their abnormal involuntary movements and plasma fatty acid levels. Abnormal movements were assessed on the AIMS scale. This study clearly demonstrated a highly significant lowered plasma AA acid levels in men exhibiting dyskinesia compared to those men who did not exhibit any dyskinesia. Dyskinetic men had significantly elevated levels of palmitic and oleic acid levels in the cholesterol ester and phospholipid fractions and DGLA levels were elevated in the triglyceride fraction. These abnormalities were present in men who have never been exposed to neuroleptics or had any psychiatric disorder. Dyskinesia was also associated with several abnormalities in EFA levels in plasma, but the most consistent finding was of low AA levels in phospholipids, triglycerides and cholesterol. It was suggested that the impaired conversion of linoleic acid to AA may be involved in the causation of these dyskinesias.

Table 28.2. Changes in abnormal movements in total body and in various body regions, related to the administration, withdrawal, and readministration of Efamol. Rockland rating scale scores in a single subject.

Date	Treatment and treatment duration	Total body	Orofacial	Neck and trunk	Upper extremity	Lower extremity
24-Aug 95	Pre-treatment (baseline)	3	26	12	13	9
03-Apr 97	Following 6 months double-blind; 2 months on 8 caps/day and 12 months on 16 caps/day	3	20	9	10	9
24-Jul 97	Had been on no treatment for 115 days; did not start Efamol Marine until 14 Aug 97	3	23	12	14	13
28-Jan 98	Following Efamol Marine 8 caps/day for 174 days	3	19	9	10	9

VULNERABILITY FACTOR IN TD, AND EFAs

Neuroleptics are often blamed for the development of TD. However, spontaneous involuntary movements have been reported in schizophrenics who have never been exposed to neuroleptics (Owens-Cunningham et al., 1982). There is an argument, therefore, that abnormal movements seen clinically may well be an integral part of the schizophrenic disease process. Cassady et al. (1992) have suggested that chronic neuroleptic blockade may be the first step in the pathogenesis of TD, followed by some other, as yet unidentified, process. The prevalence rates in TD vary between patients who have not been exposed to neuroleptics and those who have been treated with neuroleptics, and within the latter group the incidence varies between 5% and 20% (Kane and Smith, 1982). Therefore, it must be noted that not all individuals who have been treated with neuroleptics develop TD. Little is known about the processes that confer vulnerability to the emergence of TD in any given population exposed to neuroleptics. Waddington et al. (1997) has recently drawn attention to the complexity of seeking a simple unitary vulnerability factor for TD.

It is difficult to distinguish clinically those patients who are likely to develop TD when given neuroleptics over a prolonged period. There are, however, several clinical indicators that suggest caution should be exercised when prescribing neuroleptics. These patient-related factors, such as older age, female sex, organic cerebral diseases, neurodevelopmental abnormalities, affective disorders and diabetes, have all been considered as risk factors for the development of TD. A few of these putative factors will be individually discussed in relation to EFA metabolism.

Ageing

Increasing age is one of the most consistently identified risk factors for the development of TD (Saltz et al., 1997). Other risk factors, such as cerebrovascular disease and diabetes, are more common in the elderly. The ability of animals to desaturate linoleic acid declines with age (Brenner, 1971). Levels of PGE_1, formed from the 6-desaturated LA derivatives, and DGLA, decline with age in human skin (Kassis and Sondergaard, 1983). Nilsson et al. (1996), in a general population study of 59 year-old men, showed a consistent pattern of low AA levels in all plasma fractions in subjects of this age.

It is therefore likely that reduced activity of Δ-6 desaturase with ageing would significantly reduce the metabolism of n-6 and n-3 series EFAs to their respective metabolites which are particularly important in the brain (Horrobin, 1990). Nutritional deficiencies in the elderly could also contribute to this deficiency. Supplementation with EFAs (γ-linolenic acid [GLA], EPA, DHA) would therefore help to overcome this 6-desaturase step and provide neuronal cells with necessary EFAs in the desaturated form for normal cellular functioning.

Diabetes

Studies have shown a greater prevalence of TD among neuroleptic-treated diabetic patients than in a nondiabetic control group (Mukherjee et al., 1986; Ganzini et al., 1991). Mukherjee and Mahadik (1997) proposed that insulin resistance or NIDDM, or both, can increase the risk of TD, by impairing the capacity of the antioxidant defence system to cope with the increased oxidative stress that can result from the schizophrenic disease process and/or from neuroleptic treatment.

There are reports indicating reduced concentrations of DGLA and AA in spite of normal or elevated linoleic acid levels in NIDDM (Ewald et al., 1982; van Doormaal et al., 1988). This is likely to be due to decreased activity of Δ-6-desaturase and Δ-5-desaturase enzymes. These low DGLA and AA concentrations may be corrected by giving γ-linolenic acid supplementation. Diabetic neuropathy can be effectively treated by γ-linolenic acid supplementation (Horrobin, 1997a).

Impaired metabolism of EFAs could seriously affect normal cellular functioning and produce deficiency of long chain fatty acids, including AA. This could secondarily contribute to the development of TD in diabetic patients treated with neuroleptics.

Affective disorders

Mood disorders are now established as a risk factor for the development of TD (Gordos and Cole, 1997). In a study by Cole et al. (1992), unipolar depressed patients showed a vulnerability to TD comparable to that for bipolar patients; both sets of patients developed TD after significantly shorter neuroleptic exposures than did schizophrenic patients or schizoaffective disorder patients.

Lithium carbonate used in the treatment of mood disorders has been shown in a study by Cole et al. (1992) to be associated with a weak trend towards increased risk of dyskinesia. Lithium at concentrations between 0.2 mmol/l and 2 mmol/l blocks the mobilization of DGLA from cells (Horrobin and Manku, 1980). Blocking of DGLA release would lead to decreased formation of PGE_1 production. Platelet PGE_1 production is decreased in depressed patients compared to normal and manic patients (Abdulla and Hamadah, 1975). PGE_1 increases the behavioural effects of dopamine blockade (Schwartz et al., 1972) Therefore any event leading to reduced PGE_1 activity would increase the risk of development of TD. Decreased levels of α-linolenic acid (n-3 series) and EPA have been reported in serum cholesterol esters from patients with major depression compared with those with minor depression and healthy controls (Maes et al., 1996). Peet and Edwards (1997) have reported depleted total n-3 and DHA in erythrocyte membrane phospholipids from drug-free patients.

There is also an association between diabetes and depression (Gavard et al., 1993). As noted earlier, there is good evidence that there is impaired metabolism of EFAs in patients with diabetes. In depression, there are deficits particularly in n-3 EFAs. In diabetes there is evidence that insulin-binding and post-receptor events are enhanced by the availability of n-6 EFAs, especially DGLA. This effect is in part due to EFAs and in part due to their conversion to PGs (Horrobin, 1988, 1990). It is therefore not surprising to find an association between diabetes, depression and TD.

Reduced levels of both n-6 and n-3 series EFAs and reduced PGE_1 formation are likely to favour the development of dyskinesia in patients with major mood disorders who also suffer from diabetes. There are theoretical reasons to believe that treating these patients with lithium could precipitate or make their existing TD worse, though this needs to be tested.

Heavy alcohol consumption

Alcohol abuse is not uncommon in patients with mental illness. Dual disability patients who frequently abuse alcohol, illicit drugs (amphetamines) and suffer from schizophrenia or bipolar disorders are frequently seen in psychiatric clinics. Alcohol abuse has been shown to be an independent risk factor for the development of TD (Dixon et al., 1992).

High levels of alcohol affect EFA metabolism by inhibiting Δ-6 desaturase, thus reducing the formation of 6-desaturated EFAs which are vital for neural function (Horrobin, 1987). Supplementation of diet with γ-linolenic acid, bypassing the 6-desaturase step in metabolism of EFAs, improves brain functions in alcoholics (Glen et al., 1990). Alcohol, by interfering with EFA metabolism, could therefore accelerate the development of TD in neuroleptic-treated dual disability patients (e.g., mood disorder with alcohol dependence).

NEURODEVELOPMENT AND TD

Lipids contribute the major portion of the dry matter in the brain, and practically all brain lipids have structural functions in cellular and subcellular membrane structure and in myelin formation (Koletzko, 1992). The brain growth spurt phase between the 25th week of gestation and the first months after birth, is characterized by rapid multiplication of neuronal cells, their dendritic arborization with the development of synaptosomal contacts between neurones, and the myelination process. The availability of long-chain unsaturated fatty acids (EFAs) is of crucial importance for the proper functional development of the brain during this period.

In schizophrenic patients there are several studies suggesting abnormalities of membrane phospholipid metabolism (Pettegrew et al., 1993). *In vivo* brain imaging studies have shown abnormalities in cerebral structures, such as reductions in brain volume, increases in lateral ventricles and reductions in grey matter with increases in white matter (Lawrie et al., 1998).

Schizophrenic patients with negative symptoms of schizophrenia tend to develop orofacial dyskinesia at an earlier age (Liddle et al., 1993). In the schizophrenia literature, cognitive dysfunction, brain abnormalities on CT scan, and negative symptoms, show robust associations with the emergence of abnormal involuntary movements (Waddington, 1987). Type II schizophrenia with negative symptoms, is considered to be due to structural brain changes (Crow, 1980; Davis et al., 1992).

Whether these changes are neurodevelopmental, or whether they begin after the onset of schizophrenia is unclear. However, these structural abnormalities could be conceived as related to insufficient nutritional supply and/or to impaired incorporation of EFAs during foetal growth and during brain maturation, making the brain more vulnerable to the development of TD when exposed to neuroleptics in later life.

Clozapine and essential fatty acids

Clozapine, an atypical antipsychotic agent used in the treatment of schizophrenia, has been shown to have an antidyskinetic effect in patients with TD (Lieberman et al., 1991). The pharmacological actions of clozapine are similar to those of PGE_1 (Horrobin, 1978).

Clozapine has recently been shown to elevate red cell membrane AA and DHA, so promoting normal lipid composition (Horrobin, 1997b). The antidyskinetic action of clozapine might well be mediated through EFAs and PGs.

Overview

The evidence presented above suggests that in diabetes, affective disorders, alcoholism, schizophrenia and spontaneous TDs, there are underlying complex factors of impaired supply or incorporation or metabolism of EFAs of both the linoleic (n-6) and α-linolenic (n-3) series. The abnormalities could occur in different ways at various stages of metabolism affecting different enzymes (e.g., Δ-6 desaturase, Δ-5 desaturase). These could be both genetically and environmentally determined.

Antioxidant defence systems are also important to protect highly unsaturated EFAs and to prevent neuronal oxidative damage. Alpha-tocopherol supplementation as an antioxidant has been shown to be effective in amelioration of TD (Peet et al., 1993).

Therefore, supplementation with both n-6 and n-3 series EFAs, along with antioxidants, might be a useful therapeutic strategy in the treatment of dyskinesias.

ESSENTIAL FATTY ACIDS IN THE TREATMENT OF HUNTINGTON'S DISEASE

Lipid abnormalities have been described in a number of inherited neurological disorders such as Refsum disease and Fabry disease. However, little has been written about EFAs and neurodegenerative disorders. Dyck et al. (1981) reported greater than 50% reduction in AA (22:4n-6) and DHA (22:6n-3), of phosphatidylcholine and cholesterol ester, and a 20% increase in oleic acid (18:1n-9), compared to controls, in serum and erythrocyte fractions of two patients with multisystem neuronal degeneration and adrenocortical deficiency, exhibiting gait disturbance. In these patients, the levels of linoleic acid (18:2n-6) were normal, indicating a normal intake and suggesting a metabolic defect.

Similarly, research on patients with multiple sclerosis, a condition which can present with tremor and ataxia, has found lowered levels of n-3 and n-6 series EFAs in erythrocyte membranes and plasma (Cunnane et al., 1989). In a study by Sakai et al. (1991) which included some Huntington's disease (HD) patients there were significantly lowered DHA levels compared to controls. A recent ^{31}P magnetic resonance spectroscopy study in patients with HD showed decreased phosphomonoesters and phosphodiesters in the prefrontal region compared to normal individuals and patients with schizophrenia (Williamson et al., 1997).

Use of EFAs in Huntington's disease

Huntington's disease is an autosomal dominant neuropsychiatric disorder for which there is no cure. Some symptomatic relief may be obtained with dopamine blocking agents. The disease is characterized by choreiform movements, cognitive impairment and psychiatric manifestations (Penney and Young, 1993). The gene for HD has been identified, but the mechanism by which it causes neurodegeneration is not known (Ambrose et al., 1994). I have treated two HD patients with different severities of illness with large doses of EFAs in the form of Efamol™ and Efamol-Marine™ capsules (respectively providing either oil alone, containing only n-6 EFAs, or a mixture of evening primrose oil and fish oil, containing both n-6 and n-3 EFAs).

Case 1

The first patient, a Caucasian woman, was born in 1912; she had 12 children and several grandchildren. She was referred to our movement disorders clinic and was assessed by myself and the clinic neurologist. The history was obtained from her daughter and nursing home notes. She had unsteady gait and had suffered several falls over a period of at least 13 years. In 1991, she was assessed by a geriatrician who noted short-term memory deficits, athetoid movements, and NIDDM. In 1992, she was diagnosed as having HD and treatment was commenced with haloperidol 0.5 mg/day, which she took until December 1993. Her chorea, dysarthria and depression became worse and she was suicidal. She was seen in our clinic in April 1994. It was unclear from the history whether she took the haloperidol continuously. According to her daughter, she did take it, but continued to have abnormal movements and speech impairment. She was also receiving clonazepam 0.5 mg twice daily, dothiepin 50 mg daily and temazepam 10 mg nocte.

Her DNA test for HD was positive. The CAG repeats observed were 16 and 41 for two alleles. She was wheelchair-bound, frail, with severe choreiform movements of the trunk, upper limbs, and neck, and showed marked dysarthria. She was unable even to sit on the wheelchair because of these movements. A CT scan of the brain was not ordered as it was not considered clinically essential due to her poor physical state and anaesthetic risk.

In addition to haloperidol 0.5 mg bid, she was given Efamol (γ-linolenic acid, 45 mg per capsule), eight capsules daily. She was reassessed in September 1994. Her daughter reported noticeable improvement in her memory and reductions in her abnormal movements after about 8 weeks. When I examined her, there was marked reduction in her abnormal involuntary movements, with some improvement in speech, memory and general interaction. This improvement was confirmed by the nursing home staff and by her two daughters who visited her regularly. The patient herself noticed a marked improvement in her symptoms. She also gained significant weight. She was videotaped at the beginning of treatment with EFAs and at regular intervals. These tapes were blindly rated by a neurologist, who similarly noticed a significant reduction in her chorea. There was no dystonia at any stage. This clinical improvement was maintained until her death 172 weeks later (August 1997) resulting from a chest infection.

This case history highlights that when, haloperidol alone was ineffective, addition of γ-linolenic acid made a significant difference to her clinical state and improved her quality of life.

Case 2

The second patient, a 61-year-old, married male, was a quantity surveyor who ran a successful family business with his wife and other business partners. About 8 years previously his planning skills gradually started to deteriorate, as did his general work, and he had to leave the business. He subsequently worked for a wholesale nursery for 2 years. He then noticed abnormal involuntary movements in upper limbs, and repeatedly dropped objects and broke cups and glasses. He also cut himself with the razor while shaving, due to lack of coordination. His wife noted that he showed abnormal tongue movements. He developed mood swings and began to get irritable at home. He was seen by a neurologist and the possibility of HD was raised. Finally, in May 1994, his DNA test for HD was done and it proved positive.

He was seen in our clinic in August 1995, as we were doing a pilot clinical trial with EFAs. His history revealed that he had been adopted at the age of 5 years, after his biological mother, who had suffered from HD, had died. His maternal aunt had died in a psychiatric hospital at 50 years of age, and his maternal grandfather had died at 45 years of age; two uncles had died at ages of 50 and 47 years. This history was confirmed by his wife. The couple have three grown up children who have refused genetic testing. His clinical examination, done in August 1995, showed that he had abnormal involuntary movements in the orofacial region, neck, trunk and upper limb, and minimal abnormal movements in his lower limbs. His movements were videotaped and rated on the Rockland rating scale (Simpson et al., 1979). Clinical ratings of abnormal movements were repeated at 3 months and 6 months. He was given Efamol (γ-linolenic acid 45 mg), eight capsules daily. At the end of the double-blind phase of the clinical trial (he was in the active treatment group) he was noted to have made a significant improvement in his abnormal involuntary movements, which were less intense in the orofacial region and in the upper extremities, while neck and toe movements were not noticeable. He reported subjective improvement and this was confirmed by his wife. After the double-blind phase of the trial, he was continued on Efamol, the dose between April 1996 and

April 1997 being increased to eight capsules twice daily. He had reported no changes in his mood. He was able to do gardening work, dropped fewer objects, his falls became less frequent, and he was able to shave without cutting himself. At no stage in his treatment had he been given any dopamine receptor blocking agents (e.g., haloperidol or thioridazine). He had been taking Efamol (16 capsules/day) for 12 months, so he decided to stop taking it. Some 8 weeks after he ceased taking Efamol, he and his wife noticed that his movements were becoming clumsier, and by about the 12th week, he noticed an overall deterioration, including mood swings, and an increase in his abnormal limb movements. He was physically tired, knocked objects over, and stopped going out. He also reported that his skin looked unhealthy and dry. He lost 7 lb of weight during this period. He was then recommenced on Efamol-Marine 1100 mg capsules, containing both n-3 and n-6 series EFAs, namely GLA, EPA and DHA. He was given eight capsules daily in August 1997 and was videotaped at each subsequent assessment. He was seen again some 5 months later, when he again reported significant clinical improvement in his abnormal movements and mood swings, as well as regaining his 7 lb of lost weight. He was able to do gardening, had no falls, and could shave without cutting himself. He did not drop or knock over objects. He even bought exercise equipment and was actively doing exercises without losing any weight. His abnormal movement scores on Rockland scale are shown in Table 28.1.

Discussion of the case reports

Both these cases clearly illustrate that the clinical improvements in abnormal movements, and body weight, and subjective well-being, are sustained over a very long period of time on EFA treatment: in Case 1, this was for 172 weeks and in Case 2, for 82 weeks, thus far. This is unlikely to be a placebo effect over such lengthy periods, when there were both subjective and objective improvements, with no other clinically relevant interventions.

Mechanisms of EFA effects in Hungtinton's disease

The mechanisms underlying a possible therapeutic role for EFAs in HD, and perhaps in other neurodegenerative disorders, are speculative, based on our current state of knowledge and clinical experience.

There is evidence that neuroleptic agents, such as haloperidol, that are often used to treat chorea, do not favourably influence the course of HD (Feigin et al., 1995a). As the disease progresses, total functional capacity tends to decline, chorea lessens and dystonia intensifies (Feigin et al., 1995b). However, in neither of the cases presented above was there dystonia, as the chorea became less intense, and both the subjective and objective functioning improved on supplementation with EFAs. The improvements were observed within 8 weeks of commencing treatment and maintained for a long time. Feigin et al. (1995b) found no correlation between the rapid progress of disease and certain clinical factors such as early age of onset, rapid decline in weight, or paternal transmission of HD However, patients who were depressed, declined more rapidly than nondepressed patients. Our female patient was depressed and suicidal and was taking antidepressant medication. Her body weight was also low. She showed weight gain and lessening of chorea without dystonia, with improvement of speech and cognition; the expected clinical deterioration stopped abruptly.

There are several processes that could contribute to clinical improvement in HD when EFA supplementation is given.

Action on a membrane defect

It has been suggested that HD could be an expression of a generalized membrane defect (Beverstock, 1984). EFAs are important constituents of neuronal membranes, being involved in both structure and functions of the membrane and exerting a wide range of actions at second messenger levels (Nunez, 1993). Neuronal cell loss in HD is considered to be due to an N-methyl-D-aspartate (NMDA) receptor-mediated excitotoxic mechanism (Albin and Tagle, 1995). In HD patients who died early in their illness, post-mortem brain examination has shown a loss of striatal NMDA receptors with relative sparing in the hippocampus (Young et al., 1988; Feigin et al., 1995a). Activation of NMDA-receptors by glutamate released from glutaminergic nerve terminals, stimulates postsynaptic NMDA receptors. Activation of the NMDA-receptor by glutamate stimulates phospholipase A_2 to release AA (Katsuki and Okuda, 1995). AA modulates glutamate release evoked by depolarizing stimuli (Katsuki and Okuda, 1995). It is suggested that reduced availability of AA, or impaired metabolism in the AA pathway of n-6 series EFAs could lead to impaired modulation of glutamate release by AA. This, in turn, would lead to excessive or inappropriate activation of NMDA-receptors and thus to an excess of Ca^{2+} entry into cells, which would then activate a variety of enzymes including proteases, causing cell death.

AA may have distinct and opposite actions within a narrow concentration range. These actions include induction of cell death, promotion of cell survival, and enhancement of neurite extension. The neurotrophic actions are exerted by AA itself, whereas the neurotoxic action is mediated by AA-generated free radicals (Katsuki and Okuda, 1995). Therefore, the availability of adequate antioxidant operating defence system is important and supplementation with EFAs should include antioxidants (e.g., α-lipoic acid or α-tocopherol).

Action on the effects of a genetic lesion

In HD, the genetic lesion is in the human IT 15 gene (Huntington's Disease Collaborative Research Group, 1993) and it encodes a 348 kd polypeptide (huntingtin). The N-terminal portion of huntingtin contains a polyglutamine repeat (Ambrose et al., 1994) encoded by a polymorphic stretch of CAG repeats. The HD gene is not brain-specific but is widely expressed (Huntington's Disease Collaborative Research Group, 1993).

CAG/polygln expansion is not specific to HD but has been found in seven other neurodegenerative diseases (Albin and Tagle, 1995). Within the brain, the huntingtin protein is found mainly in neuronal cell bodies, dendrites and nerve terminals. It is primarily a cytosolic protein, but has also been detected in the nucleus (Hoogeveen et al., 1993). This suggests that it may have a transcriptional function (Scherzinger et al., 1997).

The mechanisms by which an elongated polyglutamine (polygln) sequence causes neurodegeneration in HD are not known. However, some possibilities have been suggested (Scherzinger et al., 1997) and high doses of EFAs administered to HD sufferers might interfere in these processes, leading to a positive therapeutic outcome.

Abnormal protein–protein interaction. It has been proposed by many investigators that HD is caused by a toxic 'gain of function' which, in turn, is caused by abnormal protein–protein interactions related to the elongated polygln. Binding of a protein to the polygln region could either confer a new property on huntingtin or alter its normal interactions, causing selective cell death, either through the specific expression patterns of interacting protein or through the selective vulnerability of certain cells (Scherzinger et al., 1997).

This protein–protein interaction could be altered by the availability of highly unsaturated lipids (long-chain EFAs) in the vicinity of the proteins, preventing or reducing their interaction and thus preventing cell death. The modulation of membranes by lipids, which can be largely independent of genes, can have profound effects on the behaviour of membrane-associated proteins (Horrobin, 1995).

Huntingtin as a transcription factor sink. Polyglutamine stretches tend to aggregate together *via* strong hydrogen bonding according to Perutz et al. (1994) and Perutz (1996), who also speculate that excessive CAG repeats might cause huntingtin to act as a sink for transcription factors, that possess polyglutamine stretches and consequently disrupt neuronal function. However, it is conceivable that a highly unsaturated lipid environment, by changing fluidity of membranes might prevent this sink-like action of huntingtin. The sink effect might be counteracted by supplementing HD patients with high continuous doses of EFAs even before the development of any symptoms of HD.

Huntingtin impairment of EFA metabolism. Huntingtin protein might be preventing a regulatory process involved in EFAs metabolism. Providing EFAs might overcome this metabolic impairment.

Toxic intraneuronal precipitate. It has also been suggested that polyglutamine aggregation might simply result in an insoluble and ultimately toxic precipitate within neurones (Albin and Tagle, 1995). EFAs might prevent this intranuclear aggregation by changing the lipid matrix in which proteins aggregate.

Genetic expression of enzymes causing neurodegeneration. Polyunsaturated fatty acids have been shown to reduce the genetic expression of many enzymes (Waters et al., 1997). It is therefore possible that large doses of EFAs might repress the HD gene expression, at least partially, and reduce the neurodegenerative effects.

Adequacy of genetic lesion hypothesis. None of the hypotheses explains the region-specific pathology in HD. However, EFA involvement at various levels explains NMDA receptor-mediated excitotoxicity and also protein interactions that lead to neuronal cell death.

CONCLUSION

EFAs are important constituents of neuronal membranes and are involved in structural and functional activities. There is accumulating evidence that there are EFA metabolism abnormalities in patients with dyskinesias. These abnormalities do not appear to be due directly to neuroleptic medication but seem to be related to the underlying disease process itself, although medication may accelerate the process. Abnormal EFA metabolism may underlie the 'vulnerability factor' which determines who will develop TD. EFAs may have a role to play in other movement disorders, such as HD. Treatment with both n-6 and n-3 series EFAs in patients with TD and HD has been shown to be therapeutically beneficial, and this improvement can be maintained for a long time. Treatment with EFAs may also have a preventive role in HD and TD. Larger controlled clinical trials using EFAs as a treatment strategy are in progress.

REFERENCES

Abdulla YH, Hamadah K. Effect of ADP on PGE formation in blood platelets from patients with depression, mania and schizophrenia. Br J Psychiatry 1975; 127: 591–595.

Albin RL, Tagle DA. Genetics and molecular biology of Huntington's disease. Trends Neurol Sci 1995; 18: 11–14.

Ambrose CM, Duyao MP, Barnes G et al. Structure and expression of the Huntington's disease gene: evidence against simple inactivation due to an expanded CAG repeat. Somat Cell Mol Genet 1994; 20: 27–38.

Beverstock GC. The current state of research with peripheral tissues in Huntington's disease. Hum Genet 1984; 66: 115–131.

Brenner RR. The desaturation step in the animal biosynthesis of polyunsaturated fatty acids. Lipids 1971; 6: 567–575.

Carlson SE, Carver JD, House SG. High fat diets varying in ratios of polyunsaturated to saturated fatty acid and linoleic to linolenic acid: a comparison of rat neural and red cell membrane phospholipids. J Nutr 1986; 116: 718–725.

Cassady S, Thakar G, Moran M, Layne J, Tamminga C. Gabaergic involvement in persistent tardive dyskinesia – a late and persistent process? Biol Psychiatry 1992; 31: 159A.

Cole JO, Gordos, G, Bowling LA, Marby D, Haskell D, Moore P. Early dyskinesia-vulnerability. Psychopharmacology 1992; 107: 503–510.

Connor WE, Lin DS, Neuringer M. Is the docosahexaenoic acid (DHA) content of brain phospholipid? FASEB J 1993; 7: A152.

Costall BM, Kelly E, Naylor RJ. The antidyskinetic action of dihomo-γ-linolenic acid in rodent. Br J Pharmacol 1984; 83: 733–740.

Crow TJ. Molecular pathology of schizophrenia. More than one disease process? Br Med J 1980; 280: 66–68.

Cunnane SC, Ho SY, Bore-Duffy P, Ells KR, Horrobin DF. Essential fatty acid and lipid profiles in plasma and erythrocytes in patients with multiple sclerosis. Am J Clin Nutr 1989; 50: 801–806.

Davidson BC, Kurstjens NP, Patton J, Cantrill RC. Essential fatty acid deprivation reduces the activity of apomorphine at presynaptic dopamine receptors modulating [³H]-dopamine release from cat caudate slices. Eur J Pharmacol 1988; 149: 317–322.

Davis EJB, Borde M, Sharma LN. Tardive dyskinesia and type II schizophrenia. Br J Psychiatry 1992; 160: 253–256.

Dixon L, Weiden PJ, Hass G, Sweeny J, Frances AJ. Increased tardive dyskinesia in alcohol-abusing schizophrenic patients. Compr Psychiatry 1992; 33: 121–122.

Dyck I, Yao J, Knickbocker DE et al. Multisystem neuronal degeneration, hepatomegaly and adrenocortical deficiency associated with reduced tissue arachidonic acid. Neurology 1981; 31: 925–934.

Ewald U, Gustafsson IB, Tuvemo T, Vessby B. Fatty acid composition of serum lipids in diabetes. Uppsala J Med Sci 1982; 87: 111–117.

Farran-Ridge C. Some symptoms referable to the basal ganglia occurring in dementia praecox and epidemic encephalitis. J Ment Sci 1926; 72: 513–523.

Farooqui AA, Horrocks LA. Metabolic functional aspects of neural membrane phospholipids. In: Horrocks LA, Kanfer JN, Porcellati G, eds. Phospholipids in the nervous system. Vol II: Physiological role. New York: Raven Press, 1985; 341–348.

Farooqui AA, Horrocks LA. Excitatory amino acid receptors, neural membrane phospholipid metabolism and neurological disorders. Brain Res Rev 1991; 16: 171–191.

Feigin A, Kieburzt K, Shoulson I. Treatment of Huntington's disease and other choreic disorders. In: Kurlan R, ed. Treatment of movement disorders. Philadelphia: JB Lippincott Co. 1995a: 337–364.

Feigin A, Kieburtz K, Bordwell K et al. Functional decline in Huntington's disease. Mov Disord 1995b; 10: 211–214.

Ganzini L, Heintz RT, Hoffman WF, Casey DE. The prevalence of tardive dyskinesia in neuroleptic treated diabetics. A controlled study. Arch Gen Psychiatry 1991; 48: 259–263.

Gattaz WF, Köllisch M, Thuren T, Virtanen JA, Kinnunen PKJ. Increased plasma phospholipase-A$_2$ activity in schizophrenic patients: reduction after neuroleptic therapy. Biol Psychiatry 1987; 22: 421–426.

Gattaz WF, Hübner CK, Nevalainen TJ, Thuren T, Kinnunen PKJ. Increased serum phospholipase-A$_2$ activity in schizophrenia: a replication study. Biol Psychiatry 1990; 28: 495–501.

Gavard J, Lustman PJ, Clouse R. Prevalence of depression in adults with diabetes. Diabetes Care 1993; 16: 1167–1178.

Glen AIM, Glen EMT, MacDonell LEF, Skinner FK. Essential fatty acids and alcoholism. In: Horrobin DF, ed. Omega-6 essential fatty acids: pathophysiology and roles in clinical medicine. New York: Wiley-Liss, 1990: 321–332.

Glen AIM, Glen EMT, Horrobin DF et al. A red cell membrane abnormality in a subgroup of schizophrenic patients: evidence for two diseases. Schizophr Res 1994; 12: 53–61.

Gordos G, Cole JO. Tardive dyskinesia and affective disorder. In: Yassa R, Nair NVP, Jeste DV, eds. Neuroleptic-induced movement disorders. Cambridge: Cambridge University Press, 1997: 69–81.

Guy W. ECEDU assessment manual for psychopharmacology. Washington, DC: US Department of Health, Education and Welfare; US Government Printing Office 1976: 76–338.

Hoogeveen AT, Willemsen R, Meyer N et al. Characterisation and localisation of the Huntington's disease gene product. Hum Mol Genet 1993; 2: 2069–2073.

Horrobin DF. Mental illness. In: Horrobin DF, ed. Prostaglandins. Physiology, pharmacology and clinical signficance. Montreal: Eden Press, 1978: 246–253.

Horrobin DF. Schizophrenia: reconciliation of the dopamine, prostaglandin and opioid concepts and the role of the pineal. Lancet 1979; i: 529–531.

Horrobin DF. Prostaglandins, essential fatty acids and psychiatric disorders: a background review. In: Horrobin DF, ed. Clinical uses of essential fatty acids. Montreal: Eden Press, 1982: 167–174.

Horrobin DF. Essential fatty acids, prostaglandins and alcoholism: an overview. Alcoholism: Clin Exp Res 1987; 11: 2–9.

Horrobin DF. The roles of essential fatty acids in the development of diabetic neuropathy and other complications of diabetes mellitus. Prostagland Leukotr Essent Fatty Acids 1988; 31: 181–197.

Horrobin DF. Essential fatty acids and psychiatric disorders: a background review. In: Horrobin DF, ed. Omega-6 essential fatty acids. Pathophysiology and roles in clinical medicine. New York: Wiley-Liss, 1990: 305–320.

Horrobin DF. DNA-protein and membrane-lipid: competing paradigms in biomedical research. Med Hypotheses 1995; 44: 229–239.

Horrobin DF. Gamma-linolenic acid in the treatment of diabetic neuropathy. In: Bolton AJM, ed. Diabetic neuropathy. Carnforth: Marius Press, 1997a; 183–195.

Horrobin DF. Clozapine: elevation of membrane unsaturated lipid levels as a new mechanism of action. Biol Psychiatry 1997b; 42: 161S.

Horrobin DF, Manku MS. Possible role of prostaglandin E1 in affective disorders and in alcoholism. Br Med J 1980; 280: 1363–1366.

Horrobin DF, Manku MS. Clinical biochemistry of essential fatty acids. In: Horrobin DF, ed. Omega-6 essential fatty acids, pathophysiology and roles in clinical medicine. New York: Wiley-Liss, 1990: 21–53.

Huntington's Disease Collaborative Research Group. A novel gene containing a trinucleotide repeat that is expanded and unstable on Huntington's disease chromosomes. Cell 1993; 72: 971–983.

Jeste DV, Caligiuri MP. Tardive dyskinesia. Schizophr Bull 1993; 19: 303–315.

Kaiya H. Prostaglandin E1 treatment of schizophrenia. Biol Psychiatry 1984; 19: 457–462.

Kane JM, Smith JM. Tardive dyskinesia: prevalence and risk factors. 1959–1979. Arch Gen Psychiatry 1982: 39: 473–481.

Kassis V, Sondergaard J. PGE_1 in normal skin: methodological evaluation, topographical distribution and data. Related to sex and age. Arch Dermatol Res 1983: 275: 9–13.

Katsuki H, Okuda S. Arachidonic acid as a neurotoxic and neurotrophic substance. Prog Neurobiol 1995; 46: 607–636.

Koletzko B. Fats for brain. Eur J Clin Nutr 1992; 46 (Suppl 1): 551–562.

Lawrie SM, Abukmeil S Uheib. Brain abnormality in schizophrenia. Br J Psychiatry 1998; 172: 110–120.

Liddle P, Barnes TRE, Speller J, Kibel D. Negative symptoms as a risk factor for tardive dyskinesia in schizophrenia. Br J Psychiatry 1993; 163: 776–780.

Lieberman JA, Saltz BL, Johns CA, Pollack S, Borenstein M, Kane J. The effects of clozapine on tardive dyskinesia. Br J Psychiatry 1991; 158: 503–510.

Maes M, Smith R, Christophe A, Cosyns P, Desnyder R, Meltzer H. Fatty acid composition in major depression: decreased ω3 fractions in cholesteryl esters and increased C20:4ω6/C20:5ω3 ratio in cholesteryl esters and phospholipids. J Affective Disord 1996; 38: 35–46.

Mellor JE, Laugharne JDE, Peet M. Schizophrenic symptoms and dietary intake of n-3 fatty acids. Schizophr Res 1995; 18: 85–86.

Mukherjee S, Mahadik S. Diabetes mellitus and tardive dyskinesia in neuroleptic-induced movement disorders. In: Yassa R, Nair NVP, Jeste DV, eds. Cambridge: Cambridge University Press, 1997: 82–98.

Mukherjee S, Bilder RM, Sackeim HA. Tardive dyskinesia and glucose metabolism. Arch Gen Psychiatry 1986; 43: 192–193.

Myers PR, Blosser J, Shain W. Neurotransmitter modulation of prostaglandin E1-stimulated increases in cyclic AMP. II: characteristics of a cultured neuronal cell line treated with dibutryl cyclic AMP. Biochem Pharmacol 1978; 27: 1173–1177.

Nilsson A, Horrobin DF, Rosengren A, Waller L, Adlerberth A, Wilhelmsen L. Essential fatty acids and abnormal involuntary movements in the general male population: a study of men born in 1933. Prostagland Leukotr Essent Fatty Acids 1996; 55: 83–87.

Nohria V, Vaddadi KS. Tardive dyskinesia and essential fatty acids: an animal model study. In: Horrobin DF, ed. Clinical uses of essential fatty acids. Montreal: Eden Press, 1982: 199–204.

Nunez EA. Fatty acids and cell signalling. Prostagland Leukotr Essent Fatty Acids 1993; 48: 1–122.

Owens-Cunningham DG, Johnstone EG, Firth DC. Spontaneous involuntary disorders of movement. Their prevalence, severity and distribution in chronic schizophrenics with and without treatment with neuroleptics. Arch Gen Psychiatry 1982; 39: 452–461.

Peet M, Edwards RhW. Lipids, depression and physical diseases. Curr Opin Psychiatry 1997; 10: 477–480.

Peet M, Laugharne J, Rangarajan N, Reynolds GP. Tardive dyskinesia, lipid peroxidation, and sustained amelioration with vitamin E treatment. Int Clin Psychopharmacol 1993; 8: 151–153.

Peet M, Laugharne JDE, Rangarajan N, Horrobin DF, Reynolds G. Depleted red cell membrane essential fatty acids in drug treated schizophrenic patients. J Psychiatr Res 1995; 29: 227–232.

Penney JB, Young AB. Huntington's disease. In: Jankovic J, Eduardo T, eds. Parkinson's disease and movement disorders. 2nd edition. Williams and Wilkins: 1993.

Perutz MF. Glutamine repeats and inherited neurodegenerative diseases: molecular aspects. Curr Opin Struct Biol 1996; 6: 848–858.

Perutz MF, Johnston T, Suzuki M, Finch JT. Glutamine repeats as polar zippers; their possible role in neurodegenerative diseases. Proc Natl Acad Sci USA 1994; 91: 5355–5358.

Pettegrew JW, Keshavan MS, Panchalingam K et al. Alterations in brain high-energy phosphate and membrane phospholipid metabolism in first-episode drug-naïve schizophrenics. A pilot study of the dorsal prefrontal cortex by in vivo phosphorus-31 nuclear magnetic resonance spectroscopy. Arch Gen Psychiatry 1991; 48: 563–568.

Pettegrew JW, Keshavan MS, Minshew NJ. ^{31}P nuclear magnetic resonance spectroscopy: neurodevelopment and schizophrenia. Schizophr Bull 1993; 91: 35–53.

Piomelli D, Pilon C, Giros B, Sokoloff P, Martres M-P, Schwartz JC. Dopamine activation of the arachidonic acid cascade as a basis for D_1/D_2 receptor synergism. Nature 1991; 353: 164–167.

Porcellati G. Phospholipid metabolism in neural membranes. In: Sun GY, Bazan N, Wu JY, Porcellati G, Sun AY, eds. Neural membranes. New York: Humana Press, 1983: 3–35.

Sakai T, Antoku Y, Iwashika H, Goto I, Nagamatsu K, Shii H. Chorea-acanthocytosis: abnormal composition of covalently bound fatty acids of erythrocyte membrane proteins. Ann Neurol 1991; 29: 664–669.

Saltz B, Kane JM, Woerner MG, Liberman JA, Jose MA, Alvir PH. Ageing and tardive dyskinesia. In: Yassa R, Nair NVP, Jeste DV, eds. Neuroleptic-induced movement disorders. Cambridge: Cambridge University Press, 1997: 13–25.

Scherzinger E, Lurz R, Turmane M et al. Huntingtin-encoded polyglutamine expansions form amyloid-like protein aggregates *in vitro* and *in vivo*. Cell 1997; 90: 549–558.

Schwartz RD, Uretsky NJ, Bianchine JR. Prostaglandin inhibition of apomorphine-induced circling in mice. Pharmacol Biochem Behav 1972; 17: 1233.

Shimuzu T, Wolfe LS. Arachidonic acid casade and signal transduction. J Neurochem 1990; 55: 1–15.

Simpson GM, Lee JH, Zoubok B, Gordos G. A rating scale for tardive dyskinesia. Psychopharmacology 1979: 64: 171–179.

Vaddadi KS. Penicillin and essential fatty acid supplementation in schizophrenia. Prostagland Med 1979; 12: 77–80.

Vaddadi KS. Essential fatty acids and neuroleptic drug induced tardive dyskinesia – preliminary clinical observations. IRCS Med Sci 1984; 12: 678–679.

Vaddadi KS, Courtney P, Gilleard CJ, Manku MS, Horrobin DF. A double-blind trial of essential fatty acid supplementation in patients with tardive dyskinesia. Psychiatry Res 1989; 27: 313–323.

Van Doormaal JJ, Idema IG, Muskiet FAJ, Martini IA, Dorenbos H. Effects of short-term high dose intake of evening primrose oil on plasma and cellular fatty acid compositions, α-tocopherol levels and erythropoiesis in normal and type I (insulin-dependent) diabetic men. Dibetologia 1988; 31: 576–584.

Waddington JL. Tardive dyskinesia in schizophrenia and other disorders: associations with ageing, cognitive dysfunction and structural brain pathology in relation to neuroleptic exposure. Hum Psychopharmacol 1987; 2: 11–22.

Waddington JL, O'Callaghan E, Buckley P, Madigan C, Larkin C, Kinsella A. Vulnerability to tardive dyskinesia in schizophrenia: an exploration of individual patient factors. In: Yassa R, Nair NVP, Jeste DV, eds. Neuroleptic-induced movement disorders. Cambridge: Cambridge University Press, 1997: 56–65.

Waters KM, Miller WC, Ntambi JM. Localization of a polyunsaturated fatty acid response region in stearoyl-COA desaturase gene 1. Biochim Biophys Acta 1997; 1349: 33–42.

Williamson PC, Malla A, Stoessl AJ, Drost D, Stanley JA. Phosphorus 31 magnetic resonance spectroscopy in patients with Huntington's disease. Arch Gen Psychiatry 1997; 54: 186–187.

Young AB, Greenamyre JT, Hollingsworth Z et al. NMDA receptor losses in putamen from patients with Hungtinton's disease. Science 1988; 241: 981–983.

Part X

THE EVOLUTIONARY CONTEXT

A Speculative Overview: The Relationship Between Phospholipid Spectrum Disorders and Human Evolution

David F. Horrobin

INTRODUCTION

Schizophrenia is a disease with a distribution like no other. In all known populations it has a lifetime prevalence of somewhere between 0.5% and 1.5% when diagnosed according to WHO-standardized criteria (World Health Organization, 1979). Although the course of the disease varies considerably from population to population, the relative numbers affected are about the same in all races and all continents (World Health Organization, 1979). There is now no longer any serious doubt that the disease has a genetic, and therefore a biochemical, basis, although one which can be substantially modulated by environmental factors. This means that the genetic basis must have been present in the common ancestor of all races. Australian aboriginals separated from the rest of humankind between 60 000 and 80 000 years ago, and so the genetic basis must have been present prior to that. Information about rates of mutation, particularly in mitochondrial DNA, suggests that humans became human in relatively modern form some time between 100 000 and 200 000 years ago (Vigilant et al., 1991; Goldstein et al., 1995; Horai et al., 1995). This means that the major genetic bases of schizophrenia must have developed around that time.

Crow has argued that the origins of schizophrenia are closely related to the speciation event and the origins of language and of marked cerebral asymmetries (Crow, 1991, 1993, 1995,1996a,b). His view is that schizophrenia is in some way a consequence of the event that made us human. Inherent in the brain lateralization process is some event which goes wrong in schizophrenia and which precipitates the disease. This stimulating hypothesis has not received the critical attention it deserves.

However, I intend to go further than Crow, and to postulate that the events which introduced schizophrenia into the human line are not mere accidental bystanders. My position is that, far from being unfortunate consequences of the language and cerebral asymmetry-introducing events, the biochemical features of schizophrenia are what made us human. We are human, in my view, because some members of the human race are schizophrenic, and because the related phospholipid spectrum disorders are associated with some of the most characteristic features of human behaviour.

The hypothesis is not a vague concept. Humans are very similar to other primates and hominids, and the biochemical differences which distinguish brain metabolism in humans must be both important and limited in number. I postulate specific biochemical candidates for the changes in metabolism which led to the increase in size of the human brain, and for the events which converted that brain from a larger version of any other animal type of brain into the creative structure which is characteristic of humanity at its best. The hypothesis derives from our growing understanding of what determines, in modern humans, the size of the brain and the connectivity of its individual components. These modern biochemical facts will be linked to observations which include the growth in brain size over about 2–3 million years, the lack of creativity associated with a large brain *per se*, the sudden emergence of creativity, religion, war, art, and perhaps music, somewhere between 50 000 and 100 000 years ago, the agricultural revolution, and the emergence of strong city and then national states 5000–15 000 years ago, and the dramatic increase in the apparent severity and frequency of schizophrenia over the past 200 years. I will suggest that all these events are related to perhaps three to five changes in specific lipid biochemical steps and to the environmental factors which influence these steps. This may seem implausible to those who know little about lipids. However, lipids make up around 60% of the brain by weight and are the major determinants of the richness of its microconnections. The evolution of the human brain must have a biochemical basis which has been almost totally ignored in contemporary accounts which have concentrated near exclusively on anatomical and social explanations. Given the importance of lipid biochemistry in the brain, this seems a reasonable place to start.

Inevitably, when a hypothesis of this type is proposed, there are many gaps and many areas susceptible to fierce criticism. What I am attempting to do here is to sketch out an overall concept. However, the overall picture includes pieces of evidence from many different sources and it is the combined weight of the structure which must be considered. The proposal is, as far as I am aware, the only one currently available which makes specific biochemical proposals about a limited number of steps which might have made us human. At the least, it provides a clear framework within which specific questions may be raised and answered. At the most, it provides an answer to the issue of what made us human, and indicates that schizophrenia is not just a consequence but a cause of our development of humanity.

In an outline of this type, covering many fields, it is impossible to provide primary references for every statement, since that would lead to several hundred citations. Wherever appropriate, therefore, I have referenced authoritative reviews which will allow the reader to track down the primary sources if desired. I apologise in advance to those primary source authors who may feel that key references have been omitted.

CHANGES IN BRAIN SIZE DURING EVOLUTION

When expressed as a percentage of body weight, the human brain is not particularly large or unusual. The squirrel and the human, for example, both have brains which constitute around 2% by weight of the body (Crawford and Marsh, 1989; Crawford, 1992). Many small mammals have relatively large brains. What is unusual about the human brain is that we are the only largish mammal whose brain size has kept pace with our growth in body size. Our only close competitors are the marine mammals, and from them we can learn lessons to which we will return (Crawford and Marsh, 1989; Crawford, 1992).

The primates as a group have been able to maintain larger brain sizes in relation to body mass than any mammalian group other than the marine ones. But it was only around 2.0–2.5 million years ago that the ancestors of modern humans began unequivocally to outdistance other primates (Mithen, 1996; Noble and Davidson, 1996). At first, there was enormous variability in brain size, and it is not clear whether this represented variable characteristics within interbreeding lines or whether it indicates several different species (Mithen, 1996; Noble and Davidson, 1996). There was then a slow drift upward until around 0.5 million years ago when there was another increase in the rate of brain growth which soon culminated in brains as big as, or slightly larger, than modern brains (Mithen, 1996; Noble and Davidson, 1996). The brains in the Neanderthals, a side-branch of human evolution, were actually larger than modern human brains, and we now know that it is unlikely that Neanderthals were our ancestors (Trinkaus, 1994; Krings et al., 1997). No changes in brain size were associated with the explosive developments in culture, knowledge and social organisation over the past 100 000 years. These developments must therefore be related to changes in brain function, rather than brain size.

CHANGES IN BRAIN FUNCTION DURING EVOLUTION

One of the more surprising features of human evolution is that so little change in apparent function took place over 2 million years (Mithen, 1996). The first hand axes appeared with the first spurt in human brain size around 2–2.5 million years or about 100 000 or more generations ago. There was an improvement in design about 1.6 million years ago, but then for another million years or so hand axe design remained essentially similar from Southern Africa to Northern Europe, and from Western Europe to Eastern Asia. There are, of course, small regional differences, but they are limited and it is the uniformity which astonishes (Mithen, 1996).

Around half a million years ago, coinciding with the later spurt in brain growth, there was a modest improvement in hand axe design and then again apparently little change for around 400 000 years or more. There was use of wood but not bone, and there is little or no evidence of any complex artefacts, any religion, or any culture. Our brains may have been large but they were certainly not particularly creative (Mithen, 1996).

And then, certainly more than 50 000 years ago, and perhaps as much as 100–200 000 years ago, a transformation happened. The precise date has to be uncertain because inevitably the change occurred first in one individual and then had to spread by genetic means to much larger numbers. For an unknown period of time after this initial event the populations involved must have been very small and so it is wildly improbable that we will find anything in the archaeological record. But between 30 000 and 60 000 years ago the change becomes obvious from the hard evidence of archaeological artefacts. Technology developed quickly, as shown by the presence of more and more complex weapons constructed from more varied structural elements and combinations of structural elements, such as bone and wood or stone and wood (Mithen, 1996; Noble and Davidson, 1996). Religion developed, as indicated by apparent ritual burials with grave goods and the anointing of the corpse with red ochre. Art developed, as indicated by the extraordinary cave drawings and paintings, and possibly by the finding of true musical instruments. Warfare perhaps developed, as indicated by tantalizing evidence of weapons and dismembered humans.

Then, around 10–15 000 years ago, the pace of change increased again. Farming led to settlements, which led to cities, states, the emergence of rulers governing large numbers, and to real war. Cultural, religious, linguistic and other forms of diversity became exuberant.

The brains of the humans of the last 100 000 years have clearly been functioning differently from those of the 2.5 million or so stable years before that. What happened to bring about the transformation? To begin to understand this, one needs to turn to the study of factors which we know influence brain size and connectivity.

DETERMINANTS OF MODERN BRAIN SIZE AND CONNECTIVITY

It is unlikely that our present biochemistry has differed substantially from that of primates for the past several million years, but there must be some differences in biochemistry which account for the differences in form and function. If we can understand some of the factors which determine brain size and connectivity in the present day, it is possible that these will give us clues to the factors which influenced these features over the past 3 million years.

First, consider size. The nonaqueous matter of the brain is around 60% lipid, with much of the remainder being protein. The overall structure of the brain depends on the availability of phospholipids which constitute all the membranes of the brain, both between and within neurones (Horrobin, 1998a, 1999). In particular, the connections between neurones are made by the phospholipid-rich fine endings of axons and dendrites. Within the phospholipid framework, the great majority of the molecules can be synthesized *de novo* from simple elements which are readily available within the human body. The only bulk substances contained within the brain which cannot be synthesized *de novo* are the essential fatty acids (EFAs) and the essential amino acids. The EFAs make up around 20% of the dry bulk of the brain and, of that, three-quarters is made up of arachidonic acid (AA) and docosahexaenoic acid (DHA). AA and DHA are the keys to understanding brain structure and function. They are not only involved in the development of the macro- and microstructure of the brain, but are also required for the normal behaviour of cell signalling systems which determine how neurones function.

AA can be synthesized from the dietary EFA linoleic acid (LA), and DHA can be synthesized from dietary α-linolenic acid (ALA) (Mead and Fulco, 1976; British Nutrition Foundation, 1992; Horrobin, 1992a). However, in many mammals, including humans, these reactions are slow and rate-limiting. It has been pointed out that in all mammals the EFA composition of the brain is rather similar, suggesting that this composition is an absolute requirement for the normal basic functioning of mammalian neural tissues (Crawford and Marsh, 1989; Crawford, 1992). In herbivores, only relatively low levels of these EFAs are found in tissues other than the brain, suggesting that most of the available AA and DHA is being supplied to the brain. Herbivore diets contain no AA and DHA and these animals must therefore make all the AA or DHA that they need from dietary LA and ALA. Crawford has argued that the formation of AA and DHA in herbivores is restricted, and that this limited availability of AA and DHA may limit brain size. If brain size is to grow with body size, AA or DHA must be provided, whether endogenously or from the diet. Among numerous pieces of evidence are the facts that the brains of mammalian carnivores and sea mammals are considerably larger than those of other mammals of similar sizes. In both cases the diet is relatively rich in AA and DHA (Crawford et al., 1976a). Animal and fish tissues contain substantial amounts of AA and DHA, in comparison with the complete absence of these brain EFAs from the diets of herbivores. These preformed brain constituents may allow the brain to grow to a greater size than is possible with animals which do not eat meat or other organs or marine food.

Crawford and others have also argued that the supply of AA and DHA is of critical importance in determining human brain size *in utero* and in infancy (Crawford et al., 1976b; Crawford et al., 1990; Koletzko, 1992; Carlson et al., 1993). The foeto-placental unit concentrates these two fatty acids from the mother, and in this respect behaves as a parasite. The recent demonstration that human maternal brain may shrink by 3–5% in the last trimester of pregnancy (Holdcroft et al., 1997) can very likely be explained by the fact that the maternal brain represents the largest available source of AA and DHA for the foetus. The situation continues after birth, and it is likely to be significant that human milk contains substantial amounts of AA and DHA. Infant formula does not usually contain AA and DHA and this may contribute to the consistent differences in intelligence between bottle-fed and breast-fed babies (Lucas et al., 1992).

Intervention studies in both premature and full-term bottle-fed babies support this view. Premature infants fed artificially with human breast milk have IQs an average of 8 points higher than premature infants fed artificially on formula without AA and DHA (Lucas et al., 1992). Premature infants fed formula with AA and DHA have improved brain and visual development as compared to those fed on equivalent formula without these fatty acids (Birch EE et al., 1992; Birch DG et al., 1992). Even with full term infants all being formula-fed, one randomized study has demonstrated improved visual acuity in those fed AA and DHA with the formula as compared to those fed placebo (Makrides et al., 1995), while another has shown improved cognitive function and problem-solving abilities in infants fed AA and DHA (Willats et al., 1997).

Detailed evaluation of the relationship between these fatty acids in the diet and in umbilical cord has suggested that AA specifically may be a major growth factor for the human brain. There is a close positive correlation between AA levels and infant head circumference, which at this age is a strong indicator of the size of the underlying brain (Crawford et al., 1990; Koletzko, 1992). Although DHA is equally important in brain structure, there is not the same relation between DHA levels and brain size, suggesting that, while DHA is required for a normal brain size, as are essential amino acids, it is not a factor regulating such size. AA, however, does seem to be a regulating factor, with possible consequences which will be explained later.

Brain size alone does not determine intelligence and creativity. Among modern humans – and indeed other mammals – there is little evidence of a close relationship between brain size and intelligence. Neanderthals had brain sizes rather larger than those of modern humans (Trinkaus, 1994), yet it is unlikely that they were more intelligent. Autism is associated with a somewhat larger brain size than normal (Davidovitch et al., 1996). While brain size is undoubtedly of some importance, in that it increases the potential number of neuronal units which may interact, it is clearly not what matters most.

What may matter is connectivity, the ways in which the various parts of the brain are connected together at both the macro and micro levels. It is now becoming widely accepted that, far from there being a single type of general intelligence, there are many different intelligences which can exist almost in isolation (Fodor, 1985; Gardner, 1993a,b; Cosmides and Tooley, 1994; Mithen 1996; Noble and Davidson 1996). At the extremes, this is obvious. Children with William's syndrome, for example, have overall brain sizes 10–20% below normal and a conventional IQ of 50–70, yet display an extraordinary vocabulary and facility with words (Udwin and Yule, 1990). Many sports stars are conventionally intelligent but some are not: someone with a very low conventional IQ may be able to watch a ball hit with great force by a cricket or baseball bat, calculate exactly the trajectory and speed of the ball and run 40 metres to position himself to make a catch. The computing skills involved are extraordinary. An autistic child who, in many respects, is severely intellectually disabled may, for example, be able to scan a series of library shelves within seconds and unerringly pick out the one book which is being sought. We are all familiar with individuals with specialist skills with computers, chess, drawing, language, music, mathematics, business, sociability and so on. The most impressive individuals are those who show considerable abilities across many domains, but particular specialist skills are much more common.

These skills, whether confined to a single narrow area or expressed more widely, all depend on information processing, and on a connection being made between information stored within the brain, new information coming in, and the actions which utilize such information appropriately. The richer the connections, the richer will be the possibilities for skilled action. The richness of the connections in the context of the brain depends on two main factors: the overall connections made by nerve fibre tracts between different brain areas; and the richness of the microconnections made between the fine dendritic extensions of the nerve cells. Accurate counts are almost impossible but it is likely that most individual neurones are capable of making between 10 000 and a million individual connections. It is likely to be the richness or otherwise of these microconnections which determines the level at which complex integrated functions can occur.

Of what do these microconnections consist? They are made up of myriads of tiny protrusions which are formed from phospholipids, the major constituents of which are DHA and AA. The growth cones of these protrusions, which are where the constant making and breaking of connections occurs, are rich in phospholipases, acyltransferases and cyclooxygenases, the enzymes which model and remodel the phospholipids and their fatty acid components, and which convert some of these components to cell signalling molecules (Yamagata et al., 1993; Adams et al., 1996; Kaufmann et al., 1996; Martin and Wickham, 1996; Negre-Aminou et al., 1996; Smalheiser et al., 1996). The nerve growth cones are also rich in nitric oxide, the formation of which is closely associated with the conversion of AA to cell signalling eicosanoids in neuronal tissue and which strongly influences development (Hess et al., 1993; Nelson et al., 1995; Omawari et al., 1995). The connectivity of the brain, which depends as much on appropriate synaptic pruning at the right stages (Purves and Lichtman, 1980; Huttenlocher et al., 1982; Feinberg, 1982–1983) as on synapse formation, is inextricably intertwined with the ability to regulate the metabolism of AA and DHA-rich phospholipids in the growth cones. The protein molecules which influence brain connectivity and which have received more attention (Inoue and Sanes, 1997) are embedded in a phospholipid matrix and are themselves regulated by phospholipid-derived cell signalling molecules (Jiang et al., 1995). It is difficult to avoid the conclusion that the ability to make and remodel phospholipids in the growth cones is one of the keys to the understanding of the development of the microarchitecture of the brain. Extensive connectivity, and its adjustment in response to age and synaptic activity, depend on the ability to make and remodel phospholipids which are rich in AA and DHA.

Thus, with regard to the modern brain, we know that its size is dependent on the ability to make the phospholipids which make up roughly 60% by weight of the brain, and that size may be specifically regulated by the effects of AA. Equally, the extensive microconnectivity of the brain depends on the rapid turnover of phospholipids in the growth cones of the myriad microprotrusions from individual nerve cells, and on the conversion of AA to eicosanoids by cyclooxygenase enzymes. These facts may be among the best clues that we have to understanding what drove the development of brain size and connectivity during human evolution.

THE KEY ENZYMES INVOLVED

The basic structure of a phospholipid and the elements of phospholipid synthesis and action are discussed by Horrobin (1999); see also Mead et al. (1986) and Vance and Vance, (1991). The enzyme sequences involved in phospholipid synthesis do not, however, completely determine the specific compositions of the fatty acid groups, which may be particular to each tissue. The precise composition of the phospholipids which make up the brain depends on the integration of the activity of acyltransferases which incorporate fatty acids into the 1- and 2-positions on the glycerol backbone, and the phospholipases which can break down the phospholipids (acyl simply means 'fatty acid'). These groups of enzymes remodel the basic phospholipid structure to give the precisely desired composition. Of the phospholipases, phospholipase A_2 and phospholipase C are likely to be particularly important, since they not only modify phospholipid structure but also provide key cell signalling molecules such as AA, DHA, diacylglycerol and inositol phosphates. Phospholipase D may also be involved. The acyltranferases use as substrates the coenzyme A derivatives of the fatty acids rather than the free fatty acids themselves. The first step in incorporating a fatty acid into a phospholipid is therefore an acyl-CoA synthetase. These groups of enzymes are thus keys to the determination of brain size, composition and connectivity.

There are also other proteins, which are less immediately central, but which also help to provide the background against which the above enzymes must work. These include, first, the enzymes which construct the basic structure of phospholipids which are then modified to provide the specific molecules required for the brain. It is the modification of the fatty acid groups after synthesis of the basic phospholipid molecule which determines the final structure of brain phospholipids (Mead et al., 1986; Vance and Vance, 1991). Second there are proteins which help to provide the unsaturated fatty acids, such as AA and DHA, for the brain. These fatty acids are made to some degree by endothelial cells, by glial cells and by the choroid plexus by the routes discussed by Horrobin (1999), but the major amounts of AA and DHA needed for the brain are synthesised in the liver from dietary LA or ALA or are provided by the diet to the liver where they are incorporated into lipoproteins or transferred to the many plasma proteins which can bind fatty acids to a greater or lesser degree, and which transport fatty acids in the blood (Mead et al., 1986; Vance and Vance, 1991). The most important of these carriers is the plasma albumin.

When the lipoproteins, and the proteins which bind fatty acids, reach the brain, the fatty acids can be made available in two main ways. First, lipoprotein lipase in the endothelial capillaries releases AA and DHA and other fatty acids from lipoproteins (Eckel and Robbins, 1984; Shirai et al., 1986; Tavangar et al., 1992; Enerback and Gimble, 1993; Farstad, 1993; Goldberg, 1996). Second, the brain contains various fatty acid and acyl-CoA binding proteins and fatty acid transport proteins which can bind specific fatty acids, reduce the concentration of fatty acids in the extracellular fluid and so lead to their release from plasma albumin and other blood fatty acid binding proteins and their transfer to the brain (Gossett et al., 1996; Myers-Payne et al., 1996).

THE IMPORTANCE OF THE SCHIZOPHRENIC INHERITANCE

Schizophrenia is now almost always regarded as a disaster for the affected individual, his or her family, friends, colleagues and other associates. The excesses of the anti-psychiatry Laingian concept that schizophrenia might be regarded as a sane response to an insane world have almost entirely receded. Few now have any doubts that it is schizophrenics who are disordered, with disastrous effects to themselves.

Yet even at the dawn of our present understanding of schizophrenia there were suggestions that the disease might also be associated with high achievement. It was noted that the disease which we would now call schizophrenia frequently struck members of families who were otherwise distinguished in many fields. Henry Maudsley, who toyed with the idea of eugenic control of the mentally disordered, had doubts when it came to schizophrenia-like disorders. He noted the high achievements of families afflicted with madness and feared that eugenic control might reduce the occurrence of individuals of high ability (Maudsley, 1908). Schizophrenia is important because of the damage and destruction wreaked upon schizophrenic patients themselves, and on their relatives, friends and colleagues. It is now my contention that the illness is also important because it is at the core of our humanity and provides many of the characteristics which distinguish us from our hominid ancestors.

The evidence for the value of our schizophrenic inheritance comes from three main sources; detailed studies of Icelandic families; studies of the outcome in children of schizophrenic and normal individuals who are adopted away in early life; and studies of the spectrum of psychiatric disorders in the relatives of schizophrenic patients. This spectrum includes the full range of phospholipid spectrum disorders. Taking the last of these first, the history of psychiatry is in many respects the history of struggles to produce valid diagnostic categories which, as occurs in the rest of medicine, will allow the accurate pigeon-holing into a specific disease classification of everyone who exhibits some form of disturbed behaviour (Shorter, 1997). Much effort has therefore gone into determining what specifically distinguishes schizophrenia from the other disorders associated with it. The fight has been between the splitters, who wish to distinguish a very large number of individual diseases, and the lumpers who want to put psychiatric disorders into much larger groups. For the moment the splitters are in the ascendant with the American Psychiatric Association Diagnostic and Statistical Manual of Mental Disorders (DSM-IV) listing over 400 specific psychiatric disorders (American Psychiatric Association, 1994). This manual is the dominant guide to research efforts around the world and it is almost obligatory for all research studies on patients to define the DSM-IV category into which the patients fall.

But it is possible that DSM-IV is simply an example of what happens when hundreds of different individuals attempt to reach a compromise (Kirk and Kutchins, 1992). The result is a less than happy and less than rigorous mish-mash of fundamentally incongruent views. Several cogent critics, notably Crow (1985, 1987) and Kendell (1987, 1989) have argued that, while it may be reasonable to distinguish between the psychoses and neuroses, there is little solid evidence of any demarcation lines between the two great Kraepelinian divisions of psychotic disorders into schizophrenia and manic-depression. While the severe schizophrenic with a relentlessly progressive psychosis can be relatively easily distinguished from the high functioning manic-depressive with occasional episodes, at the other end of each diagnostic spectrum where the two come close together it becomes much more difficult to be certain about differentiation. Indeed as early as the 1930s, a third diagnostic category, that of schizoaffective psychosis, was introduced to describe those individuals who could not readily be put into either major psychosis category but exhibited features of both (Kasanin, 1933). Thus, when the full range of behaviour is examined, and when genetic studies are taken into account, it is impossible to state with any certainty where, if anywhere, any dividing lines may sensibly be drawn. The view has therefore been taken by the authors quoted that there is indeed only one psychosis. This fits well with the concept of phospholipid spectrum disorders discussed in this book.

Others, looking at the psychological and psychiatric characteristics of some nonpsychotic family members where at least one individual is schizophrenic, or indeed looking at the general population, have gone further (Claridge, 1985, 1994, 1997). They have pointed out that there are many individuals who are not formally mentally ill who have a spectrum of personality deviations which may be classed as schizotypal. These represent schizophrenia-like features but which are much milder than those in truly psychotic individuals. There may be an excess of suspiciousness, a trace of paranoia, a difficulty in making easy social contact, the hearing of voices, great interest in religion and a good deal of eccentricity and magical thinking. Many people with schizotypal personalities are also dyslexic (Richardson, 1994). Claridge has argued that not only is there a continuum of illness between schizophrenia and manic-depression, there is also a continuum between schizophrenia, schizotypal personality and normality (Claridge, 1985, 1994, 1997; Raine et al., 1995). If susceptibility to schizophrenia has a genetic basis, then many apparently near-normal people must be carrying the genes that convey that susceptibility.

The adopted away studies and the Icelandic studies both point in the same direction. When adopted away children of normal parents are compared with adopted away children at least one of whose parents is schizophrenic, striking differences emerge (Heston, 1966; Rosenthal and Kety, 1968; Kety et al., 1994). Adopted away children of nonpsychiatric parents exhibit little psychiatric disorder of any kind, apart from modest levels of anxiety and depression typical of any population. They also exhibit little evidence of unusual ability or achievement. The children of schizophrenics could hardly be more different. As expected, substantially more of them grow up to be schizophrenic than is true of the children of apparently normal parents. But, in addition, much of the manic-depression, the alcoholism, the severe depression, the mental retardation and the psychopathy, criminality or sociopathy are to be found in the adopted away children of schizophrenics as compared to the children of nonpsychiatric people. That sounds an appalling inheritance until one looks at other aspects of the life histories of these individuals. Creative achievement of any sort was almost entirely confined to the children of the schizophrenics. This expressed itself in many ways but perhaps the most striking was in music: 15% of children of schizophrenics, but no children of normal individuals, demonstrated high calibre professional or near-professional musical skills (Heston, 1966, 1970). A similar imbalance was found with respect to religion. None of the children of normal parents was intensely religious whereas one in eight of the children of schizophrenics were highly religious (Heston, 1966, 1970).

A similar picture emerges from the unique population of Iceland (Karlsson, 1966, 1974). Because of the existence of excellent records, a small and isolated population, and an intense interest in family history, it is possible to identify a very high proportion of those individuals, who for the last two centuries, were mad, bad and dangerous to know, or gifted, creative, energetic and charismatic. Karlsson has conducted a remarkable series of investigations of this population. The thing which stands out most clearly is that the families where one or more members were schizophrenic were also the families in which almost all the other psychiatric disorders were found. But these families were also the ones which contained many of the high achieving and creative Icelanders. Madness, badness, creativity and leadership all seemed to go together in the same family trees. Families without madness were also usually families of steady ordinary people without high or unusual achievement.

Although the adopted away and Icelandic studies provide the most convincing evidence, most other studies of the relatives of schizophrenic probands provide the same picture. The relatives of schizophrenics have a higher than usual risk of schizophrenia itself, but also of alcoholism, manic-depression, sociopathy, borderline personality and other personality disorders (Alanen, 1958; Kay et al., 1975; Stephens et al., 1975; Silverton, 1988; Varma et al., 1997).

Thus there seems to be a continuum not only between schizophrenia and manic-depression but between schizophrenia and normality and schizophrenia and high achievement. Individuals of all these types seem to be grouped in the same families. The adoption away studies argue that this grouping is not simply the result of similar family and social conditioning but represents a phenomenon with a biochemical basis in the genes. These same families, of course, contain substantial numbers of normal individuals as well as the disturbed and the high achievers.

When such a continuum is demonstrable, and when a strong genetic basis is also clear, there are two broad categories of genetic explanation which may be valid. One is that a single gene is modulated over a wide range by the impact of the gene's environment. That environment may be the genetic environment, the presence or absence of other genes which influence the first gene, or it may be the external environment, the presence or absence of external factors which influence the degree of impact exerted by the gene. These explanations can be broadly summarized as the variable penetrance concept. A good example of this may be type II diabetes which is clearly a genetic disorder and which may be primarily due to one gene, but where the gene is to a substantial degree expressed only in those individuals who adopt a Western type of diet. The possibility that this is also true of schizophrenia cannot be ruled out. The WHO (World Health Organization, 1979) study showed that the prevalence of the disease was similar everywhere, but that its impact was much more severe in some countries than others. Christensen and Christensen (1988) have pointed out that severity of outcome in the WHO study is associated with a Western-style diet and have argued that, like diabetes, schizophrenia may be a genetic disease whose degree of expression is heavily influenced by the type of nutrition available. The possible importance of this concept will become more apparent later in this chapter.

The other possible explanation for continuous variations is that several genes are involved, as is the case, for example, with human height. The variable presence or absence of several genes will usually produce a continuous variation in a parameter with no obvious cutoff points. It will be argued that schizophrenia and the related conditions which together make up phospholipid spectrum disorder represent a situation where more than one gene is involved and where the expression of the genes can be substantially influenced by environmental factors.

To date, as far as I am aware, no specific biochemical candidates for the genetic changes which made us human have been proposed. Almost all the 'explanations' for recent hominid evolution over the past 3 million years are variants of social hypotheses relating to the pressures produced by factors such as food gathering, hunting, scavenging, home-base behaviour, defence against carnivores, and the need to communicate within relatively large social groups (Aiello and Dunbar, 1993; Foley, 1995; Mithen, 1996; Noble and Davidson, 1996; Rose and Marshall, 1996, among others). These hypotheses almost always include at some point a statement along the lines of 'these selective pressures would have driven the evolution of a large and effective brain.' To my mind this is somewhat akin to making the statement 'and then a miracle occurs.' It seems to me that a larger and more effective brain is likely to be of value to almost any species of animal yet in most animal lineages we do not see selective pressures forcing development in this direction. The real question which must be answered is 'What specific biochemical changes allowed the possibility of improvement in brain function, and so made human ancestors particularly well placed to respond to the selective pressures which are generally applicable to all primate species (and indeed to all animal species)?' Selective pressures are irrelevant unless there are desirable variants available which can be selected.

The thesis which will be developed in this chapter is that the biochemical variants related to changes in lipid metabolism, and that some of those changes are the ones which can be identified today in the range of high achieving and disordered individuals to be found in the families where schizophrenia is present.

POSSIBLE LIPID ABNORMALITIES IN SCHIZOPHRENIA AND RELATED DISORDERS

Elsewhere, I and colleagues have argued that abnormal phospholipid, essential fatty acid and eicosanoid metabolism are central to the understanding of the pathogenesis of schizophrenia and related disorders. The evidence is set out in detail in earlier chapters of this book and other publications but, briefly, it is suggested that there are two major types of biochemical abnormality and that the expression of these abnormalities may then be influenced by other factors (Horrobin, 1977, 1979, 1992b, 1996, 1997, 1998a,b, 1999; Horrobin et al., 1978a, 1994, 1995; Gattaz et al., 1990; Pettegrew et al., 1993; Glen et al., 1994, 1996; Peet et al., 1994, 1996, 1997a,b; Gattaz and Brunner, 1996; Mahadik and Gowda, 1996; Hudson et al., 1996, 1997; Mahadik and Evans, 1997; Ross et al., 1997; Ward et al., 1998).

There is substantial evidence that in schizophrenia there is increased activity of one or more of the phospholipases which remove unsaturated fatty acids, particularly AA and DHA, from membrane phospholipids. The main candidate is phospholipase A_2 which liberates these fatty acids directly. An alternative candidate is phospholipase C which achieves a similar result but less directly. The concept is discussed extensively in other chapters of this book but the main points may be briefly summarized.

1. Increased circulating phospholipase activity has been reported in schizophrenia (Gattaz et al., 1990; Gattaz and Brunner, 1996), and there is evidence of increased phospholipid breakdown on *in vivo* ^{31}P magnetic resonance imaging (Pettegrew et al., 1993).

2. Reduced levels of AA and DHA are observed in red cell membranes, consistent with increased PLA_2 activity (Glen et al., 1994; Peet et al., 1994, 1996, 1997a; Mahadik and Gowda, 1996; Mahadik and Evans, 1997; Ward et al., 1998).

3. Reduced skin flushing in response to oral or topical niacin which produces the effect by stimulating the conversion of AA to PGD_2, is seen in schizophrenic patients compared with control subjects (Ward et al., 1998). If AA is unavailable then the likelihood of flushing is reduced (Horrobin, 1980; Horrobin et al., 1995; Hudson et al., 1997; Ward et al., 1998; Glen et al., unpublished data).

4. Abnormalities occur in the numbers of poly-A repeat sequences in the vicinity of the promoter

region of the PLA₂ gene on chromosome 1, and in the BAN-1 site adjacent to the PLA₂ gene (Hudson et al., 1996; Ramchand et al., 1999). Such abnormalities indicate genetic variations in the regulation of phospholipase synthesis rather than in the structure of the enzyme. Because many different alleles exist there is the possibility of multiple variants of the control of enzyme synthesis.

If such phospholipase A or C abnormalities exist, they will increase the rate at which AA and DHA are removed from membrane phospholipids. If these abnormalities are relatively mild, then the increased phospholipase activity itself will not change membrane composition but only the rate of membrane turnover (Horrobin et al., 1994, 1995). A change in membrane turnover involving phospholipases will consequentially involve related enzymes like cyclooxygenases and nitric oxide synthetases which are intimately involved in the regulation of nerve growth cones and microconnectivity (Purves and Lichtman, 1980; Feinberg, 1982–1983; Huttenlocher et al., 1982; Hess et al., 1993; Yamagata et al., 1993; Jiang et al., 1995; Nelson et al., 1995; Omawari et al., 1995; Adams et al., 1996; Kaufmann et al., 1996; Martin and Wickham, 1996; Negre-Aminou et al., 1996; Smalheiser et al., 1996; Inoue and Sanes, 1997). Such changes in neuronal membrane turnover are thus strong and plausible candidates for biochemical steps which might offer selective advantages in brain development.

Another type of change which could lead to alterations in neuronal turnover might be in one or more of the groups of enzymes which incorporate AA and DHA into phospholipids, the acyl-CoA synthetase (Laposata et al., 1985) and acyltransferase families. I and colleagues have argued that such an abnormality may occur in dyslexia (Horrobin et al., 1995). The evidence is less persuasive than in the case with schizophrenia itself, but is increasing steadily. The main items are that dyslexic individuals tend to have poor night vision, a problem which can be corrected by feeding large amounts of DHA (Stordy, 1995, 1996). The peripheral retina absolutely requires membranes containing high levels of DHA for normal function, and the observation suggests that dyslexic individuals may not be able to incorporate the DHA rapidly enough because of a minor deficit in one of the acyltransferases. A second piece of evidence is that on ³¹P magnetic resonance imaging, dyslexic individuals have abnormalities consistent with impaired synthesis of phospholipids (Richardson et al., 1997).

INTER-RELATIONSHIPS BETWEEN SCHIZOPHRENIA, MANIC-DEPRESSION, DYSLEXIA AND SCHIZOTYPAL PERSONALITY

Whereas the evidence for an inherited basis for schizophrenia is strong, that for single gene involvement is weak. As discussed earlier, it is difficult to draw any precise dividing line between schizotypy, schizophrenia, manic-depression and cyclothymic personality. Schizotypy is closely related to dyslexia, with many dyslexic individuals scoring highly on scales of schizotypy (Richardson, 1994). My proposed solution to this problem is to suggest that all of these problems are related to disordered phospholipid metabolism in the ways outlined below.

Manic-depression is associated with increased activity of one of the phospholipase group of enzymes which will lead to increased formation of free AA and DHA and of the eicosanoids formed from AA. There are also likely to be increased rates of formation of related fatty acids which can give rise to eicosanoids such as dihomo-γ-linolenic acid (DGLA) or eicosapentaenoic acid (EPA). There are various pieces of evidence related to this. First, lithium is effective in treating manic-depression, and lithium, among other actions, inhibits the release of AA and the formation of prostaglandins and also inhibits the phosphatidyl-inositol cycle and decreases the rate of arachidonate turnover in brain phospholipids (Horrobin et al., 1978b; Horrobin and Manku, 1980; Chang et al., 1996). This suggests that in untreated manic-depression there may be increased release of AA and DHA. Second, there is recent evidence that niacin, on either oral or topical administration, causes excessive flushing in manic-depressive individuals (Hudson et al., 1997; Ward et al., 1998). This indicates excessive release of AA and formation of PGD₂, events consistent with increased activity of a phospholipase. It is suggested that the increased activity is modest and is compensated by an overall increase in the rate of membrane turnover, so that in manic-depression actual concentrations of AA and DHA in membranes do not change, although their flux does.

Dyslexia, in contrast, is associated with a reduced rate of incorporation of AA and DHA into membrane phospholipids. The most likely reason is a modestly reduced activity of one of the acyltransferase group of enzymes, or of the enzymes which activate fatty acids by making coenzyme A derivatives. Such derivatives are required before fatty acids can be synthesized into complex lipids such as phospholipids. Arachidonyl-CoA synthetase would be an example of this group (Laposata et al., 1985).

Schizophrenia occurs when both of these abnormalities are present together. As a consequence of their combined presence there is a much more important defect in membrane metabolism and structure, because one of the defects reduces incorporation of AA and DHA, and the other leads to excessive removal. As a result, the defects in membrane function are considerably more severe, leading not only to changes in flux but to actual changes in concentration. In schizophrenia there is evidence both of increased phospholipase activity and of reduced incorporation of fatty acids into phospholipids (Yao et al., 1996).

What will happen as a result of these deviations from the usual? There will be changed microconnectivity as a result of changes in neuronal sprouting and synaptic pruning, changed cell signalling as a result of the changed availability of membrane AA and DHA, and changed membrane structure which will lead to changes in configuration of membrane-bound proteins and hence to changes in function of these proteins.

At present, little is known about phospholipid abnormalities in the other conditions shown to be associated with schizophrenia on the basis of family studies, notably psychopathy, sociopathy, schizotypy, paranoia, mental retardation and alcoholism, on the one hand, or creativity, energy, high achievement and charismatic leadership on the other. There is evidence of interactions between alcoholism and lipid metabolism, but this is at an early stage (Glen et al., 1987; Horrobin, 1987; Glen, 1997). There is good evidence that manic-depression is associated with an unusual degree of creativity in many fields and also with periods of extraordinary productivity and energy (Hershman and Lieb, 1988; Goodwin and Jamison, 1990; Milligan and Clare, 1993; Jamison, 1995; Ludwig, 1995). Dyslexia is also associated with considerable skills in visualizing space such that dyslexics often make good architects. Einstein, Edison and Leonardo da Vinci all show evidence of having been dyslexic (Davis, 1995).

OTHER STEPS IN LIPID METABOLISM WHICH MAY INFLUENCE THE PRIMARY ABNORMALITIES

I have proposed that the primary abnormalities in the spectrum of disorders associated with schizophrenia and manic-depression lie in the incorporation into membrane phospholipids, and removal from these phospholipids, of AA and DHA, and also perhaps DGLA and EPA. However, these primary abnormalities will, in turn, be influenced by the rates at which the key fatty acids are supplied to the brain. If AA, DHA, DGLA and EPA are available in some abundance then the impact of changes in the rates of incorporation and removal will be minimized. An increased rate of removal, for example, will be readily compensated if there are abundant supplies of the relevant fatty acids. On the other hand, the primary abnormality will lead to more severe changes in brain function if the key fatty acids are in short supply.

Mammals have absolute requirements for the parent EFAs, LA and ALA. LA and ALA are relatively widely available from vegetable sources. Mammals can also convert LA to DGLA and AA, and ALA to EPA and DHA, but these reaction sequences do not always appear to occur at sufficient rates to meet the body's needs, especially the needs of the brain (Crawford and Marsh, 1989). This may be particularly true at the extremes of life when the enzymes involved have either not yet fully matured or have lost some of their functions (Horrobin, 1981; Takahashi et al., 1991).

Although brain cells and associated tissues, such as choroid plexus and endothelium (Bourre et al., 1997; Delton-Vanddenbroucke et al., 1997) may be able to make small amounts of AA and DHA from LA and ALA, the bulk of such synthesis occurs in the liver. The AA, DHA and related fatty acids are then transported into other tissues in two main ways. They may be incorporated into lipoproteins or bound to plasma albumin or other fatty acid binding proteins in the blood. When they reach a particular tissue they may be released in two main ways. The fatty acids may be released from lipoproteins by lipoprotein lipase, mainly in the endothelium cells. Alternatively, specific tissue fatty acid binding proteins or acyl-CoA binding proteins may accumulate fatty acids or their acyl-CoA derivatives, so producing local concentration gradients which prompt the release of the equivalent molecules from the binding proteins in the plasma (Gossett et al., 1996; Myers-Payne et al., 1996).

Lipoprotein lipase is an enzyme of considerable interest. It is found throughout the brain, but is especially high in concentration in the hippocampus, a part of the brain known to be particularly affected in schizophrenia (Shirai et al., 1986; Tavangar et al., 1992; Enerback and Gimble, 1993; Goldberg, 1996). Lipoprotein lipase is regulated by thyroid hormone which, as exemplified by cretinism, is important in brain growth and connectivity (Gavin et al., 1987). It is also regulated by prolactin the levels of which are elevated by all traditional neuroleptic drugs used in schizophrenia (Enerback and Gimble, 1993; Bourre et al., 1997; Hang and Rillema, 1997). Its functions are also modulated by gonadal hormones, with major changes occurring around puberty; this is of interest because of the common emergence of the first signs of schizophrenia around this time (Bucher et al., 1997). Lipoprotein lipase is of critical importance in the regulation of the supply of fatty acids to adipose tissue and to the breast. Along with the brain, the differences in adipose tissue and in the breast are among the most striking differences between humans and our nearest primate relatives (Morgan, 1994, 1997). The gene for lipoprotein lipase is located at 8p22 (Murthy et al., 1996), one of the known vulnerability loci for schizophrenia (Kendler et al., 1996). Polymorphisms in lipoprotein lipase appear important in regulating obesity and the response to starvation (Jemaa et al., 1997), biochemical characteristics which may be related to the ability to survive during periods of poor food supply.

Lipoprotein lipase and fatty acid-binding and fatty acid transport proteins are important in delivering the key fatty acids to the brain, no matter whether the AA or DHA come from endogenous synthesis in the liver and other tissues or from the diet. Although not well understood, there also appears to be a close interaction between iron, delivery of EFAs to the brain and brain growth (Oloyede et al., 1992). The effects of a limited supply of EFAs in retarding brain growth are dramatically exaggerated when there is coincident iron deficiency. The dietary supply of preformed AA, DHA, DGLA and EPA is also likely to be important given the relatively limited capacity of mammals to make these fatty acids on their own. As discussed later, there are only four practical sources of these EFAs: eggs; meat (and especially organ meat); algae of marine or alkaline lake origin; and water-based animals, fish, crustacea or molluscs higher up in the food chain which directly or indirectly consume the algae. If diets rich in these foods are being consumed, as may well have occurred in East Africa during hominid evolution, the impact of changes in brain phospholipid metabolism may be attenuated. It may be significant that almost all presumed human ancestor fossil sites are associated with water (Morgan, 1994, 1997) and that such waters would have been rich in foods, providing the EFAs required for brain function (Broadhurst et al., 1998). Such waters are also likely to be rich in iodine and zinc which are also required for normal brain development.

THE INTERACTION BETWEEN LIPID METABOLISM AND HUMAN EVOLUTION

So far, this chapter has presented a series of observations from archaeology, from brain biochemistry, from the genetics and the classification of psychiatric disease, and from the biochemistry of such disease. These observations may now be brought together to present a coherent hypothesis concerning the biochemical basis of human evolution.

Changes in brain size

There appear to have been two major spurts in brain size, one around 2 million and the other around half a million years ago, although during the whole period there was an upward drift. The recent evidence from infant development suggests that AA is not only an important component of the brain in itself but may itself be a factor which actually regulates brain size. Iron may interact with AA in this respect (Oloyede et al., 1992). It is therefore a plausible hypothesis that the two surges in brain size may have come from an increase in the availability of AA and iron for the brain. There is a relatively limited number of processes which could have led to increased availability of AA for the brain, and to an increase in brain size. One of these processes may have been primarily responsible for the first brain spurt, and another for the second.

Increased external supply of AA in the diet

There are only four substantial sources of AA from the diet. These are egg yolks, the meat and organs of animals, water-based food, and algae which grow in mineral-rich lakes. It is unlikely that, in the absence of domestication, there could ever be anything other than a seasonal supply of egg yolk, and so eggs are unlikely long-term sources. Animal carcasses are realistic sources, especially since most archaeologists date the onset of serious human hunting to around the time of the first brain growth surge, around 2 million years ago. Such carcasses would also provide iron, which is scarce in vegetable foods. Water-based foods, including algae, molluscs, crustacea, fish, birds and mammals would have been readily available to lakeshore, river and seaside dwellers. It is interesting that Elaine Morgan and others have emphasized the possible importance of an earlier semi-aquatic or littoral stage in human evolution which might have predisposed humans to take advantage of water-based foods (Verhaegen, 1985; Roede et al., 1991; Morgan, 1994, 1997). Even today the lakes of East Africa are rich in AA-producing algae, as are the freshwater animals and birds which consume such algae (Broadhurst et al., 1998). The food of a hunter/gatherer, especially one living in a waterside environment, would have been important in providing the AA, iron and probably the iodine required. It is interesting that the iodine/thyroid hormone deficient human nails are remarkably similar to the normal nails of the chimpanzee (O'Donovan, 1996a,b).

Increased incorporation of AA into brain phospholipids

The enzymes which perform this reaction are the acyltransferases which must work with activated fatty acids provided by acyl-CoA synthetases. One or more mutations increasing the rate of transfer of AA into phospholipids could have stimulated brain growth.

Increased transport of AA into the brain

This could have come about in two main ways: either by increased affinity for AA of one of the brain fatty acid or acyl-CoA binding proteins, or fatty acid transport proteins; or by increased activity of the endothelial lipoprotein lipase which, among other fatty acids, releases AA. Lipoprotein lipase is a particularly interesting candidate in view of its importance in brain, breast and adipose tissue metabolism and in resistance to starvation. It is possible that a single change in lipoprotein lipase could have contributed to four of the features which distinguish humans from our nearest primate relatives: i.e., the large amounts of subcutaneous adipose tissue; the ready variability of that adipose tissue in response to varying food supplies; the fatty female breast; and the increased size of the brain. Such parsimony of explanation is very appealing. Other good candidates would be the fatty acid binding proteins which have already been shown to be important in neurogenesis in the avian brain (Rousselot et al., 1997).

Increased conversion of dietary LA to AA

The sequence of reactions by which dietary LA is converted into AA has been described in Chapter 1 of this book. It is relatively slow in humans and has two key rate limiting steps: that governing the conversion of LA to γ-linolenic acid; and that regulating the conversion of DGLA to AA. A change in the activity of this enzyme sequence could have modified the supply of AA for the brain.

Changes in brain symmetry

Apart from brain size, another problem which must be solved is the development of brain asymmetry which may be greater in humans than in related hominids (Crow, 1991, 1993, 1995, 1996a,b). This may have been caused by a specific mutation. Alternatively it may have simply been due to the exaggeration of pre-existing but less marked brain asymmetries which became more obvious as the brain rapidly increased in size. Either way, brain lipid metabolism is likely to have been involved. It is not widely appreciated that hemispheric differences in brain lipid metabolism are phylogenetically very old, can be demonstrated in rodents, and particularly apply to activity of phospholipases (Pediconi and Rodriguez de Turco, 1984; Ginobili de Martinez et al., 1985; Ginobili de Martinez and Barrantes, 1988).

Changes in brain connectivity

Whilst size alone of the brain is important in providing sufficient neuronal elements to interact to produce a complex network, it is the richness and specificity of the fine connections of that network which determine the complexity of the information processing which can occur. Connectivity depends on the presence of cellular guiding and adhesion factors, including molecules such as the cadherins. The growth cones of nerve cells are extremely rich in phospholipases which can release AA and DHA from membrane phospholipids and they are also rich in cyclooxygenase 2 which can take the fatty acids and convert them to other cell-signalling molecules (Purves and Lichtman, 1980; Feinberg, 1982–1983; Huttenlocher et al., 1982; Hess et al., 1993; Yamagata et al., 1993; Jiang et al., 1995; Nelson et al., 1995; Omawari et al., 1995; Adams et al., 1996; Kaufmann et al., 1996; Martin and Wickham, 1996; Negre-Aminou et al., 1996; Smalheiser et al., 1996; Inoue and Sanes, 1997). My proposal is that a mutation in the phospholipases (either A_2 or C), or possibly in the cyclooxygenases, enhanced the turnover of phospholipids and increased the rate at which connections were made and broken down. This led to the formation of many more abundant microconnections and also to parts of the brain being connected which had not been connected before. It would also lead to changes in the rates of dendritic pruning during development and puberty, which are also important in determining the connectivity of the adult brain.

Other possible mutations would be in the acyltransferases or acyl-CoA synthetases. These also would lead to changes in phospholipid turnover, and to changes in the formation and pruning of neuronal connections.

Implications for evolution

Social and environmental pressures may have provided the background against which evolution occurred but they cannot provide specific explanations for the 'then a miracle occurred' stages of human evolution. These stages must have had specific biochemical causes. I suggest that there are three major events which require explanation, not just in social and environmental terms but in biochemical terms. Without the biochemistry, social and environmental pressures could have achieved nothing. The three major events are: the increase in brain size, which alone could not have produced creativity but could have provided the background against which creativity might emerge; the creativity which led to the hand axe cultures and the emergence of complex co-operative behaviour; and the creativity of a quite different sort which emerged somewhere between 50 and 200 000 years ago and which was responsible for making us truly human. Each of these events may have been modified in many minor ways, but I suggest that if we can explain these great events we will have gone a long way to accounting for what happened in the past 2.5 million years.

My hypothesis is that each of these events was related to something new happening in lipid metabolism. I propose that the increase in brain size was related to an increase in the availability of EFAs, and especially of AA, for the brain. The adoption of a water-based food chain, and of hunting, would have provided the background against which the supply of EFAs (and also of iron, iodine and zinc) could have been achieved. But that background must have been exploited by one or more changes in the delivery systems which supply the EFAs to the brain. Good candidates – but not the only ones – are the fatty acid and acyl-CoA binding and transport proteins of blood and brain, and the lipoprotein lipase group of enzymes. I find lipoprotein lipase a particularly interesting candidate. This is because it is involved in supplying fatty acids not only to the brain but also to the breast and to adipose tissue. Our abundant subcutaneous adipose tissue, as much as our brains, distinguishes our biochemistry from that of our primate relatives. As well as adapting us to a river or lakeside or marine environment as Alister Hardy and Elaine Morgan have pointed out, adipose tissue also provides us with the defences against starvation which could have represented major competitive advantages at many stages of our evolutionary history.

Big brains do not, however, necessarily mean better brains, and changes in connectivity would also have been required. Such changes may have been involved on at least two occasions, when humans first began making designed hand axes around 2 million years ago and when these designs increased in complexity and sophistication around half a million years ago. The abilities to visualize shapes and to conceptualize the final axe hidden within the stone represent the sorts of skills at which dyslexic individuals excel. These changes may therefore have been associated with the introduction of the genes for dyslexia. Again, there are several possible candidates, but the acyltranferases and acyl-CoA synthetases may be ones of particular significance.

Finally, in the period 50–250 000 years ago something fundamental happened which was so profound that it transformed hominid culture and made us human. My proposal for this is that it was associated with the introduction of increased activity of one or more phospholipases, or perhaps cyclooxygenases, and that this led to exuberant modelling, pruning, and remodelling of synapses with important changes in the development and pruning of microconnections. Such new mutations may have had particularly profound effects when they interacted with those present in individuals with dyslexia.

These specific hypotheses for the factors which influenced the development of brain size and connectivity offer a testable framework for the explanation of particular biochemical changes which made us human. In particular, they suggest that there will be three main groups of disorders; dyslexia-schizotypy; the alcoholism/affective disorders; and schizophrenia. The last of these three will appear in those individuals affected by both the other two and so all three groups will be detectable in families with a schizophrenic proband. The biochemical severity of the resulting problems will be profoundly influenced by the availability of the brain EFAs, and so the clinical severity will also be substantially affected by the supply of dietary AA, DHA, DGLA and EPA.

Consequences for society

The adopted away and Icelandic studies, and the studies on the spectrum of disordered mental function within families, suggest that the biochemical mutations which produced these disorders introduced into the human race a whole series of skills and behaviour patterns which are characteristic of the last 100 000 years but not of the 2–3 million years before that. The attributes present in some members of such families may include a tendency to hear voices and a tendency to be intensely interested in religion. Such experiences might have introduced a sense of the otherness of supreme beings, or a sense of the possession by unseen spirits of the animals and inanimate objects of the world. Religion and ritual may have had their origins in these individuals. Other people, without the creativity to imagine these things themselves, may have had the brain capacity to learn and partially understand them from others. Other individuals may show a tendency to have unusual spatial senses and visual art skills. The novel brain connections produced by these biochemical changes could have been the basis for the development of art.

The adoption studies clearly show that descendants of schizophrenics commonly have extraordinary musical skills. Such individuals may have been the first to listen with a new ear to the sounds of nature and to build on these sounds to create the first steps in human music.

Paranoia, psychopathy, sociopathy and leadership skills also occur in schizophrenics and their families. These characteristics are not necessarily wholly negative in their impact. All may have had creative effects in generating human societies, since all are capable of being imitated by less creative individuals with adequate brain size. A moderate degree of paranoia may have been important in creating a sense of the value of kinship and the dangers of other social groups. Psychopathy and sociopathy with their simultaneous understanding of, yet total lack of sympathy with, the needs of others are features of ruthless leadership. Paranoia and psychopathy, together, especially when associated with the energy and creativity of manic-depression, could have led to the emergence of rulers within groups, to suspicion of other groups, and to the suppression or slaughter of other groups or their enslavement by war. In short, the features associated with the presence of schizophrenic genes could have led to most of the features of human societies.

One of the frequently discussed problems of schizophrenia is why the disease has not been eliminated during evolution, because male schizophrenics in particular have much lower rates of reproduction than normal individuals. There are three explanations for this. The first is that within the schizophrenia spectrum are manic-depression and psychopathy, both of which are associated with increases in promiscuous activity and in numbers of children. The second is that schizophrenia, on the view of this hypothesis, requires the presence of two separate genes, i.e., for dyslexia and for manic-depression. Individuals with only one of these genes reproduce normally or perhaps, in the case of manic-depression, excessively: selective pressure would apply only against the combination and not against the two genes individually. Third, in the presence of an adequate hunter/gatherer/waterside diet, the adverse impact of schizophrenia on behaviour may have been much less that that with which we are familiar today.

Thus I propose that the lipid-metabolising genes which gave us increased brain size, dyslexia, manic-depression and schizophrenia also gave us the creative individuals who initiated the explosion of human culture and the noncreative individuals who nevertheless had the brain capacity to learn. I suggest that schizophrenia and its associated metabolic variants are what, in a real sense, made us human.

Impact of dietary changes

The relatively minor abnormalities in acyltransferases, phospholipases and other lipid-related enzymes which in my view are the bases of these psychiatric disorders will be substantially influenced by the availability of dietary AA, DHA, EPA and DGLA. They will also be affected by the presence of other competing fatty acids, including monounsaturated and saturated fats, which may partially displace them in phospholipids. High intakes of saturated fats may exaggerate phospholipid deficits of AA and DHA resulting from relatively minor abnormalities in lipid biochemistry.

Those eating a traditional hunter/gatherer diet, especially one supplemented with food gathered from sea or freshwater sources, may experience only a modest impact of these metabolic changes. Reduced acyltransferase activity may be compensated by an increased availability of AA and DHA. Equally, increased phospholipase activity may be similarly compensated so that there may be only a minimal impact on membrane structure and function.

On switching to an agricultural way of life, however, most of the AA and DHA will disappear from the diet. There will still be reasonable amounts of LA and ALA, but those would have to be converted within the body to AA and DHA. The availability of the brain-specific EFAs will be reduced, leading to a greater impact of the minor metabolic abnormalities. As a result, there might be generated greater structural and functional abnormalities, with increases in both creative and disturbed behaviour. Such changes may therefore have been factors in the astonishing further explosion of creativity and diversity associated with the agricultural revolution of the past 10 000 years. Farmers, and those obtaining food from farmers, have much lower intakes of AA, DHA and other brain-related EFAs than do hunter/gatherers and fisherpeople.

Finally, it is evident that in the past 200 years there has been a considerable increase in the apparent severity and prevalence of schizophrenia and related disorders (Shorter, 1997). At the same time, there has been a further increase in apparent energy and creativity of both desirable and undesirable varieties. It seems unlikely that further important mutations have occurred and spread extensively during this time and so environmental factors, including diet, must be involved. During the 19th century, supposedly improved cereal processing led to the removal of most of the EFAs from the diet, together with protective factors important in EFA metabolism, such as vitamins E and B_6. At the same time, this was compounded by a great increase in the consumption of saturated fat which, when present in excess, will displace EFAs from membrane phospholipids. These changes could have been partly responsible for the increase in severity of schizophrenia. Christensen and Christensen (1988) have shown that in modern times the severity of schizophrenia is worse in those societies with a high ratio of saturated fats to EFAs in the diet. Mellor, Laugharne and Peet have recently demonstrated that schizophrenic symptoms are attenuated in those taking increased intakes of the brain n-3 EFAs, particularly eicosapentaenoic acid (Mellor et al., 1995, 1996; Peet et al., 1997a).

CONCLUSIONS

Humans differ from other primates and hominids in their genes, but only to a limited degree. Genes express their function in terms of biochemistry, and so the differences between humans and related species must have a biochemical basis. No matter what social and environmental challenges were present during human evolution, it was not the challenges but the genetic responses to them which made us human. There is recent evidence from animal studies that induced behavioural challenges and changes in EFA biochemistry may interact to produce changes in brain structure not brought about by either agent alone (Yoshida et al., 1997a,b). This creates a plausible basis for the interaction between environmental challenge and lipid-related response in human evolution. The genetic responses must be expressed in terms of differences in the biochemistry of those tissues which clearly distinguish us from other primates, namely the brain, the breast and subcutaneous fat. In spite of the obviousness of these statements, and in spite of the vast intellectual investment in the study of human evolution, almost no attention has been paid to the biochemistry behind that evolution.

In this chapter I have argued that changes in lipid metabolism are responsible for the changes in brain size and connectivity which led to the emergence of humans from our hominid ancestors. These changes led to the extraordinary mix of creativity, drive and disturbed behaviour which characterizes both humanity in general and the families where schizophrenia and manic-depression are present in particular. These changes occurred at about the same time that schizophrenia was introduced to humans, prior to the separation of the races. As far as I am aware these are the first specific proposals for the biochemical changes which made us human. The hypothesis is undoubtedly wrong in detail, and possibly even in its broad outline, but my hope is that it will stimulate debate and precise testing in a way which is not possible within the current near biochemistry-free zone of human evolutionary studies. It may also help to provide a more positive perspective to what most people now see in almost wholly negative terms as the problem of schizophrenia (Chadwick, 1997).

ACKNOWLEDGEMENT

This is a modified version of a paper which appeared in the April 1998 issue of Medical Hypotheses (Horrobin, 1998b).

REFERENCES

Adams J, Collaco Moraes Y, de Belleroche J. Cyclooxygenase-2 induction in cerebral cortex: an intracellular response to synaptic excitation. J Neurochem 1996; 66: 6–13.

Aiello LC, Dunbar RIM. Neocortex size, group size, and the evolution of language. Curr Anthropol 1993; 34: 184–193.

Alanen O. The mothers of schizophrenic patients. Acta Psychiatr Neurol Scand 1958; 33 (Suppl 124): 5–361.

American Psychiatric Association. Diagnostic and statistical manual of mental disorders. 4th edn (DSM-IV). Washington, DC: American Psychiatric Association, 1994.

Birch EE, Birch DG, Hoffman DR, Uauy R. Dietary essential fatty acid supply and visual acuity development. Invest Ophthalmol Vis Sci 1992; 33: 3242–3253.

Birch DG, Birch EE, Hoffman DR, Uauy RD. Retinal development in very-low-birth-weight infants fed diets differing in omega-3 fatty acids. Invest Ophthalmol Vis Sci 1992; 33: 2365–2376.

Bourre JM, Dinh L, Boithias C, Dumont O, Piciotti MN, Cunnane S. Possible role of the choroid plexus in the supply of brain tissue with polyunsaturated fatty acids. Neurosci Lett 1997; 224: 1–4.

British Nutrition Foundation. Unsaturated fatty acids: nutritional and physiological significance. London: Chapman and Hall, 1992.

Broadhurst CL, Cunnane SC, Crawford MA. Rift Valley lake fish and shellfish provided brain-specific nutrition for early *Homo*. Br J Nutr 1998; 79: 3–21.

Bucher H, Rampini S, James RW et al. Marked changes of lipid levels during puberty in a patient with lipoprotein lipase deficiency. Eur J Paediatr 1997; 156: 121–125.

Carlson SE, Werkman SH, Peeples JM, Cooke RJ, Tolley EA. Arachidonic acid status correlates with first year growth in preterm infants. Proc Natl Acad Sci USA 1993; 90: 1073–1077.

Chadwick PK. Schizophrenia: the positive perspective. London: Routledge, 1997.

Chang MCJ, Grange E, Rabin O, Bell JM, Allen DD, Rapoport SI. Lithium decreases turnover of arachidonate in several brain phospholipids. Neurosci Lett 1996; 220: 171–174.

Christensen O, Christensen E. Fat consumption and schizophrenia. Acta Psychiatr Scand 1988; 78: 587–591.

Claridge G. Origins of mental illness. Oxford: Basil Blackwell, 1985.

Claridge G. Single indicator of risk for schizophrenia: probable fact or likely myth. Schizophr Bull 1994; 20: 151–168.

Claridge G. Schizotypy: implications for illness and health. Oxford: Oxford University Press, 1997.

Cosmides L, Tooley J. Origins of domain specificity: the evolution of functional organisation. In: Hirschfeld LA, Gelman SA, eds. Mapping the mind: domain specificity in cognition and culture. Cambridge: Cambridge University Press, 1994: 85–116.

Crawford MA. The role of dietary fats in biology: their place in the evolution of the human brain. Nutr Rev 1992; 50: 3–11.

Crawford MA, Marsh D. The driving force: food, evolution and the future. London: Heinemann, 1989.

Crawford MA, Casperd NM, Sinclair AJ. The long chain metabolites of linoleic and linolenic acids in liver and brain in herbivores and carnivores. Comp Biochem Physiol B 1976a; 54: 395–401.

Crawford MA, Hassam AG, Williams G. Essential fatty acids and fetal brain growth. Lancet 1976b; i: 452–453.

Crawford MA, Costeloe K, Doyle W, Leighfield MJ, Lennon EA, Meadows N. Potential diagnostic value of the umbilical artery as a definition of neural fatty acid status of the foetus during its growth: the umbilical artery as a diagnostic tool. Biochem Soc Trans 1990; 18: 761–766.

Crow TJ. The two syndrome concept. Origins and current status. Schizophr Bull 1985; 11: 471–486.

Crow TJ. Psychosis as a continuum and the virogene concept. Br Med Bull 1987; 43: 754–767.

Crow TJ. Origin of psychosis and 'The Descent of Man'. Br J Psychiatry 1991; 159 (Suppl 14): 76–82.

Crow TJ. Sexual selection, Machiavellian intelligence and the origins of psychosis. Lancet 1993; 342: 594–598.

Crow TJ. A Darwinian approach to the origins of psychosis. Br J Psychiatry 1995; 167: 12–25.

Crow TJ. Language and psychosis: common evolutionary origins. Endeavour 1996a; 20: 105–109.

Crow TJ. Sexual selection as the mechanism of evolution of Machiavellian intelligence: a Darwinian theory of the origins of psychosis. J Psychopharmacol 1996b; 10: 77–87.

Davidovitch M, Patterson B, Gartside P. Head circumference measurements in children with autism. J Child Neurol 1996; 11: 389–393.

Davis RD. The gift of dyslexia. Burlingame, California: Ability Workshop Press, 1995.

Delton-Vanddenbroucke I, Grammas P, Anderson RE. Polyunsaturated fatty acid metabolism in retinal and cerebral microvascular endothelial cells. J Lipid Res 1997; 38: 147–159.

Eckel RH, Robbins RJ. Lipoprotein lipase is produced, regulated, and functional in rat brain. Proc Natl Acad Sci USA 1984; 81: 7604–7607.

Enerback S, Gimble JM. Lipoprotein lipase gene expression: physiological regulators at the transcriptional and post-transcriptional level. Biochim Biophys Acta 1993; 1169: 107–125.

Farstad M. Metabolism of fatty acids of human blood platelets: possible relation to disease. Scand J Clin Lab Invest 1993; 53: 39–45.

Feinberg I. Schizophrenia: caused by a fault in programmed synaptic elimination during adolescence? J Psychiatr Res 1982–1983; 17: 319–334.

Fodor J. The modularity of mind. Cambridge, MA: MIT Press, 1985.

Foley RA. Causes and consequences in human evolution. J R Anthropol Soc 1995; 1: 67–86.

Gardner H. Frames of mind: the theory of multiple intelligences. New York: Basic Books, 1993a.

Gardner H. Multiple intelligences: the theory in practice. New York: Basic Books, 1993b.

Gattaz WF, Brunner J. Phospholipase A_2 and the hypofrontality hypothesis of schizophrenia. Prostagland Leukotr Essent Fatty Acids 1996; 55: 109–113.

Gattaz WF, Hübner CK, Nevalainen TJ, Thuren T, Kinnunen PKJ. Increased serum phospholipase-A_2 activity in schizophrenia: a replication study. Biol Psychiatry 1990; 28: 495–501.

Gavin LA, Cavalieri RR, Moeller M, McMahon FA, Castle JN, Gulli R. Brain lipoprotein lipase is responsive to nutritional and hormonal modulation. Metabolism 1987; 36: 919–924.

Ginobili de Martinez MS, Barrantes FJ. Ca^{2+} and phospholipid-dependent protein kinase activity in rat cerebral hemispheres. Brain Res 1988; 440: 386–390.

Ginobili de Martinez MS, Rodriguez de Turco EB, Barrantes FJ. Endogenous asymmetry of rat brain lipids and dominance of the right cerebral hemisphere in free fatty acid response to electroconvulsive shock. Brain Res 1985; 339: 315–321.

Glen AIM, Glen EMT, Horrobin DF et al. A red cell membrane abnormality in a subgroup of schizophrenic patients: evidence for two diseases. Schizophr Res 1994; 12: 53–61.

Glen AIM, Cooper SJ, Rybakowski J, Vaddadi K, Brayshaw N, Horrobin DF. Membrane fatty acids, niacin flushing and clinical parameters. Prostagland Leukotr Essent Fatty Acids 1996; 15: 9–15.

Glen EMT, MacDonell LEF, Skinner FK, Ward PE, Brayshaw N, Glen AIM. Significant effects of Li-GLA supplementation in severe alcohol dependence. Prostagland Leukotr Essent Fatty Acids 1997; 57: 197.

Glen I, Skinner F, Glen E, MacDonell L. The role of essential fatty acids in alcohol dependence and tissue damage. Alcoholism: Clin Exp Res 1987; 11: 37–41.

Goldberg IJ. Lipoprotein lipase and lipolysis: central roles in lipoprotein metabolism and atherogenesis. J Lipid Res 1996; 37: 693–707.

Goldstein DB, Ruiz Linares A, Cavalli Sforza LL, Feldman MW. Genetic absolute dating based on microsatellites and the origin of modern humans. Proc Natl Acad Sci USA 1995; 92: 6723–6727.

Goodwin FK, Jamison KR. Manic-depressive illness. Oxford: Oxford University Press, 1990.

Gossett RE, Frolov AA, Roths JB, Behnke WD, Kier AB, Schroeder F. Acyl-CoA binding proteins: multiplicity and function. Lipids 1996; 31: 895–918.

Hang J, Rillema JA. Prolactin's effects on lipoprotein lipase (LPL) activity and on LPL mRNA levels in cultured mouse mammary gland explants. Proc Soc Exp Biol Med 1997; 214: 161–166.

Hershman DJ, Lieb J. The key to genius. New York: Promethus Books, 1988.

Hess DT, Patterson SI, Smith DS, Skene JHP. Neuronal growth cone collapse and inhibition of protein fatty acylation by nitric oxide. Nature 1993; 366: 562–565.

Heston LL. Psychiatric disorders in foster-home-reared children of schizophrenic mothers. Br J Psychiatry 1966; 122: 819–825.

Heston LL. The genetics of schizophrenic and schizoid diseases. Science 1970; 167: 249–256.

Holdcroft A, Oatridge A, Hajnal JV, Bydder GM. Changes in brain size in normal pregnancy. J Physiol 1997; 498: 54P.

Horai S, Hayasaka K, Kondo R, Tsugane K, Takahata N. Recent African origin of modern humans revealed by complete sequences of hominoid mitochondrial DNAs. Proc Natl Acad Sci USA 1995; 92: 532–536.

Horrobin DF. Schizophrenia as a prostaglandin deficiency disease. Lancet 1977; i: 936–937.

Horrobin DF. Schizophrenia: reconciliation of the dopamine, prostaglandin and opioid concepts and the role of the pineal. Lancet 1979; i: 529–531.

Horrobin DF. Niacin flushing, prostaglandin E and evening primrose oil. A possible objective test for monitoring therapy in schizophrenia. J Orthomolec Psychiatry 1980; 9: 33–34.

Horrobin DF. Loss of delta-6-desaturase (D6D) activity as a key factor in aging. Age 1981; 4: 139.

Horrobin DF. Essential fatty acids, prostaglandins, and alcoholism: an overview. Alcoholism: Clin Exp Res 1987; 11: 2–9.

Horrobin DF. Nutritional and medical importance of gamma-linolenic acid. Prog Lipid Res 1992a; 31: 163–194.

Horrobin DF. The relationship between schizophrenia and essential fatty acids and eicosanoid metabolism. Prostagland Leukotr Essent Fatty Acids 1992b; 46: 71–77.

Horrobin DF. A possible relationship between dyslexia and schizophrenia, two disorders in which membrane phospholipid (PL) metabolism is disturbed. Schizophr Res 1996; 18: 156.

Horrobin DF. Overview: the role of brain lipid metabolism in schizophrenia. Prostagland Leukotr Essent Fatty Acids 1997; 57: 208.

Horrobin DF. The membrane phospholipid hypothesis as a biochemical basis for the neurodevelopmental concept of schizophrenia. Schizophr Res 1998a; 30: 193–208.

Horrobin DF. Schizophrenia: the illness that made us human. Med Hypotheses 1998b; 50: 269–288.

Horrobin DF. The phospholipid concept of psychiatric disorders and its relationship to the neurodevelopmental concept of schizophrenia. In: Glen I, Peet M, Horrobin DF, eds. Phospholipid spectrum disorder in psychiatry. Carnforth: Marius Press, 1999: 3–20.

Horrobin DF, Manku MS. Possible role of prostaglandin E1 in the affective disorders and in alcoholism. Br Med J 1980; 280: 1363–1366.

Horrobin DF, Ally AI, Karmali RA, Karmazyn M, Manku MS, Morgan RO. Prostaglandins and schizophrenia: further discussion of the evidence. Psychol Med 1978a; 8: 43–48.

Horrobin DF, Mtabaji JP, Manku MS, Karmazyn M. Lithium as a regulator of hormone-stimulated prostaglandin synthesis. Relevance to manic-depressive illness. In: Johnson FN, Johnson S, eds. Lithium in Medical Practice. Baltimore: University Park Press, 1978b; 243–246.

Horrobin DF, Glen AIM, Vaddadi K. The membrane hypothesis of schizophrenia. Schizophr Res 1994; 13: 195–207.

Horrobin DF, Glen AIM, Hudson CJ. Possible relevance of phospholipid abnormalities and genetic interactions in psychiatric disorders: the relationship between dyslexia and schizophrenia. Med Hypotheses 1995; 45: 605–613.

Hudson CJ, Kennedy JL, Gotowicc A et al. Genetic variant near cytosolic phospholipase A2 associated with schizophrenia. Schizophr Res 1996; 21: 111–116.

Hudson CJ, Lin A, Cogan S, Cashman F, Warsh JJ. The niacin challenge test: clinical manifestation of altered transmembrane signal transduction in schizophrenia? Biol Psychiatry 1997; 41: 507–513.

Huttenlocher PR, deCourten C, Garey LJ, van der Loos H. Synaptogenesis in human visual cortex: evidence for synapse elimination during normal development. Neurosci Lett 1982; 33: 247–252.

Inoue A, Sanes JR. Lamina-specific connectivity in the brain: regulation by N-cadherin, neurotrophins, and glycoconjugates. Science 1997; 276: 1428–1431.

Jamison KR. An unquiet mind: a memoir of moods and madness. London: Picador, 1995.

Jemaa R, Tuzet S, Betoulle D, Apfelbaum M, Fumeron F. Hind III polymorphism of the lipoprotein lipase gene and plasma lipid response to low calorie diet. Int J Obes 1997; 21: 280–283.

Jiang WG, Hiscox S, Hallett MB, Horrobin DF, Mansel RE, Puntis MCA. Regulation of the expression of E-cadherin on human cancer cells by gamma-linolenic acid (GLA). Cancer Res 1995; 55: 5043–5048.

Karlsson JL. The biologic basis of schizophrenia. Springfield, Illinois: Thomas, 1966.

Karlsson JL. Inheritance of schizophrenia. Acta Psychiatr Scand Suppl 1974; 274: 1–116.

Kasanin J. The acute schizoaffective psychoses. Am J Psychiatry 1933; 90: 97–126.

Kaufmann WE, Worley PF, Pegg J, Bremer M, Isakson P. COX-2, a synaptically induced enzyme, is expressed by excitatory neurons at postsynaptic sites in rat cerebral cortex. Proc Natl Acad Sci USA 1996; 93: 2317–2321.

Kay D, WK, Roth M, Atkinson MW, Stephens DA, Garside RF. Genetic hypotheses and environmental factors in the light of psychiatric morbidity in the families of schizophrenics. Br J Psychiatry 1975; 127: 109–118.

Kendell RE. Diagnosis and classification of functional psychoses. Br Med Bull 1987; 43: 499–513.

Kendell RE. Clinical validity. Psychol Med 1989; 19: 45–55.

Kendler KS, Maclean CJ, O'Neill A et al. Evidence for a schizophrenia vulnerability locus on chromosome 8p in the Irish study of high-density schizophrenia families. Am J Psychol 1996; 153: 134–154.

Kety SS, Wender PH, Jacobsen B et al. Mental illness in the biological and adoptive relatives of schizophrenic adoptees. II. Replication of the Copenhagen study in the rest of Denmark. Arch Gen Psychiatry 1994; 51: 442–455.

Kirk SA, Kutchins H. The selling of DSM: the rhetoric of science in psychiatry. New York: Aldine and Gruyter, 1992.

Koletzko B. Fats for brains. Eur J Clin Nutr 1992; 46 (Suppl 1): S51–S62.

Krings M, Stone A, Paabo S. Neandertal DNA sequences and the origin of modern humans. Cell 1997; 90: 19–30.

Laposata M, Reich EL, Majerus PW. Arachidonyl-CoA synthetase. Separation from non-specific acyl-CoA synthetase and distribution in various cells and tissues. J Biol Chem 1985; 260: 11016–11020.

Lucas A, Morley R, Cole TJ, Lister G, Leeson-Payne C. Breast milk and subsequent intelligence quotient in children born preterm. Lancet 1992; 339: 261–264.

Ludwig AM. The price of greatness. New York: Guilford Press, 1995.

Mahadik SP, Evans DR. Essential fatty acids in the treatment of schizophrenia. Drugs Today 1997; 33: 5–17.

Mahadik SP, Gowda S. Antioxidants in the treatment of schizophrenia. Drugs Today 1996; 32: 553–565.

Makrides M, Neumann M, Simmer K, Pater J, Gibson R. Are long-chain polyunsaturated fatty acids essential nutrients in infancy? Lancet 1995; 345: 1463–1468.

Martin RE, Wickham JQ. Membrane docosahexaenoic acid content influences A-type phospholipase activity in PC12 cell nerve growth cones. Soc Neurosci 1996; 22: 37.

Maudsley H. Heredity, variation and genius. London: Bale and Daniellson, 1908.

Mead JF, Fulco AJ. The unsaturated and polyunsaturated fatty acids in health and disease. Springfield, Illinois: Charles C. Thomas, 1976.

Mead JF, Alfin-Slater RB, Howton DR, Popjak G. Lipids: chemistry, biochemistry, and nutrition. New York: Plenum Press, 1986.

Mellor JE, Laugharne JDE, Peet M. Schizophrenic symptoms and dietary intake of n-3 fatty acids. Schizophr Res 1995; 18: 85–86.

Mellor JE, Laugharne JDE, Peet M. Omega-3 fatty acid supplementation in schizophrenia patients. Hum Psychopharmacol 1996; 11: 39–46.

Milligan S, Clare A. Depression and how to survive it. London: Ebury Press, 1993.

Mithen S. The prehistory of the mind: a search for the origins of art, religion and science. London: Thames and Hudson, 1996.

Morgan E. The descent of the child. London: Souvenir Press, 1994.

Morgan E. The aquatic ape hypothesis. London: Souvenir Press, 1997.

Murthy V, Julien P, Gagne C. Molecular pathobiology of the human lipoprotein lipase gene. Pharmacol Ther 1996; 70: 101–135.

Myers-Payne SC, Hubell T, Pu L et al. Isolation and characterization of two fatty acid binding proteins from mouse brain. J Neurochem 1996; 66: 1648–1656.

Negre-Aminou P, Nemenoff RA, Wood MR, de la Houssaye BA, Pfenninger KH. Characterization of phospholipase A_2 activity enriched in the nerve growth cone. J Neurochem 1996; 67: 2599–2608.

Nelson RJ, Demas GE, Huang PL et al. Behavioural abnormalities in male mice lacking neuronal nitric oxide synthase. Nature 1995; 378: 383–386.

Noble W, Davidson I. Human evolution: language and mind. Cambridge: Cambridge University Press, 1996.

O'Donovan DK. Hypothyroid nails and evolution. Lancet 1996a; 348: 750–751.

O'Donovan DK. Hypothyroid nails and evolution. Lancet 1996b; 348: 1261–1262.

Oloyede OB, Folyan AT, Odutuga AA. Effects of low-iron status and deficiency of essential fatty acids on some biochemical constituents of rat brain. Biochem Int 1992; 27: 913–922.

Omawari N, Mahmood S, Dewhurst M, Stevens EJ, Tomlinson DR. Deficient nitric oxide is responsible for reduced nerve blood flow in diabetic rats: prevention by essential fatty acids. Br J Pharmacol 1995; 116: 63.

Pediconi MF, Rodriguez de Turco EB. Free fatty acid content and release kinetics as manifestations of cerebral lateralization in mouse brain. J Neurochem 1984; 43: 1–7.

Peet M, Laugharne JDE, Horrobin DF, Reynolds GP. Arachidonic acid: a common link in the biology of schizophrenia? Arch Gen Psychiatry 1994; 51: 665–666.

Peet M, Laugharne JDE, Mellor J, Ramchand CN. Essential fatty acid deficiency in erythrocyte membranes from chronic schizophrenic patients, and the clinical effects of dietary supplementation. Prostagland Leukotr Essent Fatty Acids 1996; 55: 71–75.

Peet M, Laugharne JDE, Ahluwalia N, Mellor J. Fatty acid supplementation in schizophrenic patients. Schizophr Res 1997a; 24: 209.

Peet M, Poole J, Laugharne J. Infant feeding and the development of schizophrenia. Schizophr Res 1997b; 24: 255.

Pettegrew JW, Keshavan MS, Minshew NJ. ^{31}P nuclear magnetic resonance spectroscopy: neurodevelopment and schizophrenia. Schizophr Bull 1993; 19: 35–53.

Purves D, Lichtman JW. Elimination of synapses in the developing nervous system. Science 1980; 210: 153–157.

Raine A, Lencz T, Mednick SA. Schizotypal personality. Cambridge: Cambridge University Press, 1995.

Ramchand CN, Wei J, Lee KH, Peet M. Phospholipase A_2 gene polymorphism and associated biochemical alterations in schizophrenia. In: Glen I, Peet M, Horrobin DF, eds. Phospholipid spectrum disorder in psychiatry. Carnforth: Marius Press, 1999: 31–37.

Richardson AJ. Dyslexia, handedness and syndromes of psychosis-proneness. Int J Psychophysiol 1994; 18: 251–263.

Richardson AJ, Cox IJ, Sargentoni J, Puri BK. Abnormal cerebral phospholipid metabolism in dyslexia indicated by phosphorous-31 magnetic resonance spectroscopy. NMR Biomed 1997; 10: 309–314.

Roede M, Wind J, Patrick J, Reynolds V. The aquatic ape: fact or fiction? London: Souvenir Press, 1991.

Rose L, Marshall F. Meat eating, hominid sociality, and home bases revisited. Curr Anthropol 1996; 37: 307–338.

Rosenthal D, Kety S. The transmission of schizophrenia. Oxford: Pergamon, 1968.

Ross BM, Hudson C, Erlich J, Warsh JJ, Kish SJ. Increased phospholipid breakdown in schizophrenia: evidence for the involvement of a calcium-independent phospholipase A_2. Arch Gen Psychiatry 1997; 54: 487–494.

Rousselot P, Heintz N, Nottebohm F. Expression of brain lipid binding protein in the brain of the adult canary and its implications for adult neurogenesis. J Comp Neurol 1997; 385: 415–426.

Shirai K, Saito Y, Yoshida S, Matsuoka N. Existence of lipoprotein lipase in rat brain microvessels. Tohoku J Exp Med 1986; 149: 449–450.

Shorter E. A history of psychiatry: from the era of the asylum to the age of Prozac. New York: John Wiley, 1997.

Silverton L. Crime and the schizophrenia spectrum. Acta Psychiatr Scand 1988; 78: 72–81.

Smalheiser NR, Dissanayake S, Kapil A. Rapid regulation of neurite outgrowth and retraction by phospholipase A_2-derived arachidonic acid and its metabolites. Brain Res 1996; 721: 39–48.

Stephens DA, Atkinson MW, Kay DWK, Roth M, Garside RF. Psychiatric morbidity in parents and sibs of schizophrenics and non-schizophrenics. Br J Psychiatry 1975; 127: 97–108.

Stordy BJ. Benefit of docosahexaenoic acid supplements to dark adaptation in dyslexics. Lancet 1995; 346: 385.

Stordy BJ. Dark adaption, docosahexaenoic acid and dyslexia. International Conference on highly unsaturated fatty acids in nutrition and disease prevention. Barcelona, Spain, 4–6 November, 1996.

Takahashi R, Ito H, Horrobin DF. Fatty acid composition of serum phospholipids in an elderly institutionalized Japanese population. J Nutr Sci Vitaminol (Tokyo) 1991; 37: 401–409.

Tavangar K, Murata Y, Patel S et al. Developmental regulation of lipoprotein lipase in rats. Am J Physiol 1992; 262: E330–E337.

Trinkaus E. The Neanderthals. London: Pimlico, 1994.

Udwin O, Yule W. Expressive language of children with William's syndrome. Am J Med Genet Suppl 1990; 6: 108–114.

Vance DE, Vance J. Biochemistry of lipids, lipoproteins and membranes. Amsterdam: Elsevier, 1991.

Varma SL, Zain AM, Singh S. Psychiatric morbidity in first-degree relatives. Am J Med Genet 1997; 74: 7–11.

Verhaegen M. The aquatic ape theory: evidence and a possible scenario. Med Hypotheses 1985; 16: 17–32.

Vigilant LM, Stoneking M, Harpending H, Hawkes K, Wilson A. African populations and the evolution of human mitochondrial DNA. Science 1991; 253: 1503–1507.

Ward PE, Sutherland J, Glen EMT, Glen AIM. Niacin skin flush in schizophrenia: a preliminary report. Schizophr Res 1998; 29: 269–274.

Willats P, Forsyth JS, DiModugno MK, Varma S, Colvin M. Improved problem solving at 10 months by infants fed a formula supplemented with long-chain polyunsaturated fatty acids. Prostagland Leukotr Essent Fatty Acids 1997; 57: 188.

World Health Organization. Schizophrenia: an international follow-up study. New York: John Wiley and Sons, 1979.

Yamagata K, Andreasson KI, Kaufmann WE, Barnes CA, Worley PF. Expression of a mitogen-inducible cyclooxygenase in brain neurons: regulation by synaptic activity and glucocorticoids. Neuron 1993; 11: 371–386.

Yao JK, van Kammen DP, Gurklis JA. Abnormal incorporation of arachidonic acid into platelets of drug-free patients with schizophrenia. Psychiatry Res 1996; 60: 11–21.

Yoshida S, Miyazaki M, Takeshita M et al. Functional changes of rat brain microsomal membrane surface after learning task depending on dietary fatty acids. J Neurochem 1997a; 68: 1269–1277.

Yoshida S, Yasuda A, Kawazato H et al. Synaptic vesicle ultrastructural changes in the rat hippocampus induced by a combination of α-linolenate deficiency and a learning task. J Neurochem 1997b; 68: 1261–1268.

INDEX

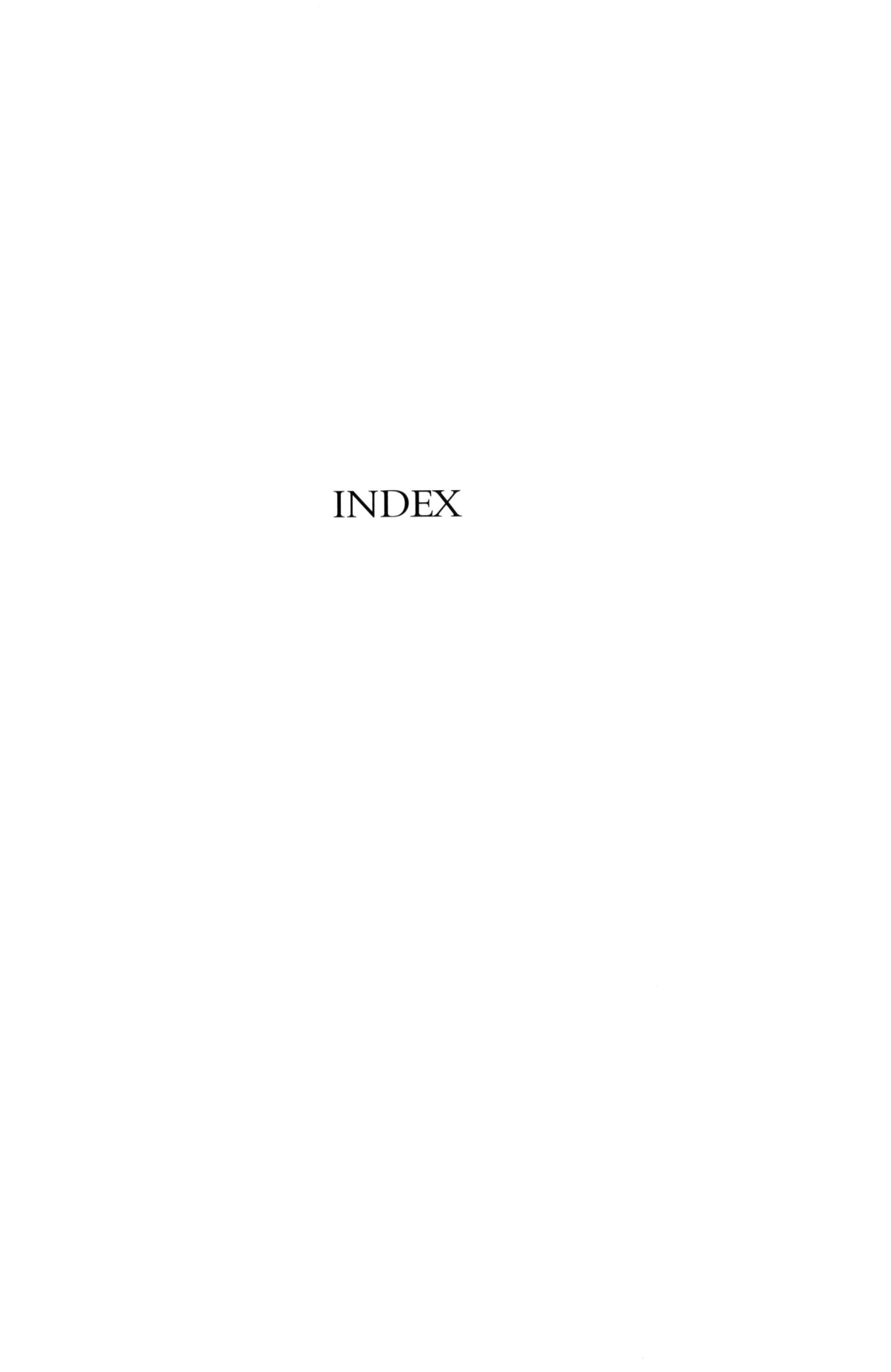

Note: for indexing purposes, ω (as in ω-3, ω-6) has been indexed as n.

ABC Movement Assessment Battery for Children, 256–257
Abnormal Involuntary Movement Scale (AIMS), 82–83, 191, 280, 286, 287
Absolute total energy intake (ATE), 215–216
Acetylcholine, 3
Achievement, 304, 308
Action potential, 81
Acyl
  bond, 32
  chains, 199
  CoA derivatives, 308
  CoA synthetase, 303, 307, 311
  groups, 5, 6
Acyltransferases, 7, 16, 302, 303, 307, 310, 311, 312
Adenine nucleotide status, 77
Adenosine triphosphate (ATP), 45, 49, 50, 76, 244
Adenosine triphosphatase systems, 153, 154
Adipose
  scores, 202
  tissue, 211, 309, 310,
Adolescence, 4
Adopted away studies, 305, 311
Adrenal medullary cells, 195
Adrenergic systems, 196
Adrenic acid (AdrA) (*see also*: 22:4n-6), 7, 35, 58, 251
Affective disorders (*see also*: Depression; Mania; Manic-depressive disorder), 3, 202, 288, 289, 290, 361
After effect
  motion, 123, 127
  tilt, 123, 127
  visual, 123
Age, 10, 12, 13, 200, 280, 288
Aggression, 197, 198, 201, 205, 214
Aging, 12, 288
Agitation, 183
Alanine, 90, 91, 93
Albumin, 9, 15, 78, 79, 80, 303, 304, 308
Alcohol, 84, 91, 100, 102, 147, 148, 149, 171, 173, 200, 202, 214, 217, 251, 281, 282, 289
  withdrawal, 202
Alcoholic hallucinosis, 145
Alcoholism, 90, 145, 197, 198, 201, 202, 280, 290, 305, 308, 311
  onset, 198
Aldosterone, 146
Alkanes, 192
Allergies, 254, 264

Alzheimer's disease, 3, 26, 52, 105, 275–278
Amino acid
  balance, 90
  transport, 90, 92
Amino acids, 3, 31, 77, 90, 91
  aromatic, 89
  brain uptake, 96
  essential, 89
  branched-chain, 89
  large neutral (LNAAs), 89, 90, 92, 95
  nonessential, 89
α-Aminobutyrate, 90, 93
γ-Aminobutyric acid (*see*: GABA)
Aminophospholipids, 60
Amphetamine, 27
Amyotrophic lateral sclerosis, 105
Anandamide, 154, 272
Anger, 205
Anhedonia, 182
Anorexia, 201
Antioxidant
  capacity, 78, 79, 100
  cofactors, 10
  defence, 100, 101, 103, 106
  defence system (AODS), 57, 77, 78, 80, 84, 103, 289, 290, 293
  effects, 114, 115
  efficiency, 84
  enzymes, 31, 79
  potential, 99, 101
  properties, 103
  supplements, 107
  systems, 12, 78
  treatment, 84, 104, 107
Antioxidants, 10, 16, 80, 99, 106–107, 115, 150, 151, 167–186, 204, 256, 267, 286, 287, 290, 293
  adjunctive use, 107
  dietary, 84, 103
  exogenous nonenzymatic, 106
  hydrophilic, 10
  plasma, 80
  primary lipophilic, 10
Anti-Parkinsonian drugs, 3
Antipsychotic drugs (*see also*: Neuroleptics), 99, 100, 102
Anxiety, 162, 183, 202, 217
  social, 237
Amacrine cells, 123
Amine metabolites, 146,
Amphetamines, 134, 289
Amygdala, 271
Amyloid plaque, 277

Index

Amyloidogenesis, 277
Amyloidogenic peptides, 275
Apathy, 95, 201
Apomorphine, 27, 42
Apoptosis, 4
    control, 12
    selective, 12
Appetite, 202
Aqueous methyl nicotinate (AMN) (*see also*: Niacin), 142–143
Arachidonates (*see also*: Arachidonic acid)
    mobilization, 140
    pathway, 140
    turnover, 307
Arachidonic acid (AA) (*see also*: 20:4n-6), 5, 8–16, 57, 63, 64, 65, 100, 113, 115, 126, 127, 139, 141, 146, 150, 154, 165, 168, 181, 187, 201, 204, 225, 226, 227, 232, 251, 253, 264, 265, 267, 271, 280, 281, 282, 285, 287, 293, 301, 303, 306, 309, 311, 312
    accumulation, 10
    administration, 13
    bimodal distribution, 76, 147, 150
    brain, 31
    breast milk, 13
    cascade, 106
    cell signalling, 11
    concentration, 76, 77, 159, 289
    conversion, 11
    decreases, 69, 76
    deficit, 163
    esterification, 67
    foetal supply, 13
    formation, 13, 14
    free, 307
    incorporation into phospholipids, 13, 62, 64, 68, 127, 308, 310
    levels, 11, 13, 69, 104, 124, 125, 126, 143, 147, 149, 150, 154, 160, 162, 169, 282, 306
    loss, 15, 244
    metabolic pathways, 64, 67
    metabolism, 126, 145
    metabolites, 65, 123–126, 285
    mobilization, 11
    neuronal production, 9
    oestrogen effects, 13
    oxidative damage, 77, 80
    platelet, 64
    platelet turnover, 23
    production, 10
    red cell membrane, 11, 62
    release, 8, 10, 15, 26, 32, 33, 65, 66, 77, 187, 272, 307, 310
    removal rate, 15
    supplementation, 160
    synthesis, 12, 64, 159
    transport, 310
    unavailability, 139
Arachidonyl CoA-synthetase, 307
Arginine, 90, 93
Art, 301, 312
Arthritis, 11
Ascorbic acid (*see*: Vitamin C)
Aspartate, 90, 93
Atopy, 226, 251
Attention, 4, 14, 127, 182, 229, 230, 254
    defects, 14
    deficit disorder (ADD), 252
    deficit hyperactivity disorder (ADHD), 14, 123, 128, 196, 226, 228, 230, 232, 251, 253, 254, 257, 258, 263
    deficits, 15
    disorder, 122
    sustained, 128
Attentional
    abnormalities, 256
    disorders, 226
    problems, 227, 237
Atypical phasic psychosis, 67
Auditory
    association area, 228
    function, 183, 231
    pathways, 228
    system, 228
    temporal coding, 220
Autism, 52, 254, 302
Autoimmune
    attack, 229
    disorders, 226, 227, 254
    dysfunctions, 57
    functions, 228, 231
Asperger's syndrome, 228, 271–273
Asthma, 226, 264
Axonal growth, 229

Ban-I
    digestion, 34
    dimorphic site, 34, 35
    site, 307
Basal ganglia, 26, 49, 51, 102
Batten's disease, 258
Bayley Scales, 161
Beck Depression Inventory, 215
Behaviour, 75, 198–200
    exploratory, 201

Behavioural
    changes, 69, 212
    disturbances, 80, 81, 189, 196, 197
    dysfunction, 264
    effects, 160
    problems, 15, 23, 163, 230, 265
    rating scores, 61
Beliefs, 187, 227, 238, 244
Bilirubin, 79, 80
Biogenic amine function, 195
Bipolar disorder (*see also*: Affective disorder; Mania; Depression; Manic-depressive disorder), 15, 52, 82–83, 139, 152, 153, 274
Birth
    order, 168, 171, 174
    seasonality, 4–5, 14, 168, 171,
    weight, 159, 161, 162, 173, 229
Blood–brain barrier, 9, 81, 90, 93–95, 106, 199
Blood pressure, 217, 218
Blunted affect, 90
Body weight, 202, 292
Bond dissociation energy, 102
Borderline
    handicap, 145, 147, 151, 153
    personality disorder, 305
Bottle-fed babies, 10
Brain, 211, 213
    abnormalities, 290
    asymmetry, 16
    connectivity, 310
    development, 12, 14, 15, 103, 104, 145, 154, 165, 167, 173, 174, 175, 229, 302, 307
    dysfunction, 170
    function, 96, 198–200, 263, 265, 267, 289, 300–301
    growth, 13, 159, 308, 309
    lateralization (*see also*: Cerebral lateralization), 299
    metabolism, 299
    morphology, 4, 12, 25–26
    size, 16, 300, 301–303, 309, 310, 311, 312
    structure, 229, 313
    temperature, 15
    tissue, autopsied, 58
    volume, 290
Breast, 309, 311, 313
    feeding, 4, 10, 13, 14, 15, 159–166, 173, 174, 230, 302, 310
    milk (*see*: Milk)
Brief Psychiatric Rating Scale (BPRS), 51, 61, 82–83
    anxiety–depression subscale, 51
    hostility–suspicious subscale, 52
British Ability Scales (BAS), 231, 234

Bromide, 145
Bunney-Hamburg scale, 61

Cadherins, 310
Calcium, 8, 32, 62, 292
    binding, 146
    channels, 203, 286
    dynamics, 64
    dysregulation, 84
    intracellular, 285
    related cell signalling, 114
    mobilizers, 32
Calmodulin, 114
Caloric intake, 81, 100, 102, 106, 150, 168, 173
Cancer, 174
Cannabis psychosis, 145, 154
Cannabinoid receptors, 145, 154
Carbohydrates, 77, 149, 173
Carbonyl moieties, 77
Cardiolipin, 78
Cardiovascular
    disease, 174, 217–218
    function, 229
β-Carotene, 10, 78, 80, 101, 105, 149, 150, 151, 168
Carrier molecules, 90
Catalase (CAT), 78, 79, 100, 101
Catatonic stupor, 146
Catecholamine
    function, 195
    metabolism, 103
Catecholamines, 10, 13
    oxidation, 77
Caudate nucleus, 76, 78
Cell adhesion molecules (CAMS), 12
Cell
    death, 78, 80, 81, 105, 292, 293
    differentiation, 62
    proliferation, 62
    signalling, 3, 5, 8, 10, 11, 113, 303, 308, 310
Cellular
    antioxidant defence, 100, 101
    defence systems, 267
    dysfunction, 218
    oxygen, 77
    toxicity, 77
    transport processes, 31
    uptake, 8
Cerebral ventricles, 105
Cerebellum, 160, 229, 271
Cerebral
    asymmetry (*see also*: Handedness; Laterality), 244, 299
    lateralization, 182, 226, 228

Cerebrospinal fluid (CSF), 19, 102, 103, 146, 197, 198, 199, 200, 201
Cerebrovascular disease, 288
Childhood
  behaviour, 14
  functional abnormalities, 4
Chlorpromazine, 65, 94, 103, 114, 125, 134, 145, 146, 148, 149, 187, 189
Cholesterol, 3, 5, 79, 145, 149, 150, 168, 197, 198–200, 213, 214, 216, 281, 287
  acyltransferase, 114
  concentrations, 199
  esters, 3, 7, 289, 290
  induced condensation, 199
  intake, 196, 199
  level, 196, 198, 204–205
  lowering, 196
Choline, 5, 6
Choreiform movements, 290
Choreoathetoid movements, 286
Choroid plexus, 308
Chromosome
  1, 11, 153, 307
  6, 15, 227
  8, 9
  21 trisomy, 105
Chromosomal abnormalities, 153
Chronic oxidative stress (*see* Oxidative stress)
Clomipramine, 213
Clonazepam, 291
Clozapine, 11, 103, 113–119, 181, 187, 189, 290
Clumsiness (*see also*: Dyspraxia), 271
Cocaine
  addicts, 134
  users, 26–27
Coenzyme A (CoA), 7, 303
  derivatives, 307
Cognitive
  deficits, 163, 229
  development, 160–162, 230, 238, 248
  disorganization, 234, 237
  dysfunction, 290
  function, 225, 229, 231, 265
  impairment, 277
  performance, 275
  processing capacity, 129
  skills, 81
  style, 227
Communication, 122
Comprehension, 183
Comprehensive Psychopathological Rating Scale (CPRS), 91
Computerised tomography (CT), 163, 290

Confusion, 234
Conjugated dienes, 80
Connectivity, 228, 301–303, 308, 310, 311
Conners Parent Rating Scale, 257, 264
Contrast sensitivity, 125–127
Coordination (*see also*: Motor coordination), 16
Corn oil, 159, 191, 201, 204–205
Coronary artery disease, 196
Corpus callosum, 52
Cortex, 26, 101
  cingulate, 51
  dorsal prefrontal, 49, 50, 103
  frontal, 23, 26, 39, 49, 58, 76, 78, 80, 104, 105, 160, 195, 197, 199, 200, 275, 277
  fronto-parietal, 49
  motor, 51
  parietal, 49, 51, 275, 277
  parieto-occipital, 47, 51
  prefrontal, 25, 42, 49–52, 80, 89
  temporal, 23, 25, 26, 49, 51, 80, 104
  temporoparietal, 49
Corticotrophin releasing factor (CRF), 200, 201
  antagonists, 201
  secretion, 200
Cortisol, 13
Cot deaths, 160
Cranial capacity (*see also*: Brain), 204
Creatinine kinase activity, 96
Creativity, 299, 302, 305, 308, 311, 312
Cretinism, 308
Cyclic nucleotides, 8
Cyclic adenosine monophosphate (cAMP), 181, 285
Cyclooxygenase, 65, 67, 153, 272, 286, 302, 303, 307, 310, 311
  pathway, 142, 151, 154
  products, 67
  system, 126, 146
Cyclooxygenase 2 (COX-2), 12
  expression, 12
Cysteine, 90, 93
Cytidine diphosphate (CDP), 63
Cytoarchitectonic abnormalities, 229
Cytochrome-c oxidase, 78
Cytokine production, 35
Cytoskeleton, 60
Cytotoxic products, 39, 42

Dark adaptation, 126–128, 133, 134, 135, 230, 244, 254–256
  testing, 127, 128

Deacylation, 187
Death
   sudden, 160
   violent, 195
Delusions, 121, 122, 145, 182, 227
Dendrites, 5, 159
Dendritic
   growth, 229
   pruning, 310
   spines, 105
Depression, 96, 152, 153
   lipid hypothesis, 212–216
   postpartum, 202
   premorbid, 201
   psychotic (*see also*: Affective disorder; Bipolar disorder), 52, 57, 141, 142, 143, 146, 154, 195–210, 211–221, 227
Depressive disorder (*see also*: Bipolar disorder), 65
Desaturase, 251
   Δ-5, 289, 290
   Δ-6, 288, 289, 290
Desaturation, 229, 251, 258, 266
Desipramine, 213
Dexamethasone suppression test (DST), 142, 200
Diabetes, 107, 174, 216, 217, 251, 280, 281, 282, 288, 289, 290, 291, 305
Diacylglycerol (DAG), 3, 6, 8, 32, 62, 63, 64, 65, 100, 175, 303
   accumulation, 66, 67
   kinase, 66, 67
   membrane-permeant, 62
   phosphorylation, 66
   thrombin-stimulated increase, 66
Diazepam receptor, 31
Diencephalon, 80
Diet (*see also*: Food), 11, 15, 64, 79, 80, 81, 104, 106, 107, 128, 147, 148, 149, 160, 190, 197, 204, 211, 212, 214–216, 256, 265, 266, 280, 301, 306, 309, 310, 311
   cultural differences, 167–180
   high-calorie, 84
   low calorie, 84
   maternal, 159, 160
   socioeconomic differences, 167–180
   vegetarian, 251
Dietary
   changes, 312–313
   deficiency, 33
   deprivation (*see also*: Starvation), 160
   factors, 84
   patterns, 170
   questionnaire, 148
   restraint, 259
   stress, 147
Digestive enzymes, 32
Dihomo-γ-linolenic acid (DGLA) (*see also*: 20:3n-6), 7, 8–11, 13, 57, 141, 191, 281, 282, 285, 286, 288, 289, 307, 308, 311, 312
   breast milk (*see also*: Milk), 13
   neuronal production, 9
   release from Sn2 position, 10, 15
Dinucleotide repeat sequence, 33
Diphenylacetic acid, 42
Distractibility, 129, 254
Disulphhydryl groups, 101
DNA, 77, 100, 299
   breakdown, 105
   oxidation, 99, 101
   peroxidative breakdown, 100, 101
   repair, 78
Docosahexanoate, 277
Docosahexaenoic acid (DHA) (*see also*: 22:6n-3), 7, 8–15, 35, 57, 102, 107, 115, 124, 126, 127, 133, 134, 149, 165, 168, 182, 187, 190, 191, 192, 195, 199, 200, 201, 204, 211, 212, 213, 215, 218, 225, 226, 233, 238, 244, 248, 251, 253, 254, 255, 256, 259, 264, 265, 267, 287, 301, 302, 303, 306, 307, 309, 311, 312
   accumulation, 160
   bimodal distribution, 76, 147, 150
   brain, 31, 212
   breast milk, 13
   cell signalling, 11
   circulating, 159
   concentrations, 159, 217
   deficiencies, 126, 127, 173, 212, 217
   deficit, 163
   depletion, 214, 252
   formation, 14
   free, 307
   incorporation, 13, 127, 308
   levels, 11, 104, 105, 147, 150, 154, 159, 160, 161, 162, 169, 175, 190, 196, 202, 213, 216, 271, 306
   loss, 15, 127, 244
   neuronal production, 8
   oestrogen effects, 13
   red cell membrane, 11, 62
   reduction, 290
   release, 8, 10, 310
   removal rate, 15
   retina, 212
   sperm, 212
   supplementation, 126, 160, 161, 212, 256, 286–287, 230

supply, 129
synthesis, 159
Docosapentaenoic acid (DPA) (*see also*: 22:5n-6), 58, 217
Dopamine (DA), 3, 89, 92, 106, 123, 181, 195, 285
    abnormalities, 123
    activity, 123
    autoinhibitory actions, 286
    autoreceptors, 212, 285
    autoxidation, 77
    blockade, 113, 114, 289, 290
    downregulation, 125
    dysfunction, 121
    function, 27, 81, 134
    impaired, 81
    levels, 122, 123, 128
    loss, 127
    mediated toxicity, 77
    metabolism, 77, 89, 90, 189, 285
    metabolites, 125, 126, 146
    neurones, 89, 93
    receptor sensitivity, 32, 39, 42
    receptor synergism, 106
    receptors, 26, 134, 175, 189, 285, 286
    regulation, 121
    release, 32, 39, 42, 285
    sensitive adenylate cyclase, 42
    synthesis, 32, 39, 93, 95, 129
    system, 26, 134
    turnover, 89
    uptake, 105
Dopaminergic
    activity, 27, 42, 135
    control, 128
    functions, 286
    hyperresponsivity, 53
    mechanisms, 113
    overactivity, 285
    potentiating effects, 26
    signalling, 26
    transmission, 27, 39, 42, 89, 93, 134
Down's syndrome, 105, 151
Drugs of abuse, 173
Duration of illness, 63
Dutch famine, 13, 163
Dyskinesia
    orofacial, 290
    spontaneous, 279
Dyskinesias, 161, 285–296
Dyslexia, 12, 14, 15, 124, 126, 127, 128, 181–188, 225–241, 243–249, 251–260, 305, 307, 311, 312
    gene, 15

Dysphasia, 228
Dyspraxia, 14, 161, 226, 228, 251–260, 272

Eating habits, 215–216
Ectopias, 228, 229, 253
Eczema, 226, 251, 264
Edinburgh Postpartum Depression Scale, 202
Efalex™, 231, 256
Efamol™, 286, 291
Efamol Marine™, 288, 290
Efavit™, 286
Egg yolks, 10
Eicosanoid
    cascade, 32, 64
    imbalances, 195
    metabolism, 306
    production, 32, 267
    synthesis, 24
Eicosanoids, 8, 12, 263, 265, 272, 285, 306, 307
    biosynthesis, 67–68
    formation, 68
Eicosapentaenoic acid (EPA) (*see also* 20:5:n-3), 7, 8, 9, 11–13, 15, 57, 107, 190, 195, 196, 200, 201, 212, 251, 253, 265, 267, 285, 287, 307, 308, 311, 312, 313
    brain, 31
    breast milk, 13
    deficiency, 186
    loss from Sn2 position, 10
    neuronal production, 8
    supplementation, 286
Elation, 146
Electron transport chain, 77, 78
Electroretinogram (ERG), 11, 123, 124, 129, 133–136, 160, 163
    a-wave, 123, 124, 133, 135
    amplitude, 133
    b-wave, 133, 134, 135
    oscillatory potentials, 134
    response variability, 134
    responsiveness, 134
    temporal pattern, 133
Elongation, 229, 251, 258, 266
Elongase, 251
Emotional withdrawal, 95
Endoperoxides, 67
Endoplasmic reticulum, 266–267
Energy, 308, 312
    intake, 215
    metabolism, 244
    supply, 258
Environment–gene interactions, 8

Environmental factors, 3, 10
Epilepsy, 115, 271, 272
Epinephrine, 195
Erythema (see also: Flushing), 141
Essential amino acids, 301
Essential fatty acids (EFAs) (see also: Fatty acids;
    Long-chain polyunsaturated fatty acids;
    Polyunsaturated fatty acids), 5, 6–16, 133–136,
    167–180, 197, 214–216, 225–241, 231,
    263–269, 285–296, 301, 306, 311
  abnormalities, 14, 279
  availability, 11, 145
  basal levels, 16
  bimodal distribution, 145
  brain supply, 15, 16
  brain-specific, 9, 14, 15
  coenzyme A derivatives, 15
  deficiency, 10, 124, 183, 228, 229, 232, 233, 234,
    237, 238, 244, 258, 264, 266, 267
  depletion, 13
  dietary, 11, 15, 103
  estimation, 125
  formation, rate, 15
  free form, 10
  incorporation, 13, 14, 15
  intake, 11, 16, 64, 211–224
  metabolism, 12, 229, 254, 258, 264, 286, 288, 289,
    293, 294, 313
  mobilization, 13
  oxidation, 10
  peroxidative breakdown, 104
  release, 16
  removal, 15
  schizophrenia, 31–32
  supplementation, 76, 84, 124, 214, 226, 230, 286
  supply, 12, 14, 15, 16
  synthesis, 13
  treatment, 14, 292
  unsaturated, 125
  utilization, 103
Essential polyunsaturated fatty acids (EPUFAs) (see:
    Polyunsaturated fatty acids)
Ethanolamine, 5, 6
Evening primrose oil, 191, 206, 265, 291
Evoked potentials, 162
  visual (VEPs), 122, 124, 128
Evolution, 204, 299–317
Extrapyramidal
  effects, 113, 189
  motor signs, 89
  symptoms, 182, 286

Eye
  development, 14
  movement disorder, 121
  movement dysfunction (EMD), 122

Fabry disorder, 290
Family size, 168, 171, 174
Fat
  consumption, 173
  dietary, 167
  intake, 171
  subcutaneous, 313
Fats, 84
Fatty acid
  abnormalities, 147
  abundance, 26
  availability, 12
  composition, 58, 248
  defects, 61, 77
  deficiency, 227, 230, 232
  desaturation, 58, 59
  elongation, 58, 59, 60
  esterification, 26
  hydroxy, 32
  incorporation, 12, 26, 62
  intake, 265
  levels, 280, 287
  loss, 10, 11
  metabolism, 64, 143, 225, 226, 227, 238, 254, 267
  oxidation, 11, 12, 258
  release, 8, 39
  removal, 11
  schizophrenia, 23–29, 31–32, 57–71
  status, 265, 267
  supplementation, 135, 141, 248, 254–257, 265
  trafficking, 9
  turnover, 26, 60
  unsaturation index, 59, 60, 61
  uptake, 12
Fatty acids (see also: Essential fatty acids;
    Polyunsaturated fatty acids), 4, 5, 6, 16, 113,
    229, 303, 308, 309
  bimodal distribution, 147, 150–151
  brain, 16
  decreased, 76
  erythrocyte, 32, 35
  free, 24, 32, 62, 272, 275
  neuronal membrane, 31
  nonessential, 7
  red cell, 115
  saturated, 5, 7, 11, 61, 64, 146, 199, 204
  supply, 9

326

total, 58
unsaturated, 5, 7, 10, 11, 64, 121, 125, 146, 199, 204
Fenton reaction, 101
Fish
consumption, 202–205
oil, 159, 161, 191, 200, 201, 217, 255, 256, 259, 291
Flavones, 101
Fluoxetine, 213
Fluphenazine, 286
Flushing (*see also*: Niacin), 11, 306, 307
Food (*see also*: Diet), 10, 11
deprivation, 13
restriction (*see also*: Starvation), 106
Forebrain, 121
Fragile X, 151
Free radical
activity, 79
burden, 77, 78
chain reactions, 78
damage, 279
effects, 114, 115
formation, 279
generation, 85
insult, 80, 81
mediated damage, 64, 77, 81, 99
metabolism, 78, 80
pathology, 84
production, 78, 81
scavengers, 190
scavenging, 81
toxicity, 78
Free radicals, 57, 63, 75, 77, 84, 280, 293
defence against, 78
excess, 81
metabolic pathway, 78
Frontal cortex, 11

GABA, 81
receptor complex, 106
uptake, 105
GABAergic function, 286
Ganglion cells, 123
Gap junctions, 123, 125, 126, 129
Gas chromatography, 145
Gastrointestinal tract, 9
Gene
expression, 77, 146, 154, 211, 212, 306
interactions, 153
General paresis, 168
Genes
lipid-metabolizing, 312
X-linked, 228
Genetic
abnormalities, 11, 12, 14, 153
factors 3, 10
Gestalt breakdown, 122
Glial cells, 9, 303
Gliosis, 80, 105
Global oxidative stress (*see*: Oxidative stress)
Glucocorticoids, 10
Glucose metabolism, 31
Glutamate, 90, 93
Glutamate receptor
function, 5
hypofunctioning, 5, 11
Glutamine, 90, 91, 93
Glutathione, 78
oxidized, 101
Glutathione peroxidase (GSHPOD), 78, 79, 100, 101, 105
human plasma (hpGSHPOD), 79
Glutathione reductase, 101
Glycerol, 5, 6, 8
backbone, 5, 6, 303
Glycerol-3-phosphocholine (GPCh), 47–51
Glycerol-3-phosphoethanolamine (GPEth), 47–51
Glycerophosphodiesters, 23, 24
Glycerophosphorylethanolamine, 244
Glycerophosphorylcholine, 244
Glycine, 90, 93
Gonadal hormones, 368
Gray Oral Reading Test, 187
Grey matter, 52
white matter ratio, 52
Growth, 258, 264, 289
factors, 99, 176
hormones, 174
indices, 229
GTP-binding proteins (*see*: Proteins)

^{1}H-magnetic resonance imaging (*see also*: Magnetic resonance imaging; Magnetic resonance spectroscopy), 45
Haber-Weiss reaction, 101
Hallucinations, 121, 145, 227
auditory, 182, 183
olfactory, 227
tactile, 122
visual, 122, 128
Hallucinosis, 145
Haloperidol, 58, 59, 62, 63, 64, 66, 67, 68, 76, 94, 134, 286

dose, 60
  induced catalepsy, 26
  withdrawal, 60, 61
Hamilton Rating Scale, 213
Handedness (*see also*: Cerebral asymmetry; Hemisphere asymmetry), 182, 184, 185, 186, 226, 231, 244
Head circumference, 4, 13, 160, 162, 229, 302
Hemisphere
  asymmetry, 253
  size, 16
  structure, 16
Hepoxilin-A_2, 68
Highly unsaturated fatty acids (HUFAs), 279
Hippocampus, 4, 9, 16, 81, 101, 105, 114, 160, 271, 292, 308
  abnormalities, 6
  lipase levels, 9
  ventral, 53
Histidine, 90, 91, 93
Homicide, 196
Homovanillic acid (HVA), 42, 89, 92, 93, 197, 198
Horizontal cells, 125, 126, 129, 134
Hormonal state, 104
Hormone
  levels, 15
  receptors, 212
Hormones, 99
Hostility, 196, 197, 201, 204, 205
Huntington's disease, 285, 290–293
Hydrogen peroxide, 77, 78, 81, 101
  autoxidation, 77, 78
Hydroperoxides, 78
12-Hydroperoxy-5,8,10,14-eicosatetraenoic acid (12-HPETE), 64, 68
Hydroxy
  metabolites, 129
  radicals, 78, 101
Hydroxyacids, 3, 8
4-Hydroxyalkylenals, 102
5-Hydroxyindole acetic acid (5-HIAA), 92, 93, 197, 198, 199, 200
5-Hydroxytryptamine (5HT), 3, 66, 81, 89, 189, 199
  binding, 196
  brain, 199
  depletion, 20
  levels, 195
  metabolites, 146
  modulation, 196
  receptor density, 197
  receptor number, 199–200
  receptors, 199
  turnover, 200

6-Hydroxydopamine, 27, 40
12-Hydroxy-5,8,10,14-eicosatetraenoic acid (12-HETE), 64, 65, 67, 68
12-Hydroxy-5,8,10-heptadecatrienoic acid (HHT), 64, 65, 67, 68
Hydroxyl radicals, 77, 78, 81
Hyperactivity, 146, 197
Hypercalcaemia, 203
Hyperdopaminergic state, 26
Hyperinsulinaemia, 217
Hypertension, 107, 174, 217–218
Hypodopaminergic activity, 42, 95
Hypomanic
  tendencies, 217
  traits, 248
Hypothalamic control system, 153
Hypothalamic–pituitary–adrenal axis, 195, 200, 201
Hypothalamus, 200
Hypotonia, 212, 271
Hypoxia, 4
  neonatal, 173
  perinatal, 4, 13, 15
Hypoxia–reperfusion models, 81

Icelandic studies, 305, 311
Imidazole, 67
Imipramine, 94
Immune
  disorders, 174
  functions, 200
  neuroendocrine interactions, 201
  neuroendocrine system, 200–201
  system, 229
Immunoglobulins, 164
Impulse control, 198
Impulsive behaviour, 195, 196, 197, 198, 254
Indomethacin, 26, 27, 67
Inflammatory
  mediators, 32
  response, 140
Information processing, 134, 161
Inositol (I), 5, 8, 63
  cycle, 114
  phosphates, 23, 32, 114, 175, 247, 303
  phospholipid hydrolysis, 62
  polyphosphate, 100
Insulin, 12, 16, 94, 202–203
  binding, 202, 289
  coma, 89
  effects, 89
  resistance, 217, 289
  therapy, 12, 89
  1,4,5-triphosphate, 63

Intelligence (*see* IQ)
Interferon, 10
Interleukin-1b (IL-1b), 200, 201
Interneuronal communication, 23
Iodine, 265, 309, 311
Ion
    channels, 8, 31, 57, 211, 285
    pumps, 105
IQ, 14, 151, 152, 161, 163, 164, 174, 212, 251, 265, 302
Iron, 77, 78, 81, 100, 101, 106, 149, 263, 265, 309, 311
Ischaemia, 16, 81
Isoleucine, 90, 91, 93
Isoniazid, 145
Isoproterenol, 94

12-Keto-5,8,10,14-eicosatetraenoic acid (12-KETE), 68
Kirunal™, 191

Language, 183, 185, 234, 235, 236, 237, 238, 253
    development, 16
    disorders, 226
    skills (*see also*: Verbal skills), 4, 14, 231
Laterality (*see also*: Cerebral asymmetry; Handedness), 184–185
Lazaroids, 80, 81, 106
L-DOPA, 3, 95–96
Leadership, 305, 308, 312
Learning, 212, 229, 230, 252, 253, 258, 263
    ability, 160
    difficulty, 152
    disorders, 162
Leucine, 90, 91, 93
Leukotriene
    B4, 200
    derivatrives, 229
Leukotrienes, 3, 8, 23, 32, 200, 285
Life
    span (*see*: Longevity), 84
    style, 99, 100, 102
Light adaptation (*see also*: Dark adaptation), 134, 135
Lingusitic function (*see also*: Language), 231
Linoleic acid (LA) (*see also*: 18:2n-6), 7, 9, 10, 12, 14, 64, 68, 141, 149, 159, 168, 198, 204, 211, 229, 251, 253, 258, 266, 282, 286, 287, 288, 289, 301, 310
    blood levels, 14, 15
    conversion rate, 8
    decrease, 76
    deficiency, 64
    desaturation, 64
    dietary EFA precursor, 9

    elongation, 64
    formula milk, 10, 14
    synthesis, 12
α-Linolenic acid (ALA), 7, 9, 10, 11, 12, 159, 189, 191, 211, 229, 251, 258, 266, 301
    conversion rate, 8
    deficiency, 212
    dietary EFA precursor, 9
    formula milk, 10, 14
    levels, 14, 15, 289
    supplementation, 286
γ-Linolenic acid (GLA), 253, 282, 286, 291, 310
    supplementation, 289
Linseed oil, 191
Lipid
    abnormalities, 154, 211, 217
    bilayer microviscosity, 31
    chemistry, 114
    derivatives, 211
    hydroperoxide, 102
    levels, 103
    loss, 78
    mediators, 265
    metabolism, 113–116, 216, 228, 248, 271, 309–313
    peroxide levels, 169
    peroxidation, 63–64, 77, 78, 79, 80, 81, 84, 99, 100–107, 146, 154, 202, 203
    peroxidation byproducts, 102
    peroxide intermediates, 63
    peroxides, 102, 103, 105
    peroxyl radical, 102
    profile, 31
    radical, 102
    synthesis, 230
    turnover, 230
Lipids, 77, 150, 264, 301, 312
Lipofiscin, 80
Lipoic acid, 10, 84, 293
Lipoprotein
    lipase, 9, 12, 15, 16, 113, 114, 303, 309
    lipase gene, 15
    triglycerides, 9
Lipoproteins, 9, 15, 303, 308
Lipoxygenase, 65, 68, 126
Lithium, 15, 57, 94, 146, 213, 289, 307
Liver, 9, 16, 266, 303, 308, 309
Locomotion, 39–42, 160
Locus coeruleus, 201
Long-chain polyunsaturated fatty acids (LCPUFAs) (*see also*: Essential fatty acids; Polyunsaturated fatty acids), 195–210, 225, 229, 251–260

deficiency, 259
status, 159
supplementation, 257, 267
synthesis, 160
Longevity, 81, 84
L-system, 89, 90, 91
    amino acid carrier, 90
    capacity, 92
Lymphocytes, 90
Lysine, 90, 91, 93
Lysophosphatidic acid (LPA), 63
Lysophosphatidylcholine (LPC), 39, 42, 62
    concentration, 39
Lysophospholipase, 24, 277
Lysophospholipid, 24, 32
    acceptors, 26
Lysophospholipids, 62, 275

Magnesium, 45, 49, 50
Magnetic resonance imaging (MRI), 11, 12, 23, 25, 105, 163, 254, 306, 307
Magnetic resonance spectroscopy (MRS), 45–55, 126–127, 181, 230, 231, 243–249, 287, 290
    chemical shift (CS) imaging, 46, 49
    depth-resolved surface coil spectroscopy (DRESS), 46, 49, 50
    fast rotating gradient spectroscopy (FROGS), 46, 49, 50
    image-selected *in vivo* spectroscopy (ISIS), 46, 49
    proton-decoupled chemical shift imaging (pd-CSI), 49, 50, 51
    rotating-frame methods, 46
    simulated echo acquisition mode (STEAM), 46, 49
    surface coil (SC) technique, 46, 49
Magnesium, 263, 266
Magnocellular
    deficits, 186
    ganglion cells, 254
    hypothesis, 228
    neurones, 228
    pathways, 253
    stream of visual processing, 184, 244
    system, 182, 230
Malar
    thermal circulation index, 140
    temperature change, 140, 141
Male sex, 12
Malonyldialdehydes (MDA), 80, 100, 102, 103
Malnutrition, 265
Manganese superoxide dismutase (*see also*: Superoxide dismutase), 80
Mania (*see also*: Bipolar disorder), 60, 153, 154

Manic-depressive illness, 143, 145, 146, 147, 148, 151, 153, 216, 304, 307–308, 312
Manic patients, 123, 128
MAX-EPA™, 287
McCarthy scale, 161
Meat, 10, 81, 106
Mellitin, 27
Membrane
    abnormalities, 31, 80, 89–97
    biosynthesis, 23
    damage, 57, 79, 84
    damage products, 77
    defects, 57, 68, 76, 292
    deficits, 75–79, 80, 84, 85
    destabilized, 212
    disturbance, 75
    dynamics, 57, 60
    dysfunction, 57, 75, 80, 81, 95, 96, 146, 212, 217
    EPUFAs, 105, 175
    fatty acids, 78, 150
    first passage, 90
    fluidity, 60, 63, 81, 143, 146, 175, 196, 198, 212, 213, 214, 216, 285
    fragility, 229
    function, 60, 93, 95, 189, 212, 258, 308, 312
    fusion, 5
    hyperpolarization, 123
    hypothesis, 52, 75
    insensitivity, 202
    instability, 63
    lipid changes, 107
    lipid loss, 78
    lipid status, 103
    lipids, 60, 75, 76–77, 99, 101, 105, 113, 115, 145, 285
    metabolism, 208
    morphology, 60
    order, 195
    outer segment disc, 124
    oxidation mechanisms, 115
    packing properties, 199
    pathology, 77, 80, 84, 105, 106, 189
    permeability, 63, 285
    peroxidation, 31, 99–111
    phospholipids, 10, 12, 52, 76, 103, 104, 113–119, 127, 140, 146, 167, 182, 187, 213, 214, 276, 287, 306, 310, 313
    protective strategies, 75–88
    proteins, 60, 106
    receptors, 211
    second passage, 90
    shapes, 5

 stability, 81
 structure, 8, 114, 195, 308, 312
 third passage, 90
 transport, 146, 153, 154
 turnover, 23, 307
 viscosity, 199
Membranes, 3, 92, 145, 199
 brain, 266
 cell, 173, 244
 dendritic, 3
 mictochondrial, 3, 78
  neuronal, 3, 5, 13, 33, 39, 57, 62, 75, 78, 101–102, 167, 191, 196, 198, 199, 200, 229, 238, 285–286, 292, 293
 nuclear, 3
 pial–glial, 229
 postsynaptic, 64
 presynaptic, 64
 red blood cell, 60
 retinal, 266
 synaptic, 3, 32, 39, 201, 213, 214, 254
 synaptic vesicle, 3
 synaptosomal, 203
Memory, 182, 286
 deficits, 291
 short-term, 254
 working, 231, 245
Menstrual cycle, 90
Mental retardation, 308
Metabolic blocks, 58
Metabolism
 inborn errors, 90
Metarhodopsin II, 199, 213
Methionine, 90, 91, 93
3-Methoxy-4-hydroxy-phenylglycol (MHPG), 92, 93
Methyl nicotinate, 271
Microconnections, 302, 307, 308, 310
Micronutrients, 100, 286
Microsomes, 251
Migration, 171, 174–175
Milk
 breast, 10, 11, 13, 14, 159, 174, 212, 229, 251, 252, 265
 cow's, 161
 DHA concentration, 174
 formula, 10, 13, 14, 105, 159, 174, 199, 229, 230, 251, 252, 302
 mammalian, 174
Mini Mental State Examination (MMSE), 275
Mitochondria, 77, 80, 195, 251, 266
Mitochondrial
 abnormalities, 77

 activity, 101
 damage, 78
 DNA, 78
 dysfunction, 78, 84
 electron transport, 101
 error, 101
 membranes, 78
 oxidative phosphorylation, 78
Mobile phospholipids (*see*: Phospholipids)
Monoacylglycerol (MAG), 63
Monoamine
 metabolism, 89
 metabolites, 90, 91, 92
 oxidase activity, 195
 oxidases, 101
Mononucleotide repeat sequence, 33–34
Moro reflex, 212
Morphine, 145
Motor
 coordination, 183, 185, 226, 228, 234, 235, 238, 254, 258
 function, 231, 253
 nerves, 96
 skills, 4, 81
 problems, 236, 237
Movement
 abnormalities, 162
 disorders, 226, 285–296
Movements
 abnormal involuntary, 279–283
 perioral, 286
Muller cells, 133
Multiple gene hypothesis, 153
Multiple sclerosis (MS), 162, 200, 202, 290
Muscle
 activity, 90
 biopsies, 96
 cells, 96
 receptors, 275, 277
Myelin, 51
 formation, 289
 sheaths, 243
Myelination, 4, 12, 159, 290
Myocardial infarction, 201
Myoinositol, 6
Myotonic dystrophy, 96

NADPH-dependent oxidases, 77
Nails, 310
National Adult Reading Test (NART), 151, 152
Neanderthal, 302
Neocortex, 9

Nerve
  conduction, 121, 285
  growth, 258
  growth cones, 303, 307
  terminals, 106
Neural
  ceroid lipofuscinosis, 267
  development, 81
  function, 121
  timing, 229
Neuroadaptive mechanisms, 213
Neurodegenerative
  diseases, 174, 290, 293
  pathophysiology, 105
Neurodevelopment, 159–166, 229, 289
  aberrant, 23
Neurodevelopmental
  abnormalities, 173, 175, 288
  disorders, 225, 244, 248
  pathology, 105
Neuroendocrine functioning, 195, 198
Neuroleptics, 10, 12, 25, 50, 62, 63, 66, 68, 79, 89, 95,
    96, 99, 100, 103, 104, 113–119, 122, 125, 128,
    135, 139, 146, 148, 149, 186, 187, 190, 191,
    280, 285, 288, 289, 292, 308
Neurological
  disorders, 162
  dysfunctions, 163, 264
Neuromuscular abnormalities, 96
Neuronal
  abnormalities, 4
  activity, 101
  cell signalling, 114
  death, 99
  degeneration, 290
  development, 9, 162
  disorganization, 105
  dysfunction, 80
  function, 7, 8, 75, 99, 167, 212, 213
  growth, 7, 9, 254
  injury, 81
  interconnections, 14
  loss, 80
  membrane order, 205
  membrane structure, 102
  migration, 228
  modelling, 7
  oxidative damage, 103, 290
  remodelling, 7, 8
  sprouting, 308
  structure, 7, 8
  surface potentials, 31
  survival, 99
  transmembrane potentials, 31
  volume, 26
Neurones, 159, 211
  bipolar, 123
  horizontal, 123, 125
  retinal, 133
Neuropeptides, 57, 153
Neuroprotective
  agents, 107
  strategies, 99
Neuropsychiatric disorders, 77
Neuropsychological functions, 42, 52
Neurotransmission, 13, 68, 75, 195, 212, 254
  decreased, 78
  glutamatergic, 13
  noradrenergic, 195
  serotonergic, 195, 205
Neurotransmitter, 3, 8
  breakdown, 195
  dysfunction, 31
  function, 195–196
  metabolism, 230
  receptor binding, 75
  release, 5, 121, 285
  secretion, 212
  systems, 57, 113, 211
  turnover, 213
  synthesis, 146, 195
Neurotransmitters, 62, 65, 75, 77, 99, 121, 123, 134,
    145, 176, 197, 213, 263
Niacin, 139–144
  flushing, 31, 139–144, 271
  oral, 11
  topical, 11
Nicotinamide, 10
Nicotinic acid, 255
Night vision (see also: Dark adaptation), 124, 307
Nitric oxide, 77, 303
N-methyl-D-aspartate (NMDA), 292
  receptors, 292, 293
Nonsteroidal anti-inflammatory drugs (NSAIDs),
    139, 142
Noradrenaline (see also: Norepinephrine), 3, 89
  depletion, 211
Norepinephrine, 195
  metabolites, 146
  release, 200
Nuclear magnetic resonance (NMR) spectroscopy,
    31, 39, 42, 104, 147, 276
Nucleotide triphosphates (NTP), 243, 244, 246, 247
Nucleotides, 164

Nutrients, 266
Nutrition (*see also*: Food), 146, 173, 230, 301
   impaired, 147
   maternal, 159, 181
   palaeolithic, 34
Nutritional
   deficiencies, 288
   deprivation (*see also*: Starvation), 195
   factors, 147

Obesity, 309
Obstetric complications, 4, 13
Oculomotor function, 122
Oestrogen, 10, 174
Olanzapine, 75, 103, 189
   levels, 13
Oleamide, 272
Oleic acid, 290
Olive oil, 231
Oral contraceptives, 90
Ornithine, 90, 93
Oscillatory potentials, 133
Oxford–Liverpool Inventory of Feelings and Experiences, 234
Oxidant systems, 12
Oxidants, 16
β-Oxidation, 266
Oxidative
   damage, 103, 105
   injury, 100, 101, 103, 105, 106, 107
   lipid peroxides, 102
   metabolism, 78
   stress, 26, 77, 78, 79–80, 84, 85, 99, 100–103, 105, 106, 107, 169, 190, 289
Oxyradicals, 101, 102, 105

^{31}P Magnetic resonance imaging (*see* Magnetic resonance imaging)
^{31}P Magnetic resonance spectroscopy (MRS) (*see* Magnetic resonance spectroscopy)
Pain, 181, 271, 272
   resistance to, 11
   tolerance, 160
Palmitic acid, 281
Panic disorder, 52
Paraldehyde, 145
Paranoia, 145, 304, 408, 312
Parkinson's disease, 3, 105, 123, 134, 285
Parkinsonian symptoms, 57, 281, 282
Parkinsonism, 83, 89
Parvocellular system, 228
Pentane, 80, 103, 104

Peptic ulcer, 168
Perception
   auditory, 254
   anomalous, 234
   flicker, 228, 244
   motion, 228, 231, 244
Perceptual
   distortions, 182
   style, 227
Perinatal events, 4, 13
Peroxidation, 147, 150, 172
Peroxidative
   breakdown, 169
   damage, 80
Peroxisomal
   biogenesis, 212
   diseases, 267
   disorders, 271
Peroxisomes, 251, 267
Peroxy-radicals, 63
Peroxyl radicals, 81
Personality
   disorder, 197
   disturbance, 96
pH, 45, 247
Phenothiazines, 114, 146, 190
Phenylalanine, 89, 90, 91, 93, 96
Phenylketonuria, 159, 161
Phonological
   problems, 228
   skills, 182, 225, 228, 245
Phosphatases, 50, 247
Phosphate, 76
Phosphatidic acid (PA), 6, 63, 66
   phosphohydrolase (PAP), 63
   thrombin-induced formation, 67
Phosphatidylcholine (PC), 6, 23, 57, 60, 63, 65, 66, 101, 114, 160, 243, 247, 290
   arachidonyl, 32
   concentration, 39
   levels, 45, 76
Phosphatidylethanolamine (PE), 6, 23, 25, 60, 65, 66, 81, 101, 114, 150, 160, 243, 247
   decrease, 58, 76
   levels, 45, 76, 104
Phosphatidylinositol (PI), 6, 8, 23, 63, 65, 66, 101, 114
   4-5-bisphosphate, 63
   cycle, 3
   increase, 77
   levels, 76, 104
   4-phosphate, 63

platelet pathway, 67
response, 67
turnover, 66, 45, 65
Phosphatidylserine (PS), 6, 45, 60, 65, 66, 101, 114, 195, 201, 213, 243
  levels, 76, 104
Phosphocholine (PCh), 47, 49, 51
Phosphocreatinine (PCr), 45, 49, 50, 243, 244, 246, 247
  β-ATP ratio, 51
Phosphodiesterase, 247
Phosphodiesters (PDE), 23, 26, 39, 45–53, 76, 103, 243, 244, 246, 247, 248, 276
Phosphoethanolamine (PEth), 47, 51
Phosphohydrolase, 114
Phopholipase
  activation, 308, 312
  activity, 16, 23–29
  expression, 12
  structure, 15
Phospholipase A, 303, 307
Phospholipase A$_1$, 6, 7
  activity, 50
Phospholipase A$_2$ (PLA$_2$), 6, 7, 8, 10, 11, 12, 15, 16, 23–29, 31–37, 39–43, 62, 63, 113, 114, 115, 127, 140, 142, 145, 147, 150, 153, 163, 181, 187, 190, 244, 271, 275–278, 287, 292, 303, 307
  activation, 62
  activity, 24, 26, 31, 33, 39, 50, 62, 63, 77
  assay system, 24
  calcium-dependent, 24, 25, 26, 32, 190
  calcium-independent, 24, 25, 26, 32, 63
  cell surface receptors, 32
  cytosolic (cPLA$_2$), 32
  deficiency, 26
  distribution, 26
  downregulation, 27
  expression, 26, 32
  extracellular, 63
  gene studies, 33–35
  gene polymorphism, 31–37
  hydrolysis, 39
  intracellular membrane-bound, 63
  neuroleptic drug effects, 25
  plasma, 39
  platelet, 39
  schizophrenia, 31–37, 39–43
  secretory (sPLA$_2$), 32
  serum, 39, 45, 53, 62
  signal tranduction, 32–33
  subtypes, 24, 25

transduction mechanisms, 32
  types, 32, 33
Phospholipase B (PLB), 6
Phospholipase C (PLC), 6, 7, 8, 11, 15, 63, 66, 113, 115, 247, 271, 303, 307
Phospholipase D (PLD), 6, 63, 303
Phospholipases, 3, 6, 10, 60, 65, 153, 271–273, 302, 303, 306, 310
Phospholipid
  abnormalities, 80, 127, 145, 182, 223, 227, 237, 247
  acyl chain, 199
  acyltransferase, 114
  breakdown, 5, 6, 23, 45, 63, 182
  changes, 169
  concentrations, 75
  degradation, 62
  depletion, 203
  disorders, 153
  dysfunction, 146
  exchange proteins, 60
  hydrolysis, 175
  incorporation, 14, 15
  mechanisms, 4
  metabolism, 3, 5, 12–16, 23–29, 39, 42, 45–55, 68, 103, 113, 145, 168, 182, 225, 227, 230, 237, 285, 287, 290, 307, 309
  metabolites, 104
  remodelling, 5, 7, 15
  storage disorder, 114
  structure, 3, 5, 211, 303
  synthesis, 5, 6, 7, 12, 15, 45, 104, 114, 303, 307
  turnover, 62, 64, 67, 310
  vesicles, 8
Phopholipids (PL), 65, 101, 145, 160, 189, 197, 213, 215, 266, 267, 279–283, 285, 301, 302, 303, 307, 308
  alterations, 76
  availability, 13
  brain, 9, 45–55
  choline-containing, 60
  conversion to eicosanoids, 12
  DHA-rich, 124
  EFA-rich, 8
  hippocampal, 9
  hypothalamic, 213
  membrane, 39, 50, 52, 60, 67
  mobile (MP), 49, 51
  platelet, 12, 67
  roles, 8
  total, 58
Phosphomonoesters (PME), 23, 39, 45–53, 76, 104, 127, 243, 244, 246, 247, 248, 276

Phosphorus (*see also*: Phosphate), 5, 45, 243, 246, 247
Phosphorylcholine, 243
Phosphorylethanolamine, 243
Phosphorylserine, 243, 247
Photophilic behaviour, 134
Photopigments, 123
Photoplethysmography, 140
Photoreceptors, 123, 124, 129, 133, 134, 135, 229
Phototransduction, 123
Physical
    abnormalities, 4, 14
    diseases, 217–218
Planum temporale, 228, 244
Platelet activating factor (PAF), 32, 63
    production, 32
Plexiform cells, 123, 134
Pollution, 81, 84
Polyamine levels, 31
Polymerase chain reaction (PCR), 33, 34
Polyunsaturated fatty acids (PUFAs) (*see also*: Essential fatty acids; Fatty acids; Long-chain polyunsaturated fatty acids), 31, 76, 99, 102, 150, 159, 160, 161, 211
    autoxidation, 63
    changes, 68
    decreased, 61, 76
    defects, 57, 61, 68
    depletion, 160, 161
    deprivation, 160
    esterified, 103–104
    levels, 76, 159, 160
    loss, 103
    n-3, 32, 33, 59, 76, 105, 107, 124, 133, 134, 135, 159, 160, 163, 167, 168, 170, 172, 174, 181, 186, 189–192, 195, 196, 199, 200, 201, 202, 205, 211, 212, 214, 215, 216, 217, 227, 229, 230, 232, 237, 248, 251, 252, 253, 256, 258, 264, 265, 267, 271, 285, 286, 287, 288, 289, 290, 294, 313
    n-6, 32, 33, 58, 59, 107, 141, 159, 160, 168, 170, 196, 204, 211, 214, 227, 229, 251, 253, 256, 263, 264, 265, 285, 286, 287, 288, 289, 290, 292, 294
    n-9, 59, 64
    18:1n-9, 127
    18:2n-6 (*see also*: linoleic acid), 57, 58, 59, 150, 197
    18:3n-3, 127, 197, 215, 216
    18:3n-6 (*see also*: γ-linoleic acid), 58, 127, 216
    18:4n-3, 150
    20:2n-6, 150
    20:3n-6 (*see also*: dihomo-γ-linolenic acid), 57, 58, 59, 141, 150, 216
    20:3n-9, 64, 266
    20:4n-6 (*see also*: arachidonic acid), 57, 58, 59, 141, 150, 195, 197, 202, 265, 267
    20:5n-3 (*see also*: eicosapentaenoic acid), 57, 197, 215
    22:0, 59
    22:1n-9, 58
    22:4n-6 (*see also*: adrenic acid), 58, 59, 127
    22:5n-3, 58, 59, 150, 215, 216
    22:5n-6 (*see also*: docosapentaenoic acid), 58, 150, 197, 216
    22:6n-3 (*see also*: docosapentaenoic acid), 57, 58, 59, 141, 150, 195, 197, 202, 203, 215, 216, 265, 267
    24:0, 59
    24:1n-9, 59
    oxidation, 77
    status, 149, 168, 173
    supplementation, 191
    therapeutic efficacy, 31
    total, 77
Positive and Negative Symptom Scale (PANSS), 191, 287
Positron emission tomography (PET), 94, 95, 96
Postreceptor signalling systems, 3
Potassium channels, 286
Pregnancy, 4, 5, 13, 14, 159, 160, 163, 175
Prematurity, 13
Prolactin, 12, 308
    secretion, 113
Proline, 90, 93
Promiscuous activity, 312
Pro-oxidant
    effects, 81
    processes, 77
    systems, 78
Pro-oxidants, 10, 106, 114, 150
Propagated spike potential, 123
Propranolol, 94
Prostaglandin (PG), 64
    availability, 143
    D_2, 11, 126, 139, 140, 143, 271, 306, 307
    E, 140
    E analogue, 115, 181
    E_1, 285, 286, 289, 290
    E_2, 200
    formation, 140
    G_3, 64
    H_2, 64, 140
    metabolism, 31
    production, 26, 81
    receptors, 115

schizophrenia, 32
synthesis, 57, 68
synthesis inhibition, 27
Prostaglandins, 3, 8, 23, 27, 32, 121, 139, 146, 200, 229, 271, 285, 286, 307
Protein, 149, 173, 216, 265, 301
  β-amyloid, 277
  amyloid precursor (APP), 275
  amyloidogenic, 275
  conformation, 31
  conformational changes, 212
  kinase C (PKC), 62, 65, 213
  kinases, 8, 213–214
  kinetics, 31
  modification, 77
  oxidation, 99, 101
  peroxidative breakdown, 100
  synthesis, 89, 96
  translocase, 114
Proteins, 3, 5, 15, 77, 100, 101
  acyl-CoA-binding, 303, 308, 310, 311
  breakdown, 105
  farnosylated, 3
  fatty acid binding (FABPs), 9, 12, 15, 16, 304, 308, 309, 311
  fatty acid transport (FATPs), 8, 303, 309, 310, 311
  G, 129, 199, 211, 213
  GTP-binding, 32
  huntingtin, 293
  interaction, 212
  intrinsic, 212
  membrane-associated, 7, 10, 293
  membrane-bound, 7, 229, 308
  myristoylated, 3
  palmitoylated, 3
  phorbol ester-induced, 90
  peroxidative breakdown, 101
  presynaptic, 51
  prenylated, 3
  quaternary folding, 3, 8
  tertiary structure, 8
Proteolipids, 51
Psychopathology, 61
Psychopathy, 308–312
Psychotic behaviour, 203
Puberty, 4, 5, 9, 12, 13, 15, 309, 310
Putamen, 25
Pyramidal cells, 81
Pyrexia, 181
Pyridine nucleotide status, 77
Pyroxidine, 10

Quality of life, 202
Quetiapine, 189
Quick test, 151, 152
Quinacrine, 27
Quinones, 101, 106

Reactive oxygen species (ROS), 77, 99, 102, 167, 169
  brain levels, 102
  mediated pathology, 99, 100
  metabolism, 101
  scavenger activity, 103
Reacylation, 187
Reading, 182, 183, 185, 225, 231, 232, 233, 234, 236, 238, 245, 253, 254, 263
Receptor
  binding, 68
  blocking, 113
  dysfunction, 211
  function, 64, 146, 212, 230, 263
  insensitivity, 217
  interaction, 92
  modulation, 189, 190
  number, 203
Receptors, 8, 31, 57, 65, 285
Red blood cell
  fatty acids, 61
  ghost membranes, 60, 64, 76
Refsum disease, 290
Relapse, 61
Religion, 301
Research Diagnostic Criteria (RDC), 91
Retina, 123, 160, 307
Retinal
  cells, 230
  damage, 134
  function, 121–131, 133, 160
  tissue, 213
Retinitis pigmentosa, 124, 133, 134, 258, 267
Retinoblastoma cells, 203
Retinol, 106, 149
Retinyl esters, 106
Revised Adult Dyslexia Checklist, 232, 233
Rheumatoid arthritis, 200
Rhodopsin, 124, 125, 129, 199, 213
Riboflavin, 255
Rotational behaviour, 39–42

S-adenosylmethionine (SAM), 6
Salivation, 115
Scale for the Assessment of Negative Symptoms (SANS), 51, 52, 61, 82–83, 182, 183, 184

Index

Scale for the Assessment of Positive Symptoms (SAPS), 52, 79, 182, 183, 184
Schizoaffective disorder, 62, 65, 147, 153, 154, 289, 304
Schizophrenia, 3–20, 23–29, 31–38, 39–43, 45–55, 57–71, 75–88, 89–97, 99–111, 121–131, 133–136, 139–144, 159–166, 167–180, 189–192, 226–227, 228, 254, 271, 285, 286, 289, 304–313
   aetiology, 93, 286
   antioxidant treatment, 84
   autopsied brain, 25
   biochemical alterations, 31–38
   biological markers, 122, 127
   chronic, 76, 77, 79, 102, 107
   diagnosis, 25, 143, 147
   dopamine hypothesis, 113, 189
   dyskinetic syndrome, 279–280
   family studies, 145–156
   fatty acids, 23, 57–71
   first-episode, 63, 76, 77, 79, 80, 102, 104
   genetic aetiology, 33
   genetic vulnerability, 122
   genomic DNA, 33
   hypofrontality hypotheses, 39–43
   L-DOPA treatment, 95–96
   lipid hypothesis, 227
   magnetic resonance spectroscopy, 45–55
   membrane hypothesis, 121, 122, 190, 192, 225, 244, 247
   membrane-protective strategies, 75–88
   monitoring, 143
   negative symptoms, 51, 57, 61, 79, 104, 122, 129, 139, 146, 147, 154, 182, 185, 227, 248, 279, 287, 290
   neurodevelopmental concept, 3–20
   neuropathology, 99–111
   pathogenesis, 89
   pathology, 107
   pathophysiology, 99
   phospholipase activity, 23–29
   phospholipid metabolism, 23, 45–55
   positive symptoms, 61, 79, 122, 145, 154, 181, 182, 185, 187, 191, 227, 248, 280, 287
   postmenopausal, 13
   prostaglandin deficiency hypothesis, 139
   relapse, 143
   remission, 181–188
   risk, 4, 9, 13, 14, 15, 164
   risk factor, 163
   severity, 13
   time of onset, 13
   viral theory, 168

Schizophrenic-like syndrome, 13
Schizophreniform disorder, 60, 62, 65
Schizotypal personality, 15, 227, 237, 238, 244, 304–305, 307–308
Schizotypy, 15, 182, 227, 234, 311
School functioning, 79
Second messengers, 32, 62, 64, 65–66, 67, 68, 77, 175, 189, 211, 212, 213–214, 292
Secretion, 64
Sedentary lifestyle, 81
Seizures, 212
Selenium, 10, 78
Sensory
   dysfunction, 264
   perceptual processes, 123
Serine, 5, 6, 90, 93
Serotonin (*see*: 5-Hydroxytryptamine)
Serotonergic
   activity, 197
   depletion, 211
   function, 198, 200, 286
   mechanisms, 113
Sex differences, 4, 10, 12, 13, 15, 171, 227–228, 288
Signal
   transduction, 32, 35, 39, 57, 62, 64, 68, 75, 99, 105–110, 175, 195, 198, 285
   transmission, 212
Skin, 139–144
   macrophages, 139
   temperature, 139, 141
Sleep, 154, 201, 202, 271
Smoking, 81, 84, 100, 102, 103, 106, 147, 148, 149, 171, 173, 214, 217, 280, 281, 282
Smooth pursuit eye movements (SPEM), 122
Snack foods, 215, 216, 251, 258
Social
   anxiety, 182
   adjustment, 162
   class, 161
   development, 4
   difficulties, 198
   functioning, 197
   interaction, 162
   skills, 15
   withdrawal, 182, 201
Sociopathy, 305, 308, 312
Sodium transport, 146
'Soft' neurological signs, 57, 226
Space visualization, 308
Spatial frequencies (SFs), 125, 126
Speech, 183, 185
Spelling, 183, 185, 231, 232, 233, 234, 245, 253, 263

Sphingomyelin, 60, 114
Spinal cord, 211
Spiperone, 189
Starch, 149
Starvation, 4, 15, 90, 309, 310
Steady-state anisotropy (S_r), 60
Stereotyped behaviour, 39–42
Steroids, 9
    ovarian, 9
    testicular, 9
Stereotypy, 160
Sterols, 199
Stress, 10, 12, 13, 16, 53, 168, 170, 172, 173, 174, 175, 201, 203–204
    dietary, 147
    emotional, 203
    illness-related, 100
    immobilization, 203
    mental, 214
Stressors, 63, 168, 175
Striatum, 26, 27, 191, 192
Sulphhydryl groups, 77
Sugar, 149
Suicidal
    acts, 197
    ideation, 197
Suicide, 195, 196, 292
    attempts, 198, 200, 201
    risk, 201
    victims, 200
Sulpiride, 94, 182
Sunflower oil, 195
Superoxide dismutase (SOD), 78, 79, 80, 81, 100, 101, 204
    polyethylene glycol conjugated (PEG-SOD), 81
Synapse formation, 303
Synapses, 229
Synaptic
    connectivity, 159
    contacts, 105
    efficiency, 80
    junctions, 121
    loss, 26
    membrane, 31
    modelling, 12, 311
    pruning, 229, 303, 308, 311
    release, 195
    remodelling, 5, 229, 311
Systemic lupus erythematosus (SLE), 228

Tardive dyskinesia, 10, 57, 79, 80, 82–83, 84, 107, 190, 191, 279, 286, 287, 288–290, 294

rating scale, 82–83, 104
Taurine, 90, 91, 92, 93
Temporal processing, 228, 229
Terbutaline, 94
Thalamus, 53, 105
Thiamin, 255
Thiobarbituric acid (TBA), 102
    reactive substances (TBARs), 77, 80, 82–83, 102, 103, 203–204
Thought, 183
    abnormalities, 15
Threonine, 90, 93
Thrombin, 64, 65, 67
    induced formation of eicosanoids, 67
Thromboxane (Tx), 64
    A_2, 64, 67
    B_2, 64, 65, 67
    synthetase, 67
Thyroid hormone, 308
Tirilazad, 81
α-Tocopherol (*see*: Vitamin E)
Total antioxidant status (TAS) (*see also*: Antioxidant), 80
Tourette's syndrome, 228
Toxins, 84
Transducin, 129
Transduction mechanisms, 31
Transition metals, 101
Transmembrane potentials, 31
Transmitter (*see also*: Neurotransmitter)
    functions, 121
    dysfunction, 99
    metabolites, 198
    systems, 195
Transport mechanisms, 121
Triacylglycerol (TAG), 65
Trienoic acids, 64
Triglycerides, 9, 196, 281, 287
Tryptophan, 89, 90, 93, 199
    hydroxylase, 195
Tyrosine, 89–97
    concentration, 94
    loading, 95
    plasma, 94, 95
    transport, 89–97
    transport velocity (V_{max}), 92
    uptake, 92

Ubiquinone zinc, 10
Unsaturation index, 125, 126, 143
Urate, 101
Uric acid, 78, 79, 80
Uterus, 159

Valine, 90, 91, 93
Vasodilatation, 140, 142
Vegetable oils, 106, 204
Vegetables, 106
Vegetarianism, 253, 256, 259
Ventricles, 173, 290
Ventricular
    enlargement, 105
    size, 4
Verapamil, 203
Verbal skills, 4, 14
Vertical axons, 51
Violent behaviour, 196, 198, 199, 200
Viral infections, 4, 10, 12, 14, 15, 16, 57, 96, 181
Viruses, 172
Vision, 230
    scotopic, 255
Visual
    acuity, 14, 124, 126, 129, 161, 251
    attention, 161
    capacity, 251
    channels, 123
    deficits, 186, 229, 230, 244
    development, 230, 238, 248, 302
    distortions, 121, 122
    dysfunction, 182
    function, 162, 183, 229, 231, 237, 248, 265
    impairment, 212
    information processing, 122
    magnocellular system, 229
    masking, 122, 123, 128
    motion sensitivity, 184
    perception, 182
    perceptual abnormalities, 121–123
    pigment density, 133
    processing, 252, 253, 254
    responses, 121
    search, 231
    sensitivity, 123, 125
    symptoms, 234, 235, 236, 237, 238
    system, 121, 123, 228, 251, 254
Visuomotor
    coordination, 182
    problems, 244
    sensitivity, 186
Vitamin
    A, 106, 129, 168, 171–172, 255, 256, 265
    B_6, 266, 313
    C, 78, 79, 101, 106, 149, 150, 151, 168, 171–172, 255
    D, 259
    E, 10, 78, 79, 80, 81, 82–83, 84, 101, 104, 106, 107, 149, 150, 168, 171–172, 190, 267, 279, 282, 290, 293, 313
Vitamins, 16, 84, 100, 107
Vocabulary, 183

Wakefulness, 154
War, 301, 312
Wheat germ, 106
Wide Range Achievement Test, 232
Wilkins Sustained Attention Test, 127
William's syndrome, 302
Word skills (*see* Verbal skills)
Writing, 225, 254

Zellweger syndrome, 212, 258
Zinc, 16, 263, 266, 309, 311
    deficiency, 251, 255